Difficult Decisions in Surgery: An Evidence-Based Approach

Series Editor
Mark K. Ferguson
Department of Surgery
University of Chicago
Chicago, IL, USA

The complexity of decision making in any kind of surgery is growing exponentially. As new technology is introduced, physicians from nonsurgical specialties offer alternative and competing therapies for what was once the exclusive province of the surgeon. In addition, there is increasing knowledge regarding the efficacy of traditional surgical therapies. How to select among these varied and complex approaches is becoming increasingly difficult. These multi-authored books will contain brief chapters, each of which will be devoted to one or two specific questions or decisions that are difficult or controversial. They are intended as current and timely reference sources for practicing surgeons, surgeons in training, and educators that describe the recommended ideal approach, rather than customary care, in selected clinical situations.

Konstantin Umanskiy • Neil Hyman
Editors

Difficult Decisions in Colorectal Surgery

Second Edition

Springer

Editors
Konstantin Umanskiy
Medical Center
University of Chicago
Chicago, IL, USA

Neil Hyman
Medical Center
University of Chicago
Chicago, IL, USA

ISSN 2198-7750 ISSN 2198-7769 (electronic)
Difficult Decisions in Surgery: An Evidence-Based Approach
ISBN 978-3-031-42302-4 ISBN 978-3-031-42303-1 (eBook)
https://doi.org/10.1007/978-3-031-42303-1

This Springer imprint is published by the registered company Springer Nature Switzerland AG
The registered company address is: Gewerbestrasse 11, 6330 Cham, Switzerland

Paper in this product is recyclable.

"To my wife, Regina, and to my daughters,
Tina, Leah, and Ilana:
You are my sparkling fountain of inspiration,
encouragement, and never-ending love."
–Konstantin Umanskiy

"With love to Naomi, EJ, and Seth—thanks
for making me feel every day like I am the
luckiest guy on the planet"
—Neil Hyman

Preface from First Edition

Colon and rectal surgery may very well be on the cusp of a golden age. Our specialty is thriving and our ACGME approved training programs are extremely popular among the best and brightest general surgery residents. Breathtaking advances in minimally invasive surgery have occurred over the past quarter century including laparoscopic bowel resection, robotic surgery, endoscopic techniques such as endoscopic mucosal/submucosal resection, and transanal approaches such as transanal endoscopic microsurgery and transanal minimally invasive surgery. Innovation in these areas has made surgery safer for many of our patients, enabled sphincter preservation, and reduced the period of disability that many experience after treatment. However, in addition to the obvious benefits of these disruptive technologies, many long-standing questions persist and new ones have been raised.

1. What is the most appropriate use of this new and often more expensive technology? Does the evidence really support that notion that everything new is really better?
2. Considering the primacy of patient safety, how do we decide who should be credentialed to do what?
3. Should **any** surgeon be able to use any technique they wish, irrespective of cost, efficacy, and demonstrated competence?
4. Should these new technologies be evaluated first by a select group of high volume/experienced surgeons in a controlled and measured environment before more widespread adoption?
5. Do we really have adequate hypotheses and frameworks of understanding for the common diseases we treat?
6. Without them, can we really devise rational treatment approaches for these maladies?
7. As such, are almost all our treatments largely empiric and lacking in the basic scientific underpinnings that would move us beyond therapeutic "hail Mary's"?

With this state of affairs, the practice of colon and rectal surgery has largely been driven by expert opinion and the practice of thought leaders—it is often the best we have. In this book, we have put together a select and highly respected group of leaders in our field and asked them both to critically review the evidence in a controversial area which they have typically contributed to and investigated during their career. We also asked them to supplement this with their clinical insights and personal experience. This is not a comprehensive textbook of colon and rectal surgery which attempts to review the basic anatomy and physiology of the vast spectrum of problems one may encounter in the small intestine, colon rectum, and anus. Many excellent textbooks like this already exist. Rather, we have selected a broad array of difficult and often controversial problems that the surgeon who deals with colorectal disease often encounters. We asked our experts to imagine that they received a phone call from a busy surgeon in the surgeon's lounge who wanted to know how a particular challenging patient management issue should be handled. The goal was NOT to list every treatment that has ever been described or utilized.

1. What are my best options?
2. What is the best evidence for/against these options in the literature?
3. How do I decide?
4. What do you think and what do you do?

The reader will be able to see what the highest quality evidence available exists to guide our management decisions. However, it will be evident that there is always going to be considerable room for alternative opinions and approaches. A different acknowledged expert with considerable clinical experience and knowledge of the applicable evidence may see things differently and approach the same problem using a very different algorithm. Indeed, as much as we like to talk about evidence based approaches, the "evidence" for much of what we do is often lacking and meager. We hope that the reader will find real help and a sense of perspective from this book. We particularly hope that we inspire our trainees and junior colleagues to uncover new paradigms of care, contribute high quality evidence to the literature, and advance the scientific underpinnings of our management decisions. Our patients deserve no less!

Chicago, IL, USA — Neil Hyman

Preface

It is truly remarkable to reflect on how much has changed, yet how much has stayed the same since our initial edition of this book in 2017. On the one hand, our specialty continues to thrive, and we continue to attract the very best and brightest general surgery residents to colon and rectal training programs. Technologic advances make our operations safer, and we are appropriately focusing on a more rapid recovery and quality of life considerations more generally.

On the other hand, there was COVID. The impact of the pandemic on many aspects of our personal and professional life was profound. We became even more siloed and disconnected and yearned for the collegial interactions that make colon and rectal surgery so special and rewarding. The reader will forgive my indulgence in what may be considered hyperbole, but I really do consider my professional colleagues to be heroes. No administrator will ever understand what it is like to share the burdens we take on when we care for our patients and their families. We worry constantly about their well-being and whether they are recovering properly. Why is this lab abnormal? How concerned should I be about this imaging finding? Could this anastomosis be leaking? We cannot and do not walk away from our patients when things go astray…and there really is no "off switch." There is an awful lot for colorectal surgeons to be proud of and we should make sure that our colleagues get the support and advocacy they richly deserve. Our steadfast commitment to our patients and professionalism should not be used as weapons against us and taken for granted.

We were very gratified by the response to the first edition and pleased to have the opportunity to work on this second edition, under the very capable leadership of Dr Konstantin Umanskiy. Best we can tell, this book has been used by many to study for their colorectal board examinations and by others who seek a clear, concise, and evidence based approach for the complex/controversial issues that we encounter in the management of colorectal disease. Again, this book is NOT intended as a comprehensive colorectal textbook that describes routine anatomy, pathophysiology and provides a complete list of potential treatments. Rather, we asked the expert authors to imagine that they were sipping coffee between cases in the OR lounge and got a call from a colleague, asking their opinion on the management of a vexing problem they have just encountered.

How should I be thinking about this case?
What are my options?
What is the best evidence for/against these options in the literature?
How do you decide in this particular circumstance what makes the most sense?
What would you do if this was your patient?

In some cases, there will be good evidence to guide decisions; in others, one must rely almost entirely on expert opinion. In this light, it is important to understand that we have asked the authors to give their own assessment of the relevance/value of the literature and what the best approach is. Undoubtedly other experts will not agree and would provide very different advice on how the situation should be managed—this is fine and the reader should keep this in mind. We do not always get the answer we are comfortable with when we "phone a friend"; in the end, each surgeon needs to decide what is best for their patient in the unique circumstances that they present.

Indeed, we really hope that readers will be inspired to identify the gaps in our collective knowledge and choose to dig deeper into the literature and even perhaps plan their own study to address these gaps. We continue to be awed and amazed at the brilliance and commitment we see every day from our junior colleagues, fellows, and residents. It is impossible not to be optimistic about the future of our specialty.

Chicago, IL, USA

Neil Hyman

Introduction

> It does not take much strength to do things, but it requires great strength to decide on what to do.
>
> Elbert Hubbard

The Clinical Challenge: Reasoning, Decision-Making, and Action

One day in the not-so-distant future, all clinical decisions will be aided by artificial intelligence. This will undoubtedly improve patient care, limit mistakes in judgment, and reduce errors of omission. For the time being, however, we, as clinicians, must continue to do all the work to arrive to the best decisions for our patients.

Surgeons make complex, high-stakes, and time-sensitive decisions when diagnosing a patient, assessing risk factors, selecting and performing an operation, and managing complications. Surgical decision-making is primarily based on hypothetical deductive reasoning and individual judgment. In the most straightforward clinical scenarios, the surgeon may recognize a pattern and base their decision on prior experience or knowledge. In cases where the diagnosis is not clear or the clinical information is limited, the clinician might rely on intuition by integrating blocks of knowledge and previous experience to arrive at the decision. This is further influenced by the patient's values and emotions, patient–surgeon interactions, decision-making volume and complexity, time constraints, and uncertainty.

Patient-centered care does not allow for a one-size-fits-all guideline of optimal decision-making. Clinical decisions are ultimately informed by patients and caregivers' goals for care and what they value most in life. Decision-making based on patients' values can improve patient satisfaction and compliance. However, surgeons' decision-making may also be negatively influenced by patients' and caregivers' apprehension about surgical diseases or complications. Patients' emotions can influence a surgeon's perception of risks and benefits and may create pressure to perform unnecessary operations.

Further, surgical decision-making is often affected by uncertainty due to missing or incomplete data. This occurs when decisions regarding an urgent condition must be made before all relevant data can be gathered and analyzed. Non-urgent decisions, too, may be hindered by time constraints and uncertainty owing to sheer

Table 1 Bias in surgical decision-making

Source of bias	Example
Framing effect	A hospital medicine provider presents a clinical scenario to a surgeon in different context than the surgeon would have perceived during an independent assessment
Overconfidence bias	A surgeon falsely believes that weaknesses and failures disproportionately affect their peers
Commission bias	A surgeon tends toward surgical intervention when non-operative management may be preferable, especially in the context of overconfidence bias
Anchoring bias	Patients are informed of expected outcomes using data from aggregate patient populations without adjusting for their personalized risk profile
Recall bias	Recent experiences, particularly negative, with a certain patient population or operation disproportionately affect surgical decision-making relative to remote experiences
Confirmation bias	Excessive reliance on personal experience. Outcomes are predicted using a set of beliefs rather than evidence-based guidelines

Adapted from: Loftus et al. [1]

decision-making volume, the time-consuming nature of data acquisition, and complex team dynamics. Even when data collection and analysis are complete, high decision-making volume begets decision fatigue, manifesting as procrastination, frustration when facing adversity, decreased physical stamina, and lower quality and quantity of diagnostic and clinical output [1].

Under the increased pressure of time constraints and uncertainty, decision-making may be affected by heuristics or cognitive shortcuts. Heuristics may lead to bias or predictable and systematic cognitive lapses, as described in Table 1.

There is a wealth of clinical-decision support tools, risk calculators, clinical guidelines, and evidence-based scientific publications to aid surgeons with clinical decision-making. The challenge of seeking answers in available resources, however, is identifying what is true and what is not. In recent years, our traditional trusted source of "truth" (published peer-reviewed literature) has come under increased scrutiny. Although we hope that scientific misconduct is uncommon, its actual incidence is unknown. "Mistakes," ranging from benign errors to outright fraud, are detected with alarming frequency. Methodological flaws and interpretive shortcomings compromise much of the biomedical literature. False-positive research findings are ubiquitous, reflecting flawed treatment effect size, underpowered studies, improper statistical analysis, flagrant data-mining, overfitting, and a lack of confirmatory studies. These issues are exacerbated by publication bias and an archaic system of editorial peer review process. Even when based on thoroughly vetted evidence, a typical textbook merely lists the outcomes of surgical trials that focus on conventional variables, such as perioperative mortality or disease-free survival, but these may not directly inform clinical decisions [2].

The Difficult Decisions in Surgery: An Evidence-Based Approach Series, and this textbook in particular, provides clinicians with an expert appraisal of available literature, augmented by an assessment of the quality of the evidence and personal recommendations by the authors. A unique feature of this series is the focus on individual author's perspectives to a series of specific clinical scenarios the surgeons face in their practice.

We would like to extend our sincere gratitude to the authors for their invaluable contributions to this publication. Your time, expertise, and thoughtful advice will help many of your colleagues to provide better care for their patients. Thank you!

References

1. Loftus TJ, et al. Artificial intelligence and surgical decision-making. JAMA Surg. 2020;155(2):148–58.
2. Matthews JB. Truth and truthiness: evidence, experience and clinical judgement in surgery. Br J Surg. 2021;108(7):742–4.

University of Chicago
Chicago, IL, USA

Konstantin Umansky

Contents

Contributors

Mohammad Abbass Division of Gastrointestinal Surgery Northwestern Medicine, Feinberg School of Medicine, Chicago, IL, USA

Maria Abou Khalil McGill University Health Center, Montreal, QC, Canada

Evan D. Adams Department of General Surgery, Cedars-Sinai Medical Center, Los Angeles, CA, USA

Karim Alavi UMass Chan Medical School, Department of Surgery, Division of Colon & Rectal Surgery, Worcester, MA, USA

Wyeth Alexander Department of Surgery, Division of Colon and Rectal Surgery, UC San Diego Health, La Jolla, CA, USA

William Allen Department of Surgery, University of Louisville, Louisville, KY, USA

Alison Althans Department of Surgery, University of Pittsburgh Medical Center, Pittsburgh, PA, USA

Allison M. Ammann University of Cincinnati College of Medicine, Surgery, Cincinnati, OH, USA

Athanasios Angistriotis, MD Division of Colorectal Surgery, Columbia University Irving Medical Center-New York Presbyterian Hospital, New York, NY, USA

Rodrigo Areán-Sanz, MD Division of Colon and Rectal Surgery, Department of Surgery, Beth Israel Deaconess Medical Center, Harvard Medical School, Boston, MA, USA

Elliot Arsoniadis Division of Colon and Rectal Surgery, University of Minnesota, Minneapolis, MN, USA

Glenn T. Ault Keck School of Medicine of USC, Los Angeles, CA, USA

Division of Colon and Rectal Surgery, Keck School of Medicine, Los Angeles, CA, USA

Kristen A. Ban Cleveland Clinic Foundation, Cleveland, OH, USA

Paulo Vitor Barreto Guimaraes Department of Urology, University of Chicago, Chicago, IL, USA

Brian L. Bello Medstar Medical Center, Washington, DC, USA

Natalie F. Berger Department of Surgery, NYU Langone Hospital, New York, NY, USA

Marco Bertucci Zoccali, MD, FACSa Division of Colorectal Surgery, Columbia University Irving Medical Center-New York Presbyterian Hospital, New York, NY, USA

Himani Bhatt Department of Surgery, Mayo Clinic, Rochester, MN, USA

Joshua I. S. Bleier Division of Colorectal Surgery, Department of Surgery, University of Pennsylvania, Perelman School of Medicine, Philadelphia, PA, USA

Sonja Boatman Division of Colon and Rectal Surgery, University of Minnesota, Minneapolis, MN, USA

Liliana G. Bordeiano Section of Colon and Rectal Surgery, Division of General and Gastrointestinal Surgery, Department of Surgery, Massachusetts General Hospital, Boston, MA, USA

Sarah Choi Division of Colon and Rectal Surgery, Department of Surgery, Keck School of Medicine, University of Southern California, Los Angeles, CA, USA

Kathryn E. Chuquin Washington, DC, USA

Robert R. Cima Mayo Clinic, Division of Colon and Rectal Surgery, Rochester, MN, USA

Kyle G. Cologne Division of Colon and Rectal Surgery, Department of Surgery, Keck School of Medicine, University of Southern California, Los Angeles, CA, USA

L. Cunningham Department of Surgery, The Ohio State University College of Medicine, Columbus, OH, USA

Aneel Damle Colon and Rectal Surgery Associates, University of Minnesota School of Medicine, Minneapolis, MN, USA

Scott C. Dolejs Indiana Colon and Rectal Specialists, Indianapolis, IN, USA

Gideon Dosunmu Section of Hematology/Oncology, Department of Medicine, University of Chicago, Chicago, IL, USA

Samuel Eisenstein Department of Surgery, Division of Colon and Rectal Surgery, UC San Diego Health, La Jolla, CA, USA

Ahmed A. Eltahir Washington University St. Louis, St. Louis, MO, USA

Oliver S. Eng Division of Surgical Oncology, Department of Surgery, University of California, Orange, CA, USA

Russ Farmer Division of Colon and Rectal Surgery, Department of Surgery, University of Louisville, Louisville, KY, USA

Linda Ferrari Guy's and St Thomas' NHS Foundation Trust, London, UK

Alessandro Fichera Division of Colon and Rectal Surgery, Baylor University Medical Center, Dallas, TX, USA

Fergal J. Fleming Division of Colorectal Surgery, Department of Surgery, University of Rochester Medical Center, Rochester, NY, USA

Bhuwan Giri DeWitt Daughtry Family Department of Surgery, University of Miami Leondard M. Miller School of Medicine, Miami, FL, USA

Jackson Health System, Miami, FL, USA

Paolo Goffredo Division of Colon & Rectal Surgery, University of Minnesota, Minneapolis, MN, USA

Emre Gorgun Department of Colorectal Surgery, Digestive Disease and Surgery Institute, Cleveland, OH, USA

Ga-ram Han Department of General Surgery, Division of Colon and Rectal Surgery, Mayo Clinic, Phoenix, AZ, USA

Traci L. Hedrick Chief, Division of General Surgery, Department of Surgery, University of Virginia Health, Charlottesville, VA, USA

Susanna S. Hill Division of Colon and Rectal Surgery, Department of Surgery, University of Minnesota School of Medicine, Minneapolis, MN, USA

Jennifer Holder-Murray Division of Colon and Rectal Surgery, Department of Surgery, University of Pittsburgh Medical Center, Pittsburgh, PA, USA

Alex L. Huang Mount Sinai Hospital, New York, NY, USA

E. Huang Department of Surgery, The Ohio State University College of Medicine, Columbus, OH, USA

Roger D. Hurst Department of Surgery, University of Chicago, Chicago, IL, USA

Alexandra Jones Department of Surgery, University of Louisville, Louisville, KY, USA

Scott R. Kelley Mayo Clinic, Colon and Rectal Surgery, Rochester, MN, USA

Sergey Khaitov Mount Sinai Hospital, New York, NY, USA

Erin King-Mullins Colorectal Wellness Center, Fayetteville, GA, USA

Ervin Kocjancic Department of Urology, University of Chicago, Chicago, IL, USA

Reconstructive Urology and Trans Health, Chicago, IL, USA

Julia Kohn Division of Colon and Rectal Surgery, University of Minnesota, Minneapolis, MN, USA

Nathan Kohrman Keck School of Medicine of USC, Los Angeles, CA, USA

John Konen Rush University Medical College, Department of Surgery, Division of Colon & Rectal Surgery, Chicago, IL, USA

Monika A. Krezalek Department of Surgery, Division of Colon and Rectal Surgery, NorthShore University Health System, Evanston, IL, USA

Samuel H. Lai University of Colorado Surgery, Aurora, CO, USA

Sean J. Langenfeld Division of Colon and Rectal Surgery, Department of Surgery, University of Nebraska Medical Center, Omaha, NE, USA

Jonathan Laryea Division of Colon and Rectal Surgery, Department of Surgery, University of Arkansas for Medical Sciences, Little Rock, AR, USA

Jennifer A. Leinicke Omaha, NE, USA

Chih-Yi Liao Section of Hematology/Oncology, Department of Medicine, University of Chicago, Chicago, IL, USA

Sender Liberman McGill University Health Centre, Colon & Rectal Surgery, Montreal, QC, Canada

Amy L. Lightner Department of Colorectal Surgery, Digestive Disease Surgical Institute, Cleveland Clinic, Cleveland, OH, USA

Anthony Loria Division of Colorectal Surgery, Department of Surgery, University of Rochester Medical Center, Rochester, NY, USA

Henry J. Lujan, M.D., F.A.C.S., F.A.S.C.R.S. Jackson South Medical Center, Colon and Rectal Surgery, Miami, FL, USA

Victor Maciel, MD Allegheny General Hospital/St. Vincent Hospital, Colon and Rectal Surgery, Pittsburgh, PA, USA

Kellie Mathis Department of Surgery, Mayo Clinic, Rochester, MN, USA

Nicholas P. McKenna Mayo Clinic, Division of Colon and Rectal Surgery, Rochester, MN, USA

Evangelos Messaris, MD, PhD, MBA Division of Colon and Rectal Surgery, Department of Surgery, Beth Israel Deaconess Medical Center, Harvard Medical School, Boston, MA, USA

Maxwell D. Mirande Mayo Clinic, General Surgery, Rochester, MN, USA

Nitin Mishra Department of Colon and Rectal Surgery, Mayo Clinic, Phoenix, AZ, USA

Yusuke Miyatani Inflammatory Bowel Disease Center, The University of Chicago Medicine, Chicago, IL, USA

Matthew G. Mutch Washington University St. Louis, Colon and Rectal Surgery, St. Louis, MO, USA

Valentine N. Nfonsam LSU Health Department of Surgery, Louisiana State University, New Orleans, LA, USA

Cory Nonnemacher Atrium Health Navicent, Department of General Surgery, Macon, GA, USA

Megan Obi Department of General Surgery, Digestive Disease Surgical Institute, Cleveland Clinic, Cleveland, OH, USA

Kinga S. Olortegui Section of Colon & Rectal Surgery, Department of Surgery, UChicago Medicine, Chicago, IL, USA

Arsha Ostowari Department of Surgery, University of California, Orange, CA, USA

Ian M. Paquette Chief of the Division of Colon and Rectal Surgery, University of Cincinnati College of Medicine, Cincinnati, OH, USA

Nell Maloney Patel Rutgers Robert Wood Johnson Medical School, Colon and Rectal Surgery, Westfield, NJ, USA

Terrah J. Paul Olson Division of Colorectal Surgery, Department of Surgery, Emory University, Atlanta, GA, USA

Kayla Polcari University of Chicago, Chicago, IL, USA

Vitaliy Poylin Division of Gastrointestinal Surgery Northwestern Medicine, Feinberg School of Medicine, Chicago, IL, USA

Northwestern University Feinberg School of Medicine, Northwestern Medical Group, Chicago, IL, USA

Felipe F. Quezada-Diaz Colorectal Unit, Department of Surgery, Complejo Asistencial Doctor Sótero del Río, Santiago, RM, Chile

Omer Raheem Department of Urology, University of Chicago, Chicago, IL, USA

Shahrose Rahman, MD Department of Surgery, Oregon Health & Science University, Portland, OR, USA

Ray Ramirez Rutgers Robert Wood Johnson Medical School, Surgery, New Brunswick, NJ, USA

Tobi J. Reidy Indiana Colon and Rectal Specialists, Indianapolis, IN, USA

Jeffrey L. Roberson Department of Surgery, Hospital of the University of Pennsylvania, Philadelphia, PA, USA

Gustavo A. Rubio Jackson Health System, Miami, FL, USA

Atsushi Sakuraba RUSH Center for Crohn's and Colitis, RUSH University Medical Center, Chicago, USA

Nicole M. Saur Division of Colon and Rectal Surgery, Department of Surgery, Hospital of the University of Pennsylvania, Philadelphia, PA, USA

Cimarron E. Sharon Department of Surgery, University of Pennsylvania, Perelman School of Medicine, Philadelphia, PA, USA

Benjamin D. Shogan University of Chicago, Chicago, IL, USA

Hillary Simon Division of Colon and Rectal Surgery, Department of Surgery, University of Louisville, Louisville, KY, USA

Bradford Sklow Cleveland Clinic Florida, Department of Colorectal Surgery, Port St. Lucie, FL, USA

J. Joshua Smith Colorectal Service, Department of Surgery, Memorial Sloan Kettering Cancer Center, New York, NY, USA

Radhika K. Smith Washington University St. Louis, St. Louis, MO, USA

Ernie Soto Division of Colon and Rectal Surgery, Department of Surgery, University of Arkansas for Medical Sciences, Little Rock, AR, USA

Melinda E. Stack Colon and Rectal Surgery Associates, Minneapolis, MN, USA

David B. Stewart Southern Illinois University School of Medicine, SIU Department of Surgery, Springfield, IL, USA

Patricia Sylla Department of Colon and Rectal Surgery, Mount Sinai Hospital, New York, NY, USA

Joseph Terlizzi Mount Sinai School of Medicine, Surgery, New York, NY, USA

Vassiliki Liana Tsikitis, MD, MBA Division of Gastrointestinal and General Surgery, School of Medicine, Oregon Health & Science University, Portland, OR, USA

Martin Uwah Department of Colon and Rectal Surgery, University of Chicago, Chicago, IL, USA

Michael A. Valente University of Arizona, Surgical Oncology, Tucson, AZ, USA

Jon D. Vogel University of Colorado Surgery, Aurora, CO, USA

Sarah A. Vogler Cleveland Clinic Florida, Martin Health, Port St Lucie, FL, USA

Thomas M. Ward Section of Colon and Rectal Surgery, Division of General and Gastrointestinal Surgery, Department of Surgery, Massachusetts General Hospital, Boston, MA, USA

Martin R. Weiser Stuart Quan Chair in Colorectal Surgery, Memorial Sloan Kettering Cancer Center, New York, NY, USA

Weill Cornell Medical College, New York City, NY, USA

Maggie L. Westfal Washington University St. Louis, Colon and Rectal Surgery, St. Louis, MO, USA

Matthew Z. Wilson Dartmouth Hitchcock Medical Center, Geisel School of Medicine at Dartmouth, Division of Colon and Rectal Surgery, Lebanon, NH, USA

Zhaomin Xu Division of Colorectal Surgery, University of Rochester, Rochester, NY, USA

Sumeyye Yilmaz Department of Colorectal Surgery, Digestive Disease and Surgery Institute, Cleveland, OH, USA

Allen T. Yu Mount Sinai Hospital, New York, NY, USA

Karen Zaghiyan Division of Colorectal Surgery, Cedars-Sinai Medical Center, Los Angeles, CA, USA

1 Evaluating Evidence

Zhaomin Xu and Bradford Sklow

Evaluating Evidence

Evidence-based medicine (EBM) is an approach to clinical decision-making that emphasizes the use of the best available evidence to guide clinical practice. The term was first coined by Gordon Guyatt from McMaster University in Canada in the 1990s. [1] EBM involves critically evaluating evidence to determine validity, relevance, and applicability to particular clinical situations.

As a starting point, there must first be a clinical question that is well defined and therefore answerable. A poorly formulated question results in wasted time and resources evaluating irrelevant evidence and sources. When considering how to formulate a good clinical question, first we must define the patient population we are interested in. Then, there has to be an exposure or action, which may include a comparison control. And finally, we must define a desired outcome. Once the clinical question has been formulated, then we can move forward with identifying relevant sources and evaluating their quality and ability to answer the question.

This chapter will provide an overview of the key steps involved in evaluating medical evidence, so the reader may formulate their own assessment of the literature and carry these practices forward in their continued education. This chapter is not meant to serve as an in-depth review of statistics, and there are numerous other

Z. Xu
University of Rochester, Division of Colorectal Surgery, Rochester, NY, USA
e-mail: zhaomin_xu@umrc.rochester.edu

B. Sklow (✉)
Cleveland Clinic Florida, Department of Colorectal Surgery, Port St. Lucie, FL, USA
e-mail: SKLOWB@ccf.org

K. Umanskiy, N. Hyman (eds.), *Difficult Decisions in Colorectal Surgery*, Difficult Decisions in Surgery: An Evidence-Based Approach,
https://doi.org/10.1007/978-3-031-42303-1_1

resources dedicated to statistics that can be referenced if readers have specific questions. For more in depth discussion of many of the topics addressed in this chapter, a useful reference is "How to Read a Paper: The Basics of Evidence-Based Medicine and Healthcare," by Dr. Trisha Greenhalgh [2]. Another useful resource for readers to reference is a recent set of guides to different statistical methods published by JAMA Surgery which is easily accessible for those who don't have a strong statistical background. [3–11]

Assessing Methodology

The study design is critical in determining the strength and quality of the evidence. A well-designed study will help to minimize bias and confounding factors. Different study designs have different strengths and weaknesses, and the design should be chosen based on the research question. The hierarchy of evidence is often used to rank studies in order of their quality with reviews and meta-analyses based on high quality randomized controlled trials (RCTs) being generally considered the gold standard. (Table 1.1) This is followed by high-quality RCTs themselves, low quality RCTs, well-designed case-control and cohort studies, and finally expert opinions at the bottom of the hierarchy. However, in some instances a large, well-designed cohort study may be more important than a poorly done meta-analysis or a methodologically questionable RCT. In addition, there are also instances where RCTs may not be the appropriate study design. [2] For example, if we were interested whether ctDNA could reliably diagnose a recurrence in a colon cancer patient, the ideal design would be a cross-sectional study, not a RCT. So, while the traditional hierarchy of evidence we are familiar with is a useful framework to being thinking about quality of evidence, it is not enough.

Table 1.1 The hierarchy of evidence

Level of evidence	Description
Level I	Evidence from a systematic review or meta-analysis of all relevant RCTs or evidence-based clinical practice guidelines based on systematic reviews of high quality RCTs.
Level II	Evidence from a well-designed RCT.
Level III	Evidence obtained from lower quality RCTs or controlled trials without randomization.
Level IV	Evidence from a well-designed case-control or cohort studies
Level V	Evidence from systematic reviews of descriptive and qualitative studies (meta-synthesis).
Level VI	Evidence from a single descriptive or qualitative study.
Level VII	Evidence from expert opinion.

RCT randomized controlled trial

There are five broad questions that should be asked of any paper when assessing the methodology:

1. Was the study original?
2. What's the patient population?
3. What are the exposures and outcomes and do they make sense?
4. Was an adequate attempt made to control for bias?
5. Was the study large enough and continued long enough to make the results useful?

Was the Study Original?

Once we start looking for relevant papers to answer our clinical question, it can suddenly become apparent that there appears to be many papers trying to answer the same question. While it may seem common sense that a question that has already been answered shouldn't be asked again, but the reality is that most papers only tell us if a hypothesis is incrementally more or less likely than before. It's rare that a single paper is enough to change clinical practice. Therefore, the question is not whether a study is completely novel, but rather does the paper add to the existing literature in any way.

A paper could add to the existing literature by providing a larger study population or a longer follow up. Or the paper may be looking at a more defined portion of the patient population that previous papers did not have the opportunity to explore, such as a specific age group or minority populations. Perhaps there were methodological flaws with the existing literature that the current paper is trying to correct. And finally, it could be that for whatever reason, despite there being robust current evidence, there is still skepticism and therefore an additional study may contribute to a future meta-analysis or review that will contribute to solidifying the literature further.

What's the Patient Population?

The patient population can be tricky. We are frequently faced with a single patient that generated the clinical question that we are investigating, so no matter how large and high quality a study may be, there's the possibility that the study can't be applied to our patient because the study population is different from our patient. Therefore, there are several questions we want to ask ourselves when looking at a study's patient population:

1. **How were the patients recruited or what was the source of the patient population?**

   For example, we may find a very robust cohort study sourced from an administrative database like the Medicare dataset. But if our original clinical question was in regards to a young patient, the results of this Medicare study may not apply to our patient no matter how high quality the study is.

The method by which patients are recruited for a study may also lead to recruitment bias. A common example of this is in survey-based studies where the sample of patients obtained is skewed in some fashion due to certain populations being more likely to respond to a particular survey.

2. **What were the inclusion and exclusion criteria?**

   Traditionally, RCTs suffer from limited patient inclusion excluding many elderly patients, minority populations, and those with poor education or are non-English speakers [12]. While having a very limited population makes for cleaner and easier studies, it makes results difficult to extrapolate for the general population. If we are evaluating a cohort study looking at any long-term outcome of rectal cancer patients, it's important to know whether any inclusions or exclusions were made based on neoadjuvant or adjuvant therapies. And in this example, some older studies may no longer be relevant despite being robust because of the differences in how rectal cancer is now managed compared to before.

3. **Was the population studied in a different environment?**

   This question address whether the study population of a paper came from an environment similar to our patients. If, for example, we practice in a low resource setting, a robust paper that heralds the newest and best technology to assist with the endoscopic treatment of large polyps may not be relevant to our practice and patients. So, while this does not invalidate the paper from a methodological standpoint and will serve a different population well, it cannot be applied to our patients

What Are the Exposures and Outcomes and Do They Make Sense?

A fundamental question when appraising a paper is what the exposure is and what is it being compared to, if any comparison is being made. At face value, this may be quite simple. For example, the authors may have stated in the paper that they compared patients who recorded their ileostomy output to those who did not. However, this begs the question of how the authors determined whether a patient did or did not measure their ileostomy output, which inherently require assumptions such as that patients who were recording, were doing it accurately. Another example would be in studies that depend on a review of medical records, an assumption is being made that medical records are accurate and reliable. These assumptions may or may not be true and could potentially impact the validity of the results. Therefore, it is important to determine whether the method by which the authors used to gather their exposure data is reliable. If not, this could skew the results of the study in the positive or negative.

Similar to exposure, the outcome has to be sensible and measurable. Binary outcomes, such as survival tend to be self-explanatory. However, the difficulty with outcomes such as survival comes down to how the outcome was captured and measured and whether this was reliable. We have to assess the methods by which the authors used to determine whether a patient was still alive and how long did the authors follow up for to determine the outcome. When evaluating a study that measures an outcome that is less concrete, such as patient-reported outcomes, it is important to confirm that the outcome measure has been objectively validated and actually measures what it claims to measure. The development of patient reported outcome measures should be done in a rigorous and protocol-driven method and can provide valuable insight into patient perspectives [6].

Was an Adequate Attempt Made to Control for Bias?

No matter how well designed a study is there can inevitably be error that impacts the validity of the results. There are two different types of error: random error and systematic error, which is also referred to as bias [13]. Regardless of the study design, a paper that aims to compare groups should aim for the groups to be as comparable as possible in order to isolate the effects of the exposure. Random error in a study is not necessarily a mistake, but a natural part of measurement that result in variability of the results when the same measurement is repeated multiple times. Random error impacts precision, which is how reproducible the results of a measurement is when taken multiple times under the same conditions. It is equally likely to be higher or lower than the true value and therefore is not typically seen as a large problem. It can be mitigated through several strategies:

1. Take repeated measurements: For example, if a paper is studying a specific lab value, there is likely random error associated with the measurement itself, so perhaps the authors ran the lab multiple times to obtain an average that more represents the true value.
2. Increase sample size: This is the most common way studies attempt to minimize random error, and is otherwise referred to as the power of the study. The larger the sample size, the greater the power. A well-designed prospective study should have a predetermined power and a power calculation that tells us the number of patients that are needed to reach that power. When evaluating a study, if the authors report no statistically significant difference between an intervention and control arm and there was no power calculation, the reader needs to examine whether the study was underpowered [14].
3. Efficient statistical analysis: Estimation of random error is typically carried out in studies through hypothesis contrast tests (p-values) and confidence intervals.

Systemic error, or bias, is directly impacted by study methodology and causes a skewing of the results that is predictable. Systematic error impacts accuracy, so unlike random error, results can be very precise and consistent, but it is not around the true value. There are many different types of bias and they can occur at any stage of a study. Bias typically falls within three major categories: selection, measurement, and confounding.

Selection bias occurs when the relationship between the exposure and outcomes changes from group to group due to systematic differences in the characteristics of the groups. In RCTs, this is typically controlled for by the randomization process, which should be blinded. Selection bias is much harder to control for in retrospective studies. A common method by which a statistical adjustment is made is to perform a propensity score analysis. However, propensity score analysis is not without criticism and in some instances may actually worsen the imbalance [15]. A more in- depth discussion of propensity score analysis is beyond the scope of text and readers should refer to other sources when faced with a paper that utilizes this technique.

Measurement bias comes in many forms and may result from a bias in the measured exposure such as recall bias, a bias over time in the way the exposure is defined such as a change in diagnostic criteria or a bias in the way the observer performing measurements.

Confounding leads to an error in the interpretation of the interaction between exposure and outcome due to inadequate control of other variables. A confounding variable is one that is associated with both the exposure and the outcome but is not found in the causal pathway between the exposure and the outcome. For example, in a study of rectal cancer patients with neoadjuvant chemoradiation being the exposure and survival being the outcome, age of the patient is a confounding variable because age is likely associated with the likelihood of neoadjuvant therapy administration and older patients are at greater risk of mortality. Confounding is an incredibly common and difficult issue in retrospective observational studies. Hence, investigators frequently use statistical models of different complexities to attempt to control for as much confounding as possible and it is the task of the reader to determine whether enough confounding is accounted for to make the reported interaction between exposure and outcome believable. [16]

Was the Study Large Enough and Continued Long Enough to Make the Results Believable?

Sample size and power was discussed earlier in the context of controlling for random error. To reiterate, a study or trial needs to be large enough to have a high chance of detecting a statistically significant difference between groups.

A study needs to be continued for long enough and participants need to have been adequately followed up on for the effect of the exposure to be seen in the outcome. This obviously depends on the type of exposure and type of outcome. If we return to a rectal cancer example, a study looking at the impact of an enhanced recovery protocol on hospital length of stay after proctectomy may only need a follow up of a couple of weeks. However, if the study was instead looking at the impact of an enhanced recovery protocol on 30-day readmission, we would expect that the majority of the patients have at least a follow up of 30 days in order to capture the event of interest. In RCTs, careful attention has to be paid to the completeness of follow up and dropout rate of participants. RCTs that exclude patients that were randomized but dropout risk biasing their results, therefore it is standard practice to analyze the results based on an intent-to-treat. This means that all patients that were randomized are analyzed as part of the original group they were randomized to. The reader should confirm that the paper clearly states an intention-to-treat analysis and also confirm the patient numbers within the results to the number of patients randomized.

Final Thoughts

We all strive to make clinical decisions based on the best clinical evidence available. The analytical process involved in determining whether a study result can be applied to clinical practice is complex and should be interpreted in the context of what is already known. This unfortunately necessitates a discussion of publication bias. Publication bias may be the most difficult bias to overcome because it relates to hidden information that the reader never gets a chance to assess. Negative studies are less likely to get published and if they are published, frequently end up in lower impact journals or never make it to manuscript from their abstract form. This unfortunately leads to a bias towards overestimation of treatment effects and is a bias that may not be correctable no matter how high quality the studies or the subsequent meta-analyses are [17].

Another common phenomenon in clinical literature is a heavy reliance on p-values and confidence intervals. This has resulted in a lack of true critical evaluation of methodology and biases. The use of p-values is increasingly being criticized because of the potential impact of sample size on it. With a large enough sample size, the p-value will almost certainly be significant, even though the effect size could be very small. Alternatively, a study with a small sample size may have insignificant p-values, but there could be a very large effect that wasn't detected. While both p-values and confidence intervals rely on statistical inference and sample size, confidence intervals at least provide more information about the degree of uncertainty. [18]

Personal View

When evaluating a study or manuscript, the first question to ask is what is the hypothesis or question the study is trying to answer? If not familiar with the evidence on the subject matter, a search of the literature might be required to determine if there is novelty of the study or if it provides a significant contribution to the literature. The other question one should ask is the study designed to answer the proposed hypothesis or question the authors are asking.

Assuming the study design is solid, we would then want to know if the study was powered adequately to show a difference or to prove or disprove the hypothesis. Was a power calculation done? In the results section, are the tables and figures formatted properly with appropriate labels? Do the results make sense and are the data relative to the hypothesis? There are some studies where there is data overload and not relative to the question being asked. Does the study suffer from any kind of bias that could affect the results (e.g. selection bias, etc)? We would also want to know if the length of follow up was appropriate to answer the proposed question. For example, most studies looking at cancer survival have at least 5 year follow up as 5 year survival is the standard in the literature.

As far as the Discussion is concerned, is the length appropriate? It is not uncommon for the Discussion section to be too long and wordy, with extraneous information provided that is not relevant. The Discussion should highlight the novelty of the findings and contain references to other previously published studies that are relevant. Lastly, are the conclusions appropriate and are they supported by the data? A study can only draw conclusions based on the data within the study and a conclusion must be supported by the data.

Conclusion

Ultimately, it is up to clinicians to weigh the risks and benefits of their decisions and apply the available evidence to each unique patient, which may be the greatest challenge to evidence-based medicine. So much of EBM is provisioned on the importance of empirical data that it is easy to forget that to an individual patient, if they are unable to benefit from the study, it doesn't matter how high quality it was. The only way to do this effectively is to have a framework of skills to evaluate the evidence, integrate knowledge, and adapt evidence to the needs of our patients.

References

1. Thoma A, Eaves FF. A brief history of evidence-based medicine (EBM) and the contributions of Dr David Sackett. Aesthet Surg J. 2015;35:NP261–3.
2. Greenhalgh T. How to read a paper: the basics of evidence-based medicine and healthcare. Wiley; 2019.
3. Arya S, Schwartz TA, Ghaferi AA. Practical guide to meta-analysis. JAMA Surg. 2020;155:430.
4. Brasel K, Haider A, Haukoos J. Practical guide to survey research. JAMA Surg. 2020;155:351.
5. Brooke BS, Kaji AH, Itani KMF. Practical guide to cost-effectiveness analysis. JAMA Surg. 2020;155:250.
6. Davidson GH, Haukoos JS, Feldman LS. Practical guide to assessment of patient-reported outcomes. JAMA Surg. 2020;155:432.
7. Dossett LA, Kaji AH, Dimick JB. Practical guide to mixed methods. JAMA Surg. 2020;155:254.
8. Merkow RP, Schwartz TA, Nathens AB. Practical guide to comparative effectiveness research using observational data. JAMA Surg. 2020;155:349–50.
9. Neuman HB, Kaji AH, Haut ER. Practical guide to implementation science. JAMA Surg. 2020;155:434.
10. Scott JW, Schwartz TA, Dimick JB. Practical guide to health policy evaluation using observational data. JAMA Surg. 2020;155:353.
11. Segev DL, Haukoos JS, Pawlik TM. Practical guide to decision analysis. JAMA Surg. 2020;155:436.

12. Van Spall HG, Toren A, Kiss A, Fowler RA. Eligibility criteria of randomized controlled trials published in high-impact general medical journals: a systematic sampling review. JAMA. 2007;297(11):1233–40.
13. Popovic A, Huecker MR. Study Bias. In: StatPearls. StatPearls Publishing; 2022.
14. Ambrosius WT. Topics in biostatistics. Humana Press; 2007.
15. Guo S, Fraser M, Chen Q. Propensity score analysis: recent debate and discussion. J Soc Soc Work Res. 2020;11:463–82.
16. Groenwold RHH, Van Deursen AMM, Hoes AW, Hak E. Poor quality of reporting confounding bias in observational intervention studies: a systematic review. Ann Epidemiol. 2008;18:746–51.
17. Guyatt GH, et al. GRADE guidelines: 5. Rating the quality of evidence—publication bias. J Clin Epidemiol. 2011;64:1277–82.
18. Greenland S, et al. Statistical tests, P values, confidence intervals, and power: a guide to misinterpretations. Eur J Epidemiol. 2016;31:337–50.

Part I

Inflammatory Bowel Disease

Surgical vs Medical Management of Symptomatic Anal Fistulas in Patients with Crohn's Disease

2

Megan Obi and Amy L. Lightner

Introduction

Crohn's disease (CD) is a chronic inflammatory disease that predominantly affects the gastrointestinal (GI) tract. Along with ulcerative colitis (UC), it is thought to affect 1.3% of the US population and has an annual incidence of 3 to 20 cases per 100,000 [1, 2]. It is characterized by transmural inflammation of the GI tract that results in intestinal wall damage. One of the most common presentations of CD is the formation of perianal fistulas which affects anywhere from 5–40% of CD patients worldwide [3]. Unlike idiopathic anal fistula that develop from occlusion and infection of the anal glands resulting in cryptoglandular abscesses, fistulas related to CD are thought to be due to the inflammatory process characteristic of CD which penetrates the mucosal lining of the GI tract [4]. Perianal fistulizing disease is quite heterogeneous in its presentation, and complete remission is notoriously challenging to achieve. Therefore, medical and surgical management are both necessary to optimize patient outcomes.

CD patients with perianal fistulizing disease report significantly impaired quality of life, overall health, and physical and sexual function [5, 6]. At presentation of perianal disease, several patients may not have an underlying diagnosis of CD, as perianal fistulas can be the initial presenting phenotype in 10% of CD patients [7]. The presence of a perianal fistula alone predicts increased utilization of medications

M. Obi
Department of General Surgery, Digestive Disease Surgical Institute, Cleveland Clinic, Cleveland, OH, USA
e-mail: Obim2@ccf.org

A. L. Lightner (✉)
Department of Colorectal Surgery, Digestive Disease Surgical Institute, Cleveland Clinic, Cleveland, OH, USA

K. Umanskiy, N. Hyman (eds.), *Difficult Decisions in Colorectal Surgery*, Difficult Decisions in Surgery: An Evidence-Based Approach, https://doi.org/10.1007/978-3-031-42303-1_2

such as steroids and immunosuppressants, frequent re-hospitalizations, and likelihood of undergoing at least one surgical procedure given that perianal disease signals a more severe phenotype of CD. Because the recurrence rate of perianal fistulas is as high as 60% [3], treatment has required a multidisciplinary approach with medicine optimizing the underlying disease process and surgery attempting to anatomically close the internal opening(s).

PICO Table

Patients	Intervention	Comparator	Outcome
Patients with fistula in ano due to Crohn's Disease	Surgery	Medical therapy	Fistula healing, fecal continence, fistula fistula recurrence

Diagnosis

Diagnosis of perianal fistulas is commonly initiated by identification of symptoms commonly associated with fistula presence. Patients can describe new onset recto-vaginal discharge, perianal erythema or skin irritation, perianal pain, air or stool in the urine, and pain with defecation. Systemic symptoms such as fever are rarely associated with perianal fistulas [8]. A thorough history and physical exam evaluating for skin tags, hemorrhoidal tissue, fissures, bleeding, and palpation and inspection of areas of fluctuance and external tract openings is the first step in diagnosis. Subsequent imaging may be a helpful next step in better characterizing the underlying fistula anatomy. In certain scenarios, this can be a useful adjunct to guide treatment.

The most common diagnostic imaging modalities include magnetic resonance imaging (MRI) and endoanal ultrasonography (EUS). MRI is typically the initial modality utilized for both diagnosis and follow-up as it is non-invasive, and can serve to help locate fistula tract openings that would otherwise be difficult to find on EUA as well as diagnose more complex fistula tracts and locate clinically "silent" fluid collections [9]. T2- weight sequencing with fat suppression is the optimal imaging technique but gadolinium-enhanced T1 weighted sequences can help differentiate fluid/ gas from granulation tissue [10]. EUS, like MRI, can help identify internal tract openings as well as provide more anatomical details of the sphincter complex. It is limited though by its inability to identify ischioanal fossa or supralevator abscesses given poor penetration [11].

Computerized tomography (CT) and fistulography are modalities that have been previously considered in the diagnosis of perianal fistulas, but have been deemed to have poor accuracy and thus are not typically recommended for diagnostic purposes. There are few exceptions when fistulography can provide additional information in the setting of particularly complex fistulas [12]. In addition, in an acute clinical setting where CT may be more readily available, it can be a useful modality to expedite diagnosis and treatment of less clinically "silent" disease.

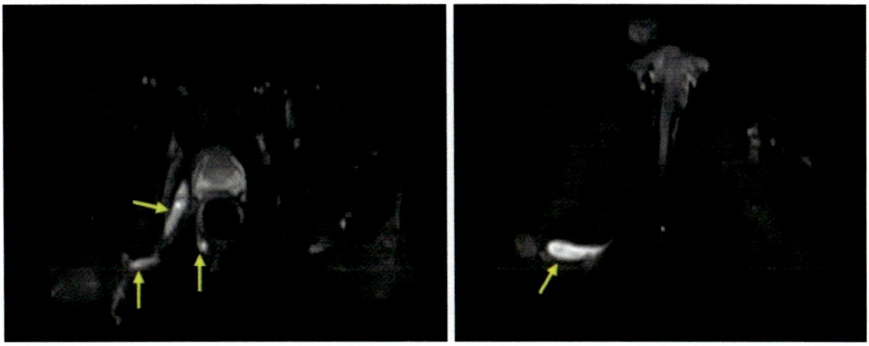

Fig. 2.1 Axial image of a T2- weighted MRI of the pelvis demonstrating a complex trans-sphincteric fistula and gluteal abscess (yellow arrows). (Adapted from Sharma et al. [14])

The gold standard for diagnosis and treatment is an exam under anesthesia (EUA). EUAs can be performed in either lithotomy or prone positioning and have the benefit of allowing for immediate treatment as well as diagnosis [12]. Experienced colorectal surgeons have been found to have up to 90% accuracy in their ability to detect and classify perianal disease [11]. Use of Hydrogen peroxide can be an adjunct with EUAs to help identify internal openings when not immediately clear, and this method can be utilized with EUS as well. The combination of imaging and EUA results in a near 100% chance of accurate diagnosis [13] (Fig. 2.1).

Park's Classification

In the setting of CD, the incidence of perianal fistulas increases as the transmural disease process extends distally, and is most common in the setting of Crohn's proctitis. Fistulas can tract to numerous locations including the perianal skin, rectum and bowel (entero-enteric), vagina (rectovaginal), bladder (entero-vesical) and intra-abdominally (entero-intra-abdominal), and can be singular or numerous in presentation [3]. Specifically in CD, anovaginal fistulas are less common than anoperineal fistulas [15–17].

In 1976, Sir Alan Park published his classification system for perianal fistulas that is still widely utilized today [17]. He described four types of fistulas: inter-sphincteric, trans-sphincteric, suprasphincteric, and extrasphincteric [18]. Intersphincteric and trans-sphincteric fistulas are the most common fistulas accounting for about 45% and 30% of all perianal fistulas respectively. Intersphincteric fistulas penetrate through the internal sphincter but spare the external sphincter whereas trans-sphincteric fistulas affect both the internal and external sphincters exiting below the level of the puborectalis muscle into the ischiorectal fossa. Suprasphincteric fistulas occur in about 20% of cases and penetrate the internal sphincter and tract between in the plane between both sphincters superiorly over the puborectalis and external sphincter before extending out to the perineum. Horseshoe abscesses form as this tract passes over the puborectalis into the supralevator space and downward into the ischiorectal fossa creating an abscess cavity round the rectum. Lastly, extrasphincteric fistulas are amongst the rarest occurring in about 5% of cases. These fistulas pass from the rectum, through the levators and ischiorectal fat encompassing the sphincter complexes, to exit via the perianal skin. Superficial fistulas were not a part of Park's original classification as they have no communication with the sphincter complex, but are more commonly associated with CD or post anorectal procedures *(i.e.* hemorrhoidectomy or sphincterotomies) [17] (Fig. 2.2).

While the Park classification remains the most widely utilized, it fails in providing information related to complexity of disease and presence of proctitis [20]. The American Gastroenterological Association (AGA) proposed a classification system in 2003 that divided fistulas into two categories: simple or complex. Complex fistulas can be high trans-sphincteric fistulas (tract runs through the upper two thirds of the external anal sphincter), have multiple external openings, multiple tracts, be associated with stricturing disease, or be related to active proctitis [21]. While this system has significant prognostic value, it does not help with determining effective individualization of treatment. Additional classifications such as the St James University Hospital Classification (1996), the Hughes- Cardiff classification (1978), and the Milligan-Morgan classification (1934) have been proposed but have not been used extensively due to their inability to translate to daily practice and lack of descriptive ability [20].

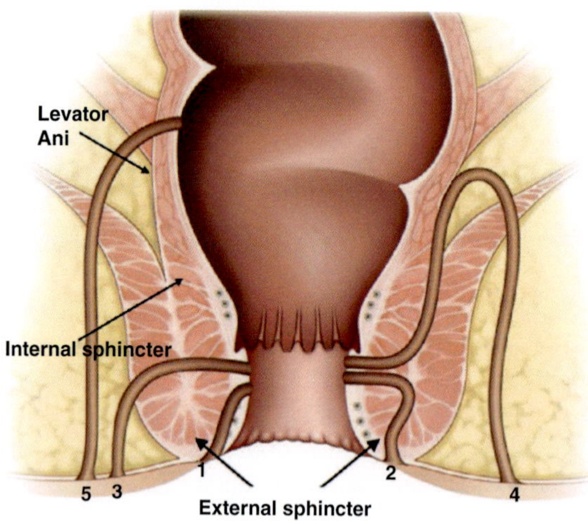

Fig. 2.2 Parks' classification of perianal fistulas. (1) Superficial Fistula (2) Intersphinteric, Parks type 1 (3) Transphincteric, Parks type 2 (4) Suprasphincteric, Parks type 3 (5) Extrasphincteric, Parks type 4. (Adapted from Park et al. [19])

Treatment Goals

The primary treatment goal is resolution of symptoms associated with the fistula (*i.e.* drainage and pain) and complete closure of the fistula tract without impairing continence. Ultimately, the goal is to improve patient quality of life while avoiding treatment complications including incontinence or major colorectal surgery that can result in stoma creation or bowel resection.

From a clinical standpoint, the Perianal Diseases Activity Index (PDAI) exists to assess quality of life and disease severity in regards to clinical improvement and response to therapy. It utilizes a 5-point Likert scale with scores of greater than 4 representing active fistula disease with an accuracy of 87% [22, 23]. The Perianal Crohn's Disease Activity Index (PCDAI) was also created to specifically assess features of perianal CD such as abscess, fistula, fissures and/or ulcers, stenosis and concomitant disease to determine disease severity as well as assess surgical success [22, 24]. Radiographic healing can also be determined in conjunction with clinical resolution. Typically, MRI is the modality of choice and healing is defined as lack of presence of a fistula tract or internal opening [25]. While complete fistula closure may remain the primary goal, in some instances symptom control may have to be enough to avoid multiple procedures that negatively affect a patient's quality of life. Thorough discussions and shared decision making between the physician and patient are thus necessary to ensure proper individual balance between remission and symptom relief.

Medical Management

Corticosteroids

Corticosteroids do not play a significant role in the treatment of fistulizing CD. Prior studies found that corticosteroids had increased risk of worsened discharge and as well as increased surgical needs [26]. Corticosteroid use has only been proposed in the treatment of luminal disease with the caveat that any concern for perianal sepsis was addressed and well controlled prior to utilization [4].

Aminosalicylate (ASA) Derivatives

Aminosalicyclates (i.e. sulfasalazine and mesalazine) have also been found to have no role in the treatment of fistulizing CD. Studies have demonstrated no clinical improvement for the treatment of CD despite their usefulness in the ulcerative colitis patient population [27].

Antibiotics

Metronidazole and ciprofloxacin are the most commonly used antibiotics for the treatment of perianal CD and remain a mainstay of treatment in acute treatment [4]. However few studies have been performed to evaluate their efficacy and use. A meta- analysis of 15 clinical trials assessing the efficacy of antibiotics was performed and noted ciprofloxacin was better than placebo (p = 0.005) in treating perianal fistulas in CD patients but not significantly effective when looking at active CD in general [28]. A subsequent randomized control trial (RCT) found that while their data was insignificant, 10 weeks of ciprofloxacin treatment for perianal CD increased remission (p = 0.41) and response (p = 0.43) as compared to those treated with metronidazole or a placebo [29]. Other broad spectrum antibiotics such as amoxicillin-clavulanic acid have been utilized [30].

Overall, antibiotics provide a good first- line therapy but treatment requires at least 6–8 weeks of therapy and more commonly patients only have symptom relief without significant fistula closure with symptom recurrence after treatment has been stopped [31, 32]. As such, antibiotics should be treated as an adjuvant therapy; additional treatment with other therapies including azathioprine [33] or infliximab [34] produce a significantly longer term healing response.

Immunomodulators

Thiopurines are purine analogues that work by deactivating key steps in T lymphocyte functioning that result in an inflammatory response [35]. The two most commonly studied with fistulizing CD are azathioprine (AZA) and 6- mercaptopurine (6-MP; an active metabolite of AZA) which have been found to have a moderate treatment effect. No direct prospective trials currently exist evaluating thiopurine effect on fistula closure but an early meta-analysis found as a secondary endpoint that those treated with thiopurines had a response rate of 54% compared to a rate of 21% found in those given a placebo [36]. A more recent systematic review found no significant improvement in clinical outcomes or steroid free remission with AZA and 6-MP as compared to placebo and methotrexate, respectively [37]. A prospective open label trial did show that, in combination with antibiotics, AZA had a significantly improved response rate [33].

Calcineurin inhibitors, which reduce interleukin synthesis and thus subsequently reduce T-cell activation, have also been utilized in the treatment of perianal CD [38]. An RCT found that oral tacrolimus resulted in a significantly higher (43% vs 8%; p = 0.004) fistula response rate but only a 10% actual closure rate which was not significant (p = 0.86) compared to placebo. In addition, nephrotoxicity was a significant adverse effect of drug usage [39]. Topical tacrolimus has demonstrated no significant benefit for fistulizing CD [40]. Although all data is observational, cyclosporine is another potential option for treatment especially in refractory disease. Early studies demonstrated significant closure rates of up to 44% but were consistently complicated by high relapse rates upon drug discontinuation and a notable number of adverse events limiting continued use [41, 42]. As such, calcineurin inhibitors have a potential role in combination therapy for refractory disease, but should be used with caution due to side effects attributed to long term use.

Little evidence exists to support the use of methotrexate, a dihydrofolate reductase inhibitor that leads to decreased nucleic acid synthesis and increased T cell apoptosis, for the treatment of fistulizing CD despite evidence of its effectiveness in luminal CD [43]. Two small retrospective reviews noted fistula response rates ranging from 44–56% with complete closure in up to 31% [44, 45]. Further prospective and larger studies still need to be done to confirm the potential role of methotrexate for the treatment of fistulizing CD.

Biologics

With the introduction of anti- tumor necrosis factor (anti- TNF) therapy in the late 1990s, the medical management of perianal fistulizing CD significantly improved and anti- TNF therapy is now considered the gold standard of care. Infliximab (a monoclonal antibody that binds to TNF-α) remains the initial and most widely studied biologic, but adalimumab and certolizumab have growing evidence for induction and maintenance of remission of fistulizing CD.

In 1999, Present et al. performed a placebo controlled trial with 5 mg/kg and 10 mg/kg dosing of infliximab as an induction agent for fistula closure. They found at least 50% closure of the fistula to have occurred in 56–68% of patients with complete closure noted in 38–55% of patients as compared to placebo with the 5 mg dosing producing higher response rates [46]. The subsequent ACCENT II trial evaluated infliximab as maintenance therapy. After 14 weeks of infliximab induction treatment with an observed 64% healing rate, those who subsequently received 5 mg/kg infliximab every 8 weeks had longer time to loss of response (>40 weeks) than placebo (14 weeks; $p = 0.001$) and achieved an additional 39% vs 19% ($p = 0.009$) complete closure rate by 54 weeks [47]. Infliximab therapy was also found to reduce hospitalizations, need for surgery, and number of procedures compared to placebo [48]. Combination therapy with antibiotics and AZA has been shown to be superior to infliximab alone for induction of steroid- free clinical remission [34, 37, 49], but this data remains conflicting as sub-group analyses of the ACCENT II trial demonstrated that concomitant immunosuppression with infliximab therapy did not improve response rates at 1 year [47].

While no dedicated control trials have been performed for adalimumab, subgroup analyses in several RCTs have demonstrated its efficacy. In the CLASSIC I trial, adalimumab's effectiveness as induction therapy was evaluating after 4 weeks of therapy. Of the 299 patients in the study, 32 had perianal fistulizing disease and at 4 weeks, the rate of fistula improvement remission weren't significantly improved although a positive trend did exist [50]. The GAIN trial evaluated CD patients who previously failed infliximab and of the 14 patients who had fistulizing disease, again at 4 weeks, no significant improvement was found with adalimumab therapy [51]. Both these trials though were likely underpowered and had limited follow-up. The

CHARM trial on the other hand evaluated 778 patients of which 117 had fistulizing disease and at 26 weeks found a 30% rate of complete fistula closure compared to 13% ($p = 0.043$) in the placebo group. Additionally, those who had complete closure underwent maintenance therapy and at 56 weeks continued to have complete closure. At 2 years, 90% had sustained closure [52, 53]. Infliximab has been found to have similar effectiveness as adalimumab in treating perianal CD and studies have also demonstrated adalimumab's effectiveness in in treating patients who lost response to infliximab [54, 55]. Combination with ciprofloxacin has also proven to be more effective than monotherapy [56].

Like adalimumab, there are no direct studies to assess the efficacy of certolizumab and overall fewer studies available. The PRECiSE trials demonstrated significant improvement in complete closure rates at 26 weeks compared to placebo (36% vs 17%, $p = 0.038$) [57]. Longer term follow-up demonstrated consistent efficacy of treatment [58].

Although anti-TNF therapy has significantly improved healing rates for fistulizing CD, work continues to be done to improve the treatment, and as such, new therapies have been developed and are under investigation. A sub-group analysis of the GEMINI II trial evaluated vedolizumab (a biologic which prevents lymphocyte adhesion to intestinal vascular endothelium) and reported a probability of fistula closure at 1 year to be 33% as well as faster time to closure. While the sample size was relatively small, the study did also find that about half of the patients had previously failed anti-TNF therapy suggesting vedolizumab could be an effective refractory treatment [59]. An ongoing study, the ENTERPRISE trial, has described a prospective trial for vedolizumab resulting in sustained improvement of fistulizing disease of up to 54% with clinically relevant improvement of fistula drainage at 2 weeks for refractory disease [60]. Ustekinumab (an anti- interleukin monoclonal antibody) is the most recent biologic agent in development. No prospective trials have been performed but a recent open label study has demonstrated promising results in regards to fistula closure [61].

Hyperbaric Oxygen Therapy: An Alternative Therapy

Studies have proposed that hypoxia contributes to the proliferation of an inflammatory response and as such it is though that improved tissue oxygenation can lead to reduction of pro-inflammatory cytokine production, increase fibroblast proliferation, upregulate the hypoxia response pathways, and promote stem cell migration to lead to improved wound healing [62, 63]. The therapy involves placing a patient in a hyperbaric chamber where they can inhale 100% oxygen at a pressure of >1 atm. A 1994 study found 50% complete healing in 10 CD patients with refractory perianal fistulizing disease after two courses of therapy [64]. A systematic review of inflammatory bowel disease patients showed an 88% response rate after therapy [62]. Adverse events have been mild and related to barometric pressure alterations and oxygen toxicity including middle ear trauma most commonly [63, 65]. In addition, concern exists that treatment effect might diminish once therapy is stopped.

While not widely utilized or recently studied, prior findings suggest hyperbaric oxygen could be considered a last-line and/or adjuvant option for perianal fistulizing CD.

Surgical Management

While medical management has improved over the years, response and remission rates with medical management alone rarely surpass 50% [4]. As such, a combined medical- surgical approach is widely viewed as the best treatment strategy. In the PREFACE study, around 90% of patients underwent at least one surgical intervention (frequently seton placement or drainage procedures) consistent with prior estimates of the eventual need for surgery in this patient population [3, 66]. There currently exists no standard medical- surgical treatment algorithm, although many have been proposed, but the consistent overall treatment pathway remains to get initial local sepsis control prior to optimal medical management [4].

It is important to note that the presence of a fistula on its own is not an indication for surgery [67]. Typically surgery is indicated if symptoms fail to respond to medical management, drainage results in poor quality of life, if they create a tract that results in malabsorption or if they have connections to the genitourinary tracts [68]. While surgery can have definitive benefits, the complication risk is also substantial with the highest risk being that of incontinence [69]. In addition, iatrogenic injury as well as poor wound healing are additional complications that must be considered and counseled for when discussing the decision to proceed with surgical management. The choice of surgical procedure is largely based on location and complexity of disease process.

Incision & Drainage (I&D)

I&Ds are the most common pre-operative intervention for the treatment of perianal fistulas [68]. Perianal abscess have been found to be present in over 80% of perianal CD fistulas [70]. It is unclear whether the abscess precedes the fistula or develops as a result of poor fistula drainage. Surgical drainage has been found to significantly minimize the risk of septic complications as compared to waiting for spontaneous drainage [71]. Typically, drainage is recommended prior to initiating any medical therapy, especially immunosuppressives [12]. I&D is usually reserved for symptomatic abscesses >1 cm that could not otherwise be treated with medication alone [72].

Seton

Setons serve to maintain patency of the fistula tract to allow for adequate drainage and decrease the risk of abscess formation and septic complications. Setons can either be cutting (any seton, i.e. silk suture a non-absorbable multifilament suture type, meant to cut through tissue either mechanically or chemically) or non-cutting (a loosely tied non-absorbable suture or vessel loop passed through the fistula tract that helps preserve integrity of the external anal sphincter). Cutting setons are typically not preferred due to their risk of anal incontinence [73]. Non-cutting setons have a low incidence of recurrent abscesses or formation of new fistulous branches [74] although some studies have reported that sole treatment with setons results in significant re-intervention rate, hence with the evolution of biologics, specifically infliximab, several studies have reported the improved efficacy and healing rate with dual therapy [20, 75, 76]. From a patient standpoint, setons have the disadvantage of being rather uncomfortable and take time to achieve adequate healing. In addition, the risk of tract epithelization exists the longer the seton remains in place and currently there is no consensus on when the optimal time is to remove a seton. The ACCENT II study suggested seton removal after 2 weeks but subsequently saw a 15% new abscess rate whereas Thornton et al. described similar long-term outcomes after over a year of seton presence [76, 77]. The recent PISA trial compared long term seton placement (1 year) vs a year of anti-TNF treatment and advancement flap vs LIFT procedure after 2 months of anti-TNF treatment and found that the long-term seton group underwent a higher rate of re-intervention suggesting chronic seton treatment is not effective in CD patients [78]. Typically, seton removal is recommended only after ongoing inflammation has subsided, a significant decrease in drainage has been demonstrated, and induction of anti-TNF treatment has been completed (Fig. 2.3).

Fistulotomy vs Fistulectomy

Fistulotomy involves identifying the internal and external openings of the fistula tract via probe placement, identifying sphincter involvement, and with cautery or sharp dissection, opening the tract along the length of the probe then with cautery,

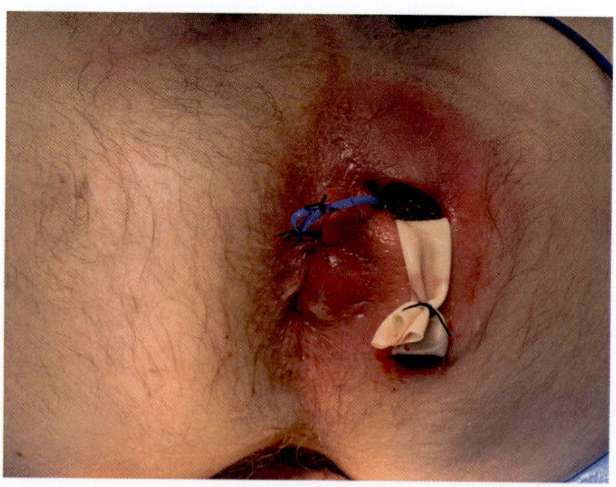

Fig. 2.3 Seton placement (blue vessel loop) and abscess drainage (penrose drain) in a CD patient with complex perianal CD

obliterating the epithelized tract and leaving the wound open to heal [79]. It is an effective treatment for superficial, low intersphincteric, and in select low trans-sphincteric fistulas with less than 33% sphincter involvement [12, 30]. Recurrence rates remain low at about 15% [30]. Healing rates have been reported to be greater than 80% in this population but decrease significantly if performed in the setting of active proctitis [80, 81]. In the setting of proctitis, primary management remains seton placement with attempts for fistula closure via fistulotomy or other methods performed only after endoscopic remission [12]. Despite high success rates, the risk of incontinence remains significant and found to be higher in patients with diarrhea, short anal canals, significant external sphincter involvement, and women with anterior fistulas (as the anterior portion of the external sphincter is shorter) [82].

For high trans-sphincteric or suprasphincteric fistulas, fistulectomy with primary sphincter reconstruction is an option. Like a fistulotomy, the fistula tract is divided but additionally excised. Once the tract is excised, the sphincter is re-approximated with absorbable sutures [79]. This procedure remains relatively new with few studies noting similar healing rates as fistulotomy, recurrence rates of 1–10%, and rates of incontinence ranging from 2–20% [83, 84]. Compared to fistulotomy, healing time has been found to be significantly longer with similar complication rates. Thus, when able, fistulotomy remains the preferred procedure [85].

Fibrin Glue and Fistula Plug

Fibrin glue and fistula plugs are beneficial treatment methods because they avoid the risk of sphincter injury. That being said, their efficacy has been challenged and are thus not often used.

Fibrin glue is a mixture of thrombin and fibrinogen that results in fibrin clot formation when injected into a fistula tract. This clot is thought to promote wound healing via angiogenesis as the clot undergoes fibrinolysis over time [4]. A large multicenter, open-label, RCT found clinical remission rates after fibrin glue injection to be 38% after 8 weeks compared to only 16% in the observation group who just had seton removal performed ($p = 0.04$). Adverse events did not differ significantly [86]. While results were promising, the limited follow-up time did not provide sufficient enough data to provide definitive recommendations regarding treatment use. Subsequent studies had demonstrated increased success rates that lasted for longer periods indicating its potential as a viable treatment for those without alternative options [87, 88].

Fistula plugs are bioprosthetic absorbable plugs made of substances such as collagen or porcine intestinal submucosa that are inserted into the internal fistula opening and occasionally sutured in place. Typically, they are only utilized after adequate drainage of the fistula tract has been done (i.e. with seton placement). Success rates vary from 20–90% dependent on ability of plug to remain in place and severity of perianal disease [12]. The 2019 ECCO guidelines noted that anal fistula plugs shouldn't be routinely utilized as a fistula closure mechanism as seton removal was found to be equally effective [88]. Two RCTs demonstrated that plug placement was no more effective than seton removal or surgeon's preference (i.e. fistulotomy, cutting seton, flap, etc.), had similar adverse events, and additionally was associated with higher costs [89, 90]. Of note, recurrence was found to be higher than with other surgical methods for fistula treatment [79]. Overall, the use of a fistula plugs is relatively safe and can be considered in certain patients bearing in mind cost and varying success rates (Fig. 2.4).

Endorectal Advancement Flap

In the setting of perianal fistula disease without active proctitis or stenosis, endorectal advancement flaps (ERAF) is an effective surgical treatment. The procedure involves coring out the fistula tract then mobilizing a rectal mucosal flap (either elliptical, rhomboid, or U-shaped) to cover the internal fistula opening thus closing of the high pressure end of the fistula. The external opening remains open to allow it to drain and heal on its own. The method attempts to avoid damage to the sphincter complex and avoids the creation of an external wound that can be more challenging to heal [12, 20]. Multiple systematic reviews have demonstrated a success rate of about 60% in CD patients, but have a 9% risk of incontinence when thicker flaps are utilized [92, 93]. Recurrence remains a significant problem but ERAFs have the benefit of being utilized in the setting of prior fistula surgery, although risk for failure increases with each additional attempt at flap creation [94]. Prior immunologic treatment as well as adequate fistula drainage have been shown to improve outcomes of ERAF [95] (Fig. 2.5).

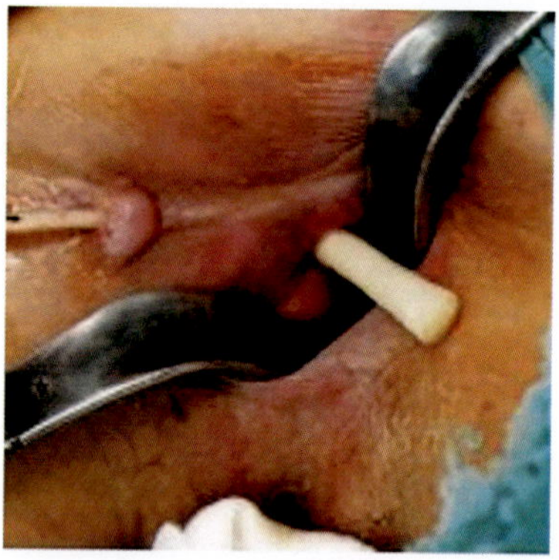

Fig. 2.4 Insertion of a fistula plug through the internal opening of an anal fistula and pulled out of the external opening until it is well seated and can subsequently be secured. (Adapted from Song [91])

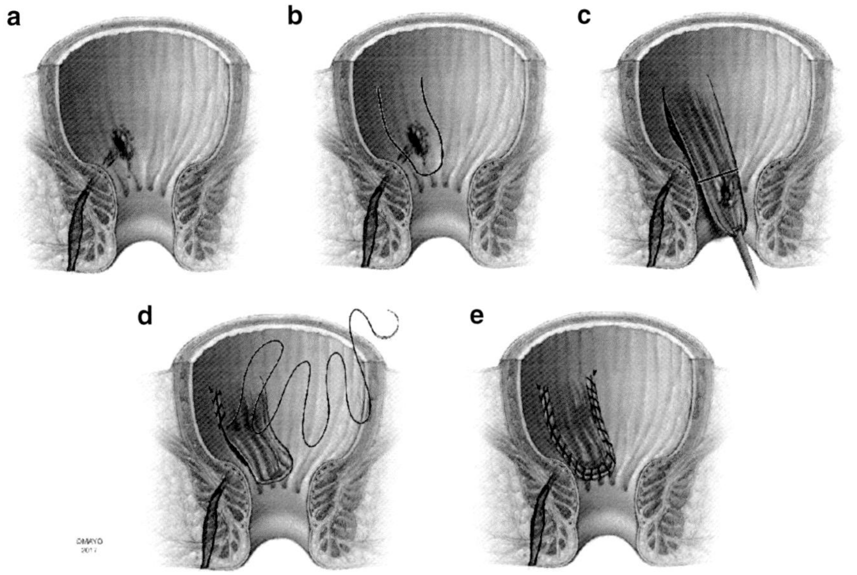

Fig. 2.5 Creation of an endorectal advancement flap. Full or partial thickness U-shaped flap of rectal tissue advanced to remove the superficial opening of a fistula tract and cover the tract. (Adapted from Lightner et al. [96])

Ligation of Intersphincteric Fistula Tract (LIFT) Procedure

The LIFT procedure was first described by Rojanasakul et al. in 2007 for the treatment of trans-sphincteric fistulas, and has subsequently been expanded to address more complex fistulas that cross the intersphincteric groove (ISG) [97]. A perineal incision at the ISG is made, the intersphincteric tract is identified, and the internal and external ends of the tract are suture ligated within the ISG. Distal to the ligation, the tract is divided, which can be confirmed via injection of saline or hydrogen peroxide into the external opening, and any tract remnant is removed. The initial incision overlying the ISG is approximated with absorbable suture [79, 97]. Retrospective studies have demonstrated healing rates of 40–90% with increased success in CD patients with concurrent small bowel disease as opposed to colonic disease [88, 98, 99]. Gingold et al. performed a prospective study on CD patients and demonstrated one-year healing rates of 67% without development of incontinence. They additionally demonstrated that long term healing was associated with lateral versus midline incision location as well as longer fistula length [100]. Recently published prospective data out of Cedars-Sinai Medical Center continues to demonstrate healing rates of 65% in CD patients after a mean follow-up of 33 months, indicating that the LIFT procedure may be a viable treatment option in this patient population [101] (Fig. 2.6).

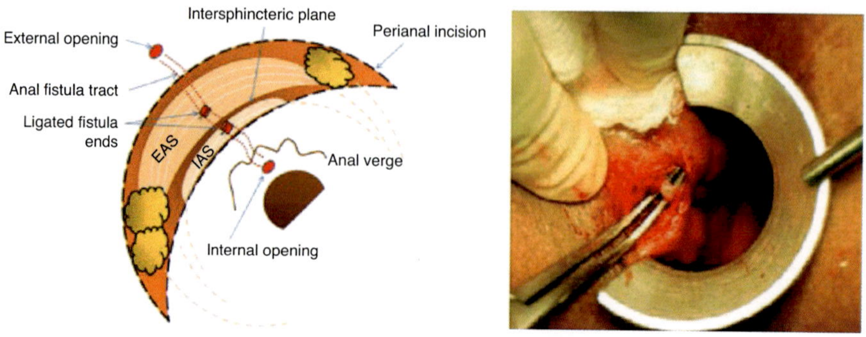

Fig. 2.6 Depiction of the dissection made in the ISG and subsequent view of the intersphincteric tract meant to be ligated during the LIFT procedure. IAS internal anal sphincter. EAS external anal sphincter. (Adapted from Lo and Sangar [102, 103])

Fecal Diversion

Healing remains the most difficult outcome for perianal CD. Fecal diversion (i.e. loop ileostomy or end colostomy) serves to divert stool thereby preventing further contamination and inflammatory response. The goal is to avoid the need for proctectomy and is indicated in severe refractory disease. A retrospective study demonstrated early remission in 81% of CD patients but also noted relapse in 68% of those patients and only about 10% of patients were able to undergo eventual stoma reversal [104]. A subsequent meta- analysis demonstrated early response rates of about 64% and similar low success (17%) of restoration of continuity with about 27% of those patients requiring re-intervention. In addition, there was no notable change in clinical response between the pre- and post-biologic eras [105]. No RCTs exist though comparing diversion with other surgical or medical interventions. Unfortunately, a high percentage (about 41%) of those who undergo diversion ultimately require a proctectomy [30].

Proctectomy

Proctectomy is considered a last resort for the treatment of perianal CD in the setting of severe, refractory disease associated with concomitant rectal involvement resulting in incontinence and worsening quality of life [68]. While biologics have slightly diminished the need for proctectomy and have improved post-diversion restoration of continuity rates, up to 40% will still undergo a proctectomy to treat perianal CD [12, 106]. One series described that patients underwent a median number of 12 operations over a median time of 6 years prior to undergoing a proctectomy. The cited risks factors for eventual proctectomy include multiple prior perineal procedures, prior fecal diversion, CD without rectal involvement, and CD with proctitis [68]. The main risks of the surgery include, pelvic nerve damage, presacral abscesses, chronic draining sinus formation and delayed wound healing

[12]. Given the high risk for perineal wound complications, an intersphincteric dissection is recommended [107]. For patients with large perineal defects, further treatment with myocutaneous advancement flaps (i.e. rectus abdominus flap transposition and gracilis interposition) have also had success. A retrospective review in CD patients with complex perianal fistulas demonstrated an overall success rate of 64% with significant long-term efficacy noted at a median of 64-month follow up [108]. Rectus abdominus flaps were found in subsequent studies to have better healing rates than gracilis flaps [109].

Emerging Therapies

Mesenchymal Stem Cells (MSCs)

Mesenchymal stem cells (MSCs) are an emerging therapy with early promising results for the treatment of perianal fistulizing CD. They are non-hematopoietic multipotent cells that are precursors of connective tissue cells commonly found in subdermal adipose tissue (obtained via liposuction) and bone marrow; no study has directly compared adipose stem cells to marrow stem cells with regard to efficacy [63, 110]. The exact mechanism of action is unknown, but MSCs are thought to have anti-inflammatory, immunomodulatory and fibroblast- like healing effects via their inhibition of T cell proliferation and promotion of T regulatory cells and formation of granulation tissue [4, 8]. They can be injected around the fistula opening directly into the rectal mucosa or they can be injected into the fistula tract along with fibrin glue. The use of this product was first described in a case report of a woman with a refractory rectovaginal fistula treated with MSCs and advancement flap with complete healing observed after 1 week and maintained at 3 months [111]. García-Olmo subsequently initiated the first phase I clinical trial in Spain evaluating 4 patients who had autologous adipose tissue-derived stem cells injected intralesionally. Complete healing occurred in 75% by week 9 and no adverse events occurred after an average of 22 months of follow up [112]. A subsequent phase II trial by the same group re-demonstrated a complete healing rate of 71% when MSCs were combined with fibrin glue as compared to 16% in the fibrin glue only cohort ($p < 0.001$) [113]. An additional phase II study also determined there to be closure rates of 82% at 8 weeks after direct injection into the fistula tract of MSCs mixed with fibrin glue. A sustained healing rate of 88% was noted after 1 year [20]. A recent phase III trial out of Europe again evaluated adipose derived MSCs and their effect on treatment- refractory, draining complex perianal fistulas in CD patients. Of the 107 patients who received MSCs, 53 (50%) compared to 34% of patients in the placebo group achieved clinical remission ($p = 0.024$). In addition, only 17% compared to 29% in the placebo group experienced treatment- related adverse events, most notable anal abscess and proctalgia [114].

Most recently ADMIRE- CD, the largest phase III, multicenter, double blinded, placebo controlled trial, is underway evaluating the efficacy and safety of adult allogeneic expanded adipose- derived stem cells for the treatment of refractory complex perianal fistulas in CD. MSCs are injected into the fistula tract walls after curettage of the internal opening. After 24 weeks, closure of all external opening without any additional collections was note in 51% of treated patients compared to 36% in the control group ($p = 0.021$). Adverse events again remained fairly mild and similar to previously reported complications. At 54 weeks follow-up, the efficacy and safety profiles remained similar [114, 115]. Out of Mayo Clinic, the STOMP trial recently found that MSCs could effectively be utilized in a bioabsorbable matrix in the setting of simple fistulas and another phase I study found that fistula plugs coated with MSCs could also promote significantly high healing rates [116, 117]. These phase I, II, and III trials have provided significant promising results in regards to expanding treatment options for patients who otherwise had limited to no other options for clinical improvement. While impactful, these early studies have largely excluded patients with active proctitis, 3 or more tracts, anal canal involvement, prior diversion, or vaginal or pouch. Recently submitted phase IB/IIA RCT data in this more severe patient population found at 1 year, clinical and radiographic healing in 70% of perianal, 37.5% of rectovaginal, and 46.2% of ileal pouch fistulas without any significant treatment- related adverse effects [118]. As such, MSCs are continuing to demonstrate significant effectiveness in the treatment of perianal fistulizing CD. As more research continues to be done and cost- effectiveness continues to be examined, this treatment option is likely to become less investigational and more widely spread amongst medical practitioners (Fig. 2.7).

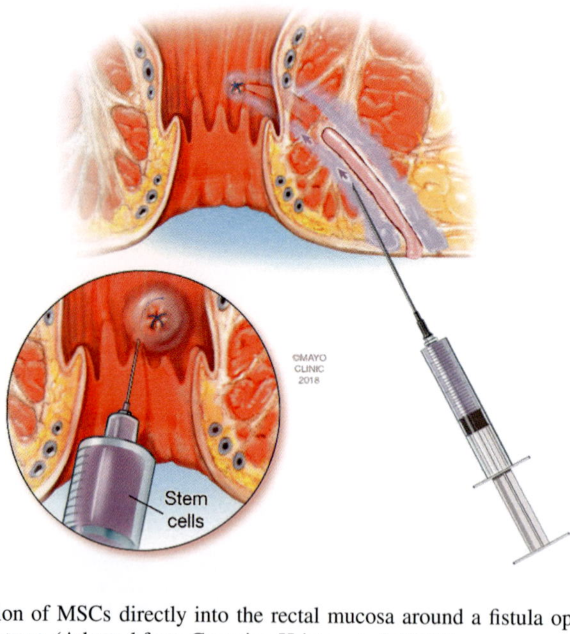

Fig. 2.7 Injection of MSCs directly into the rectal mucosa around a fistula opening as well as along the fistula tract. (Adapted from Georgiev-Hristov et al. [119])

Fistula Laser Closure (FiLaC™)

In 2006, Moy et al. described the first use of a laser, specifically a carbon dioxide laser, in the successful treatment of perianal fistula in CD patients [120]. Subsequently in 2011, Wilhelm et al. described a new technique with a radial- emitting laser probe [Fistula-tract Laser Closure (FiLaC™), Biolitec AG, Jena, Germany] that works by destroying the epithelium of the fistula tract despite lack of direct visualization of the pathway [121]. Closure of the internal opening with an endorectal advancement flap was also described. Initial studies demonstrated an overall healing rate of 64% of all fistula patients and 69% in specifically CD patients. This rate subsequently increased to 92% in the CD population after a second procedure [122]. FiLaC™ has the benefit of a faster recovery, it preserves the sphincter, and it has a relatively short learning curve to incorporate into one's practice. The cost though, can be prohibitive and because one is unable to visualize the tracts as they are treated, there is the potential for failure of treatment of secondary and more complex fistulous tracts resulting in decreased healing rates. Ultimately, this technology is still relatively new and further studies are needed to describe its efficacy and benefit related to other treatment techniques, however initial findings in CD patients has been promising [123].

Video-Assisted Anal Fistula Treatment (VAAFT)

Video-assisted anal fistula treatment (VAAFT) is a two stage procedure in which a "fistuloscope" is first inserted into the external opening of a fistula tract in order to identify the internal opening as well as any secondary tracts. Once fully explored, a special electrode is placed and cautery is used to obliterate the tract under direct visualization followed by debridement of the tract and closure of the internal opening with suture, staples, or an advancement flap. The technique was initially described in by Meinero et al. in 2011 in non-CD patients in which they described a 3 month healing rate of 73% and 1 year healing rate of 87% [124]. Subsequent studies in CD patients demonstrated consistent high healing rates. A prospective study in 13 CD patients who underwent VAAFT with and advancement flap closure demonstrated a success rate of 82% at 9 months without any associated morbidity or incontinence [125]. A subsequent study in 25 CD patients who underwent VAAFT with seton placement instead of definitive closure, demonstrated improved self-reported pain and discharge in 84% of participants [126]. Unlike FiLaC™, VAAFT has the benefit of direct visualization in addition to sphincter preservation but cost and longer learning curve are possible disadvantages. The VAAFT procedure remains a promising technique for the treatment of perianal fistulas in CD patients but further studies and comparisons between other techniques are still needed (Fig. 2.8).

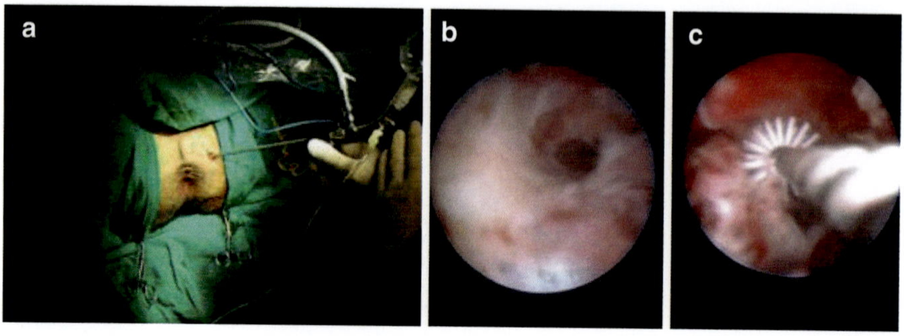

Fig. 2.8 Fistuloscope within the external opening of a fistula tract (**a**). View from fistuloscope of lumen of the fistula tract and abscess cavity before (**b**) and after (**c**) cauterization. (Adapted from El-Barbary and Yusof et al. [127, 128])

Conclusion

Fistulizing perianal CD is a challenging phenotype of CD associated with substantial morbidity. Innovative surgical and medical approaches have enriched the therapeutic options available, but more work is needed to provide an algorithm for consistent ability to achieve remission. As such, a multidisciplinary approach continues to be required in order to maximize optimal patient outcomes.

Conflict of Interest Amy Lightner: consultant for Takeda, Mesoblast, Ossium, Boomerang, Direct Biologics

References

1. Feuerstein JD, Cheifetz AS. Crohn disease: epidemiology, diagnosis, and management. Mayo Clin Proc. 2017;92(7):1088–103. https://doi.org/10.1016/j.mayocp.2017.04.010.
2. Molodecky NA, Soon IS, Rabi DM, Ghali WA, Ferris M, Chernoff G, et al. Increasing incidence and prevalence of the inflammatory bowel diseases with time, based on systematic review. Gastroenterology. 2012;142(1):46.e42–54.e42; quiz e30. https://doi.org/10.1053/j.gastro.2011.10.001.
3. Schwartz DA, Loftus EV Jr, Tremaine WJ, Panaccione R, Harmsen WS, Zinsmeister AR, et al. The natural history of fistulizing Crohn's disease in Olmsted County. Minn Gastroenterol. 2002;122(4):875–80. https://doi.org/10.1053/gast.2002.32362.
4. Geldof J, Iqbal N, Warusavitarne J, Hart A. The essential role of a multidisciplinary approach in inflammatory bowel diseases: combined medical-surgical treatment in complex perianal fistulas in CD. Clin Colon Rectal Surg. 2022;35(1):21–31. https://doi.org/10.1055/s-0041-1740035.
5. Owen HA, Buchanan GN, Schizas A, Cohen R, Williams AB. Quality of life with anal fistula. Ann R Coll Surg Engl. 2016;98(5):334–8. https://doi.org/10.1308/rcsann.2016.0136.
6. Kotze PG, Shen B, Lightner A, Yamamoto T, Spinelli A, Ghosh S, et al. Modern management of perianal fistulas in Crohn's disease: future directions. Gut. 2018;67(6):1181–94. https://doi.org/10.1136/gutjnl-2017-314918.

7. Hellers G, Bergstrand O, Ewerth S, Holmström B. Occurrence and outcome after primary treatment of anal fistulae in Crohn's disease. Gut. 1980;21(6):525–7. https://doi.org/10.1136/gut.21.6.525.
8. Zalieckas JM. Treatment of perianal Crohn's disease. Semin Pediatr Surg 2017;26(6):391–397. doi: https://doi.org/https://doi.org/10.1053/j.sempedsurg.2017.10.009.
9. Bell SJ, Halligan S, Windsor AC, Williams AB, Wiesel P, Kamm MA. Response of fistulating Crohn's disease to infliximab treatment assessed by magnetic resonance imaging. Aliment Pharmacol Ther. 2003;17(3):387–93. https://doi.org/10.1046/j.1365-2036.2003.01427.x.
10. Koelbel G, Schmiedl U, Majer MC, Weber P, Jenss H, Kueper K, et al. Diagnosis of fistulae and sinus tracts in patients with Crohn disease: value of MR imaging. AJR Am J Roentgenol. 1989;152(5):999–1003. https://doi.org/10.2214/ajr.152.5.999.
11. Schwartz DA, Wiersema MJ, Dudiak KM, Fletcher JG, Clain JE, Tremaine WJ, et al. A comparison of endoscopic ultrasound, magnetic resonance imaging, and exam under anesthesia for evaluation of Crohn's perianal fistulas. Gastroenterology. 2001;121(5):1064–72. https://doi.org/10.1053/gast.2001.28676.
12. Gecse KB, Bemelman W, Kamm MA, Stoker J, Khanna R, Ng SC, et al. A global consensus on the classification, diagnosis and multidisciplinary treatment of perianal fistulising Crohn's disease. Gut. 2014;63(9):1381–92. https://doi.org/10.1136/gutjnl-2013-306709.
13. Vogel JD, Johnson EK, Morris AM, Paquette IM, Saclarides TJ, Feingold DL, et al. Clinical practice guideline for the Management of Anorectal Abscess, Fistula-in-Ano, and rectovaginal Fistula. Dis Colon Rectum. 2016;59(12):1117–33. https://doi.org/10.1097/dcr.0000000000000733.
14. Sharma A, Yadav P, Sahu M, Verma A. Current imaging techniques for evaluation of fistula in ano: a review. Egypt J Radiol Nucl Med. 2020;51(1):130. https://doi.org/10.1186/s43055-020-00252-9.
15. Eglinton TW, Barclay ML, Gearry RB, Frizelle FA. The spectrum of perianal Crohn's disease in a population-based cohort. Dis Colon Rectum 2012;55(7):773–7. doi: https://doi.org/10.1097/DCR.0b013e31825228b0, 777.
16. Göttgens KW, Jeuring SF, Sturkenboom R, Romberg-Camps MJ, Oostenbrug LE, Jonkers DM, et al. Time trends in the epidemiology and outcome of perianal fistulizing Crohn's disease in a population-based cohort. Eur J Gastroenterol Hepatol. 2017;29(5):595–601. https://doi.org/10.1097/meg.0000000000000840.
17. Park SH, Aniwan S, Scott Harmsen W, Tremaine WJ, Lightner AL, Faubion WA, et al. Update on the natural course of Fistulizing perianal Crohn's disease in a population-based cohort. Inflamm Bowel Dis. 2019;25(6):1054–60. https://doi.org/10.1093/ibd/izy329.
18. Carr S. Fistula In Ano. In: Velasco A, editor. StatPearls [Internet]: StatPearls Publishing; 2022.
19. Park MY, Yoon YS, Lee JL, Park SH, Ye BD, Yang S-K, et al. Comparative perianal fistula closure rates following autologous adipose tissue-derived stem cell transplantation or treatment with anti-tumor necrosis factor agents after seton placement in patients with Crohn's disease: a retrospective observational study. Stem Cell Res Ther. 2021;12(1):401. https://doi.org/10.1186/s13287-021-02484-6.
20. Lee WY, Park KJ, Cho YB, Yoon SN, Song KH, Kim DS, et al. Autologous adipose tissue-derived stem cells treatment demonstrated favorable and sustainable therapeutic effect for Crohn's fistula. Stem Cells. 2013;31(11):2575–81. https://doi.org/10.1002/stem.1357.
21. Sandborn WJ, Fazio VW, Feagan BG, Hanauer SB. AGA technical review on perianal Crohn's disease. Gastroenterology. 2003;125(5):1508–30. https://doi.org/10.1016/j.gastro.2003.08.025.
22. Irvine EJ. Usual therapy improves perianal Crohn's disease as measured by a new disease activity index. McMaster IBD study group. J Clin Gastroenterol. 1995;20(1):27–32.
23. Losco A, Viganò C, Conte D, Cesana BM, Basilisco G. Assessing the activity of perianal Crohn's disease: comparison of clinical indices and computer-assisted anal ultrasound. Inflamm Bowel Dis. 2009;15(5):742–9. https://doi.org/10.1002/ibd.20826.

24. Pikarsky AJ, Gervaz P, Wexner SD. Perianal Crohn disease: a new scoring system to evaluate and predict outcome of surgical intervention. Arch Surg. 2002;137(7):774–8. https://doi.org/10.1001/archsurg.137.7.774.
25. Garg P, Kaur B, Goyal A, Yagnik VD, Dawka S, Menon GR. Lessons learned from an audit of 1250 anal fistula patients operated at a single center: a retrospective review. World J Gastrointest Surg. 2021;13(4):340–54. https://doi.org/10.4240/wjgs.v13.i4.340.
26. Jones JH, Lennard-Jones JE. Corticosteroids and corticotrophin in the treatment of Crohn's disease. Gut. 1966;7(2):181–7. https://doi.org/10.1136/gut.7.2.181.
27. Nielsen OH, Munck LK. Drug insight: aminosalicylates for the treatment of IBD. Nat Clin Pract Gastroenterol Hepatol. 2007;4(3):160–70. https://doi.org/10.1038/ncpgasthep0696.
28. Su JW, Ma JJ, Zhang HJ. Use of antibiotics in patients with Crohn's disease: a systematic review and meta-analysis. J Dig Dis. 2015;16(2):58–66. https://doi.org/10.1111/1751-2980.12216.
29. Thia KT, Mahadevan U, Feagan BG, Wong C, Cockeram A, Bitton A, et al. Ciprofloxacin or metronidazole for the treatment of perianal fistulas in patients with Crohn's disease: a randomized, double-blind, placebo-controlled pilot study. Inflamm Bowel Dis. 2009;15(1):17–24. https://doi.org/10.1002/ibd.20608.
30. Williams JL, Shaffer VO. Modern Management of Perianal Crohn's disease: a review. Am Surg. 2021;87(9):1361–7. https://doi.org/10.1177/0003134820956331.
31. Taxonera C, Schwartz DA, García-Olmo D. Emerging treatments for complex perianal fistula in Crohn's disease. World J Gastroenterol. 2009;15(34):4263–72. https://doi.org/10.3748/wjg.15.4263.
32. Brandt LJ, Bernstein LH, Boley SJ, Frank MS. Metronidazole therapy for perineal Crohn's disease: a follow-up study. Gastroenterology. 1982;83(2):383–7.
33. Dejaco C, Harrer M, Waldhoer T, Miehsler W, Vogelsang H, Reinisch W. Antibiotics and azathioprine for the treatment of perianal fistulas in Crohn's disease. Aliment Pharmacol Ther. 2003;18(11–12):1113–20. https://doi.org/10.1046/j.1365-2036.2003.01793.x.
34. West RL, van der Woude CJ, Hansen BE, Felt-Bersma RJ, van Tilburg AJ, Drapers JA, et al. Clinical and endosonographic effect of ciprofloxacin on the treatment of perianal fistulae in Crohn's disease with infliximab: a double-blind placebo-controlled study. Aliment Pharmacol Ther. 2004;20(11–12):1329–36. https://doi.org/10.1111/j.1365-2036.2004.02247.x.
35. Neurath M. Thiopurines in IBD: what is their mechanism of action? Gastroenterol Hepatol (N Y). 2010;6(7):435–6.
36. Pearson DC, May GR, Fick GH, Sutherland LR. Azathioprine and 6-mercaptopurine in Crohn disease. A meta-analysis. Ann Intern Med. 1995;123(2):132–42. https://doi.org/10.7326/0003-4819-123-2-199507150-00009.
37. Chande N, Tsoulis DJ, MacDonald JK. Azathioprine or 6-mercaptopurine for induction of remission in Crohn's disease. Cochrane Database Syst Rev. 2013;4:Cd000545. https://doi.org/10.1002/14651858.CD000545.pub4.
38. Mejia JC, Basu A, Shapiro R. Chapter 17 – Calcineurin inhibitors. In: Morris PJ, Knechtle SJ, editors. Kidney transplantation – principles and practice. 7th ed. Philadelphia (PA): W.B. Saunders; 2014. p. 231–49.
39. Sandborn WJ, Present DH, Isaacs KL, Wolf DC, Greenberg E, Hanauer SB, et al. Tacrolimus for the treatment of fistulas in patients with Crohn's disease: a randomized, placebo-controlled trial. Gastroenterology. 2003;125(2):380–8. https://doi.org/10.1016/s0016-5085(03)00877-1.
40. Hart AL, Plamondon S, Kamm MA. Topical tacrolimus in the treatment of perianal Crohn's disease: exploratory randomized controlled trial. Inflamm Bowel Dis. 2007;13(3):245–53. https://doi.org/10.1002/ibd.20073.
41. Hanauer SB, Smith MB. Rapid closure of Crohn's disease fistulas with continuous intravenous cyclosporin a. Am J Gastroenterol. 1993;88(5):646–9.
42. Present DH, Lichtiger S. Efficacy of cyclosporine in treatment of fistula of Crohn's disease. Dig Dis Sci. 1994;39(2):374–80. https://doi.org/10.1007/bf02090211.
43. Cronstein BN, Aune TM. Methotrexate and its mechanisms of action in inflammatory arthritis. Nat Rev Rheumatol. 2020;16(3):145–54. https://doi.org/10.1038/s41584-020-0373-9.

44. Soon SY, Ansari A, Yaneza M, Raoof S, Hirst J, Sanderson JD. Experience with the use of low-dose methotrexate for inflammatory bowel disease. Eur J Gastroenterol Hepatol. 2004;16(9):921–6. https://doi.org/10.1097/00042737-200409000-00018.
45. Mahadevan U, Marion JF, Present DH. Fistula response to methotrexate in Crohn's disease: a case series. Aliment Pharmacol Ther. 2003;18(10):1003–8. https://doi.org/10.1046/j.1365-2036.2003.01790.x.
46. Present DH, Rutgeerts P, Targan S, Hanauer SB, Mayer L, van Hogezand RA, et al. Infliximab for the treatment of fistulas in patients with Crohn's disease. N Engl J Med. 1999;340(18):1398–405. https://doi.org/10.1056/nejm199905063401804.
47. Sands BE, Anderson FH, Bernstein CN, Chey WY, Feagan BG, Fedorak RN, et al. Infliximab maintenance therapy for fistulizing Crohn's disease. N Engl J Med. 2004;350(9):876–85. https://doi.org/10.1056/NEJMoa030815.
48. Lichtenstein GR, Yan S, Bala M, Blank M, Sands BE. Infliximab maintenance treatment reduces hospitalizations, surgeries, and procedures in fistulizing Crohn's disease. Gastroenterology. 2005;128(4):862–9. https://doi.org/10.1053/j.gastro.2005.01.048.
49. Colombel JF, Sandborn WJ, Reinisch W, Mantzaris GJ, Kornbluth A, Rachmilewitz D, et al. Infliximab, azathioprine, or combination therapy for Crohn's disease. N Engl J Med. 2010;362(15):1383–95. https://doi.org/10.1056/NEJMoa0904492.
50. Hanauer SB, Sandborn WJ, Rutgeerts P, Fedorak RN, Lukas M, MacIntosh D, et al. Human anti-tumor necrosis factor monoclonal antibody (adalimumab) in Crohn's disease: the CLASSIC-I trial. Gastroenterology. 2006;130(2):323–33; quiz 591. https://doi.org/10.1053/j.gastro.2005.11.030.
51. Sandborn WJ, Rutgeerts P, Enns R, Hanauer SB, Colombel JF, Panaccione R, et al. Adalimumab induction therapy for Crohn disease previously treated with infliximab: a randomized trial. Ann Intern Med. 2007;146(12):829–38. https://doi.org/10.7326/0003-4819-146-12-200706190-00159.
52. Colombel JF, Sandborn WJ, Rutgeerts P, Enns R, Hanauer SB, Panaccione R, et al. Adalimumab for maintenance of clinical response and remission in patients with Crohn's disease: the CHARM trial. Gastroenterology. 2007;132(1):52–65. https://doi.org/10.1053/j.gastro.2006.11.041.
53. Colombel JF, Schwartz DA, Sandborn WJ, Kamm MA, D'Haens G, Rutgeerts P, et al. Adalimumab for the treatment of fistulas in patients with Crohn's disease. Gut. 2009;58(7):940–8. https://doi.org/10.1136/gut.2008.159251.
54. Ji CC, Takano S. Clinical efficacy of adalimumab versus infliximab and the factors associated with recurrence or aggravation during treatment of anal fistulas in Crohn's disease. Intest Res. 2017;15(2):182–6. https://doi.org/10.5217/ir.2017.15.2.182.
55. Hinojosa J, Gomollón F, García S, Bastida G, Cabriada JL, Saro C, et al. Efficacy and safety of short-term adalimumab treatment in patients with active Crohn's disease who lost response or showed intolerance to infliximab: a prospective, open-label, multicentre trial. Aliment Pharmacol Ther. 2007;25(4):409–18. https://doi.org/10.1111/j.1365-2036.2006.03232.x.
56. Dewint P, Hansen BE, Verhey E, Oldenburg B, Hommes DW, Pierik M, et al. Adalimumab combined with ciprofloxacin is superior to adalimumab monotherapy in perianal fistula closure in Crohn's disease: a randomised, double-blind, placebo controlled trial (ADAFI). Gut. 2014;63(2):292–9. https://doi.org/10.1136/gutjnl-2013-304488.
57. Schreiber S, Lawrance IC, Thomsen O, Hanauer SB, Bloomfield R, Sandborn WJ. Randomised clinical trial: certolizumab pegol for fistulas in Crohn's disease - subgroup results from a placebo-controlled study. Aliment Pharmacol Ther. 2011;33(2):185–93. https://doi.org/10.1111/j.1365-2036.2010.04509.x.
58. Vavricka SR, Spasojevic M, Rogler G, Schoepfer AM, Seibold F, Borovicka J, et al. Long-term efficacy and safety of Certolizumab Pegol in an unselected Crohn's disease population: the FACTS III survey. Dig Dis. 2017;35(5):423–32. https://doi.org/10.1159/000475494.
59. Feagan BG, Sandborn WJ, D'Haens G, Lee SD, Allez M, Fedorak RN, et al. Randomised clinical trial: vercirnon, an oral CCR9 antagonist, vs. placebo as induction therapy in active

Crohn's disease. Aliment Pharmacol Ther. 2015;42(10):1170–81. https://doi.org/10.1111/apt.13398.

60. Schwartz DA, Peyrin-Biroulet L, Lasch K, Adsul S, Danese S. Efficacy and safety of 2 Vedolizumab intravenous regimens for perianal Fistulizing Crohn's disease: ENTERPRISE study. Clin Gastroenterol Hepatol. 2022;20(5):1059–67.e9. https://doi.org/10.1016/j.cgh.2021.09.028.
61. Khorrami S, Ginard D, Marín-Jiménez I, Chaparro M, Sierra M, Aguas M, et al. Ustekinumab for the treatment of refractory Crohn's disease: the Spanish experience in a large multicentre open-label cohort. Inflamm Bowel Dis. 2016;22(7):1662–9. https://doi.org/10.1097/mib.0000000000000842.
62. Dulai PS, Buckey JC Jr, Raffals LE, Swoger JM, Claus PL, O'Toole K, et al. Hyperbaric oxygen therapy is well tolerated and effective for ulcerative colitis patients hospitalized for moderate-severe flares: a phase 2A pilot multi-center, randomized, double-blind, sham-controlled trial. Am J Gastroenterol. 2018;113(10):1516–23. https://doi.org/10.1038/s41395-018-0005-z.
63. Zabot GP, Cassol O, Saad-Hossne R, Bemelman W. Modern surgical strategies for perianal Crohn's disease. World J Gastroenterol. 2020;26(42):6572–81. https://doi.org/10.3748/wjg.v26.i42.6572.
64. Lavy A, Weisz G, Adir Y, Ramon Y, Melamed Y, Eidelman S. Hyperbaric oxygen for perianal Crohn's disease. J Clin Gastroenterol. 1994;19(3):202–5.
65. Wang X, Shen B. Advances in perianal disease associated with Crohn's disease-evolving approaches. Gastrointest Endosc Clin N Am. 2019;29(3):515–30. https://doi.org/10.1016/j.giec.2019.02.011.
66. Ferrante M, Siproudhis L, Poggioli G, Reinshagen M, Milicevic S, Roset M, et al. P801 treatment patterns of complex perianal fistula in Crohn's disease in five European countries: the PREFACE study, a retrospective chart review. J Crohn's Colitis. 2020;14(Supplement_1):S628. https://doi.org/10.1093/ecco-jcc/jjz203.929.
67. Broe PJ, Bayless TM, Cameron JL. Crohn's disease: are enteroenteral fistulas an indication for surgery? Surgery. 1982;91(3):249–53.
68. Fichera A, Michelassi F. Surgical treatment of Crohn's disease. J Gastrointest Surg. 2007;11(6):791–803. https://doi.org/10.1007/s11605-006-0068-9.
69. Keighley MR, Allan RN. Current status and influence of operation on perianal Crohn's disease. Int J Color Dis. 1986;1(2):104–7. https://doi.org/10.1007/BF01648416.
70. Solomon MJ. Fistulae and abscesses in symptomatic perianal Crohn's disease. Int J Color Dis. 1996;11(5):222–6. https://doi.org/10.1007/s003840050051.
71. Hyder SA, Travis SP, Jewell DP, Mc CMNJ, George BD. Fistulating anal Crohn's disease: results of combined surgical and infliximab treatment. Dis Colon Rectum. 2006;49(12):1837–41. https://doi.org/10.1007/s10350-006-0656-5.
72. Shenoy-Bhangle A, Nimkin K, Goldner D, Bradley WF, Israel EJ, Gee MS. MRI predictors of treatment response for perianal fistulizing Crohn disease in children and young adults. Pediatr Radiol. 2014;44(1):23–9. https://doi.org/10.1007/s00247-013-2771-5.
73. Hämäläinen KP, Sainio AP. Cutting seton for anal fistulas: high risk of minor control defects. Dis Colon Rectum. 1997;40(12):1443–6.; discussion 7. https://doi.org/10.1007/bf02070710.
74. Feroz SH, Ahmed A, Muralidharan A, Thirunavukarasu P. Comparison of the efficacy of the various treatment modalities in the Management of Perianal Crohn's Fistula: a review. Cureus. 2020;12(12):e11882.
75. Talbot C, Sagar PM, Johnston MJ, Finan PJ, Burke D. Infliximab in the surgical management of complex fistulating anal Crohn's disease. Color Dis. 2005;7(2):164–8. https://doi.org/10.1111/j.1463-1318.2004.00749.x.
76. Tanaka S, Matsuo K, Sasaki T, Nakano M, Sakai K, Beppu R, et al. Clinical advantages of combined seton placement and infliximab maintenance therapy for perianal fistulizing Crohn's disease: when and how were the seton drains removed? Hepato-Gastroenterology. 2010;57(97):3–7.

77. Thornton M, Solomon MJ. Long-term indwelling seton for complex anal fistulas in Crohn's disease. Dis Colon Rectum. 2005;48(3):459–63. https://doi.org/10.1007/s10350-004-0830-6.
78. Wasmann KA, de Groof EJ, Stellingwerf ME, D'Haens GR, Ponsioen CY, Gecse KB, et al. Treatment of perianal fistulas in Crohn's disease, Seton versus anti-TNF versus surgical closure following anti-TNF [PISA]: a randomised controlled trial. J Crohns Colitis. 2020;14(8):1049–56. https://doi.org/10.1093/ecco-jcc/jjaa004.
79. Jimenez M, Mandava N. Anorectal Fistula. In: StatPearls. Treasure Island (FL): StatPearls Publishing Copyright © 2022. StatPearls Publishing LLC; 2022.
80. Sangwan YP, Schoetz DJ Jr, Murray JJ, Roberts PL, Coller JA. Perianal Crohn's disease. Results of local surgical treatment. Dis Colon Rectum. 1996;39(5):529–35. https://doi.org/10.1007/bf02058706.
81. Nordgren S, Fasth S, Hultén L. Anal fistulas in Crohn's disease: incidence and outcome of surgical treatment. Int J Color Dis. 1992;7(4):214–8. https://doi.org/10.1007/bf00341224.
82. Halme L, Sainio AP. Factors related to frequency, type, and outcome of anal fistulas in Crohn's disease. Dis Colon Rectum. 1995;38(1):55–9. https://doi.org/10.1007/bf02053858.
83. Farag AFA, Elbarmelgi MY, Mostafa M, Mashhour AN. One stage fistulectomy for high anal fistula with reconstruction of anal sphincter without fecal diversion. Asian J Surg. 2019;42(8):792–6. https://doi.org/10.1016/j.asjsur.2018.12.005.
84. Seyfried S, Bussen D, Joos A, Galata C, Weiss C, Herold A. Fistulectomy with primary sphincter reconstruction. Int J Color Dis. 2018;33(7):911–8. https://doi.org/10.1007/s00384-018-3042-6.
85. Murtaza G, Shaikh FA, Chawla T, Rajput BU, Shahzad N, Ansari S. Fistulotomy versus fistulectomy for simple fistula in ano: a retrospective cohort study. J Pak Med Assoc. 2017;67(3):339–42.
86. Grimaud JC, Munoz-Bongrand N, Siproudhis L, Abramowitz L, Sénéjoux A, Vitton V, et al. Fibrin glue is effective healing perianal fistulas in patients with Crohn's disease. Gastroenterology 2010;138(7):2275–81, 81.e1. doi: https://doi.org/10.1053/j.gastro.2010.02.013, 2281.e1.
87. Vidon M, Munoz-Bongrand N, Lambert J, Maggiori L, Zeitoun JD, Corte H, et al. Long-term efficacy of fibrin glue injection for perianal fistulas in patients with Crohn's disease. Color Dis. 2021;23(4):894–900. https://doi.org/10.1111/codi.15477.
88. Adamina M, Bonovas S, Raine T, Spinelli A, Warusavitarne J, Armuzzi A, et al. ECCO guidelines on therapeutics in Crohn's disease: surgical treatment. J Crohns Colitis. 2020;14(2):155–68. https://doi.org/10.1093/ecco-jcc/jjz187.
89. Senéjoux A, Siproudhis L, Abramowitz L, Munoz-Bongrand N, Desseaux K, Bouguen G, et al. Fistula plug in Fistulising Ano-perineal Crohn's disease: a randomised controlled trial. J Crohns Colitis. 2016;10(2):141–8. https://doi.org/10.1093/ecco-jcc/jjv162.
90. Jayne DG, Scholefield J, Tolan D, Gray R, Edlin R, Hulme CT, et al. Anal fistula plug versus surgeon's preference for surgery for trans-sphincteric anal fistula: the FIAT RCT. Health Technol Assess. 2019;23(21):1–76. https://doi.org/10.3310/hta23210.
91. Song K. New techniques for treating an anal Fistula. J Korean Soc Coloproctol. 2012;28:7–12. https://doi.org/10.3393/jksc.2012.28.1.7.
92. Stellingwerf ME, van Praag EM, Tozer PJ, Bemelman WA, Buskens CJ. Systematic review and meta-analysis of endorectal advancement flap and ligation of the intersphincteric fistula tract for cryptoglandular and Crohn's high perianal fistulas. BJS Open. 2019;3(3):231–41. https://doi.org/10.1002/bjs5.50129.
93. Soltani A, Kaiser AM. Endorectal advancement flap for cryptoglandular or Crohn's fistula-in-ano. Dis Colon Rectum. 2010;53(4):486–95. https://doi.org/10.1007/DCR.0b013e3181ce8b01.
94. Nielsen OH, Rogler G, Hahnloser D, Thomsen O. Diagnosis and management of fistulizing Crohn's disease. Nat Clin Pract Gastroenterol Hepatol. 2009;6(2):92–106. https://doi.org/10.1038/ncpgasthep1340.

95. Bessi G, Siproudhis L, Merlini l'Héritier A, Wallenhorst T, Le Balc'h E, Bouguen G, et al. Advancement flap procedure in Crohn and non-Crohn perineal fistulas: a simple surgical approach. Color Dis. 2019;21(1):66–72. https://doi.org/10.1111/codi.14417.
96. Lightner AL, Faubion WA, Fletcher JG. Interdisciplinary Management of Perianal Crohn's disease. Gastroenterol Clin N Am. 2017;46(3):547–62. https://doi.org/10.1016/j.gtc.2017.05.008.
97. Rojanasakul A, Pattanaarun J, Sahakitrungruang C, Tantiphlachiva K. Total anal sphincter saving technique for fistula-in-ano; the ligation of intersphincteric fistula tract. J Med Assoc Thail. 2007;90(3):581–6.
98. Mujukian A, Truong A, Fleshner P, Zaghiyan K. Long-term healing after complex anal fistula repair in patients with Crohn's disease. Tech Coloproctol. 2020;24(8):833–41. https://doi.org/10.1007/s10151-020-02238-1.
99. Kamiński JP, Zaghiyan K, Fleshner P. Increasing experience of ligation of the intersphincteric fistula tract for patients with Crohn's disease: what have we learned? Color Dis. 2017;19(8):750–5. https://doi.org/10.1111/codi.13668.
100. Gingold DS, Murrell ZA, Fleshner PR. A prospective evaluation of the ligation of the intersphincteric tract procedure for complex anal fistula in patients with Crohn's disease. Ann Surg. 2014;260(6):1057–61. https://doi.org/10.1097/sla.0000000000000479.
101. Wood T, Truong A, Mujukian A, Zaghiyan K, Fleshner P. Increasing experience with the LIFT procedure in Crohn's disease patients with complex anal fistula. Tech Coloproctol. 2022;26(3):205–12. https://doi.org/10.1007/s10151-022-02582-4.
102. Lo OSH. Ligation of the Intersphincteric Fistula tract (LIFT). In: Meng WCS, Cheung HYS, Lam DTY, Ng SSM, editors. Minimally invasive Coloproctology: advances in techniques and technology. Cham: Springer International Publishing; 2015. p. 175–82.
103. Sangar P. Fistula-in-ano: how I do the LIFT procedure. Sri Lanka J Sur. 2012;29:97.
104. Yamamoto T, Allan RN, Keighley MR. Effect of fecal diversion alone on perianal Crohn's disease. World J Surg. 2000;24(10):1258–62; discussion 62–3. https://doi.org/10.1007/s002680010250.
105. Singh S, Ding NS, Mathis KL, Dulai PS, Farrell AM, Pemberton JH, et al. Systematic review with meta-analysis: faecal diversion for management of perianal Crohn's disease. Aliment Pharmacol Ther. 2015;42(7):783–92. https://doi.org/10.1111/apt.13356.
106. Bell SJ, Williams AB, Wiesel P, Wilkinson K, Cohen RC, Kamm MA. The clinical course of fistulating Crohn's disease. Aliment Pharmacol Ther. 2003;17(9):1145–51. https://doi.org/10.1046/j.1365-2036.2003.01561.x.
107. Wolff BG, Culp CE, Beart RW Jr, Ilstrup DM, Ready RL. Anorectal Crohn's disease. A long-term perspective. Dis Colon Rectum. 1985;28(10):709–11. https://doi.org/10.1007/bf02560279.
108. Maeda Y, Heyckendorff-Diebold T, Tei TM, Lundby L, Buntzen S. Gracilis muscle transposition for complex fistula and persistent nonhealing sinus in perianal Crohn's disease. Inflamm Bowel Dis. 2011;17(2):583–9. https://doi.org/10.1002/ibd.21311.
109. Collie MH, Potter MA, Bartolo DC. Myocutaneous flaps promote perineal healing in inflammatory bowel disease. Br J Surg. 2005;92(6):740–1. https://doi.org/10.1002/bjs.4872.
110. Marzo M, Felice C, Pugliese D, Andrisani G, Mocci G, Armuzzi A, et al. Management of perianal fistulas in Crohn's disease: an up-to-date review. World J Gastroenterol. 2015;21(5):1394–403. https://doi.org/10.3748/wjg.v21.i5.1394.
111. García-Olmo D, García-Arranz M, García LG, Cuellar ES, Blanco IF, Prianes LA, et al. Autologous stem cell transplantation for treatment of rectovaginal fistula in perianal Crohn's disease: a new cell-based therapy. Int J Color Dis. 2003;18(5):451–4. https://doi.org/10.1007/s00384-003-0490-3.
112. García-Olmo D, García-Arranz M, Herreros D, Pascual I, Peiro C, Rodríguez-Montes JA. A phase I clinical trial of the treatment of Crohn's fistula by adipose mesenchymal stem cell transplantation. Dis Colon Rectum. 2005;48(7):1416–23. https://doi.org/10.1007/s10350-005-0052-6.

113. Garcia-Olmo D, Herreros D, Pascual I, Pascual JA, Del-Valle E, Zorrilla J, et al. Expanded adipose-derived stem cells for the treatment of complex perianal fistula: a phase II clinical trial. Dis Colon Rectum. 2009;52(1):79–86. https://doi.org/10.1007/DCR.0b013e3181973487.
114. Panés J, García-Olmo D, Van Assche G, Colombel JF, Reinisch W, Baumgart DC, et al. Expanded allogeneic adipose-derived mesenchymal stem cells (Cx601) for complex perianal fistulas in Crohn's disease: a phase 3 randomised, double-blind controlled trial. Lancet. 2016;388(10051):1281–90. https://doi.org/10.1016/s0140-6736(16)31203-x.
115. Panés J, García-Olmo D, Van Assche G, Colombel JF, Reinisch W, Baumgart DC, et al. Long-term efficacy and safety of stem cell therapy (Cx601) for complex perianal fistulas in patients with Crohn's disease. Gastroenterology. 2018;154(5):1334–42.e4. https://doi.org/10.1053/j.gastro.2017.12.020.
116. Lightner AL, Wang Z, Zubair AC, Dozois EJ. A systematic review and meta-analysis of mesenchymal stem cell injections for the treatment of perianal Crohn's disease: Progress made and future directions. Dis Colon Rectum. 2018;61(5):629–40. https://doi.org/10.1097/dcr.0000000000001093.
117. Dietz AB, Dozois EJ, Fletcher JG, Butler GW, Radel D, Lightner AL, et al. Autologous mesenchymal stem cells, applied in a bioabsorbable matrix, for treatment of perianal fistulas in patients with Crohn's disease. Gastroenterology. 2017;153(1):59–62.e2. https://doi.org/10.1053/j.gastro.2017.04.001.
118. Lightner AL, Otero Pineiro A, Reese J, Ream J, Nachand D, Bena J, et al. One year follow up of three phase IB/IIA clinical trials of Ex Vivo expanded Allogeneic Bone marrow derived mesenchymal stem cells for the treatment of Fistulizing Crohn's Disease In Press 2022.
119. Georgiev-Hristov T, Guadalajara H, Herreros MD, Lightner AL, Dozois EJ, García-Arranz M, et al. A step-by-step surgical protocol for the treatment of perianal Fistula with adipose-derived mesenchymal stem cells. J Gastrointest Surg. 2018;22(11):2003–12. https://doi.org/10.1007/s11605-018-3895-6.
120. Moy J, Bodzin J. Carbon dioxide laser ablation of perianal fistulas in patients with Crohn's disease: experience with 27 patients. Am J Surg. 2006;191(3):424–7. https://doi.org/10.1016/j.amjsurg.2005.10.050.
121. Wilhelm A. A new technique for sphincter-preserving anal fistula repair using a novel radial emitting laser probe. Tech Coloproctol. 2011;15(4):445–9. https://doi.org/10.1007/s10151-011-0726-0.
122. Wilhelm A, Fiebig A, Krawczak M. Five years of experience with the FiLaC™ laser for fistula-in-ano management: long-term follow-up from a single institution. Tech Coloproctol. 2017;21(4):269–76. https://doi.org/10.1007/s10151-017-1599-7.
123. Alam A, Lin F, Fathallah N, Pommaret E, Aubert M, Lemarchand N, et al. FiLaC(®) and Crohn's disease perianal fistulas: a pilot study of 20 consecutive patients. Tech Coloproctol. 2020;24(1):75–8. https://doi.org/10.1007/s10151-019-02134-3.
124. Meinero P, Mori L. Video-assisted anal fistula treatment (VAAFT): a novel sphincter-saving procedure for treating complex anal fistulas. Tech Coloproctol. 2011;15(4):417–22. https://doi.org/10.1007/s10151-011-0769-2.
125. Schwandner O. Video-assisted anal fistula treatment (VAAFT) combined with advancement flap repair in Crohn's disease. Tech Coloproctol. 2013;17(2):221–5. https://doi.org/10.1007/s10151-012-0921-7.
126. Adegbola SO, Sahnan K, Tozer PJ, Strouhal R, Hart AL, Lung PFC, et al. Symptom amelioration in Crohn's perianal fistulas using video-assisted anal Fistula treatment (VAAFT). J Crohns Colitis. 2018;12(9):1067–72. https://doi.org/10.1093/ecco-jcc/jjy071.
127. El-Barbary HM. Video assisted anal Fistula treatment "VAAFT technique" for complex perianal fistulas. Open Access J Sur: Juniper Publishers. 2016;1:555571.
128. Yusof S, Zhao Y. Novel use of video-assisted anal fistula treatment (VAAFT) fistuloscope in the treatment of chronic sinus tracts following low anterior resection. Asian J Sur. 2020;43(8):851–2. https://doi.org/10.1016/j.asjsur.2020.04.015. Copyright Elsevier 2020

What Are the Treatment Options for Painful Anal Fissure in Patients with Crohn's Disease?

3

Michael A. Valente

Introduction

Perianal manifestations of Crohn's disease (CD) disease are usually chronic in nature, and often characterized by waxing and waning symptoms. The goals of treatment are typically achieved through multimodal management, which minimizes surgical intervention and preserves the sphincter complex [1–3]. While there is a broad spectrum of severity of perianal CD, even the perceived minor issue of fissuring of the anus can present the clinician and patient with difficult decisions in management.

Fissures are identified in approximately 20 to 40% of patients with CD and although they are often painless, 40–85% are associated with pain [1–3]. Additionally, persistent, unhealed fissures can lead to perianal abscess and fistulae in up to 20% of patients with CD; this presents quality of life issues for the patient and a treatment dilemma for the surgeon [2].

When chronic anal fissures in patients without CD fail to respond to conservative measures, lateral internal sphincterotomy (LIS) is performed with a high degree of success and limited morbidity. In the setting of active anorectal CD, however, even a minor anorectal procedure may carry an enhanced risk of morbidity, including wound complications, anorectal/pelvic sepsis, fistulous disease and incontinence [1, 4]. Thus, a significant degree of caution must be applied when managing the refractory painful fissure in the setting of CD.

M. A. Valente (✉)
University of Arizona, Surgical Oncology, Tucson, AZ, USA
e-mail: vnfons@lsuhsc.edu

K. Umanskiy, N. Hyman (eds.), *Difficult Decisions in Colorectal Surgery*, Difficult Decisions in Surgery: An Evidence-Based Approach,
https://doi.org/10.1007/978-3-031-42303-1_3

Search Strategy

A comprehensive literature search of EMBASE, MEDLINE, Cochrane Database of Collected Research and PubMed was performed to identify all of the English-language publications related to the treatment outcomes of anal fissure, Crohn's disease, and perianal Crohn's disease from 1990–2022. Key search terms included "anal fissure," "Crohn's disease," "perianal Crohn's disease," "inflammatory bowel disease," "lateral internal sphincterotomy," Botulinum toxin," and Botox." Table 3.1 summarizes the population, intervention, comparator, and key outcomes (PICO) for the patient population.

Results

Over the last three to four decades, there has been a paucity of studies on perianal Crohn's disease associated fissure-in-ano. A review of the most pertinent literature is summarized in Table 3.2, with the quality of the studies evaluated using the GRADE system. The studies in the literature are all retrospective with low patient numbers, with little power and no standardization of outcomes.

D'Ugo and colleagues reviewed 41 patients with Crohn's associated fissures and found that medical therapy was effective in 66% of patients over a 37-month follow-up. Fourteen patients went on to have either lateral internal sphincterotomy or botulinum toxin injection in the internal anal sphincter, with or without fissurectomy. The overall complication rate was 57%. However, in patients with confirmed active Crohn's disease of the anal canal/rectum, Botox was performed instead of LIS and therefore, there is no true comparison between Botox and LIS in known CD patients [2].

Similarly, Lozynskyy et al. reported a 75% healing rate with medical management in CD patients and reported they had not performed surgical treatment of a fissure associated with CD in the last 5 years of their study [5]. Fleshner and colleagues compared medical versus surgical management of CD anal fissures and reported a 49% fissure healing rate with medical management alone, with the majority of healing in acute and painless fissures. They then compared fissure healing rates when after patients underwent anorectal procedures versus bowel resection for proximal disease. They showed an 88% healing rate with anorectal procedures (LIS, fissurectomy) versus 43% healing rate with proximal bowel resection for active ileal or colonic CD. Additionally, the authors reported that abscess or fistula formation

Table 3.1 PICO table for Crohn's disease-associated painful anal fissure

Patient population	Intervention	Comparator	Key outcomes
Patients with Crohn's disease and painful anal fissure	Lateral internal sphincterotomy (LIS)	Conservative medical management (including Botox injection)	Morbidity, pain resolution, healing, need for additional intervention(s)

Table 3.2 Literature reported outcomes and quality of evidence

Study	Patients (n)	Interventions (n)	Outcome classification	Healing (%) medical management	Healing (%) surgical management	Morbidity (%) surgical treatment	Quality of evidence (GRADE)
D'Ugo (2013) [2]	41, CD (22 with definitive diagnosis)	Medical management (27), surgical treatment (Botox/fissurectomy vs LIS; 14)	Healing rate, complication rate	65.8	78.5% (recurrences)	57.1	Very low quality
Lozynskyy (2009) [5]	60 CD	Medical management (45), surgical treatment (Maslyak's method; 15)	Healing rate	75	NR	NR	Very low quality
Fleshner (1995) [6]	56 CD (49 symptomatic)	Medical management (35), surgical treatment (LIS, fissurectomy, bowel resection; 15 (8 anorectal))	Healing rate	50	67	NR	Low quality

arises from the base of an unhealed fissure in 26% of all patients, with no significant difference between the medical and surgical groups [6].

Several additional retrospective studies have been performed but very little outcome data exists. For example, Wolkomir et al. evaluated 25 CD patients undergoing 27 procedures for anal fissure. However, they did not directly report on the healing or complication rates in their study. They did describe a mean follow up of greater than 7 years and noted that 22 patients (88%) had a healed wound by 2 months; however, 11 patients subsequently developed anorectal pathology of whom three developed recurrent fissure and 2 went on to proctectomy (secondary to progression of primary disease, not due to surgery) [7]. Similarly, Sangwan et al. studied 21 patients with anal fissure of whom six underwent LIS and one underwent fissurectomy. However, again, no outcome data was reported in this study [8].

Although it is stated in many review articles that LIS should be reserved for patients without active anorectal CD [1, 3, 4, 9, 10], active CD simply has not been assessed as a study variable in any recent literature. This may be because it is assumed to be unsafe to proceed with LIS in the setting of active CD. However, this assumption may not be valid, especially in the era of biologic treatment for CD, and should be validated in future studies.

Recommendations

Painful anal fissures in Crohn's disease that do not respond to conservative measures may be treated with Botulinum toxin injection and/or lateral internal sphincterotomy. **(Evidence: low; Recommendation: weak)**

Surgical intervention for anal fissure may pose increased morbidity in patients with active anorectal CD. **(Evidence: low; Recommendation: weak)**

There is a paucity of literature evaluating medical versus surgical management of Crohn's disease associated fissures. Additionally, the literature to date consists of low to very low quality retrospective studies with incomplete outcome data. To further clarify the treatment algorithm in the presence of active perianal Crohn's disease, new, well-designed studies are needed, especially those comparing Botox to LIS in patients who have failed conservative medical management.

Personal View

First and foremost, the distinction between patients with a painful anal fissure that has concurrent abdominal CD versus a patient that has a painful anal fissure in the setting of active anorectal/perianal CD must be elucidated. The pathophysiology of painful anal fissures in patients with abdominal CD without active anorectal disease is similar to common fissures in the general population; they are caused by internal sphincter muscle spasm/hypertonicity, secondary to trauma to the anoderm from frequent, loose bowel movements. In patients without active anorectal disease, the treatment algorithm is essentially the same as for patients without a diagnosis of

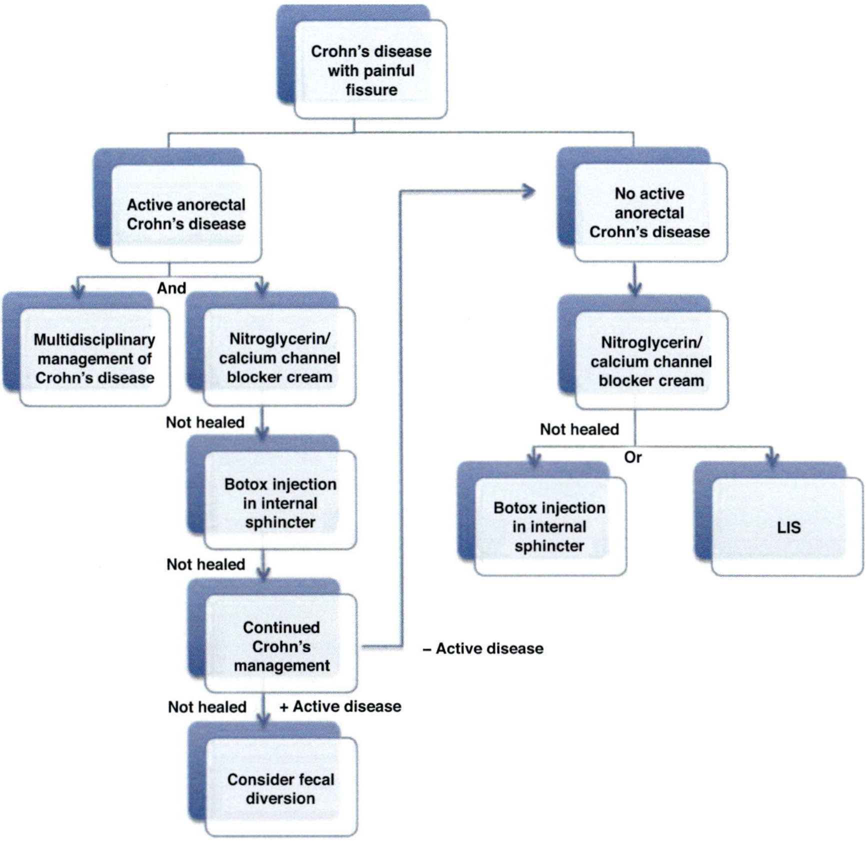

Fig. 3.1 Algorithm for management of fissure associated with Crohn's disease. (From: IBD: management of a painful anal fissure and skin tags in patients with Crohn's disease)

CD. Medical management is first line and includes optimization of bowel habits to minimize diarrhea (treat the proximal Crohn's disease, loperamide, fiber supplements) and a trial of topical calcium channel blocker or similar smooth muscle relaxant (nitroglycerin is discouraged due to poor side effect profile). In the event of an unhealed fissure, Botox injection (50–100 Units) delivered directly into the internal sphincter muscle, or LIS may be performed (Fig. 3.1). Additionally, it should be noted that *painless* anal fissures in patients with CD should not undergo surgery and biologics should be utilized, as the vast majority of these will heal after starting medical treatment.

In the setting of active anorectal CD, multidisciplinary treatment should be standard and medical management (i.e., biologics) should be considered first line treatment, in addition to the conservative management regimen as aforementioned. The majority of these painful fissures will heal with conservative measures, albeit it may take considerably longer to achieve than in typical fissure patients and recurrences are commonplace.

When a CD painful fissure has failed aggressive medical management, Botox (50–100 units) can be injected. Additionally, the injection of 40–80 mg/ml of triamcinolone (Kenalog) into any anorectal inflammatory strictures and /or inflammation is often performed. If Botox injection does not result in healing of the fissure, continued aggressive medical management should be undertaken and a repeat injection of Botox/steroid may be contemplated. Lateral internal sphincterotomy should be contemplated and performed in refractory cases that have failed all other options. Depending on the amount of active inflammation, a closed or open approach may be employed, but a closed approach is potentially more desirable due to the smaller wound that is created. The patients are begun on an antibiotic regimen post-operatively (i.e., oral metronidazole) and seen in early post-operative period for wound examination.

Consideration for temporary fecal diversion or proctectomy is considered a last resort to palliate symptoms. In the author's experience, there is often additional anal pathology present, such as severe fistulizing disease and/or anorectal stenosis, which in conjunction with painful fissures, may make fecal diversion or proctectomy necessary. However, temporary fecal diversion for these anorectal ailments is often not temporary in over 70–80% of cases, and hence, proctectomy with permeant diversion should be contemplated and discussed with the patient early on in cases of severe, refractory disease [11].

References

1. Bolshinsky V, Church J. Management of Complex Anorectal and Perianal Crohn's disease. Clin Colon Rectal Surg. 2019 Jul;32(4):255–60.
2. D'Ugo S, Franceschilli L, Cadeddu F, et al. Medical and surgical treatment of haemorrhoids and anal fissure in Crohn's disease: a critical appraisal. BMC Gastroenterol. 2013;13(1):13–47.
3. Mahmoud NN, Halwani Y, Montbrun S, Shah PM, Hedrick TL, Rashid F, Schwartz DA, Dalal RL, Kamiński JP, Zaghiyan K, Fleshner PR, Weissler JM, Fischer JP. Current management of perianal Crohn's disease. Curr Probl Surg. 2017 May;54(5):262–98.
4. Lu KU, Hunt SR. Surgical management of Crohn's disease. Surg Clin North Am. 2013;93(1):167–85.
5. Lozynskyy YS. Treatment algorithms in the case of perianal complications of Crohn's disease. Dig Dis. 2009;27(4):565–70.
6. Fleshner PR, Schoetz DJ, Roberts PL, Murray JJ, Coller JA, Veidenheimer MC. Anal fissure in Crohn's disease: a plea for aggressive management. Dis Colon Rectum. 1995;38(11):1137–43.
7. Wolkomir AF, Luchtefeld MA. Surgery for symptomatic hemorrhoids and anal fissures in Crohn's disease. Dis Colon Rectum. 1993;36(6):545–7.
8. Sangwan YP, Schoetz DJ, Murray JJ, Roberts PL, Coller JA. Perianal Crohn's disease. Results of local surgical treatment. Dis Colon Rectum. 1996;39(5):529–35.
9. Singh B, George BD, McC Mortensen NJ. Surgical therapy of perianal Crohn's disease. Dig Liver Dis. 2007;39(10):988–92.
10. Stewart DB Sr, Gaertner W, Glasgow S, Migaly J, Feingold D, Steele SR. Clinical practice guideline for the Management of Anal Fissures. Dis Colon Rectum. 2017 Jan;60(1):7–14.
11. Gu J, Valente MA, Remzi FH, Stocchi L. Factors affecting the fate of faecal diversion in patients with perianal Crohn's disease. Color Dis. 2015 Jan;17(1):66–72.

4 Elective Surgical Management in Patients with Ulcerative Colitis: How Many Stages?

Roger D. Hurst

Introduction

For the last three decades restorative proctocolectomy with J-pouch ileoanal anastomosis has been the primary treatment for ulcerative colitis patients who require surgery. While most patients requiring surgery for ulcerative colitis are young and are at baseline in good health, many are at least temporarily debilitated from either severity of disease, infection, malnutrition, obesity, or from side effects of immunosuppressant medications. These factors can greatly increase the risk for poor surgical outcomes both in the short and long term. Even when conditions are optimized, the ileoanal anastomosis is known to be a high risk anastomosis with frequent leaks and pelvic sepsis. Leak rates for the procedure are reported to be between 5 and 14% [1]. This high risk for anastomotic dehiscence was recognized early in the development of the procedure and strategies have been implemented in the hopes of diminishing the risks and consequences of poor anastomotic healing. For these reasons performing the operation multiple stages was the initial standard approach. However, the absolute need for staging has been questioned and many have advocated for a strategy of omitting the approach of multiple stages in selected cases and some have advocated for omitting staging in almost all cases [2–4]. This chapter will review the current available evidence to support the need for staging of the operations for the treatment of ulcerative colitis.

The ileo-anal procedure can be performed in either a single stage, two-step, or three-step approach [5, 6]. The decision points for the staging center around two separate issues. (Tables 4.1 and 4.2).

R. D. Hurst (✉)
Department of Surgery, University of Chicago, Chicago, IL, USA
e-mail: rhurst@surgery.bsd.uchicago.edu

K. Umanskiy, N. Hyman (eds.), *Difficult Decisions in Colorectal Surgery*, Difficult Decisions in Surgery: An Evidence-Based Approach,
https://doi.org/10.1007/978-3-031-42303-1_4

Table 4.1 Is diversion prefered with ileal pouch-anal anastomosis?

Pt population	Intervention	Comparator	Outcomes studied
Ulcerative colitis patients undergoing ileo-anal procedure	Omission of diverting stoma	Diversion of fecal stream	Anastomotic leaks, pelvic sepsis, long-term function, cost, length of hospital stay

Table 4.2 Should total colectomy with ileostomy preceed ileal pouch-anal anastomsis?

Pt population	Intervention	Comparator	Outcomes studied
Ulcerative colitis patients undergoing initial surgery	Total abdominal colectomy as initial operation	Ileo-anal anastomosis as initial operation	Anastomotic leaks, pelvic sepsis, long-term function, cost, length of hospital stay

1. When constructing the ileal pouch-anal reservoir and performing the ileoanal anastomosis should the fecal stream be diverted from the pouch and the anastomosis with a loop ileostomy to allow for healing?
2. In patients who are temporarily debilitated, should a total abdominal colectomy with end ileostomy and de-functionalized Hartmann's pouch be performed to allow for physiologic recovery prior to undertaking the more risky reservoir construction and ileoanal anastomosis?

This chapter will review each of these controversies.

Search Strategy

A Medline Ovid database search was performed on publications from 1985 through November 2022 comparing ileal pouch-anal anastomosis with or without diverting loop ileostomy. MeSH search headings utilized: restorative proctocolectomy, ileo-anal, ileo-anal anastomosis, ileal pouch, ileal reservoir, ileostomy, and loop ileostomy. References found from these articles were also searched and reviewed. Additionally "Find Citing Articles" function was utilized as a citation index to further enhance the extent of the search.

Results

Diverting Loop Ileostomy

Multiple reports have been published regarding the value of diverting loop ileostomy when performing pouch construction and creating the ileoanal anastomosis. No definitive conclusive study exists as each of these studies is flawed by either a lack of adequate numbers, poor study design, or significant bias. Many studies are retrospective reports comparing only highly selected cases. Case control studies do exist, but again in most instances these studies involve highly selected patients or

Table 4.3 Studies supporting the use of diverting stomas

Author	Date	Study type	Patients with stoma	Patients without stoma	Quality of evidence
Cohen, Z et al. [7]	1992	Retrospective, selected	87	71	Low
Tjandra, J, et al. [8]	1993	Matched controls	50	50	Moderate
Williamson, MER, et al. [9]	1997	Selected	50	50	Low
Kienle P, et al. [10]	2003	Prospective cohort, Selected	27	32	Low
Weston-Petrus [11]	2008	Meta-analysis			Moderate
Mennigen, R, et al. [12]	2011	Selected, retrospective	89	33	Low

insufficient numbers. Add to this, the results of these studies have been conflicting. Some studies suggesting an increased risk for anastomotic leaks and pelvic sepsis when the diverting stoma is omitted [7–12] while other studies suggest that the presence of the stoma does not affect the rate of anastomotic complications [13–31]. The studies supporting and opposing the use of a temporary diverting stoma are listed in Tables 4.3 and 4.4.

A common design strategy employed in many of these reports is to allow the operative surgeon to make a judgment regarding the need for the loop ileostomy (Those with "selected" study designs as designated in Tables 4.3 and 4.4). This decision by the surgeon is made as a judgment regarding the risk for anastomotic complications. The surgeon therefore decides who is at high risk and in places these patients in the diverted group and patients judged to be a low risk are placed in the un-diverted group. While this strategy may well be a reasonable approach in the management of patients undergoing surgery for ulcerative colitis, when applied to a clinical study this method of patient selection creates bias such that interpretation of the results can be difficult. Thus by design such selective cannot conclusively demonstrate that there is no benefit from the loop ileostomy. The absence of a difference between the two groups may result from the loop ileostomy effectively taking high risk patients and decreasing their risk to that of the lower risk group. So from these studies using a selected approach, one can really only claimed that patients judged to be at low risk for anastomotic complications will do as well as a high risk cohort when the loop ileostomy is omitted. Additionally, it is important to note that there are several studies with results that would indicate that even in patients selected in this manner, those without a loop ileostomy have an inferior outcome [7, 9, 12].

There is only one randomized controlled trial looking at the value of diverting loop ileostomy in restorative proctocolectomy [16]. But this study was markedly underpowered with only 23 patients in the loop ileostomy group and 22 patients in the un-diverted group. In each group there is only one incidence of anastomotic leak and even with this study the patients that were randomized had been preselected by the operating surgeon as having had a low risk for anastomotic leak.

Table 4.4 Studies supporting omission of diverting stoma

Author	Date	Study type	Patients with stoma	Patients without stoma	Quality of evidence
Everett WG, et al. [13]	1990	Selected	35	29	Low
Matikainen M, et al. [14]	1990	Consecutive	21	25	Low
Galandiuk S, et al [15]	1991	Retrospective matched controls, selected	37	37	Low
Grobler SP, et al. [16]	1992	Randomized control study, selected	23	22	Low
Sagar PM, et al [17]	1992	Consecutive, selected	28	30	Very low
Gorfine SR, et al [18]	1995	Retrospective, selected	69	74	Low
Gullberg K, et al. [19]	1995	Consecutive	7	13	Low
Hainsworth PJ, et al. [20]	1998	Selected	30	72	Low
Antos, F, et al. [21]	1999	Selected	20	23	Low
Dolgin SE, et al. [22]	1999	Consecutive, Prospective nonrandomized	14	16	Low
Mowschenson PM, et al. [23]	2000	Retrospective, selected	28	102	Low
Heuschen UA, et al. [24]	2001	Matched controls, selected	144	57	Moderate
Lepisto A, et al. [25]	2002	Retrospective	154	332	Moderate
Ikeuchi H, et al. [26]	2005	Retrospective, selected	92	150	Low
Remzi FH, et al [27]	2006	Retrospective, selected	1725	277	Low
Joyce, MR [28]	2010	Retrospective	715	120	Low
Gray BW, et al. [29]	2012	Selected	28	22	Low
Sahami, et al [30]	2016	Retrospective	305	316	Low
Olecki, et al. [31]	2022	Retrospective, selected	323	91	Low

Perhaps the best available study to suggest that loop ileostomy may not be necessary is a matched-pair controlled study conducted by Heuschen et al. [24] In this study 57 patients in the study group (no diversion) were compared to 114 matched controls. Heuschen et al. found no significant differences in early complications including pouch related septic complications. Conversely, Tjandra, et al., also reported a study with matched controls with 50 patients in each group and found a

14% risk for anastomotic leak and pelvic sepsis in patients who had not been diverted compared to 4% in the controls [8].

In 2008 Weston-Petrides, et al., published a meta-analysis for the data available from 1978 through 2005 from all comparative studies looking at restorative proctocolectomy with or without covering ileostomy [11]. This analysis indicated that restorative proctocolectomy without a diverting loop ileostomy resulted in similar long-term functional results but was associated with an increased risk for anastomotic leak and pelvic sepsis. The conclusion of the authors was that the loop ileostomy should only be omitted in carefully selected patients.

The goal of avoiding an anastomotic leak is worthwhile as poor anastomotic healing has major consequences both in the short and long term. Pelvic sepsis after ileal pouch-anal anastomosis has significant effects on long-term outcomes. For instance, patients who experience pelvic sepsis are five times more likely to require excision of their pouches when compared to those patients who avoided anastomotic leaks and pelvic sepsis [1, 32, 33]. Those patients who have pelvic sepsis but are able to retain their pouches were more likely to have anal incontinence [1].

While many of the studies looking at the value of fecal diversion focus on the risk for anastomotic leak, there are other considerations that come into play when deciding which operative strategy is best for the patient. Studies looking at the total length of stay and total costs have favored the approach of performing the ileoanal anastomosis without the loop ileostomy. While performing the operation in a single step tends to lead to a longer initial hospitalization, when the length of hospital stay for the reversal of the loop ileostomy is taken into account the total hospitalization is shorter with the one step approach [9, 12, 14, 16–18, 20, 21, 26, 28]. Additionally total costs have been shown to be lower in those patients undergoing the procedure without a diverting loop ileostomy [28].

When considering a staged approach the morbidity associated with the loop ileostomy itself must also be considered [34]. Some have suggested that the overall morbidity associated with loop ileostomy is substantial [35, 36], but others have noted that severe complications are not frequent [37]. Additionally a large study published in 2005 involving 1504 patients from the Cleveland Clinic demonstrated that closure of the ileostomy can be accomplished with an overall complication rate of 11.4% and a risk of intra-abdominal sepsis of only 1% [38]. Additionally an aggressive and coordinated approach of managing stoma patients can greatly diminish the incidence of stoma related dehydration and need for readmission [39].

Initial Colectomy Prior to IPAA

The value of an initial total abdominal colectomy prior to ileal pouch-anal anastomosis in patients with intra-abdominal sepsis or severe co-morbid disease has not been subject to comparative studies as the risks to these patients would be difficult to justify. However, reports of patients who have undergone either a two or three step approach have identified certain parameters under which a three stage approach would be prefered [40–42]. Traditionally these have included urgent surgery, sepsis, fulminate disease, anemia, hypoalbuminemia, steroids, and uncertain diagnosis [3, 5, 42, 43].

A more recent and significant controversy surrounds the risks for perioperative complications for patients who are being treated with anti-TNF and other biologic agents. In 2005 the anti-TNF antibody, infliximab, was approved for use in patients with ulcerative colitis [44]. Shortly after the widespread use of infliximab for the treatment of ulcerative colitis, the Mayo Clinic and the Cleveland Clinic both reported a substantial increase in postoperative related infectious complications in ulcerative colitis patients treated with infliximab [45, 46]. This finding is not entirely consistent across all reports and is somewhat surprising given that prior to this infliximab had been used for many years in the treatment of Crohn's disease and no significant increase in perioperative complications has been seen in these patients [47–53]. This may be explained by the fact that the ileal pouch-anal anastomosis is normally a high risk anastomosis even under ideal conditions. It may well be that infliximab generates a relatively small effect on healing in general, but that this effect is magnified with this very delicate anastomosis.

In response to the findings suggesting that anti-TNF therapy increases risk for anastomotic leaks, many surgeons have changed their approach to the surgical management by utilizing a three-step approach in patients treated with anti-TNF agents [54, 55]. In a study from the Cleveland Clinic, Gu et al. looked at patients undergoing surgery for ulcerative colitis without an initial total abdominal colectomy [54]. They found that those patients on anti-TNF therapy had a significantly greater risk for pelvic sepsis (32% versus 16%; $p = 0.012$) when the procedure is not staged with an initial total abdominal colectomy. However, they reported no difference in outcomes between the patients who had been treated with anti-TNF therapy as compared to those who had never been treated with anti-TNF agents when patients initially undergo a staged colectomy. These findings not only indicate that the use of anti-TNF therapy increases the risk for septic complications, they also indicate that utilizing an initial total abdominal colectomy can mitigate the negative effects of the anti-TNF agents.

Recommendations Based on the Data

1. A diverting loop ileostomy may be omitted in highly selected patients undergoing ileal pouch-anal anastomosis. (Weak Recommendation based upon low-quality of evidence)

   From the current available data it is difficult to give strong recommendations as to appropriateness of omitting a diverting loop ileostomy with restorative proctocolectomy. Even investigators intimately involved in the subject have had difficulties with this. For instance in 1992 Sagar, et al. initially reported a comparison of one stage versus two-stage ileoanal procedures and found no significant difference in the risk for anastomotic leaks or other complications and concluded that omission of the loop ileostomy may be a reasonable option in selected patients [17]. The same group later reported in 1997 that with further experience they found that patients undergoing a one stage restorative proctocolectomy had significantly higher risk for severe septic complications and cautioned against the routine use of a one stage proctocolectomy [9]. Additionally Tjandra et al. initially reported 1994 a matched control study and found that in equally favorable cases restorative proctocolectomy without diversion was not as safe as with diversion [8]. The same institution later reported a retrospective study indicating no difference in septic complications [27]. The senior author on both of these studies subsequently co-authored a meta-analysis indicating that restorative proctocolectomy without a diverting ileostomy was associated with an increased risk for anastomotic leak [11].

Even with these difficulties, there is general consensus among experts that the diverting loop ileostomy can be omitted in highly selected patients. And this has been the recommendation from expert panels from both Europe and North America [56, 57]. Patient selected for omission of loop ileostomy are best not to have any of the risk factors listed in Table 4.5. Despite the recommendations from expert panels that omission of the loop ileostomy is reasonable in selected patients, many practicing surgeons appear to adopt a very conservative approach to this issue. A 2009 survey of colorectal surgeons in North America indicated that 73% would perform a diverting loop ileostomy even in low risk patients. [58]

2. Ulcerative colitis patients with sepsis, severe comorbid factors, or who have been treated with anti-TNF therapy should undergo an initial total abdominal colectomy prior to ileal pouch-anal anastomosis. (Weak recommendation based upon low-quality of evidence)

   There is little controversy that the sickest of patients should undergo a three stage approach. At the same time, there is insufficient evidence to accurately delineate the circumstances in which the three stage approach is the best option.

Table 4.5 Factors that may increase risk for poor anastomoic healing

Factors that may increase risk for poor anastomotic healing
1. Severe or fulminate colitis
2. Sepsis
3. Malnutrition
4. Hypoalbuminemia
5. Obesity
6. Technical difficulties
7. Steroid use
8. Use of immunosuppressants
9. Technical concerns
10. Tension on anastomosis
11. Fecal contamination
12. Anemia
13. Anti-TNF therapy

Early evidence suggests that the use of anti-TNF therapy poses a risk for increase in anastomotic leaks and pelvic sepsis and that these risks can be diminished by utilizing a three-stage approach [54]. Further study however is required to confirm the advantage of this approach. Even less is known about the effects on healing with other biologics such as anti-integrins and JAK inhibitors.

A Personal View of the Data

Unfortunately the data on the value of staging the surgeries for the ileoanal procedure are conflicting. Thus, it is truly a difficult decision as to whether to omit the diverting loop ileostomy. Likewise it is also a difficult decision as when to perform an initial total abdominal colectomy prior to the ileoanal procedure. Ultimately it is up to the discretion of the experienced surgeon working in concert with the patient's wishes to determine the best approach for each individual case.

In the past as many as one third of this author's patients underwent an ileoanal procedure in a single step. With the advent of anti-TNF therapy this however has changed and now most patients in my practice undergo surgery with a staged approach. The reports of poor anastomotic healing with anti-TNF therapy are concerning. This combined with my personal, albeit antidotal, experience with anastomotic problems in patients receiving anti-TNF therapy has made staging in my practice much more common. Additionally, the decision to stage the operations has become somewhat more attractive with the advent of laparoscopic surgery. The decrease morbidity and enhanced recovery after laparoscopic total abdominal colectomy makes the decision for staging easier to accept as it is much better tolerated than an open procedure [59].

References

1. Farouk R, Dozois RR, Pemberton JH, Larson D. Incidence and subsequent impact of pelvic abscess after ileal pouch-anal anastomosis for chronic ulcerative colitis. Dis Colon Rectum. 1998;41:1239–43.
2. Sugerman HJ, Sugerman EL, Meador JG, Newsome HH, Kellum JM, DeMaria EJ. Ileal pouch anal anastomosis without ileal diversion. Ann Surg. 2000;232:530–41.
3. Harms BA, Myers GA, Rosenfeld DJ, Starling JR. Management of fulminant ulcerative colitis by primary restorative proctocolectomy. Dis Colon Rectum. 1994;37:971–8.
4. Metcalf AM, Dozois RR, Kelly KA, Wolff BG. Ileal pouch-anal anastomosis without temporary, diverting ileostomy. Dis Colon Rectum. 1986;29:33–5.
5. Hurst RD, Finco C, Rubin M, Michelassi F. Prospective analysis of perioperative morbidity in one hundred consecutive colectomies for ulcerative colitis. Surgery. 1995;118:748–54; discussion 54–5
6. Swenson BR, Hollenbeak CS, Poritz LS, Koltun WA. Modified two-stage ileal pouch-anal anastomosis: equivalent outcomes with less resource utilization. Dis Colon Rectum. 2005;48:256–61.
7. Cohen Z, McLeod RS, Stephen W, Stern HS, O'Connor B, Reznick R. Continuing evolution of the pelvic pouch procedure. Ann Surg. 1992;216:506–11; discussion 11–2
8. Tjandra JJ, Fazio VW, Milsom JW, Lavery IC, Oakley JR, Fabre JM. Omission of temporary diversion in restorative proctocolectomy – is it safe? Dis Colon Rectum. 1993;36:1007–14.

9. Williamson ME, Lewis WG, Sagar PM, Holdsworth PJ, Johnston D. One-stage restorative proctocolectomy without temporary ileostomy for ulcerative colitis: a note of caution. Dis Colon Rectum. 1997;40:1019–22.
10. Kienle P, Weitz J, Benner A, Herfarth C, Schmidt J. Laparoscopically assisted colectomy and ileoanal pouch procedure with and without protective ileostomy. Surg Endosc. 2003;17:716–20.
11. Weston-Petrides GK, Lovegrove RE, Tilney HS, et al. Comparison of outcomes after restorative proctocolectomy with or without defunctioning ileostomy. Arch Surg. 2008;143:406–12.
12. Mennigen R, Senninger N, Bruwer M, Rijcken E. Impact of defunctioning loop ileostomy on outcome after restorative proctocolectomy for ulcerative colitis. Int J Color Dis. 2011;26:627–33.
13. Everett WG, Pollard SG. Restorative proctocolectomy without temporary ileostomy. Br J Surg. 1990;77:621–2.
14. Matikainen M, Santavirta J, Hiltunen KM. Ileoanal anastomosis without covering ileostomy. Dis Colon Rectum. 1990;33:384–8.
15. Galandiuk S, Wolff BG, Dozois RR, Beart RW. Ileal pouch-anal anastomosis without ileostomy. Dis Colon Rectum. 1991;34:870–3.
16. Grobler SP, Hosie KB, Keighley MR. Randomized trial of loop ileostomy in restorative proctocolectomy. Br J Surg. 1992;79:903–6.
17. Sagar PM, Lewis W, Holdsworth PJ, Johnston D. One-stage restorative proctocolectomy without temporary defunctioning ileostomy. Dis Colon Rectum. 1992;35:582–8.
18. Gorfine SR, Gelernt IM, Bauer JJ, Harris MT, Kreel I. Restorative proctocolectomy without diverting ileostomy. Dis Colon Rectum. 1995;38:188–94.
19. Gullberg K, Lindquist K, Lijeqvist L. Pelvic pouch-anal anastomoses: pros and cons about omission of mucosectomy and loop ileostomy. A study of 60 patients. Ann Chir. 1995;49:527–33.
20. Hainsworth PJ, Bartolo DC. Selective omission of loop ileostomy in restorative proctocolectomy. Int J Color Dis. 1998;13:119–23.
21. Antos F, Serclová Z, Slauf P. Is covering ileostomy after pouch operations necessary? Zentralbl Chir. 1999;124(Suppl 2):50–1.
22. Dolgin SE, Shlasko E, Gorfine S, Benkov K, Leleiko N. Restorative proctocolectomy in children with ulcerative colitis utilizing rectal mucosectomy with or without diverting ileostomy. J Pediatr Surg. 1999;34:837–9; discussion 9–40
23. Mowschenson PM, Critchlow JF, Peppercorn MA. Ileoanal pouch operation: long-term outcome with or without diverting ileostomy. Arch Surg. 2000;135:463–5; discussion 5–6
24. Heuschen UA, Hinz U, Allemeyer EH, Lucas M, Heuschen G, Herfarth C. One- or two-stage procedure for restorative proctocolectomy: rationale for a surgical strategy in ulcerative colitis. Ann Surg. 2001;234:788–94.
25. Lepistö A, Luukkonen P, Järvinen HJ. Cumulative failure rate of ileal pouch-anal anastomosis and quality of life after failure. Dis Colon Rectum. 2002;45:1289–94.
26. Ikeuchi H, Nakano H, Uchino M, et al. Safety of one-stage restorative proctocolectomy for ulcerative colitis. Dis Colon Rectum. 2005;48:1550–5.
27. Remzi FH, Fazio VW, Gorgun E, et al. The outcome after restorative proctocolectomy with or without defunctioning ileostomy. Dis Colon Rectum. 2006;49:470–7.
28. Joyce MR, Kiran RP, Remzi FH, Church J, Fazio VW. In a select group of patients meeting strict clinical criteria and undergoing ileal pouch-anal anastomosis, the omission of a diverting ileostomy offers cost savings to the hospital. Dis Colon Rectum. 2010;53:905–10.
29. Gray BW, Drongowski RA, Hirschl RB, Geiger JD. Restorative proctocolectomy without diverting ileostomy in children with ulcerative colitis. J Pediatr Surg. 2012;47:204–8.
30. Sahami S, Buskens CJ, Fadok TY, et al. Defunctioning ileostomy is not associated with reduced leakage in proctocolectomy and ileal pouch anastomosis surgeries for IBD. J Crohns Colitis. 2016;10:779–85.
31. Olecki EJ, Kronfli AP, Stahl KA, King S, Razavi NC, Koltun WA. Stoma-less IPAA is not associated with increased anastomotic leak rate or long-term pouch failure in patients with ulcerative colitis. Dis Colon Rectum. 2022;65:1342–50.
32. Heuschen UA, Allemeyer EH, Hinz U, Lucas M, Herfarth C, Heuschen G. Outcome after septic complications in J pouch procedures. Br J Surg. 2002;89:194–200.

33. Gorfine SR, Fichera A, Harris MT, Bauer JJ. Long-term results of salvage surgery for septic complications after restorative proctocolectomy: does fecal diversion improve outcome? Dis Colon Rectum. 2003;46:1339–44.
34. Kaidar-Person O, Person B, Wexner SD. Complications of construction and closure of temporary loop ileostomy. J Am Coll Surg. 2005;201:759–73.
35. Metcalf AM, Dozois RR, Beart RW, Kelly KA, Wolff BG. Temporary ileostomy for ileal pouch-anal anastomosis. Function and complications. Dis Colon Rectum. 1986;29:300–3.
36. Park J, Gessler B, Block M, Angenete E. Complications and morbidity associated with loop ileostomies in patients with ulcerative colitis. Scand J Surg. 2018;107:38–42.
37. Phang PT, Hain JM, Perez-Ramirez JJ, Madoff RD, Gemlo BT. Techniques and complications of ileostomy takedown. Am J Surg. 1999;177:463–6.
38. Wong KS, Remzi FH, Gorgun E, et al. Loop ileostomy closure after restorative proctocolectomy: outcome in 1,504 patients. Dis Colon Rectum. 2005;48:243–50.
39. Nagle D, Pare T, Keenan E, Marcet K, Tizio S, Poylin V. Ileostomy pathway virtually eliminates readmissions for dehydration in new ostomates. Dis Colon Rectum. 2012;55:1266–72.
40. Nicholls RJ, Holt SD, Lubowski DZ. Restorative proctocolectomy with ileal reservoir. Comparison of two-stage vs. three-stage procedures and analysis of factors that might affect outcome. Dis Colon Rectum. 1989;32:323–6.
41. Bikhchandani J, Polites SF, Wagie AE, Habermann EB, Cima RR. National trends of 3- versus 2-stage restorative proctocolectomy for chronic ulcerative colitis. Dis Colon Rectum. 2015;58:199–204.
42. Heyvaert G, Penninckx F, Filez L, Aerts R, Kerremans R, Rutgeerts P. Restorative proctocolectomy in elective and emergency cases of ulcerative colitis. Int J Color Dis. 1994;9:73–6.
43. Hyman NH, Cataldo P, Osler T. Urgent subtotal colectomy for severe inflammatory bowel disease. Dis Colon Rectum. 2005;48:70–3.
44. Rutgeerts P, Sandborn WJ, Feagan BG, et al. Infliximab for induction and maintenance therapy for ulcerative colitis. N Engl J Med. 2005;353:2462–76.
45. Selvasekar CR, Cima RR, Larson DW, et al. Effect of infliximab on short-term complications in patients undergoing operation for chronic ulcerative colitis. J Am Coll Surg. 2007;204:956–62; discussion 62–3
46. Mor IJ, Vogel JD, da Luz MA, Shen B, Hammel J, Remzi FH. Infliximab in ulcerative colitis is associated with an increased risk of postoperative complications after restorative proctocolectomy. Dis Colon Rectum. 2008;51:1202–7; discussion 7–10
47. Marchal L, D'Haens G, Van Assche G, et al. The risk of post-operative complications associated with infliximab therapy for Crohn's disease: a controlled cohort study. Aliment Pharmacol Ther. 2004;19:749–54.
48. Schluender SJ, Ippoliti A, Dubinsky M, et al. Does infliximab influence surgical morbidity of ileal pouch-anal anastomosis in patients with ulcerative colitis? Dis Colon Rectum. 2007;50:1747–53.
49. Colombel JF, Loftus EV, Tremaine WJ, et al. Early postoperative complications are not increased in patients with Crohn's disease treated perioperatively with infliximab or immunosuppressive therapy. Am J Gastroenterol. 2004;99:878–83.
50. Krane MK, Allaix ME, Zoccali M, et al. Preoperative infliximab therapy does not increase morbidity and mortality after laparoscopic resection for inflammatory bowel disease. Dis Colon Rectum. 2013;56:449–57.
51. Kunitake H, Hodin R, Shellito PC, Sands BE, Korzenik J, Bordeianou L. Perioperative treatment with infliximab in patients with Crohn's disease and ulcerative colitis is not associated with an increased rate of postoperative complications. J Gastrointest Surg. 2008;12:1730–6; discussion 6–7
52. Sewell JL, Mahadevan U. Infliximab and surgical complications: truth or perception? Gastroenterology. 2009;136:354–5.
53. Ferrante M, D'Hoore A, Vermeire S, et al. Corticosteroids but not infliximab increase short-term postoperative infectious complications in patients with ulcerative colitis. Inflamm Bowel Dis. 2009;15:1062–70.

54. Gu J, Remzi FH, Shen B, Vogel JD, Kiran RP. Operative strategy modifies risk of pouch-related outcomes in patients with ulcerative colitis on preoperative anti-tumor necrosis factor-α therapy. Dis Colon Rectum. 2013;56:1243–52.
55. Geltzeiler CB, Lu KC, Diggs BS, et al. Initial surgical management of ulcerative colitis in the biologic era. Dis Colon Rectum. 2014;57:1358–63.
56. Pellino G, Sciaudone G, Canonico S, Selvaggi F. Role of ileostomy in restorative proctocolectomy. World J Gastroenterol. 2012;18:1703–7.
57. Holubar SD, Lightner AL, Poylin V, et al. The American Society of Colon and Rectal Surgeons clinical practice guidelines for the surgical management treatment of ulcerative colitis. Dis Colon Rectum. 2021;64:783–804.
58. de Montbrun SL, Johnson PM. Proximal diversion at the time of ileal pouch-anal anastomosis for ulcerative colitis: current practices of north American colorectal surgeons. Dis Colon Rectum. 2009;52:1178–83.
59. Gu J, Stocchi L, Remzi FH, Kiran RP. Total abdominal colectomy for severe ulcerative colitis: does the laparoscopic approach really have benefit? Surg Endosc. 2014;28:617–25.

Which Patients with Ulcerative Colitis Benefit from Ileal Pouch-Anal Anastomosis?

5

Rodrigo Areán-Sanz and Evangelos Messaris

Given the long-term bowel function and patient satisfaction rates, proctocolectomy with ileal pouch-anal anastomosis (IPAA) is considered the standard procedure for the surgical treatment of ulcerative colitis (UC), with 10-20% of patients undergoing IPAA due to failure of medical treatment or dysplasia. [1–3] However, short- and long-term complications (e.g. pouchitis, pouch failure, increased stool frequency, anal stenosis, and incontinence) are reported in up to 50% of patients [4–6], making it essential to determine which patients are at higher risk and could benefit from an alternative, non-restorative procedure (i.e. proctocolectomy with end ileostomy). The most vulnerable groups are patients with obesity and those with increased risk of incontinence, mainly elderly patients and individuals with a history of sphincter abnormalities [7].

PICO Table:

Population:	Intervention:	Comparator:	Outcome:
Patients with ulcerative colitis treated with total proctocolectomy and ileal pouch-anal anastomosis	Ileal pouch-anal anastomosis	Patients with ulcerative colitis treated with total proctocolectomy and end ileostomy	Mortality, complications, quality of life, costs.

R. Areán-Sanz (✉) · E. Messaris
Division of Colon and Rectal Surgery, Department of Surgery, Beth Israel Deaconess Medical Center, Harvard Medical School, Boston, MA, USA
e-mail: rareansa@bidmc.harvard.edu; emessari@bidmc.harvard.edu

K. Umanskiy, N. Hyman (eds.), *Difficult Decisions in Colorectal Surgery*, Difficult Decisions in Surgery: An Evidence-Based Approach,
https://doi.org/10.1007/978-3-031-42303-1_5

Search Strategy

Referenced publications were identified through a comprehensive search of Pubmed, Medline, and Cochrane using the following search terms: "ulcerative colitis", "restorative surgery", "ileal pouch-anal anastomosis", "ileostomy", "pouch", and "proctocolectomy". Articles published from 1985 to 2022 were reviewed for the present book chapter. Studies comparing IPAA to ileostomy for UC as well as publications on factors associated with poor short- and long-term outcomes were synthesized and compared. Papers that analyzed patients diagnosed with Crohn's disease or any other colorectal condition were only included if a subgroup analysis of patients diagnosed with UC was performed. Additional studies deemed relevant for inclusion in this chapter were identified via review of the included publications' references.

Results

IPAA has been the preferred procedure for surgical management of UC for many years as it allows for restoration of gastrointestinal continuity with outcomes that are comparable or superior to total proctocolectomy with end ileostomy. As a result, there have not been many recent studies that directly compare the outcomes of IPAA versus those with end ileostomy in terms of morbidity and quality of life. (Table 5.1).

Most studies that have used validated quality of life scales have found that there are no major differences between IPAA and total proctocolectomy with end ileostomy in terms of patient quality of life. [8–16] However, a study by Emblem et al. [8] found that patients who underwent ileostomy for UC had higher rates of urinary and sexual dysfunction, whereas patients who underwent IPAA used antidiarrheal agents more frequently. O'Birchere et al. [11] found that diet changes and altered bowel habits were the only outcomes that were superior for ileostomy patients. On the other hand, social functioning and emotional functioning, as measured by the SF-36 and IBDQ questionnaires respectively, were significantly better in patients who underwent IPAA [12].

Similarly, Kuruvilla et al. [14] conducted a cross-sectional study comparing 35 IPAA patients and 24 ileostomy patients, and found no significant difference in disease-specific and health-related quality of life at 1 year, as measured by five validated scores: EQ-5D-3L, Short Quality of Life in Inflammatory Bowel Disease Questionnaire, Cleveland Global Quality of Life, Fecal Incontinence Quality of Life Scale, and Stoma Quality of Life Scale.

In line with the superior quality of life reported for restorative procedures, medical care costs that take surgical and long-term management into account are higher for patients who undergo ileostomy. A study by Van der Valk et al. [15] compared care costs and quality of life between the two surgical options during a follow-up of 2 years and found that ileostomy patients needed to visit a specialized nurse and surgeon more frequently and required more hospitalizations than IPAA patients.

Table 5.1 Included publications and main findings

Study	No. of patients (IPAA v Ileostomy)	Outcome evaluated	Results	Quality of evidence
Emblem et al. (1988) [8]	14 v 22	Dietary restrictions Use of antidiarrheal Urinary dysfunction Sexual dysfunction	No difference 79% v 9% ($p < 0.01$) 0% v 32% ($p < 0.05$) 0% v 36% ($p < 0.05$)	Low
McLeod et al. (1991) [9]	37 v 28	TTOT DQO	No difference No difference	Moderate
Liddell et al. (1995) [10]	25 v 10	Overall satisfaction (subdivided by specific activity satisfaction)	No difference	Low
O'Birchere (2000) [11]	30 v 30	SF-36 Body image (VAS) Altered bowel emptying (VAS) Odor (VAS) Noise (VAS) Sexual relationship Clothes Diet	No difference No difference 8.0 vs 5.0 No difference No difference No difference No difference 5.5 vs 2.0	Moderate
Nordin et al. (2002) [12]	57 v 42	SF-36 – Social functioning – Rest of components IBDQ – Emotional functioning – Rest of components	70.2 v 89.3 ($p < 0.05$) No difference 64.8 v 72.2 ($p < 0.01$) No difference	Moderate
Camilleri-Brennan et al. (2003) [13]	19 v 19	IBDQ SF-36	No difference No difference	High
Kuruvilla et al. (2012) [14]	35 v 24	EQ-5D-3L SIBDQ scores CGQL score (Fazio score) FIQL scale SQOL scale	No difference No difference 0.9 v 0.8 ($p < 0.05$) No difference IPAA > Ileostomy[a]	Moderate
van der Valk et al. (2015) [15]	81 v 48	Costs IBDQ	3-fold higher costs for ileostomy No difference	Moderate
Hassab et al. (2022) [16]	95 v 297	30-day readmission Other 30-day complications	29.5 v 16.8 ($p < 0.05$) No difference	Moderate

SIBDQ Short Quality of Life in Inflammatory Bowel Disease Questionnaire, *CGQL* Cleveland Global Quality of Life, *FIQL* Fecal Incontinence Quality of Life Scale, *SQOL* Stoma Quality of Life Scale, *TTOT* Time Trade-Off Technique, *DQO* Direct Questioning of Objections, *SF36* Short-Form 36, *VAS* Visual analogue scale, *IBDQ* Inflammatory Bowel Disease Questionnaire

[a] IPAA was superior than ileostomy in: sexuality/body, work/social function, and skin irritation

However, ileostomy patients reported needing less medication. Despite this, healthcare costs were three times higher for ileostomy patients than for IPAA patients. In terms of quality of life, the study found no difference when using the overall IBDQ score, but bowel symptoms-related IBDQ subscores were lower in IPAA patients. Median QALY was higher for IPAA patients, as ileostomy patients reported more frequent mobility-related problems.

According to a study by Hassab et al. [16] using data from the American College of Surgeons National Surgical Quality Improvement Program (ACS-NSQIP), restorative procedures were found to have a higher rate of readmissions compared to non-restorative procedures. However, the study found that there were no significant differences in other 30-day complications, including mortality rates, between the two groups.

Recommendations

Most patients diagnosed with ulcerative colitis who have failed medical therapy should be offered total proctocolectomy with ileal pouch-anal anastomosis with the aim of maintaining gastrointestinal tract continuity, taking into account the comparable rate of postoperative complications, similar quality of life parameters, and potential lower care costs.

However, certain groups of patients such as the elderly, patients with obesity, patients with multiple comorbidities, patients with a diagnosis of indeterminate colitis or Crohn's disease, and those with previous bowel or sphincter dysfunction may not be suitable candidates for IPAA surgery due to an increased risk of complications and poorer quality of life outcomes. For these patients, a total proctocolectomy with end ileostomy is an alternative that has similar surgical and quality of life outcomes. In patients in which IPAA surgery is contraindicated and an end-ileostomy is either refused or contraindicated, an ileo-rectal anastomosis (IRA) is an alternative procedure.

It's important to note that, despite a potentially higher incidence of surgical complications and inferior quality of life outcomes than primary pouch creation, a revisional procedure, or re-do IPAA, can still benefit patients who failed primary IPAA surgery.

Personal View

Total proctocolectomy with IPAA should be the procedure of choice in most cases; however, it's vital to keep complications and populations at risk in mind when selecting candidates for this procedure. Multiple studies have been published that evaluate the predictive factors for short- and long-term complications, poor quality of life measures, and mortality for patients with UC who underwent IPAA as curative treatment.

In a retrospective review of 116 patients followed for 10 years, the authors reported a 30-day complication rate of 16.4%. Fifty-seven percent of patients presented late adverse events —chronic pouchitis being the most frequent (23.3%), followed by intestinal obstruction (17.2%) and perianal fistula (13%)—. The study also evaluated functional outcomes using the Öresland scale and the Cleveland Global Quality of Life Scale. The results indicate that 75% of the study cohort reported that their social life was not compromised by the procedure and 92.7% of patients were satisfied with the results and would recommend the procedure to other patients who might benefit from it [17].

Male sex, older age, higher body-mass index, and extraintestinal manifestations have been associated with failure of IPAA. (1,7) Moreover, the use of steroids before colectomy may be a risk factor for anastomotic leak, fistula formation, and pouch failure [6].

Using the IBD-disability index, Kayal et al. [2] reported that 37.2% of patients who underwent an IPAA creation for UC had moderate to severe disability. Certain aspects, such as overall health, sleep, energy, regulating defecation, and pain were found to be particularly affected when compared to patients receiving medical treatment alone. The study also found that certain patient groups were more likely to experience higher levels of disability, such as women, patients with active symptoms, and those with public insurance.

Patients with Obesity

Up to 32% of patients diagnosed with UC have a BMI > 30 and this population has been traditionally considered at high risk for complications and failure of IPAA. Although there is no consensus on whether functional outcomes such as incontinence, frequency of bowel movement, pad usage, and pouchitis are significantly different between patients with obesity and patients without, studies have found that the former are more likely to undergo open IPAA surgery and have longer operative times, greater rates of complications (mainly surgical site and urinary tract infections), as well as more blood transfusion requirements and longer length of stay [18]. Furthermore, studies using the ACS-NSQIP database of patients who underwent IPAA for UC have found that obesity is an independent factor associated with higher rates of organ space sepsis and readmission for infectious complications [19, 20]. Similar findings were reported by Abd el Aziz et al. [21] which also found higher rates of postoperative organ space infections in patients with obesity. In contrast, all the other complications included in their multivariate analysis showed no difference when compared with patients with a BMI < 30. The poor surgical outcomes in this population are mainly due to intraoperative technical difficulties such as a short mesentery length (due to adiposity or inflammation, regarded as the most common direct cause), as well as a limited working space in a narrow pelvis, which can sometimes lead to deferring the surgery until after the patient has lost excess weight [1, 21].

More recently, a retrospective multivariable analysis of 2202 patients found that patients with obesity had longer surgical times, lower pouch survival and, most importantly, they found that obesity was the strongest independent predictor of pouch failure (HR 4.24). Global quality-of-life scores were also lower than in patients without. The authors did not, however, find an independent association between obesity and postoperative complications (defined as a composite outcome of any complication), in-hospital length of stay or anastomotic leak. [22]

Taking the aforementioned reports into account, patients with a BMI < 30 should be offered IPAA surgery, whereas caution should be taken when deciding whether or not this procedure is recommended for patients with a BMI between 30 and 35. For patients with a BMI over 35, other than carefully selected exceptions, pouch surgery should not be offered given the higher risk of complications and negative quality of life impact. On the other hand, weight loss management can convert these high-risk patients to low-risk when BMI becomes <30 or < 35 in some cases.

Elderly Patients

There is still no consensus in terms of an age cut-off at which IPAA should not be recommended, given that there are multiple factors associated with complications and/or failure, and age alone does not seem to impact as much as previously thought. Nonetheless, there still seems to be a tendency to recommend end ileostomy procedure to elderly patients. When comparing rates of procedure choice (IPAA vs ileostomy), Cohan et al. [23] found that older age patients received ileostomy more often than IPAA, given the notion that the risks of the latter are higher; however, more elderly patients have been undergoing IPAA over time.

In 2016, Bollegala et al. [24] published a comparative analysis of postoperative outcomes in patients diagnosed with IBD and found that 30-day mortality among elderly patients was almost 10 times higher than in non-elderly patients (5.3% vs 0.5%); in-hospital mortality was also found to be significantly higher for this group of patients (3.3% vs 0.4%). The authors reported higher rates of postoperative complications in elderly IBD patients. Emergent surgery in elderly patients diagnosed UC presented five-fold risk mortality rates in comparison to the non-elderly group. Still, this study's findings are limited given a lack of information regarding disease severity and previous medical treatments; moreover, as mentioned by Piper et al. [25], it is unclear whether the findings of Bollegala et al's study correspond to specific risks posed by the surgical treatment of IBD, or if they are those inherent to abdominal surgical procedure in the elderly population. This study's results are not consistent with previous and more recent reports. For instance, Cohan et al. [26] published an ACS-NSQIP analysis comparing patients aged 50 or younger against patients aged 51–60 and > 60, as well as based on frailty trait count. They found no significant differences in terms of complication rate other than a 0.8-day longer length-of-stay at the hospital for the >60 group, which, although statistically significant, is not clinically relevant. Frailty trait count showed no association with either complication rates or length of stay.

More recently, Lightner et al. [27] published an analysis of 1875 patients with a median follow-up of 16.1 years after IPAA. For patients aged 65 or older who had undergone IPAA surgery, 47% reported complete lack of incontinence, 36% presented occasional incontinence, and only 17% reported frequent incontinence throughout the day. At night, rates of no, occasional, and frequent incontinence episodes were 25%, 43%, and 33%, respectively.

When it comes to differences among elderly subgroups, Minagawa et al. [28] compared functional outcomes in patients aged 65–69 vs aged 70 and older and found no significant difference regarding stool frequency, and daytime/nighttime soiling.

Age should not be the sole factor in determining whether a patient is suitable for ileal pouch-anal anastomosis (IPAA) surgery, as multiple studies and a systematic review published in 2021 have found. The review, conducted by Pedersen in 2021 [29], analyzed 13 studies and found no statistically significant difference between elderly (65 and older) and non-elderly patients in terms of short-term and long-term complications after IPAA surgery. Instead, other factors such as comorbidities, functional status, pre-operative bowel function, and patient preference should be considered when making the decision to proceed with IPAA surgery.

Sphincter Abnormalities

The restorative nature of IPAA surgery poses the benefit of preserving sphincter function; still, up to 30% of patients report some degree of fecal incontinence. Certain patient populations, such as the elderly and those with a history of obstetric complications, may be at higher risk for continence issues following the surgery. This is likely due to potential preoperative sphincter abnormalities in these groups [7]. A retrospective study that included patients who had had pouch surgery for over 30 years found that patients older than 80 years of age did not have higher rates of fecal incontinence but did report increased episodes of seepage and more frequent use of pads during both day and night [30].

An anorectal manometry is not always required, but a digital rectal examination should be performed to evaluate sphincter tone before determining suitability for an IPAA procedure. Patients with preoperative altered sphincter tone may be better suited for a non-restorative procedure; however, this decision should be made after a thorough discussion of postoperative expectations with the patient [7]. If a permanent stoma is not accepted by the patient, an IRA is a viable option in this group of patients.

Primary Sclerosing Cholangitis

The outcomes of IPAA for patients with both ulcerative colitis (UC) and primary sclerosing cholangitis (PSC) are not well understood. While these patients may have a higher rate of pouch dysfunction and pouchitis, there does not appear to be a significant difference in surgical complications when compared to other groups. However, a study by Pavlides et al. [31] found that patients with UC and PSC reported significantly higher rates of nighttime bowel movements. On the other hand, a large cohort study comparing restorative procedures for patients with UC and PSC found no statistically significant difference in terms of pouch failure, with failure rates of 4%, 11%, and 18% at 1, 3, and 5 years, respectively [32]. Patients with UC and PSC should be treated as patients with UC and without PSC.

Patients with Indeterminate Colitis or Crohn's Disease

Patients who underwent pouch surgery can develop postoperative inflammation of the pouch with features similar to Crohn's disease (CD), a complication controversially referred to as "CD of the pouch" [33, 34]. However, it is important to distinguish between actual CD of the pouch (i.e., a patient with preoperative diagnosis of CD or a patient with a preoperative diagnosis of UC or indeterminate colitis (IC) whose colectomy specimen was diagnosed as CD) versus a pouch with CD-like features. Suggestive features for the former include pre-pouch ileitis; development of fistulas and abscesses 6–12 months after ileostomy takedown; strictures, segmental or skip lesions affecting the pouch or small intestine; and non-caseating granulomas in the pouch or cuff [34, 35]. Postoperative (*de novo*) CD has been reported in up to 15.9% of patients who undergo IPAA for UC, and their outcomes differ from those patients where CD diagnosis was already established [36, 37].

Patients with a preoperative diagnosis of CD who undergo pouch creation have a risk of complications such as fistulas, strictures, and abscesses, and end-ileostomy is the preferred procedure in most cases where colectomy is needed. However, certain patients may benefit from IPAA surgery, mainly those without perianal or small bowel involvement (occurring in up to 20% of cases) [35, 38]. Information on patients preoperatively diagnosed with CD who have undergone IPAA is limited and most studies report results of patients with original diagnosis of UC or indeterminate colitis (IC) [36]. The risk of pouch failure is higher in patients with CD and has been reported in up to 15% of patients, a rate significantly higher than that of patients with UC. Due to this, some experts prefer IRA over IPAA in patients with indeterminate colitis without rectal involvement to avoid the potential pouch failure if the patient is postoperatively diagnosed with CD. However, other complications and long-term functional outcomes appear to be similar to those reported for patients with UC [37]. Therefore, patients with a preoperative CD diagnosis with no perianal or small bowel disease who undergo IPAA should be closely monitored for adverse events and complications. Specifically, for patients with CD in which the pouch did not fail, complication rates and functional outcomes are comparable to those in patients with UC [38]. Biologic medications can be used to maintain the disease in remission and increase IPAA retention.

Re-doing IPAA after a failed primary restorative procedure in patients with preoperative CD may be a viable option for specific patients given acceptable quality of life outcomes, although complication rates are higher for this group compared to re-doing IPAA in patients with UC [39].

Patients of Childbearing Age

There have been reports of higher infertility rates after IPAA surgery in patients of childbearing age, although the evidence behind this has been inconclusive. Some surgeons offer these patients an IRA as an alternative to IPAA with the same purpose of restoring the GI tract while lowering the risk of postoperative infertility [40]. However, the proposed advantage in fertility supporting IRA is debatable, with some studies showing no difference between the two procedures. For instance, a recent large observational study compared the impact of IPAA and IRA in pregnancy rates, and also compared them with a control group of people who had undergone appendectomy. After adjusted analysis, they found that both procedures for UC increased the rate of infertility versus the control population, yet reported no difference between IPAA and IRA [41]. It's important to note that any restorative procedure for UC can decrease fertility. Patients may choose to delay restoration with IPAA or IRA until after they no longer wish to have more children.

Redo IPAA

There is limited information available on the effectiveness of re-doing an IPAA procedure for patients who have previously failed primary IPAA surgery. The main indication for this is patients with failed IPAA with a significant aversion to living with a permanent stoma. Moreover, if re-do IPAA surgery is unsuccessful, another attempt at a restorative procedure may be considered. The long-term outcomes in patients who have undergone an IPAA revision after failed re-do IPAA appear to be similar to re-do IPAA procedures in terms of pouch survival rate and patient quality of life, making revision after a failed re-do IPAA a safe and viable option for this patient population [42]. It's worth noting that pouch excision after a failed IPAA creation is also linked with increased morbidity and reduced quality of life. [43] For selected patients, re-do of the IPAA is the best option in order to preserve the gastrointestinal continuity.

Conclusion

In conclusion, total proctocolectomy with ileal pouch-anal anastomosis offers comparable postoperative complications, quality of life, and potentially lower care cost to patients in need of surgery for ulcerative colitis as measured against total proctocolectomy and end ileostomy and should be offered to most patients with an indication for surgical treatment of ulcerative colitis. The decision-making process should take into account several patient characteristics which could affect the surgical morbidity and overall quality of life of patients undergoing restorative proctocolectomy.

References

1. Frese JP, Gröne J, Lauscher JC, Konietschke F, Kreis ME, Seifarth C. Risk factors for failure of ileal pouch-anal anastomosis in patients with refractory ulcerative colitis. Surgery. 2022;171:299–304.
2. Kayal M, Ungaro RC, Riggs A, Kamal K, Agrawal M, Cohen-Mekelburg S, et al. Ileal pouch anal anastomosis for the management of ulcerative colitis is associated with significant disability. Clin Gastroenterol Hepatol. 2022;20:e761–9.
3. Holubar SD, Lightner AL, Poylin V, Vogel JD, Gaertner W, Davis B, et al. The American Society of Colon and rectal surgeons clinical practice guidelines for the surgical management of ulcerative colitis. Dis Colon Rectum. 2021;64:783–804.
4. Lee GC, Deery SE, Kunitake H, Hicks CW, Olariu AG, Savitt LR, et al. Comparable perioperative outcomes, long-term outcomes, and quality of life in a retrospective analysis of ulcerative colitis patients following 2-stage versus 3-stage proctocolectomy with ileal pouch-anal anastomosis. Int J Color Dis. 2019;34:491–9.
5. Baker DM, Folan AM, Lee MJ, Jones GL, Brown SR, Lobo AJ. A systematic review and meta-analysis of outcomes after elective surgery for ulcerative colitis. Color Dis. 2020;23:18–33.
6. Lim MH, Lord AR, Simms LA, Hanigan K, Edmundson A, Rickard MJFX, et al. Ileal pouch-anal anastomosis for ulcerative colitis: an Australian institution's experience. Ann Coloproctol. 2021;37:318–25.
7. Chang S, Shen B, Remzi F. When not to pouch: important considerations for patient selection for ileal pouch-anal anastomosis. Gastroenterol Hepatol (N Y). 2017;13(8):466–75. PMID: 28867978; PMCID: PMC5572960
8. Emblem R, Larsen S, Torvet SH, Bergan A. Operative treatment of ulcerative colitis: conventional proctectomy with Brooke ileostomy versus mucosal proctectomy with ileoanal anastomosis. Scand J Gastroenterol. 1988;23:493–500.
9. McLeod RS, Churchill DN, Lock AM, Vanderburgh S, Cohen Z. Quality of life of patients with ulcerative colitis preoperatively and postoperatively. Gastroenterology. 1991;101:1307–13.
10. Liddell A, Pollett WG, MacKenzie DS. Comparison of postoperative satisfaction between ulcerative colitis patients who chose to undergo either a pouch or an ileostomy operation. Int J Rehabil Heal. 1995;1:89–96.
11. O'Bichere A, Wilkinson K, Rumbles S, Norton C, Green C, Phillips RK. Functional outcome after restorative panproctocolectomy for ulcerative colitis decreases an otherwise enhanced quality of life. Br J Surg. 2000;87:802–7.
12. Nordin K, Påhlman L, Larsson K, Sundberg-Hjelm M, Lööf L. Health-related quality of life and psychological distress in a population-based sample of Swedish patients with inflammatory bowel disease. Scand J Gastroenterol. 2002;37:450–7.
13. Camilleri-Brennan J, Munro A, Steele RJ. Does an ileoanal pouch offer a better quality of life than a permanent ileostomy for patients with ulcerative colitis? J Gastrointest Surg. 2003;7:814–9.
14. Kuruvilla K, Osler T, Hyman NH. A comparison of the quality of life of ulcerative colitis patients after IPAA VS ileostomy. Dis Colon Rectum. 2012;55:1131–7.
15. van der Valk ME, Mangen M-JJ, Severs M, van der Have M, Dijkstra G, van Bodegraven AA, et al. Comparison of costs and quality of life in ulcerative colitis patients with an ileal pouch-anal anastomosis, ileostomy and anti-TNFα therapy. J Crohn's Colitis. 2015;9:1016–23.
16. Hassab T, McKinney D, D'Adamo CD, Svoboda S, Katlic M, Wolf JH. Short-term outcomes for restorative and non-restorative proctocolectomy in older adults. J Surg Res. 2022;269:11–7.
17. Carcamo L, Miranda P, Zuniga A, Alexander E, Molina ME, Urrejola G, et al. Ileal pouch-anal anastomosis in ulcerative colitis: outcomes, functional results, and quality of life in patients with more than 10-year follow-up. Int J Color Dis. 2020;35:747–53.
18. McKenna NP, Mathis KL, Khasawneh MA, Dozois EJ, Larson DW, Pemberton JH, et al. Obese patients undergoing ileal pouch-anal anastomosis. Inflamm Bowel Dis. 2017;23:2142–6.
19. McKenna NP, Glasgow AE, Cima RR, Habermann EB. Risk factors for organ space infection after ileal pouch anal anastomosis for chronic ulcerative colitis: an ACS nsqip analysis. Am J Surg. 2018;216:900–5.

20. McKenna NP, Habermann EB, Glasgow AE, Mathis KL, Lightner AL. Risk factors for readmission following ileal pouch-anal anastomosis: an American College of Surgeons National Surgical Quality Improvement Program analysis. J Surg Res. 2018;229:324–31.
21. Abd El Aziz MA, Calini G, Grass F, Behm KT, D'Angelo A-L, Shawki S, et al. Minimally invasive ileal pouch-anal anastomosis for patients with obesity: a propensity score-matched analysis. Langenbeck's Arch Surg. 2021;406:2419–24.
22. Leeds IL, Holubar SD, Hull TL, Lipman JM, Lightner AL, Sklow B, et al. Short- and long-term outcomes of ileal pouch anal anastomosis construction in obese patients with ulcerative colitis. Dis Colon Rectum. 2022;65:e782–9.
23. Cohan JN, Bacchetti P, Varma MG, Finlayson E. Impact of patient age on procedure type for ulcerative colitis. Dis Colon Rectum. 2015;58:769–74.
24. Bollegala N, Jackson TD, Nguyen GC. Increased postoperative mortality and complications among elderly patients with inflammatory bowel diseases: an analysis of the National Surgical Quality Improvement Program cohort. Clin Gastroenterol Hepatol. 2016;14:1274–81.
25. Piper MS, Waljee AK, Stidham RW. Operate or medicate: understanding surgical risks in the elderly with inflammatory bowel disease. Gastroenterology. 2016;151:1029–30.
26. Cohan JN, Bacchetti P, Varma MG, Finlayson E. Outcomes after ileoanal pouch surgery in frail and older adults. J Surg Res. 2015;198:327–33.
27. Lightner AL, Mathis KL, Dozois EJ, Hahnsloser D, Loftus EV, Raffals LE, et al. Results at up to 30 years after ileal pouch-anal anastomosis for chronic ulcerative colitis. Inflamm Bowel Dis. 2017;23:781–90.
28. Minagawa T, Ikeuchi H, Kuwahara R, Horio Y, Sasaki H, Chohno T, et al. Functional outcomes and quality of life in elderly patients after restorative proctocolectomy for ulcerative colitis. Digestion. 2019;101:737–42.
29. Pedersen KE, Jia X, Holubar SD, Steele SR, Lightner AL. Ileal pouch-anal anastomosis in the elderly: a systematic review and meta. Äêanalysis Color Dis. 2021;23:2062–74.
30. Lightner AL, Steele SR, McMichael JP, Jia X, Qazi T, Click BH, et al. Pouch function over time and with advancing age. Dis Colon Rectum. 2022;65:254–63.
31. Pavlides M, Cleland J, Rahman M, Christian A, Doyle J, Gaunt R, et al. Outcomes after ileal pouch anal anastomosis in patients with primary sclerosing cholangitis. J Crohn's Colitis. 2014;8:662–70.
32. Nordenvall C, Olén O, Johan Nilsson P, Ekbom A, Bottai M, Myrelid P, et al. Restorative surgery in patients with primary sclerosing cholangitis and ulcerative colitis following a colectomy. Inflamm Bowel Dis. 2018;24:624–32.
33. Shehab M, Alrashed F, Charabaty A, Bessissow T. Biologic therapies for the treatment of post-ileal pouch anal anastomosis surgery chronic inflammatory disorders: systematic review and meta-analysis. J Can Assoc Gastroenterol. 2022;5:287–96.
34. Akiyama S, Dyer EC, Rubin DT. Diagnostic and management considerations for the IPAA with Crohn's disease-like features. Dis Colon Rectum. 2022;65:S77–84. https://doi.org/10.1097/dcr.0000000000002547.
35. Shaffer SR, Bernstein CN. Controversies in Crohn's disease before and after pouch surgery. Dis Colon Rectum. 2022;65:S45–9. https://doi.org/10.1097/dcr.0000000000002550.
36. Lopez NE, Zaghyian K, Fleshner P. Is there a role for ileal pouch anal anastomosis in Crohn's disease? Clin Colon Rectal Surg. 2019;32:280–90.
37. Lightner AL, Jia X, Zaghiyan K, Fleshner PR. IPAA in known preoperative Crohn's disease: a systematic review. Dis Colon Rectum. 2020;64:355–64.
38. Connelly TM, Lincango E, Holubar SD. Crohn's of the pouch: now what? Clin Colon Rectal Surg. 2022;35:475–86.
39. Lavryk OA, Stocchi L, Shawki S, Aiello A, Church JM, Steele SR, Hull TL. Redo IPAA after a failed pouch in patients with crohn's disease: is it worth trying? Dis Colon Rectum. 2020;63:823–30.
40. Faye AS, Oh A, Kumble LD, Kiran RP, Wen T, Lawlor G, Lichtiger S, Abreu MT, Hur C. Fertility impact of initial operation type for female ulcerative colitis patients. Inflamm Bowel Dis. 2019;26:1368–76.

41. Challine A, Voron T, O'Connell L, Chafai N, Debove C, Collard M, Parc Y, Lefèvre JH. Does an ILEO-anal anastomosis decrease the rate of successful pregnancy compared to an ileorectal anastomosis? A national study of 1,491 patients. Ann Surg. 2022;277:806–12. https://doi.org/10.1097/sla.0000000000005569.
42. Esen E, Lynn PB, Da luz Moreira A, Erkan A, Aytac E, Grieco MJ, et al. Operative, long-term and quality of life outcomes after salvage of failed re-do ileal pouch anal anastomosis. Color Dis. 2022;24:790–2.
43. Carpenter H, Hotouras A, English WJ, Taylor FG, Andreani S. Revisional ileoanal pouch surgery: a systematic literature review assessing outcomes over the last 40 years. Color Dis. 2021;23:52–63.

Persistent Posterior Sinus After Ileal Pouch-Anal Anastomosis

6

Kathryn E. Chuquin and Brian L. Bello

Introduction

Ileal pouch-anal anastomosis (IPAA) is the preferred reconstructive option to maintain continence after proctocolectomy for inflammatory bowel disease or familial adenomatous polyposis syndrome. IPAA has many documented complications, one of which is formation of a posterior sinus tract. This is a blind-ending tract usually in the presacral space originating from the pouch-anal anastomosis that most frequently forms as a sequela of a contained anastomotic leak. Incidence of posterior sinus after IPAA has been reported to range from 2–8% [1–3], with persisting sinus a significant predictor of pouch failure [2]. Pouch sinus is routinely diagnosed when performing a Gastrografin enema (or pouchoscopy) prior to consideration of diverting loop ileostomy closure. Management of a posterior sinus can be difficult and ranges from observation to pouch excision depending on the size and complexity of the sinus, patient symptoms, and surgeon expertise.

Search Strategy

A comprehensive search of PubMed, EMBASE, MEDLINE and Cochrane Database was performed to include the last 25 years (1997–2022). Results were limited to English language and peer-reviewed publications. Additional studies were identified using the references sections from the initially identified papers. Search terms

K. E. Chuquin
Washington, DC, USA

B. L. Bello (✉)
Medstar Medical Center, Washington, DC, USA
e-mail: brian.l.bello@medstar.net

K. Umanskiy, N. Hyman (eds.), *Difficult Decisions in Colorectal Surgery*, Difficult Decisions in Surgery: An Evidence-Based Approach,
https://doi.org/10.1007/978-3-031-42303-1_6

included “ileal pouch-anal anastomosis”, “ileal pouch”, “IPAA”, “anastomotic leak” and “sinus”.

PICO table

Patient population	Intervention	Comparator	Outcome
Patients with ileal pouch-anal anastomosis who developed a posterior sinus	Observation	Operative intervention	Sinus tract healing, pouch retention

Results

Overall, there is no high-quality literature on pouch sinus management, and the studies that exist are small and observational or descriptive in nature. Most of the literature focuses on the treatment of asymptomatic sinus tracts. Reported treatment methods include watchful observation, sinus tract debridement, tract unroofing, fibrin glue, and revising or creating a new pouch. Many patients need more than one treatment to achieve healing. Ultimately, if these methods fail, this may lead to the need for pouch excision or permanent fecal diversion. Although there is literature reporting the success rates of various interventions, little exists in the way of guidance on choosing one particular intervention over another.

Delay Ostomy Closure/Watchful Observation

Delay of ostomy closure and observation alone have been shown to have a reasonable healing rate, particularly in the setting of an asymptomatic sinus. If a contained sinus is detected on pouchogram, observation is usually recommended as the initial strategy. In the series reported by Ahmed Ali [2], observation alone with delay of ostomy closure was successful in achieving sinus healing in 65% of patients, although this was higher in asymptomatic sinus (79%) versus symptomatic sinus (44%). Slightly lower rates of sinus healing were reported by Akbari [4] who found that 52.6% of patients treated with delay in ostomy closure and observation alone ultimately achieved sinus healing without the need for further procedures.

When considering ileostomy reversal and pouch retention, Nyam et al [5] reported a series of 41 patients with pouch sinuses who were observed for 3- to 6-month periods before repeat pouchogram. All 41 patients eventually had their ileostomy reversed, although 2 patients required repeat diversion for recurrent sinus prior to ultimately having their second ileostomy closed. Of the 41 patients in this series, only one patient ultimately had pouch failure requiring pouch excision.

Debridement

After watchful observation, approximately 62% of patients require additional treatment [2]. Exam under anesthesia with irrigation and debridement can be done safely with mechanical debridement usually with curettage. The success of tract debridement is reported by Akbari [4]. Of 6 patients who underwent EUA with tract debridement, 4 patients subsequently underwent successful ileostomy closure. Debridement may also be used in conjunction with other interventions at the time of operative intervention including during the use of fibrin glue[6] and during tract unroofing [7].

Fibrin Glue

Swain and Ellis [6] published a series of 7 patients with persistent low pelvic anastomotic sinuses including both patients with IPAA and patients with low colorectal anastomosis done for rectal cancer. All patients were asymptomatic. After mechanical debridement of the sinus, fibrin glue was injected to obliterate the sinus tract. At 11 months, 100% of the patients had achieved complete healing of the sinus.

The series reported by Ahmed Ali [2] included 3 patients treated with fibrin glue, although use of glue was employed only as the second or third intervention. Of these 3 patients, 2 achieved sinus healing. No comment is made on which patients ultimately received treatment with fibrin glue and whether or not they were symptomatic.

Unroofing

Unroofing of a sinus involves dividing the common wall of the sinus and adjacent pouch. Sinus tract unroofing has success rates varying from 50% to 100% [7–10], with multiple techniques for sinus tract unroofing have been described.

Whitlow [7] reported outcomes of a cohort of 6 patients with sinuses including both patients with IPAA and with low colorectal anastomosis. In all patients, the sinus tract was unroofed using laparoscopic scissors to divide the septum between the sinus and the bowel. All six patients achieved sinus tract healing at 1 year, with 5 of those patients achieving healing at 1 month.

Use of a laparoscopic stapler to divide the septum between the bowel and the sinus tract has also been described. Although not specific to IPAA, Alsanea & Alabbad [8] report 100% healing of sinus tract using this method in 4 patients with sinus after low colorectal anastomosis.

Treatment using endoscopic sinusotomy has also been described by Lan [9] in a series that included 109 patients with IPAA sinus tracts. This is performed using an endoscopic needle knife to divide the septum before placing endoscopic clips along the edges of the opened sinus to marsupialize the sinus. Additionally, the sinus tract is treated with topical doxycycline +/−50% dextrose to encourage fibrosis. Using this technique, complete healing was achieved in 49.5% of these patients, and partial healing was reported in 18.3%. The majority of patients did require more than 1 treatment, and sinus recurrence was found in 15% of patients treated with endoscopic sinusotomy alone.

Ileostomy Closure with Persistent Sinus

In some instances, ileostomy closure has been reported despite the presence of a persistent asymptomatic sinus. In the series published by Nyam [5], 6 patients ultimately had their ileostomies reversed despite a persistent sinus after a prolonged period of expectant management. All of these patients were asymptomatic, and at the time of ileostomy closure, the sinus tract was either stable in size or smaller than at the time of initial diagnosis. None of these 6 patients developed symptoms after ileostomy closure, and pouch function was not different than in patients who had demonstrated sinus healing prior to ileostomy closure.

Redo Pouch

In the absence of sinus healing after more conservative measures, pouch redo may offer a chance at pouch retention. In the series by Ahmed Ali [2], 3 patients were ultimately treated with pouch redo with 2 of 3 patients achieving sinus healing and the remaining patient eventually requiring pouch excision.

In a series by Lan [10] comparing endoscopic sinusotomy to redo pouch surgery, redo pouch had an initial healing rate of 94.1%, however, there was a 32.5% sinus recurrence rate. Of the patients that had a sinus recurrence, 73% went on to demonstrate complete healing after additional treatments for an overall healing rate in the redo pouch group of 85.9%. Although the healing rate was high in the redo pouch group, the authors point out that the rate of postoperative morbidity was high in the redo pouch group at 43.5%.

Study	Number of patients included	Intervention	Outcome	Success rate	Quality of evidence
Ali et al [2]	45	Observation, drainage, unroofing, Closure, Diversion	Sinus healing	60%	Low
Akbari et al [4]	22	Observation, Debridement	Ileostomy reversal	95.5%	Low
Alsanea & Alabbad [8]	4	Unroofing (stapler)	Sinus healing	100%	Low
Lan et al [10]	226	Unroofing (endoscopic), Redo pouch	Sinus healing	53.2%, 94.1%	Low
Lan & Shen [9]	109	Unroofing (endoscopic)	Sinus healing	49.5%	Low
Nyam et al [5]	41	Observation	Pouch retention	97.6%	Low
Swain et al [6]	7	Fibrin glue	Sinus healing	100%	Low

Study	Number of patients included	Intervention	Outcome	Success rate	Quality of evidence
Whitlow et al [7]	6	Sinus unroofing (scissors)	Sinus healing	100%	Low
Zhuo [3]	20	Observation, Debridement, Unroofing	Sinus healing, Ileostomy reversal	80%, 80%	Low

Recommendations

All reported evidence quality is low given that all data regarding pouch-sinus management comes from small observational studies. Given this, all recommendations based on that data are weak recommendations.

1. Management of pouch sinus should be individualized based on symptoms, presence of diverting ileostomy, and prior interventions.
2. Observation with delay of ileostomy reversal is an acceptable initial management of an asymptomatic pouch sinus.

Personal View of the Data

Anastomotic complications can lengthen the path to recovery after complex surgery. A pouch sinus from a contained leak demands a measured approach to avoid any future failures. Most of the literature regarding this topic is focused on the treatment of the asymptomatic sinus and is limited to observational studies and case series. Thus, the recommendations should be interpreted with caution. The initial approach should be watchful waiting and delaying three to six months for a repeat pouchogram since a significant amount of these tracts resolve or get smaller [2, 4, 5]. Debridement, fibrin glue, and unroofing can then be considered with not any single approach showing any distinct advantage. Decision on approach is individualized and based on sinus characteristics and surgeon expertise. If a persistent sinus is still present after initial treatment and remains asymptomatic despite the above strategy, ileostomy closure can be considered. A redo pouch can also be carefully considered depending on level of expertise as repeat pouch creation may be more problematic due to adhesions, inherent difficulty in operating in a redo pelvis, and dealing with possible reach issues. A redo pouch has good success, yet recurrent sinus is a possibility [10]. Pouch excision and redo also comes with a higher morbidity rate than the index procedure. Further comparative studies are needed to elucidate success rates of these different approaches. Unfortunately, up to 33% patients ultimately have pouch failure despite above treatments and require permanent diversion [2].

References

1. Kiely JM, Kiran RP. Leak, fistula, sepsis, sinus, portal vein thrombosis. Semin Colon Rectal Surg. 2019;30(1):7–9. https://doi.org/10.1053/j.scrs.2019.01.003.
2. Ali UA, Shen B, Remzi FH, Kiran RP. The management of anastomotic pouch sinus after IPAA. Dis Colon Rectum. 2012;55(5):541–8. https://doi.org/10.1097/dcr.0b013e318244087c.
3. Zhuo C, Trencheva K, Maggiori L, Milsom JW, Sonoda T, Shukla PJ, Vitellaro M, Makino T, Lee SW. Experience of a specialist centre in the management of Anastomotic sinus following leaks after low rectal or ileal pouch-anal anastomosis with diverting stoma. Color Dis. 2013;15(11):1429–35. https://doi.org/10.1111/codi.12436.
4. Akbari RP, Madoff RD, Parker SC, Hagerman G, Minami S, Bullard Dunn KM, Mellgren AF. Anastomotic sinuses after ileoanal pouch construction: incidence, management, and outcome. Dis Colon Rectum. 2009;52(3):452–5. https://doi.org/10.1007/dcr.0b013e31819a20e0.
5. Nyam D. Does the presence of a pre-ileostomy closure asymptomatic pouch-anastomotic sinus tract affect the success of ileal pouch-anal anastomosis? J Gastrointest Surg. 1997;1(3):274–7. https://doi.org/10.1016/s1091-255x(97)80120-5.
6. Swain BT, Ellis CN. Fibrin glue treatment of low rectal and pouch-anal anastomotic sinuses. Dis Colon Rectum. 2004;47(2):253–5. https://doi.org/10.1007/s10350-003-0040-7.
7. Whitlow CB, Opelka FG, Gathright BJ, Beck DE. Treatment of colorectal and ileoanal anastomotic sinuses. Dis Colon Rectum. 1997;40(7):760–3. https://doi.org/10.1007/bf02055427.
8. Alsanea N, Alabbad S. Use of the endostapler for the treatment of non-healing sinus secondary to a dehisced colorectal anastomosis. Tech Coloproctol. 2010;14(3):249–51. https://doi.org/10.1007/s10151-010-0600-5.
9. Lan N, Shen B. Endoscopic treatment of ileal pouch sinus. Inflamm Bowel Dis. 2018;24(7):1510–9. https://doi.org/10.1093/ibd/izy029.
10. Lan N, Hull TL, Shen B. Endoscopic sinusotomy versus redo surgery for the treatment of chronic pouch anastomotic sinus in ulcerative colitis patients. Gastrointest Endosc. 2019;89(1):144–56. https://doi.org/10.1016/j.gie.2018.08.004.

How to Manage Pouch-Perineal and Pouch-Vaginal Fistula After Ileal Pouch–Anal Anastomosis

7

Melinda E. Stack and Monika A. Krezalek

Introduction

Total proctocolectomy with ileoanal pouch anastomosis is the main surgical treatment for patients who require surgery with a history of ulcerative colitis or those with familial adenomatous polyposis [1–6]. While many patients who have undergone IPAA have a high quality of life, some patients will develop complications, such as pouch vaginal or perineal fistulae. While an uncommon problem with incidence rates ranging from 2.9–16.7% [7–19], PVF is a source of considerable morbidity for the patient and a technical challenge for the surgeon. Patients who develop a PVF face high pouch failure rates of 21–30% [7].

PVFs typically present in the first year after surgery; however, a late presentation might occur even after 10 years from surgery. Due to the relative paucity of published data, optimal management is still debated. However, most agree the management strategy needs to take into account factors related to the etiology of the fistula (surgical related, disease related, or sepsis related), as well as the location of the fistula in relation to the anastomosis. For example, it is important to note that a stapled anastomosis is going to be more cephalad, therefore making a pouch advancement flap to the dentate line a more viable remedial option when PVF complicates a stapled anastomosis. Conversely, following an index handsewn anastomosis, pouch advancement may not be a viable option. As for pouch type, Wexner et al. found no difference in the incidence of PVF for different pouch types [15].

M. E. Stack (✉)
Colon and Rectal Surgery Associates, Minneapolis, MN, USA

M. A. Krezalek
Department of Surgery, Division of Colon and Rectal Surgery, NorthShore University HealthSystem, Evanston, IL, USA
e-mail: mkrezalek@northshore.org

K. Umanskiy, N. Hyman (eds.), *Difficult Decisions in Colorectal Surgery*, Difficult Decisions in Surgery: An Evidence-Based Approach,
https://doi.org/10.1007/978-3-031-42303-1_7

Clearly, surgical technique and post operative sepsis are major contributors to the development of PVF, reemphasizing the need for appropriate technique at the index operation [18, 20–25]. As inflammation often plays a role in the pathogenesis of PVF, careful review of appropriate histopathologic materials by an expert gastrointestinal pathologist may be crucial to future management options. This step is especially true for the 2–3% of patients who undergo IPAA for UC only to find the long-term diagnosis is Crohn's disease (CD). Lee et al. [23] found a high correlation between PVF and CD, with 12 of the 23 women (52%) with a preoperative diagnosis of UC eventually diagnosed with CD. It is worth noting that the average time to development of a PVF is typically longer in patients with CD, and these patients suffer from a significantly higher rate of pouch failure and ultimately excision. Often biologics with TNF-alpha inhibitors may be considered in those patients with Crohn's disease [45]. In addition, patients who undergo IPAA for indeterminate colitis also have a high rate of pouch complications including PVF and pouch failure [26]. However, patients whose indication for surgery is familial adenomatous polyposis present with a significantly lower rate of PVF when compared to IBD patients [27, 28].

Patients with PVF may be asymptomatic or present with minor symptoms. They may also present with severe symptoms such as vaginal discharge of fecal material or gas, recurrent vaginitis, and vulvar irritation. Some cases of asymptomatic PVF are found on routine pouchography prior to ileostomy closure. Once PVF is suspected, further investigation is needed to confirm the diagnosis and establish its nature. This will also be important in helping to decide the next course of action. As noted above, the surgeon should request the pathology slides for expert pathology review. If not clinically evident, a perineogram and a water-soluble contrast pouchogram may help to diagnose the presence and the level of the fistula tract.

Imaging with computed tomography (CT) scan, ideally with contrast enema, may also help to identify fistulous tracts, although magnetic resonance imaging (MRI) T1 weighted with fat suppression and IV gadolinium is preferable. In expert hands, endoanal ultrasound is also helpful in detecting sphincter deformity, especially in women with a history of vaginal delivery. However, the reliability of endoanal ultrasound is poor for fistula detection because the fistulous tracts in PVF are short and wide.

Although clinical examination in the office will often confirm the diagnosis, careful examination under anesthesia (EUA) may be preferable. EUA allows access to the fistula and excludes associated sepsis while overcoming the potential limitations of patient discomfort. It also allows identification of the level of the internal opening, its relation to the anastomosis (usually the staple line), the direction of the tract, and the location of the external orifice in relation to the vaginal wall, vaginal fourchette, labia, or perineum. While most tracts are short and straight, they can be complex and branched, and a low PVF can mask the presence of a higher fistula from the pouch-body to the mid-body of the vagina. If necessary, introduction of dye such as methylene blue into the pouch, with white swabs placed in the vagina to identify staining, is useful. Alternatively, for low fistulae, hydrogen peroxide gently instilled into the anus may demonstrate bubbles as they emerge from the vaginal opening. Lastly, patients should typically undergo anal manometry to assess the sphincter pressures, and a pudendal nerve terminal motor latency study to assess for neural impairment, especially in women after childbirth.

Table 7.1 Search strategy

P (patients)	I (Intervention)	C (comparator)	O (outcomes)
Patient who underwent restorative proctocolectomy with ileal pouch anal anastomosis and developed a pouch-vaginal or pouch-perineal fistula	See Table 1	Not applicable	Fistula healing, pouch retention

Search Strategy (See Table 7.1)

A literature search was carried out to identify articles on PVF. The search was done on the electronic databases PubMed, Embase, and Medline, from 1980 to December 2022. The main search terms used were 'pouch-vaginal fistula', 'ileoanal pouch-vaginal fistula,' 'anal pouch-vaginal fistula,' 'ileoanal pouch fistula' OR 'anal pouch fistula.'

Results

Many procedures have been proposed for the treatment of PVF, most of them adopted from rectovaginal fistula repairs [29, 30]. The procedures can be divided into those performed via a perineal approach or via an abdominal approach. All studies provide level IV evidence, with small numbers of patients and significant heterogeneity. There are no randomized controlled trials and only three systematic reviews with one meta-analysis on the management of PVF. Pooled results for the different types of PVF repair are presented in Table 7.2.

Table 7.2 Pooled results for the different types of PVF repair

Type of repair	Success rate
Perineal approach	
Seton	5/15 (33%)
Fistulectomy	3/22 (14%)
Biological Collagen plug [33, 46] Fibrin glue [31, 42]	1/14 (7%) 2/6 (33%)
Transanal ileal advancement flap [9, 10, 14, 15, 18, 23, 31, 34, 46]	95/196 (48%)
Transvaginal [10, 12–15, 18, 35, 36, 46]	49/83 (58%)
Gracilis muscle interposition [15, 31, 37–39, 49, 51]	57/91 (62%)
Transanal pouch advancement [19, 41]	2/4 (50%)
Abdominoperineal approach	
(a) Abdominoperinal approach [10, 15, 16, 18, 19, 31, 42–44, 46]	Overall success 50–75%
Pouch advancement	8/16 (50%)
Redo pouch	38/65 (58%)
(b) Pouch excision 60/401 (15%)	100%

(a) Some studies not indicating different success rates for pouch advancement vs redo pouch
(b) Number represents percentage of patients eventually requiring pouch excision

Perineal Approach

Seton Drain

A draining seton is mainly used for controlling pelvic sepsis and for defining the fistula tract. One study [12] reported a success rate of 25% in patients with the use of a seton as definitive treatment. However, Wexner et al. (0/2) [15], Mallick et al. (0/3) [10] and Shah et al. (0/5) [18] all reported 100% failure rates. Tsujinaka et al. [31] showed complete healing in one patient with an asymptomatic fistula. To date, there is no evidence to support seton use except for initial control of sepsis before definitive repair. Most studies chose not to include patients treated with setons in their final analysis, instead focusing on patients undergoing procedures with a clear intent to close the fistula. Despite the widespread use of seton drain placement before attempting a definitive repair of PVF, there are no studies showing definitive data impacting the outcome.

Fistulectomy

The coring out of the fistula tract with repair of the internal opening at the pouch level has been described with disappointing results [12, 14, 15]. With little evidence available to support its use in the management of PVF, more recent studies have not included it as an option in their approach.

Biological Therapy

The use of a collagen plug to treat PVF was first reported by Gonsalves et al. [32]. While initial healing rates of 57% at 16 weeks (4/7) were promising, long term results showed 0/11 PVF successfully healed at 2 years [33]. Early success was probably related to the persistence of the collagen plug within the tract, but failure of local tissue in-growth coupled with the relatively short length of PVF led to long-term failure. Sapci et al. had success in 1/3 (33%) patients with use of a fistula plug, though this was limited to patients with a fistula distal to the anastomosis [46]. Tsujinaka et al. [31] reported the instillation of fibrin glue in the fistula tract with complete healing in one patient with a minimally symptomatic fistula and failure in 2/3 symptomatic patients who eventually required pouch advancement and a redo pouch.

Transanal Ileal Advancement Flap

An ileal pouch advancement involves mobilizing a flap of mucosa and submucosa from the ileal pouch, excising the internal opening, and then advancing the flap beyond the internal fistula opening where it is sutured in place. Mallick et al. [10] reported healing rates of 42% (20/48) when advancement flap was performed as a primary procedure and 66% (4/6) when performed secondarily after a different procedure. Tsujinaka et al. [31] showed healing rates of 60% (6/10), while Shah et al. [18] and Ozuner et al. [34] reported success rates of 44% (17/39) and 45% (15/24), respectively. Lee et al. [23] had a slightly higher success rate of 50% (10/20), with the rate increasing to 83% (10/12) when excluding patients with CD. Wexner et al. [15] reported successful fistula healing in 8/16 patients with this approach in a survey of North American colorectal units, whereas Groom et al. [14] reported only one success in 10 attempts. Sapci et al. reported a success of 14/23 (61%) of patients, with most of these fistulae located below the anastomosis (18/23) [46]. Pellino et al. performed a meta-analysis including 34 total articles with 770 total patients and reported an overall recurrence rate with this technique at 56.9% [47].

Advantages of the ileal pouch advancement flap include the relative simplicity of the procedure with more distal mobility of the flap [9]. The disadvantages of this approach include the suboptimal exposure, the risk of damage to the sphincters in patients with borderline incontinence, and the fact that the flap lies on the high-pressure side of the PVF.

Transvaginal Repair

Transvaginal repair is commonly one of the first interventions used for treatment of low PVF. These fistulas are usually the result of ileal-anal anastomotic disruption or inclusion of the vaginal wall in the anastomosis at the time of pouch creation. Advantages of the transvaginal approach include improved exposure compared to the transanal approach, decreased risk of damage to the anal sphincters, and less tension on the repair. The procedure can be repeated if necessary and yields satisfactory results with relatively less morbidity. The repair can also be augmented by placement of a biologic mesh between the pouch and the vagina. Possible complications include bleeding and hematoma development due to the vascularity of the vagina. However, this risk can be minimized with meticulous technique, drainage, and use of a vaginal packing [13, 18]. Dyspareunia is another possible complication.

The largest series published by Mallick et al. reported results for transvaginal approach in 32 patients. The healing rate was 55.5% (15 of 27 patients) when done as a primary procedure and 40% (2 of 5 patients) when performed after a failure of another approach. Authors noted that postoperative diagnosis of Crohn's disease was the only factor associated with failure of the repair [10]. Sagar et al. [35] reported the results of transvaginal repair for PVF in 11 patients, each of whom had previously undergone an attempt to close the fistula with a collagen button plug. Nine (81%) were successful at a median follow-up of 14 (6–56) months and the remaining two patients described symptomatic improvement. Sapci et al. reported a success rate in 1 of 4 patients (25%) [46].

Burke et al. [36] published the St. Mark's Hospital experience with transvaginal repair for PVF in 14 patients. They reported total success in 11/14 patients (78%), although 8 required multiple attempts to achieve long-term success. O'Kelly et al. [13] reported successful repair in 5/7 patients (71%) with this approach, and once again some patients in this series required more than one attempt before complete healing was achieved. Others have reported success rates of 0% (0/1) [18, 31], 27% (3/11) [15], and 100% (1/1) [12, 14]. A systematic review published in 2020 by Machin et al. included 13 retrospective cohort studies, 2 prospective cohort studies, eight case series, three case reports and a case-control study. 143 patients in this review underwent a transvaginal approach with a success rate of 51% [47]. The meta-analysis by Pellino et al. found an overall recurrence rate of 52.3% [46].

Muscle Interposition Flap

Muscle interposition flaps are particularly useful after previously failed repairs, in setting of poor quality of native tissues, as well as when abdominal procedures are contraindicated. The expected perioperative morbidity is 33–50% and includes perineal wound infection, urethral stricture, fever, urinary retention, and perineal bleeding [38, 40]. Perhaps because of the technical challenge, the procedure seems to have been underused. This procedure should be preceded by fecal diversion. At present, the low reported numbers and the relative complexity of the procedure prevent it from being strongly recommended as a first-line treatment. Another form of flap used for treating rectovaginal fistulas is the martius flap; however, results with treating PVF have not been published.

Gorenstein et al. [37] reported successful repair in two women with PVF. Previous attempts at local repair had failed in both patients and a simultaneous diverting loop ileostomy was constructed. Anterior sphincteroplasty was performed in one patient for associated incontinence. Wexner et al. [15] reported results of a multicenter study including treatment of PVF in 26 patients, 4 of whom underwent gracilis interposition flap with a 50% success rate. In a later publication, Wexner et al. [38] published results of gracilis flap in 53 patients, two of whom for the indication of PVF. One patient had complete healing and the patient who did not heal was eventually diagnosed with CD and opted to have a permanent ileostomy. Zmora et al. [39] published their experience with the gracilis interposition flap in 9 patients. Only one patient had a PVF and the fistula ultimately completely healed.

Another report by Tsujinaka et al. [31] described one patient with a failed gracilis interposition. Hull et al. reported on two patients undergoing gracilis muscle interposition as a subsequent repair following prior unsuccessful attempts. Both patients were diverted ahead of time and both healed successfully, however both also developed surgical site infections [49]. Machin et al. in their systematic review included 13 patients treated with various muscle transposition procedures (majority of which used gracilis muscle) with a success rate of 76.9% [48]. Yellinek et al. reviewed 11 cases of PVF repair with gracilis muscle transposition as part of a bigger cohort of complex perianal fistula repairs [50]. Although the authors do not report the success rate for these 11 patients separately, one interesting finding is that bed rest of >3 days was associated with flap failure. Frontali et al. had an overall success rate of 7 out of 10 (70%) patients with gracilis muscle interposition for PVF, and interestingly found that found that failure in PVF and RVF patients was significantly associated with lack of postoperative antibiotics prophylaxis [51].

Transanal Pouch Advancement

The technique of transanal disconnection of the ileal pouch from the IPAA, advancement of the pouch, and re-suture at the dentate line can be employed in patients with PVF, especially in slimmer patients with demonstrable mobility of the pouch above the level of the anastomosis. The advantage of this procedure is that it allows healthy, full thickness tissue to be delivered to the perineum. This operation should be offered after creation of a diverting ostomy. Both Fazio et al. [41] and Heriot et al. [19] showed that this procedure was successful in 50% of their patients. Sapci et al. reported success in 14/23 patients (61%), including 4 out of 5 patients having successful closure of a fistula above the anastomosis [46]. Machin et al. in their systematic review included 64 pouch advancement procedures with an overall success rate of 48.4% [48].

Abdominoperineal Approach

A "high" PVF that arises from the mid-body of the ileal pouch requires a transabdominal approach. This approach may also be selected after failed local repairs and in patients with ongoing pelvic sepsis due to abscess cavities with granulation tissue that cannot be completely removed using a local approach. The pouch needs to be carefully mobilized down to the level of the pelvic floor with attention given to the anterior wall of the pouch and the posterior wall of the vagina.

There are basically three surgical options: pouch advancement, pouch redo with a new handsewn IPAA, and pouch excision. The reported overall success rates for treating a PVF via the abdominoperineal approach are approximately 50–75% [10, 15, 16, 18, 19, 31, 42–44, 46]. Machin et al. in their systematic review included 161 transabdominal approaches with an overall success rate of 60.2% [48] The authors note that excision and reconstruction of the pouch was used in 107 patients with a 65.4% success rate. Sapci et al. demonstrated a simultaneous transabdominal and transperineal approach with pouch reconstruction and closure of the PVF had the highest success rate of closure at 69% overall and 71% for PVFs located distal to the anastomosis [46]. The authors specifically believe that if the tissue of fistula origin is retained at the rectum/ anal transition zone, removal should be considered for a successful outcome. The authors caution that due to complexity of the operation, these should be undertaken by experts with high volume of pouch redo surgeries. This is precisely why it should be noted that transabdominal revision of the pouch is technically demanding and carries a significant risk of loss of the pouch [10, 16, 18]. In addition, failed attempt at pouch revision may result in significant loss of small bowel with the risk of short gut syndrome. The patient needs to be fully counseled about these risks and preferably referred to a center of excellence in this field.

Diversion

A diverting ileostomy is commonly used in patients with PVF to control pelvic sepsis, relieve symptoms, or to divert fecal material away from the repair. Some authors have reported healing with the ileostomy alone [15, 31]. However, most authors describe construction of a diverting ileostomy either before or at the time of PVF repair [10, 18, 23]. Lee et al. [23] found higher success rates (60% vs. 45%) when a diverting ileostomy was performed before a transanal pouch advancement. Sapci et al. also showed improved success of PVF closure procedures with a diverting stoma in place (65.3% versus 27.7%), favoring diversion of all patients when operating to close PVFs [46]. However, much of the data is mixed in showing that a diverting ileostomy improves the chance of PVF healing. A permanent diversion, with or without pouch excision, is recommended when all other attempts have failed.

Recommendations

As noted above, all studies provide low quality data, providing weak recommendations.

1. Patients presenting with pelvic sepsis should undergo EUA and seton drainage.
2. A diverting ileostomy should be considered for all patients before or at the time of repair.

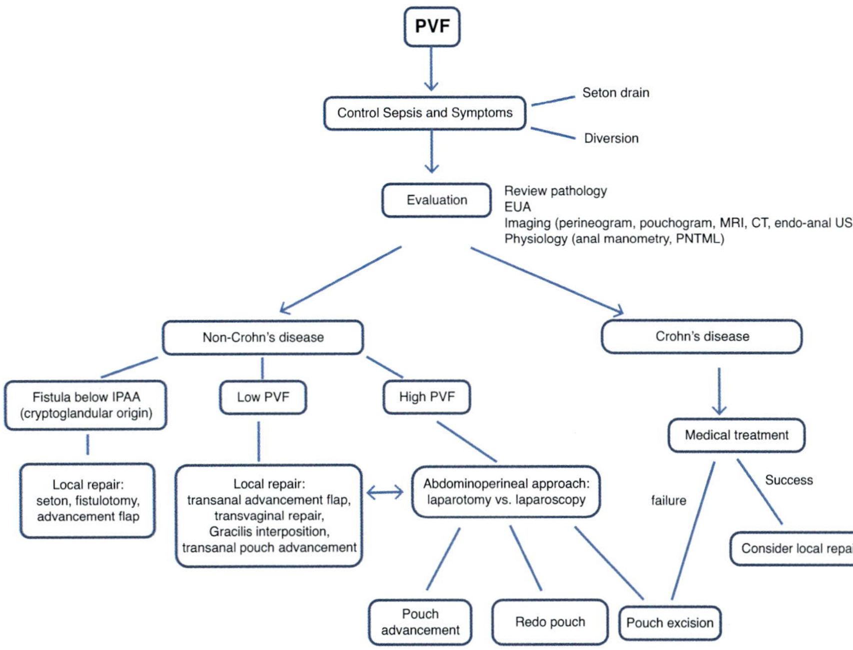

Fig. 7.1 Suggested treatment algorithm

3. Local repair should be attempted first for low PVFs.
4. An abdominoperineal approach should be reserved for "high" PVF and failed attempts at local repair.

A suggested algorithm based on results and recommendations is presented in Fig. 7.1.

Personal View of the Data

The management of pouch complications such as pouch perineal and pouch vaginal fistula presents a major challenge for the surgeon and the patient. It is our view that these patients should ideally be referred to large volume experienced centers for a more optimal outcome. It is essential for the surgeon to review all of the patients' prior relevant history including pathology and operative reports, as well as physiologic and imaging studies. In reviewing the data of multiple management strategies, it is clear that one's approach should be tailored to each individual patient. It is important to counsel patients that successful treatment often requires several operations over a long time period in order to achieve healing. Most studies had an average over 2.5 operations per patient prior to success. In addition, patients with CD should also be aware of the higher rate of pouch failure.

Local repair via the perineal approach should be considered when dealing with a low PVF, with the transanal ileal advancement flap, gracilis interposition, and pouch advancement all viable options. The abdominoperineal approach should be used for high fistulas and those that have failed previous local attempts. A diverting loop ileostomy before or at the time of repair offers the patient symptom relief, better sepsis control, and in our view an increased chance of successful healing. It seems that no single procedure is optimal for all cases of PVF. Therefore, the surgeon should be familiar with the existing armamentarium of treatment options and be continually updated on their success rates.

References

1. Parks AG, Nicholls RJ. Proctocolectomy without ileostomy for ulcerative colitis. Br Med J. 1978;2(6130):85–8.
2. Utsunomiya J, Iwama T, Imajo M, Matsuo S, Sawai S, Yaegashi K, et al. Total colectomy, mucosal proctectomy, and ileoanal anastomosis. Dis Colon Rectum. 1980;23(7):459–66.
3. Heald RJ, Allen DR. Stapled ileo-anal anastomosis: a technique to avoid mucosal proctectomy in the ileal pouch operation. Br J Surg. 1986;73(7):571–2.
4. McGuire BB, Brannigan AE, O'Connell PR. Ileal pouch-anal anastomosis. Br J Surg. 2007;94(7):812–23.
5. Bach SP, Mortensen NJ. Ileal pouch surgery for ulcerative colitis. World J Gastroenterol. 2007;13(24):3288–300.
6. Wong WD, Rothenberger DA, Goldberg SM. Ileoanal pouch procedures. Curr Probl Surg. 1985;22(3):1–78.
7. Lolohea S, Lynch AC, Robertson GB, Frizelle FA. Ileal pouch-anal anastomosis-vaginal fistula: a review. Dis Colon Rectum. 2005;48(9):1802–10.
8. Maslekar S, Sagar PM, Harji D, Bruce C, Griffiths B. The challenge of pouch-vaginal fistulas: a systematic review. Tech Coloproctol. 2012;16(6):405–14.
9. Gaertner WB, Witt J, Madoff RD, Mellgren A, Finne CO, Spencer MP. Ileal pouch fistulas after restorative proctocolectomy: management and outcomes. Tech Coloproctol. 2014;18(11):1061–6.
10. Mallick IH, Hull TL, Remzi FH, Kiran RP. Management and outcome of pouch-vaginal fistulas after IPAA surgery. Dis Colon Rectum. 2014;57(4):490–6.
11. Radcliffe AG, Ritchie JK, Hawley PR, Lennard-Jones JE, Northover JM. Anovaginal and rectovaginal fistulas in Crohn's disease. Dis Colon Rectum. 1988;31(2):94–9.
12. Keighley MR, Grobler SP. Fistula complicating restorative proctocolectomy. Br J Surg. 1993;80(8):1065–7.
13. O'Kelly TJ, Merrett M, Mortensen NJ, Dehn TC, Kettlewell M. Pouch-vaginal fistula after restorative proctocolectomy: aetiology and management. Br J Surg. 1994;81(9):1374–5.
14. Groom JS, Nicholls RJ, Hawley PR, Phillips RK. Pouch-vaginal fistula. Br J Surg. 1993;80(7):936–40.
15. Wexner SD, Rothenberger DA, Jensen L, Goldberg SM, Balcos EG, Belliveau P, et al. Ileal pouch vaginal fistulas: incidence, etiology, and management. Dis Colon Rectum. 1989;32(6):460–5.
16. MacLean AR, O'Connor B, Parkes R, Cohen Z, McLeod RS. Reconstructive surgery for failed ileal pouch-anal anastomosis: a viable surgical option with acceptable results. Dis Colon Rectum. 2002;45(7):880–6.
17. Schoetz DJ, Coller JA, Veidenheimer MC. Can the pouch be saved? Dis Colon Rectum. 1988;31(9):671–5.

18. Shah NS, Remzi F, Massmann A, Baixauli J, Fazio VW. Management and treatment outcome of pouch-vaginal fistulas following restorative proctocolectomy. Dis Colon Rectum. 2003;46(7):911–7.
19. Heriot AG, Tekkis PP, Smith JJ, Bona R, Cohen RG, Nicholls RJ. Management and outcome of pouch-vaginal fistulas following restorative proctocolectomy. Dis Colon Rectum. 2005;48(3):451–8.
20. Hicks CW, Hodin RA, Bordeianou L. Possible overuse of 3-stage procedures for active ulcerative colitis. JAMA Surg. 2013;148(7):658–64.
21. Meagher AP, Farouk R, Dozois RR, Kelly KA, Pemberton JH. J ileal pouch-anal anastomosis for chronic ulcerative colitis: complications and long-term outcome in 1310 patients. Br J Surg. 1998;85(6):800–3.
22. Reilly WT, Pemberton JH, Wolff BG, Nivatvongs S, Devine RM, Litchy WJ, et al. Randomized prospective trial comparing ileal pouch-anal anastomosis performed by excising the anal mucosa to ileal pouch-anal anastomosis performed by preserving the anal mucosa. Ann Surg. 1997;225(6):666–76. –discussion 676–7
23. Lee PY, Fazio VW, Church JM, Hull TL, Eu KW, Lavery IC. Vaginal fistula following restorative proctocolectomy. Dis Colon Rectum. 1997;40(7):752–9.
24. Neilly P, Neill ME, Hill GL. Restorative proctocolectomy with ileal pouch-anal anastomosis in 203 patients: the Auckland experience. Aust N Z J Surg. 1999;69(1):22–7.
25. Luukkonen P, Järvinen H. Stapled vs hand-sutured ileoanal anastomosis in restorative proctocolectomy. A prospective, randomized study. Arch Surg. 1993;128(4):437–40.
26. Koltun WA, Schoetz DJ, Roberts PL, Murray JJ, Coller JA, Veidenheimer MC. Indeterminate colitis predisposes to perineal complications after ileal pouch-anal anastomosis. Dis Colon Rectum. 1991;34(10):857–60.
27. Paye F, Penna C, Chiche L, Tiret E, Frileux P, Parc R. Pouch-related fistula following restorative proctocolectomy. Br J Surg. 1996;83(11):1574–7.
28. Dozois RR, Kelly KA, Welling DR, Gordon H, Beart RW, Wolff BG, et al. Ileal pouch-anal anastomosis: comparison of results in familial adenomatous polyposis and chronic ulcerative colitis. Ann Surg. 1989;210(3):268–71. –discussion 272–3. Lippincott, Williams, and Wilkins
29. Mazier WP, Senagore AJ, Schiesel EC. Operative repair of anovaginal and rectovaginal fistulas. Dis Colon Rectum. 1995;38(1):4–6.
30. Rothenberger DA, Christenson CE, Balcos EG, Schottler JL, Nemer FD, Nivatvongs S, et al. Endorectal advancement flap for treatment of simple rectovaginal fistula. Dis Colon Rectum. 1982;25(4):297–300.
31. Tsujinaka S, Ruiz D, Wexner SD, Baig MK, Sands DR, Weiss EG, et al. Surgical management of pouch-vaginal fistula after restorative proctocolectomy. J Am Coll Surg. 2006;202(6):912–8.
32. Gonsalves S, Sagar P, Lengyel J, Morrison C, Dunham R. Assessment of the efficacy of the rectovaginal button fistula plug for the treatment of ileal pouch-vaginal and rectovaginal fistulas. Dis Colon Rectum. 2009;52(11):1877–81.
33. Gajsek U, McArthur DR, Sagar PM. Long-term efficacy of the button fistula plug in the treatment of Ileal pouch-vaginal and Crohn's-related rectovaginal fistulas. Dis Colon Rectum. 2011;54(8):999–1002.
34. Ozuner G, Hull T, Lee P, Fazio VW. What happens to a pelvic pouch when a fistula develops? Dis Colon Rectum. 1997;40(5):543–7.
35. Sagar RC, Thornton M, Herd A, Brayshaw I, Sagar PM. Transvaginal repair of recurrent pouch-vaginal fistula. Color Dis. 2014;16(12):O440–2.
36. Burke D, van Laarhoven CJ, Herbst F, Nicholls RJ. Transvaginal repair of pouch-vaginal fistula. Br J Surg. 2001;88(2):241–5. Blackwell Science Ltd
37. Gorenstein L, Boyd JB, Ross TM. Gracilis muscle repair of rectovaginal fistula after restorative proctocolectomy. Report of two cases. Dis Colon Rectum. 1988;31(9):730–4.
38. Wexner SD, Ruiz DE, Genua J, Nogueras JJ, Weiss EG, Zmora O. Gracilis muscle interposition for the treatment of rectourethral, rectovaginal, and pouch-vaginal fistulas: results in 53 patients. Ann Surg. 2008;248(1):39–43.

39. Zmora O, Tulchinsky H, Gur E, Goldman G, Klausner JM, Rabau M. Gracilis muscle transposition for fistulas between the rectum and urethra or vagina. Dis Colon Rectum. 2006;49(9):1316–21.
40. Zmora O, Potenti FM, Wexner SD, Pikarsky AJ, Efron JE, Nogueras JJ, et al. Gracilis muscle transposition for iatrogenic rectourethral fistula. Ann Surg. 2003;237(4):483–7.
41. Fazio VW, Tjandra JJ. Pouch advancement and neoileoanal anastomosis for anastomotic stricture and anovaginal fistula complicating restorative proctocolectomy. Br J Surg. 1992;79(7):694–6.
42. Johnson PM, O'Connor BI, Cohen Z, McLeod RS. Pouch-vaginal fistula after ileal pouch-anal anastomosis: treatment and outcomes. Dis Colon Rectum. 2005;48(6):1249–53.
43. Zinicola R, Wilkinson KH, Nicholls RJ. Ileal pouch-vaginal fistula treated by abdominoanal advancement of the ileal pouch. Br J Surg. 2003;90(11):1434–5. John Wiley & Sons Ltd
44. Fazio VW, Ziv Y, Church JM, Oakley JR, Lavery IC, Milsom JW, et al. Ileal pouch-anal anastomoses complications and function in 1005 patients. Ann Surg. 1995;222(2):120–7. Lippincott, Williams, and Wilkins
45. Haveran LA, Sehgal R, Poritz LS, Mckenna KJ, Stewart DB, Koltun WA. Infliximab and/or azathioprine in the treatment of crohn's disease-like complications after IPAA. Dis Colon Rectum. 2011;54:15–20.
46. Sapci I, Akeel N, DeLeon MF, Stocchi L, Hull T. What is the best surgical treatment of pouch-vaginal fistula? Dis Colon Rectum. 2019;62:595–9.
47. Pellino G, Celentano V, Vinci D, Romano FM, Pedone A, Vigorita V, Signoriello G, Selvaggi F, Sciaudone G. Ileoanal pouch-related fistulae: a systematic review with meta-analysis on incidence, treatment options and outcomes. Dig Liver Dis. 2023;55(3):342–9.
48. Machin M, Younan HC, Slesser AAP, Mohsen Y. Systematic review on the management of ileoanal pouch-vaginal fistulas after restorative proctocolectomy in the treatment of ulcerative colitis. Color Dis. 2021;23(1):34–51.
49. Hull TL, Sapci I, Lightner AL. Gracilis flap repair for reoperative rectovaginal fistula. Dis Colon Rectum. 2023;66:113–7.
50. Yellinek S, Barros Sousa C, Gilshtein H, Strassmann V, da Silva G, Wexner SD. Gracilis muscle interposition for treatment of complex anal fistula: experience with 119 consecutive patients. Dis Colon Rectum. 2021;64:881–7.
51. Frontali A, Rottoli M, Chierici A, Poggioli G, Panis Y. Rectovaginal fistula: risk factors for failure after graciloplasty – a bicentric retrospective European study of 61 patients. Color Dis. 2021;23(8):2113–8.

Ileal Pouch–Anal Anastomosis Failure: What to Do?

8

Wyeth Alexander and Samuel Eisenstein

Introduction

First described by Parks and Nicholls in 1978 [1], restorative proctocolectomy with ileal pouch-anal anastomosis (IPAA) has been widely adopted as the treatment of choice for management of Familial Adenomatous Polyposis (FAP), medically refractory Ulcerative Colitis (UC), and more recently adopted for management of highly selected patients with medically refractory Crohn's disease. Over four decades of development, the creation of a double loop stapled "J-shaped" pouch with anastomosis between the apex of the pouch and the anus has become the standardized approach with an abundance of literature demonstrating low mortality and excellent patient satisfaction when compared to creation of an end ileostomy.

Despite these promising end results, high rates of post-operative complications have plagued the IPAA with morbidity ranging between 15% and 70% [2–4]. Furthermore, "pouch failure" has been reported to occur in roughly 3.5–18% with the broad range of occurrence largely owing to difference in follow up time [2–4]. While exact terminology varies between studies, for the purpose of this chapter, pouch failure will be broadly defined as need for indefinite de-functioning fecal diversion in the presence of IPAA with or without pouch excision.

While the IPAA has been widely adopted in the modern-day colorectal surgeon's tool belt, little data exists to guide management of pouch failure. Additionally, existing literature lacks broad use of standardized vocabulary, protocols, or endpoint data between institutions making comparisons difficult. Given the seemingly inevitability of practitioners to encounter IPAA pouch failure, this chapter will aim to

W. Alexander · S. Eisenstein (✉)
Department of Surgery, Division of Colon and Rectal Surgery, UC San Diego Health, La Jolla, CA, USA
e-mail: walexander@ucsd.edu; seisenstein@ucsd.edu

K. Umanskiy, N. Hyman (eds.), *Difficult Decisions in Colorectal Surgery*, Difficult Decisions in Surgery: An Evidence-Based Approach,
https://doi.org/10.1007/978-3-031-42303-1_8

Table 8.1 PICO diagram for Ileal pouch failure

Patients	Intervention	Comparator	Outcome
Patients s/p IPAA with subsequent pouch failure	Creation of defunctioning ileostomy with pouch left in-situ	Creation of ileostomy with pouch excision	Health-related quality of life (HRQOL)

provide a succinct review of data driven recommendations to answer the question: Ileal-anal pouch anastomosis failure- what to do.

PICO Diagram (Table 8.1)

Search Strategy

A Medline Ovid database search was performed on publications from 1985 through July 2022 detailing operative strategies for management of pouch failure. Search phrases utilized: "ileal-anal anastomosis", "ileal pouch", "J-pouch", "proctocolectomy". Articles were omitted if they were not in the English language or if they were conducted at pediatric centers. The literature search was further broadened with review of references of resulted articles.

Results

When considering management of a failed pouch, the two common interventions include creation of a defunctioning ileostomy with pouch left in-situ vs ileostomy creation with pouch excision. The creation of a continent ileostomy can additionally be considered however for simplicity, and due to the relative rarity of this procedure in the modern era, discussion of this approach will be deferred. Despite nearly four decades since the advent of the IPAA, few studies have analyzed the difference in patient safety and health-related quality of life outcomes of these two approaches. Furthermore, as previously mentioned, early studies are plagued by the absence of common nomenclature or validated quality of life metrics. More recently, the Cleveland Global QOL [5] and Short Form (SF)-36 [6] questionaries have been widely adopted as validated measures of patient quality of life following IPAA.

Interestingly, the two available studies offering direct comparisons of pouch left in-situ vs pouch excision via validated quality of life questionnaires come to conflicting conclusions. In their retrospective comparison of 22 patients with pouch left in situ compared to 31 patients with pouch excisions, Das et al. found little difference in overall health related quality of life metrics between the two groups [7]. The study does note a trend towards higher quality of life scores among the pouch-excision group by the Cleveland Clinic Foundation QoL however this trend did not reach statistical significance in any of the included questionnaire domains. The group went on to include additional metrics of urinary and sexual function and found that pouch excision was associated with higher incidence of urinary and sexual complications hypothesized to be related to pelvic nerve damage related to the excision. They additionally included added metrics of stoma function citing increased risk of stoma retraction in the pouch excision group which likely stems from the creation of end ileostomies with pouch excision compared to creation of diverting ileostomies with pouches left in situ. The group concludes that a defunctioning ileostomy with pouch left in-situ offers similar outcomes with reduced risk of complication related to pouch excision.

In a slightly larger retrospective study, Kiran et al. compared the health-related quality of life of 31 patients who underwent ileostomy creation with pouch left in-situ to 105 patients who underwent pouch excision [5]. Despite the slightly larger population size, the group relied on less validated measures of outcome including a non-descript quality of life and quality of health questionnaire and an abbreviated SF-12 questionnaire. Additionally they included the Cleveland Global QoL. In direct disagreement with the findings present by Das et al., Kiran et al. report significantly higher QoL scores of the pouch excision group in all domains with the exception of urinary function and sexual function. Kiran et al. note that anal pain and anorectal seepage within the pouch left in-situ group were the main morbidities driving the worse QoL scores among the population. The authors conclude that while pouch excision adds to the operative complexity with theoretical risk of increased morbidity, it offers increased long term health related quality of life and should be pursued when appropriate (Table 8.2).

Data for direct comparisons of pouch left in situ vs pouch excision is extremely sparse, including only studies with small population sizes and variable outcome metrics. In attempt to further understand the topic, additional insight can be gleaned from literature available reporting morbidity and patient satisfaction of each approach individually without direct comparisons.

Table 8.2 Direct comparison of Pouch Excision to Diversion

	Type of Study	Study size (N)	Reason for pouch failure (IS vs PE)	Follow up (median years, range)	Quality of Life Measure	Results IS vs PE	Quality of evidence
Kiran et al. (2012) [5]	Retrospective	IS: 31 PE: 105	Septic event: 48.4% vs 37.1% Outlet obstruction: 19.4% vs 13.3% Pouchitis: 12.9% vs 21.9% Poor function: 9.7% vs 14.3% Other: 9.7% vs 13.3%	IS: 9.9 (2.3–21.5) PE: 9.8 (1.3–24.8)	QOL QOH Energy level CGQL score SF-12 MCS SF-12 PCS Urinary function Sexual function	6.5 vs 8.1 (P = 0.005) 6.4 vs 7.9 (P = 0.008) 5.6 vs 7.1 (P = 0.026) 0.6 vs 0.8 (P = 0.005) 38.8 vs 48.8 (P = 0.004) 38.4 vs 46.6 (P = 0.014) No significant difference No significant difference	Moderate
Das et al. (2006) [7]	Retrospective	IS: 22 PE: 31	Sepsis (including fistula): 64% vs 68% Poor function: 32% vs 26% Pouchitis: 4% vs 6%	IS: 6 (1–20) PE: 4 (0–15)	SF-36 CCF QoL Stoma function Bladder function Sexual function	No significant difference No significant difference Stoma retraction 7% vs 47% (P = 0.003). No significant difference Ability to maintain erection worse in male patients after PE (P = 0.05).	Moderate

Outcomes after direct comparison of pouch excision to diversion

IS Pouch left in-situ, *PE* Pouch excision, *QoL* quality of life, *QoH* quality of health, *CGQL* Cleveland Clinic Global Quality of Life score, *SF-12 MCS* San Francisco Mental Component Summary, *SF-12 PCS* San Francisco Physical Component Summary, *SF-36* San Francisco-36 Survey

Creation of Diverting Loop Ileostomy with Pouch Left In-Situ

As mentioned previously, creation of a diverting loop ileostomy is the least invasive management approach for pouch failure. While a diverting loop ileostomy may be created with the intent of permanent defunctioning diversion, it allows for continued possibility of restoration of continuity while also allowing for pouch excision based on resulting clinical outcomes. When considering the potential downfalls of leaving the pouch in-situ at the time of initial operation of failed pouch management, patient quality of life and concerns for potential malignant transformation of the remnant mucosa have been considered. Prior studies have suggested that chronic inflammation of the ileal pouch following IPAA may result in dysplasia with potential progression to adenocarcinoma with other studies reporting rare cases of malignancy developing following IPAA [8–12].

Patient Satisfaction of Pouch Left In-Situ

In their series of 460 patients, Foley et al. report 21 cases requiring defunctioning ileostomy creations [13]. Of these 21 patients, 5 ultimately went on to have successful restoration of continuity, all in the absence of Crohn's disease. It should be noted that all 5 of the successfully restored patients required additional procedures prior to ileostomy takedown as diversion alone was not sufficient to eradicate the underlying complications. Of the remaining 16 patients who had pouch failure, 7 underwent pouch excision; 5 for extensive fistulation related to Crohn's disease, 1 for infarcted pouch related to mesenteric injury, and 1 with persistent anal incontinence despite re-diversion. The remaining 9 patients were adequately treated with permeant ileostomy diversion alone with good patient satisfaction.

Of 620 patients who underwent IPAA, Bengtsson et al. identified 56 pouch failures including 23 pouch excisions, 22 defunctioned pouches in-situ, and 11 pouches converted to continent ileostomy [14]. Of the 22 defunctioning procedures with pouch in-situ, patients had a median follow up time of 3.5 years with twenty patients reporting minor mucous discharge per anus and two patients reporting anal pain. Of note, no patients requested further operative management and a majority were reported to have had "satisfactory ileostomy function".

The available literature highlights the comparable patient satisfaction of defucntioning ileostomy without pouch excision while maintaining a theoretical possibility of restoring intestinal continuity. These conclusions, however, are limited by the lack of standardized quality of life measures such as the Short-Form 36-item quality-of-life questionnaire and lack of comparison to alternative forms of management. While maintaining patient satisfaction, fecal diversion with pouch left in-situ mitigates the considerable morbidity associated with pouch excision [15–17]. However, when considering the risks and benefits of primary defunctioning ileostomy, findings by Foley et al. highlight the need for consideration of the underlying disease process (e.g. Crohn's disease) when counseling patients on best initial management approach and likelihood of need for future procedures and/or pouch-excision [13] (Table 8.3).

Table 8.3 Outcomes after Pouch Diversion

	Type of study	Study size (N)	Etiology of pouch failure (IS vs PE)	Follow up (median years, range)	Quality of life measure	Results IS vs PE	Quality of evidence
Foley et al. (1995) [13]	Prospective	IS: 14[a] PE: 7	Pouch fistula: 57% Pouchitis: 19% Anastomotic stricture: 14% Anastomotic separation: 14% Miscellaneous: 9.5%[b]	Unspecified	Not included	Pouch excision selectively reserved for patients with extensive perianal sepsis or fistulization persisting after re-diversion. Unable to make meaningful comparisons given population differences	Poor
Bengtsson et al. (2007) [14]	Prospective	IS: 22 PE: 23	Pelvic sepsis: 41% vs 39% Poor function: 36% vs 48% Pouchitis: 4.5% vs 22% Fissure: 4.5% vs 4.3%	14 (0.5–22)[c]	Not included	No functional results of PE reported for comparison	Poor

Outcomes after pouch diversion when not compared directly to pouch excision
IS Pouch left in-situ, *PE* Pouch excision
[a] Continuity restored in 5 of 14
[b] Etiology of pouch failure not subdivided to IS vs PE
[c] Median follow up data provided for IS only

Morbidity of Pouch Left In-Situ

Bengtsson et al. report that of the 22 patients with defunctioning ileostomy with pouch left in-situ, thirteen completed endoscopic evaluation of the retained pouch (mean pouch age 13.8 years, mean time after diversion 8.2 years) [14]. Of this group, no cases of dysplasia or carcinoma was found. One patient was seen to have atypia however this was interpreted as reactive due to severe inflammation. The authors concluded that a retained pouch results in high patient satisfaction and carries little malignant potential without need of additional routine surveillance. These findings are further supported by Kiran et al. who found that none of 18 patients with pouch in situ and long term follow up developed pouch dysplasia or cancer [5].

Ileostomy Creation with Pouch Excision

Patient Satisfaction of Pouch Excision

In their relatively small study, Tan et al. investigated the differences in quality of life between patients who underwent proctocolectomy with initial conventional ileostomy creation and IPAA failure requiring ileostomy creation with pouch excision [18]. Utilizing the Short-Form 36-item quality-of-life questionnaire, Tan et al. conclude that the two groups demonstrate comparable quality of life with the pouch excision group only reporting increased troublesome bowel symptoms (though no significant difference in systemic symptoms, functional impairment, social impairment, emotional impairment, or global score). Lepisto et al. expanded on this body of data by comparing Short-Form 36-item quality-of-life questionnaire scores between pouch excision, intact IPAA, and the healthy population [19]. The group conclude that the pouch excision group had significantly decreased physical function ($P < 0.003$), energy ($P < 0.01$), and social function ($P < 0.05$) when compared to intact IPAA control group. This data should be taken with careful consideration as it is generally accepted that patients with pouch failure have increased morbidity due to the underlying pathology (including Crohn's) related to pouch failure; this observed difference may be a product of this morbidity over the morbidity related to ileostomy creation and pouch excision. While the available data on patient satisfaction following IPAA failure with pouch excision is invaluable in setting patients' expectations, it provides little guidance in directly management of pouch failure given the absence of comparison to defunctioning ileostomy with pouch left in situ and continent ileostomy creation (Table 8.4).

Recommendations Based on the Data

1. Permanent diversion of ileal pouch carries minimal risk of pouch-related neoplasia. (Strong Recommendation based upon low-quality of evidence)

Table 8.4 Outcomes after Pouch Excision

	Type of study	Study size (N)	Reason for pouch failure (IS vs PE)	Follow up (median years, range)	Quality of life measure	Health-related quality of life (HRQOL): PE vs control	Quality of evidence
Tan et al. (1998) [18]	Retrospective	PE: 9 Control (proctocolectomy with initial end ileostomy): 14	–	–	SF-36	Bowel function: 5.64 vs 6.13 (P = 0.03) Otherwise no significant difference	Weak
Lepiesto et al. (2002) [19]	Retrospective	PE: 18 Control: (successfull IPAA): 18	Fistula: 21% [5] Pouchitis: 12.5% [3] Pouchitis with fistula: 8.3% [2] Incontinences: 21% [5] Crohns: 17% [4] Other: 21% [5]	2–16 years	SF-36	Physical function 73 vs 93 (P = 0.003) Energy 51 vs 65 (P = 0.01) Role function (physical) 55 vs 83 (P = 0.05) No significant difference in remaining domains	Weak

Outcomes after pouch excision when not compared directly to pouch diversion
PE pouch excision

2. Pouch excision carries a greater risk of operative morbidity than diversion alone. (Weak Recommendation based upon low-quality of evidence)
3. Pouch excision may impart better long-term quality of life than diversion alone for patients who experience QoL limiting symptoms from their diverted pouch. (Weak Recommendation based upon low-quality of evidence)

Personal View

Patients who are experiencing pouch failure have often suffered a significant insult by the time they are prepared to undergo definitive intervention. The patients are often malnourished, anemic, on immunosuppressive medications, and experiencing significant pain as well as other systemic symptoms. The goal will always be to maximize the patient's quality of life while exposing them to a surgery with an acceptable risk profile. While pouch revision may be an option for some patients, we have chosen to omit that population for the purpose of this chapter understanding that the question being asked is whether to divert or excise the pouch once a patient has exhausted their other options. Often times the answer is yes to both of these options.

Pouch excision in and of itself can be an incredibly morbid procedure in a sick patient and thus the definitive options is often a step-wise process where the pouch is diverted first and the patient is allowed to recover. Pouch diversion can be seen as a bridge to allow the patient to both recover their health and to remember that an ileostomy can impart an improvement in the quality of life while allowing time for making important decisions about what their future will hold. The potential for reversibility is often important when a patient makes the decision to undergo diversion from a poorly functioning pouch. When diverting the pouch, it is important to ensure that the surgeon leaves themselves maximal flexibility for a patient's future needs and depending on the etiology of the pouch failure. If there is a possibility for a redo IPAA, it is important to construct the ileostomy in such a way that it can be used in a future pouch, about 20 cm proximal to the pouch inlet [20].

Ultimately, many patients will either opt not to restore continence or will not have the option to restore continence given the etiology of their pouch failure. For these patients the question is whether it is in their best interest to have their pouch excised. Generally, in this patient population there is no imperative to ultimately go on to pouch excision as it has been demonstrated that there is no increased risk of neoplasia in the diverted pouch [5, 7, 14] and the decision to move beyond simple diversion is made to improve quality of life when the patient has problems with either their pouch or their diversion.

There are several issues to consider when making the decision about definitive management including the quality of the patient's ileostomy, the amount of drainage the patient is experiencing from their anus, and potential pelvic inflammation from a diseased pouch or cuff, all weighed against the risks of the surgery including non-healing perineal wounds and the myriad of other complications which spring up around redo pelvic surgery.

The loop ileostomy in the setting of an IPAA is often imperfect. Tension along the mesentery pulls in 2 directions with the origin of the blood supply being tethered cephalad and the pouch being tethered caudally. This can lead to problems getting an adequate stoma eversion for effective pouching, particularly in those patients who have short mesenteries or thick abdominal walls. In a truly sick patient, it is sometimes unavoidable to make an imperfect stoma with an understanding that either revision or pouch excision may ultimately be necessary once the patient recovers. In those patients who are unlikely to have restoration of intestinal continuity in the future, an end ileostomy is the best option, dividing the ileum as close to the pouch as possible preserve proximal ileum length. Another option may be separating the proximal and distal ends of the stoma or considering an end-loop configuration. This maneuver, however should not be employed in patients with distal strictures as they could dehisce the distal suture line. Ultimately to obtain a high-quality end ileostomy it is often necessary to perform a pouch excision, freeing up the caudal tension and allowing a stoma to come up more easily.

A common complaint of the diverted pouch patient is anal mucus drainage. This can be uncomfortable, leading to significant anal pruritus, as well as embarrassment in social situations necessitating use of a pad or disposable undergarment. While this may seem trivial, it was a significant complaint in the largest comparative series, with 12/31 (38.7%) of patients who were diverted complaining of problematic seepage or anal pain [6]. It is certainly reasonable to consider pouch excision in acceptable risk patients for this indication as the QoL does seem to be better for those patients whose pouches are excised [5].

While QoL is likely higher after pouch excision if things go well, there is significant risk of morbidity from these procedures with morbidity rates from excision ranging from 44% to 62% in larger series [2, 15, 16, 21]. While postoperative ileus and pelvic abscesses are recoverable, perineal nerve injury can lead to significant sexual and urinary dysfunction. Perineal wound complications are likely the most significant issues faced by this population. Kiran, et al. reported 51% delayed perineal wound healing and 39.8% persistent pouch sinus [22]. These are important issues to counsel your patient on prior to undertaking such a significant procedure, particularly when the patients have already experienced significant morbidity because of their pouch failure.

Unfortunately for our patients the quality of data on this issue is not the highest. Most studies are retrospective in nature and demonstrate a significant selection bias. That being said, having a thoughtful approach based on a variety of patient factors is key to maximizing QoL. Generally, when we see patients with pouch failure it is important to understand their current QoL, what their long-term goals for continence are, and what their risk factors are for surgical intervention. If restoration of continuity is a priority in the future, then a loop ileostomy is often a good first step for improving both the health and satisfaction of the patient. This should be done in such a way that pouch revision is possible, but also with the understanding that many patients will not ultimately seek out pouch revision once their QoL is restored. Once the patients have recovered and resumed their usual life, the decision to excise the pouch should be made on symptoms alone. If the patient is satisfied there is no imperative to expose them to a potentially morbid procedure. If the pouch or stoma related symptoms dictate that there is a possibility that pouch excision will improve their QoL, then this approach is reasonable after counseling the patient on the potential risks of the procedure, understanding that there is data support a higher QoL after pouch excision in symptomatic patients.

References

1. Nicholls RJ, Pescatori M, Motson RW, Pezim ME. Restorative proctocolectomy with a three-loop ileal reservoir for ulcerative colitis and familial adenomatous polyposis. Ann Surg. 1984;199:383–8.
2. Hueting WE, Buskens E, van der Tweel I, et al. Results and complications after ileal pouch anal anastomosis: a meta-analysis of 43 observational studies comprising 9,317 patients. Dig Surg. 2005;22:69–79.
3. de Zeeuw S, Ali UA, Donders RART, et al. Update of complications and functional outcome of the ileo-pouch anal anastomosis: overview of evidence and meta-analysis of 96 observational studies. Int J Color Dis. 2012;27:843–53. https://doi.org/10.1007/s00384-011-1402-6.
4. Heuthorst L, Wasmann KATGM, Reijntjes MA, Hompes R, Buskens CJ, Bemelman WA. ileal pouch-anal anastomosis complications and pouch failure: a systematic review and meta-analysis. Ann Surg Open. 2021 June;2(2):e074. https://doi.org/10.1097/AS9.0000000000000074.
5. Kiran RP, Delaney CP, Senagore AJ, O'Brien-Ermlich B, Mascha E, Thornton J, Fazio VW. Prospective assessment of Cleveland Global Quality of Life (CGQL) as a novel marker of quality of life and disease activity in Crohn's disease. Am J Gastroenterol. 2003 Aug;98(8):1783–9. https://doi.org/10.1111/j.1572-0241.2003.07592.x. PMID: 12907333.
6. Lins L, Carvalho FM. SF-36 total score as a single measure of health-related quality of life: scoping review. SAGE Open Med. 2016 Oct 4;4:2050312116671725. https://doi.org/10.1177/2050312116671725. PMID: 27757230; PMCID: PMC5052926.
7. Das P, Smith JJ, Tekkis PP, Heriot AG, Antropoli M, John NR. Quality of life after indefinite diversion/pouch excision in ileal pouch failure patients. Color Dis. 2007 Oct;9(8):718–24. https://doi.org/10.1111/j.1463-1318.2007.01216.x. Epub 2007 Aug 31. PMID: 17764535.
8. Hultén L, Willén R, Nilsson O, Safarani N, Haboubi N. Mucosal assessment for dysplasia and cancer in the ileal pouch mucosa in patients operated on for ulcerative colitis–a 30-year follow-up study. Dis Colon Rectum. 2002 Apr;45(4):448–52. https://doi.org/10.1007/s10350-004-6218-9. PMID: 12006923.
9. Börjesson L, Willén R, Haboubi N, Duff SE, Hultén L. The risk of dysplasia and cancer in the ileal pouch mucosa after restorative proctocolectomy for ulcerative proctocolitis is low: a long-term term follow-up study. Color Dis. 2004 Nov;6(6):494–8. https://doi.org/10.1111/j.1463-1318.2004.00716.x. PMID: 15521942.
10. Veress B, Reinholt FP, Lindquist K, Löfberg R, Liljeqvist L. Long-term histomorphological surveillance of the pelvic ileal pouch: dysplasia develops in a subgroup of patients. Gastroenterology. 1995;109(4):1090–7, ISSN 0016-5085
11. Setti Carraro P, Talbot IC, Nicholls RJ. Longterm appraisal of the histological appearances of the ileal reservoir mucosa after restorative proctocolectomy for ulcerative colitis. Gut. 1994 Dec;35(12):1721–7. https://doi.org/10.1136/gut.35.12.1721. PMID: 7829009; PMCID: PMC1375260.
12. Gullberg K, Ståhlberg D, Liljeqvist L, Tribukait B, Reinholt FP, Veress B, Löfberg R. Neoplastic transformation of the pelvic pouch mucosa in patients with ulcerative colitis. Gastroenterology. 1997 May;112(5):1487–92. https://doi.org/10.1016/s0016-5085(97)70029-5. PMID: 9136826.
13. Foley EF, Schoetz DJ Jr, Roberts PL, Marcello PW, Murray JJ, Coller JA, Veidenheimer MC. Rediversion after ileal pouch-anal anastomosis. Causes of failures and predictors of sub-

sequent pouch salvage. Dis Colon Rectum. 1995 Aug;38(8):793–8. https://doi.org/10.1007/BF02049833. PMID: 7634973.

14. Bengtsson J, Börjesson L, Willén R, Oresland T, Hultén L. Can a failed ileal pouch anal anastomosis be left in situ? Color Dis. 2007 Jul;9(6):503–8. https://doi.org/10.1111/j.1463-1318.2007.01308.x. PMID: 17573744.
15. Karoui M, Cohen R, Nicholls J. Results of surgical removal of the pouch after failed restorative proctocolectomy. Dis Colon Rectum. 2004 Jun;47(6):869–75. https://doi.org/10.1007/s10350-004-0536-9. Epub 2004 Apr 19. PMID: 15108024.
16. Prudhomme M, Dehni N, Dozois RR, Tiret E, Parc R. Causes and outcomes of pouch excision after restorative proctocolectomy. Br J Surg. 2006 Jan;93(1):82–6. https://doi.org/10.1002/bjs.5147. PMID: 16288450.
17. Lightner AL, Dattani S, Dozois EJ, Moncrief SB, Pemberton JH, Mathis KL. Pouch excision: indications and outcomes. Color Dis. 2017 Oct;19(10):912–6. https://doi.org/10.1111/codi.13673. PMID: 28387059.
18. Tan HT, Morton D, Connolly AB, Pringle W, White M, Keighley MR. Quality of life after pouch excision. Br J Surg. 1998 Feb;85(2):249–51. https://doi.org/10.1046/j.1365-2168.1998.00582.x. PMID: 9501828.
19. Lepistö A, Luukkonen P, Järvinen HJ. Cumulative failure rate of ileal pouch-anal anastomosis and quality of life after failure. Dis Colon Rectum. 2002 Oct;45(10):1289–94. https://doi.org/10.1007/s10350-004-6412-9. PMID: 12394424.
20. Schwartzberg DM, Esen E, Remzi FH. Thoughtful ileostomy creation in patients undergoing redo IPAA. Dis Colon Rectum. 2020 Jan;63(1):117–20. https://doi.org/10.1097/DCR.0000000000001535. PMID: 31804276.
21. Esen E, Grieco MJ, Erkan A, Aytac E, Sutter AG, Lynn PB, Esterow J, da Luz MA, Kirat HT, Remzi FH. Management, functional outcomes, and quality of life after development of pelvic sepsis in patients undergoing re-do Ileal pouch anal anastomosis. Dis Colon Rectum. 2022 Aug 1;65(8):e790–6. https://doi.org/10.1097/DCR.0000000000002337. Epub 2022 Jul 5. PMID: 34840297.
22. Nisar PJ, Turina M, Lavery IC, Kiran RP. Perineal wound healing following ileoanal pouch excision. J Gastrointest Surg. 2014 Jan;18(1):200–7. https://doi.org/10.1007/s11605-013-2340-0. Epub 2013 Oct 22. PMID: 24146336.

Perioperative Steroid Management in IBD Patients Undergoing Colorectal Surgery

9

Evan D. Adams and Karen Zaghiyan

Introduction

Perioperative management of patients with inflammatory bowel disease (IBD) is paramount to surgical success. Steroids, as potent anti-inflammatory agents, play a central role in the management of IBD symptoms and disease progression. However, chronic steroid use may suppress the hypothalamic-pituitary adrenal (HPA) axis, thereby hindering the natural physiologic stress response to surgery. This has led physicians to be wary of surgery-induced adrenal insufficiency (AI). Colorectal surgeons, therefore, must be familiar and confident with perioperative steroid management in this complex patient population.

The concept of prophylactic administration of supra-physiologic doses of glucocorticoids to prevent an Addisonian crisis arose from case reports of rapid postoperative death after uneventful surgeries in the 1950s [1, 2]. The initial cases were young patients with long term corticosteroid use for rheumatologic conditions who underwent orthopedic procedures, and subsequently developed unexplained cardiovascular collapse. At no point did these patients receive basic aspects of modern critical care including aggressive fluid resuscitation, vasoactive support, and invasive hemodynamic monitoring. At least one had their cortisone abruptly halted two days prior to operation. While no serum cortisol was drawn, the observation on autopsy of atrophied adrenal glands and/or large adrenal hemorrhages was concluded to represent a need for supra-physiologic "stress-dose" steroids to compensate for adrenal insufficiency induced by surgical stress. This practice became

E. D. Adams (✉)
Department of General Surgery, Cedars-Sinai Medical Center, Los Angeles, CA, USA
e-mail: Evan.Adams@cshs.org

K. Zaghiyan (✉)
Division of Colorectal Surgery, Cedars-Sinai Medical Center, Los Angeles, CA, USA

K. Umanskiy, N. Hyman (eds.), *Difficult Decisions in Colorectal Surgery*, Difficult Decisions in Surgery: An Evidence-Based Approach,
https://doi.org/10.1007/978-3-031-42303-1_9

widely adopted, as physicians were understandably wary of overlooking a preventable etiology of calamitous postoperative demise. Based on these anecdotal reports, stress-dose or high-dose perioperative steroids became standard practice in any steroid-dependent patient undergoing surgery.

Stress-dose steroids typically consists of hydrocortisone 100 mg intravenous (IV) preoperatively then every 8 hours postoperatively for the first 24 hours, followed by a taper down to the basal preoperative dose over the subsequent 2–3 days [3]. Current guidelines are variable, but generally recommend an individualized decision to utilize stress-dosing depending on the home dose, duration of steroid use, time since last use, and anticipated physiologic burden of the operation. However, they note the decision to stress-dose must be weighed against the negative aspects of supra-physiologic steroid administration [4–6].

While suppression of the HPA axis is known to occur with chronic steroid supplementation [7], the dosage and duration of steroid exposure required to induce suppression is unknown. Further, the duration of time to recover from HPA axis dysfunction is not known [8]. Historically, HPA axis dysfunction was speculated to persist for up to 1 year [9], thus stress-dose steroids have been recommended in patients treated with corticosteroids within the past year. However, perioperative high-dose steroids are not without consequence and have been associated with hyperglycemia, impaired wound healing, anastomotic leak, hypertension, electrolyte imbalance, immunosuppression and psychological impairments [7]. These risks are further potentiated and associated with increased perioperative morbidity if accompanied with malnutrition, advanced age, or concomitant use of immunosuppressive medications [10].

Despite the potential for AI and perioperative cardiac decompensation, a standardized preoperative evaluation algorithm for adrenal insufficiency is not established. Furthermore, the clinical significance of diagnostic tests for adrenal insufficiency is currently debated [11]. Over the past 6 decades, several large case series have been conducted in both IBD and non-IBD patients challenging the practice of stress-dose steroid administration. Recent recommendations lean towards avoiding perioperative stress-dose steroids [5, 12]. Still, there remains great variability in perioperative steroid dosing for IBD patients undergoing colorectal surgery [13]. In this chapter, we review the literature and evidence surrounding perioperative steroid dosing followed by our recommendations for steroid management in patients with IBD undergoing colorectal surgery.

Search Strategy

Relevant PICO (Population, Intervention, Comparator, Outcome) questions were generated (Table 9.1). A Medline and PubMed search was conducted for publications in the English language between January 1952 and July 2022 using the following search terms: (‘inflammatory bowel disease’ or ‘IBD’ or ‘ulcerative colitis’ or ‘Crohn’s’ or ‘organ transplant’ or ‘transplant’ or ‘steroid-treated’) and (‘corticosteroid’ or ‘steroid’) and (‘colorectal’ or ‘colorectal surgery’ or ‘surgery’ or ‘surgical’

Table 9.1 PICO questions

P (Patients)	I (Intervention)	C (Comparator)	O (Outcomes)
Steroid-treated patients with or without IBD undergoing colorectal or non-colorectal surgery	Low-dose perioperative steroids	High-dose or stress-dose perioperative steroids	Perioperative hemodynamic instability, adrenal insufficiency, morbidity, mortality, infectious complications
Patients with or without IBD, previously treated with steroids within 1 year undergoing colorectal or non-colorectal surgery	No corticosteroids	High-dose or stress-dose perioperative steroids	Perioperative hemodynamic instability, adrenal insufficiency, morbidity, mortality, infectious complications

or 'operation' or 'operative' or 'perioperative') and ('stress-dose' or 'high-dose' or 'low-dose' or 'dosing' or 'previous steroid') and ('adrenal insufficiency' or 'hemodynamic' or 'outcome' or 'complication' or 'morbidity' or 'mortality'). We additionally searched the reference section of each relevant article to identify additional articles pertaining to this topic. Retrospective and prospective, observational and randomized studies were included. Given the paucity of studies investigating IBD patients undergoing colorectal surgery, the search was expanded to include organ transplant recipients and other non-IBD steroid treated patients undergoing non-colorectal surgery.

Results

Several studies have been performed over the past 60 years to assess the clinical utility and optimal dosage of perioperative steroids in steroid-treated or steroid-dependent patients undergoing surgery (Table 9.2). The concept of reducing or omitting high-dose or stress-dose steroids in steroid-treated patients is not novel, particularly given serious concerns about surgical wound healing. In the early trials, steroid-treated patients underwent surgery without perioperative steroids and clinical parameters and HPA function were tested. In 1962, Solem and Lund reported 30 patients whose steroids were stopped more than 4 weeks before a variety of surgical procedures (IBD undergoing major colorectal surgery, n = 4) without perioperative steroid dosing and showed no severe hemodynamic collapse to suggest clinically relevant AI in any of these patients [14]. Two studies from the 1970s further investigated the consequence of perioperative steroid omission in steroid-treated patients undergoing surgery. They similarly implemented HPA axis testing and correlated them with clinical parameters and found that hypotension attributed to AI in only 4 out of 125 patients combined [15, 16]. In a series of 104 patients, Kehlet and Binder followed steroid-treated patients undergoing major and minor operations. Home-dose steroids were stopped 48 h before surgery and restarted 24 h after minor cases and 48 h after major cases. In these patients, who did not receive high-dose, stress-dose, nor any perioperative steroids, clinical adrenal insufficiency was minimal with

Table 9.2 Studies evaluating perioperative steroid dosing

First author (year)	Patients studied	Intervention	Study design	N	Outcome	Quality of evidence
Solem (1962) [14]	Patients previously treated with steroids/ various surgeries (n = 4 IBD/ CRS).	No periop steroids	R	30	No unexplained death attributed to AI	Very low
Jasani (1968) [15]	RA/anterior synovectomy	No periop steroids	PO	21 steroid-treated vs. 20 controls	1 patient with abnormal preop ACTH had hypotension responsive to steroids.	Very low
Kehlet (1973) [16]	Steroid-treated patients undergoing various major/minor operations	No periop steroids	PO	104	3 patients with hypotension and low cortisol thought to be AI	Low
Knudsen (1981) [18]	IBD/CRS	200 with no periop steroids, 50 received steroids	R	250	11 cases of hypotension treated with steroids/possible AI	Very low
Lloyd (1981) [19]	RA/ Orthopedic surgery	Stress-dose vs. usual daily dose	PO	61	No difference in periop steroid supplementation between the 2 groups	Very low
Symreng (1981) [20]	Various patients (n = 7 IBD, n = 16,CRS)	If impaired ACTH stim test>HC 25 mg IV preop then 100 mg IV/24 hrs. If normal ACTH stim test: No periop steroids. Return to usual daily dose postop	PO	14 steroid-treated patients and 8 steroid-naïve controls	No hemodynamic instability	Very low

Table 9.2 (continued)

First author (year)	Patients studied	Intervention	Study design	N	Outcome	Quality of evidence
Bromberg (1991) [22]	Renal transplant patients admitted w/ significant physiologic stress	Usual daily dose	PO	40	No unexplained hemodynamic instability	Very low
Bromberg (1995) [23]	Renal transplant patients/ various surgeries	Usual daily dose	PO	52	No clinical or laboratory evidence of adrenocortical insufficiency	Very low
Friedman (1995) [24]	Renal-transplant or RA/major orthopedic surgery	Usual daily dose	PO	28	All patients with endogenous adrenal function. No unexplained hemodynamic instability.	Very low
Glowniak (1997) [26]	Various (colorectal n = 2) with positive ACTH stim test	Stress-dose vs. placebo. Return to usual daily dose postop	RCT	18	No episodes of AI. One in each group with hypotension.	Very low
Thomason (1999) [27]	Organ transplant/ gingival surgery	Stress-dose vs. placebo. Return to usual daily dose postop	RCT	20	No hemodynamic instability	Very low
Mathis (2004) [25]	Organ transplant/ lymphocele drainage	Stress-dose vs. no steroid. Return to usual daily dose postop	R	58	No hypotension, arthralgia, ileus, mental status changes. Blood glucose higher with stress-dose	Very low
Zaghiyan (2012) [31]	IBD/CRS previously on steroids within 1 year	No periop steroids	R	49	No difference in hemodynamic instability	Low
Zaghiyan (2012) [32]	IBD/CRS	HDS vs. LDS	RO	32	No unexplained hemodynamic instability	Very low
Zaghiyan (2011) [33]	IBD/CRS	HDS vs. LDS	R	97	No difference in hemodynamic instability	Moderate

(continued)

Table 9.2 (continued)

First author (year)	Patients studied	Intervention	Study design	N	Outcome	Quality of evidence
Aytac (2013) [34]	IBD/CRS	Stress-dose vs. usual daily dose	R	235	More tachycardia with stress-dose otherwise no difference in hemodynamic instability	Moderate
Zaghiyan (2014) [36]	IBD/CRS	HDS vs. LDS	RCT	92	Non-inferiority of LDS vs. HDS with respect to postural hypotension; no difference in hemodynamic instability. More infections with HDS.	High
Ritter (2019) [35]	IBD/CRS	Stress dose with rapid IV taper vs. PO taper	R	686	Postoperative oral steroid taper associated with pelvic sepsis	Low

IBD Inflammatory bowel disease, *CRS* Colorectal Surgery, *RA* Rheumatoid arthritis, *ACTH* Adrenocorticotropic hormone, *HDS* High-dose steroids, *LDS* Low-dose steroids, *R* Retrospective, *PO* Prospective observational, *RO* Retrospective observational, *RCT* Randomized controlled trial

only 3 patients (2.8%) exhibiting unexplained hypotension and abnormal adrenocorticotropin hormone (ACTH) testing. However, each of these patients recovered spontaneously without the administration of steroids [16].

The utility and clinical relevance of preoperative ACTH testing has been an area of interest. In theory, preoperative testing could be utilized to identify potential steroid-treated patients with HPA suppression who may require perioperative steroids to prevent AI. It may also be used to identify patients whose HPA axis has recovered, thereby sparing these patients from the side effects of unnecessary steroids. In practice, the link between biochemical HPA axis suppression and clinical practice has been opaque. In a prospective study of perioperative HPA axis function, ACTH testing correlated with preoperative HPA function in 48 steroid-treated patients undergoing elective surgery (colorectal, n = 7) without perioperative steroids. While 17 of the 48 steroid-treated patients exhibited a normal response to both ACTH stimulation and postoperative HPA axis testing, none exhibited any symptoms consistent with AI or hemodynamic instability and none required steroid administration including the 31 patients with abnormal ACTH responses [17]. Thus, while normal HPA testing indicates the safety of foregoing steroids, this may still be possible in those with abnormal HPA testing.

Further studies investigated if the timing of steroids impacted the requirement for perioperative steroids. In 1981, Knudsen and colleagues performed a retrospective study evaluating 250 steroid-treated IBD patients undergoing major colorectal surgery [18]. The study included 3 groups of patients: (1) patients on steroids at the time of surgery (n = 48); (2) patients whose steroids were stopped 1 week to 2 months before surgery (n = 76); and (3) patients with steroid cessation greater than 2 months before surgery (n = 126). Intraoperative hypotension occurred in 29 patients overall (11.6%) but was less common in those furthest from steroid use (>2 months, 5.6%). In 9 patients, intraoperative rescue hydrocortisone was given, however none of these patients had biochemically proven AI. These early studies elaborated on the inconsistency between positive ACTH testing and clinically significant AI and reinforced the need for perioperative steroids in some patients, though the optimal patient cohort and steroid dose remained unclear.

Subsequent studies evaluated various perioperative steroid dosing regimens consisting of low-dose steroids or maintaining patients on their preoperative steroid dose without the addition of a stress-dose steroid. In 1981, Lloyd completed a prospective observational trial of 61 arthritic patients requiring orthopedic surgery comparing a single preoperative stress-dose of steroids (hydrocortisone 100 mg intramuscular) against omission of any stress-dose steroids [19]. They found no significant difference in the need for perioperative rescue steroids in patients treated with preoperative stress-dose steroids (24%) compared to those patients without stress dose steroids (17%). These findings provide evidence that steroid-treated patients may not require rescue medication despite receiving no stress-dose steroids. Furthermore, they showed that the physiologic requirement for perioperative steroid supplementation may be lower than expected. Further justification for low-dose perioperative steroid safety was evidenced by Symreng in a small study of 14 steroid-treated patients (IBD, n = 7) compared to 8 steroid-naïve controls undergoing various operations (major colorectal surgery, n = 16) [20]. They report that steroid-treated patients with abnormal preoperative ACTH-stimulation testing (n = 6) may be managed with low-dose steroids (hydrocortisone 15 mg IV upon induction of anesthesia followed by 100 mg IV over the next 24 h) followed by reinstitution of the preoperative dose, whereas patients with normal ACTH- stimulation testing may be managed without steroids on the day of the surgery.

In the 1990s, Shapiro and colleagues prospectively observed 13 pediatric transplant patients whose home-dose steroid regimen were either weaned or abruptly stopped before an allograft nephrectomy [21]. The range of overall steroid use was broad (range: 21 days to 5 years) and although 6 patients, had evidence of HPA-axis dysfunction on preoperative ACTH testing, no patient in the entire series developed signs or symptoms of AI. This indicates the potential for adrenal reserve regardless of immunosuppression duration. Bromberg and colleagues later performed two prospective cohort studies evaluating renal transplant recipients admitted with significant physiologic stress (n = 40) or for various operations (n = 52), both managed with continuation of their home-dose steroid dosing [22, 23]. Almost all patients had normal urinary cortisol levels and no clinical expression of hemodynamic compromise yet ACTH-stimulation testing appeared to overestimate adrenal dysfunction in a majority of patients. Friedman and colleagues prospectively evaluated 28 renal-transplant or rheumatoid arthritis patients on an average prednisone dose of

10 mg/day undergoing major orthopedic surgery [24], and similarly found that all patients had endogenous adrenal function and no episodes of clinically significant adrenal insufficiency. Further, another retrospective study of 58 pancreas and kidney transplant recipients undergoing lymphocele drainage showed no difference in hypotension, arthralgia, mental status changes, ileus, or wound healing in patients treated with stress-dose steroids or not, but patients treated with stress-dose steroids had more hyperglycemia [25].

Several years later, Glowniak and Loriaux conducted a randomized double-blind study of 18 steroid-treated patients with positive ACTH stimulation tests undergoing various surgical procedures (colorectal, n = 2) managed with either stress-dose steroids or placebo plus the patient's baseline steroid dose and observed no episodes of hypotension related to AI [26]. Their conclusion was that patients with secondary AI do not manifest symptoms consistent with cardiovascular collapse when given, at minimum, their preoperative steroid dose. Another randomized double-blind crossover study of 20 organ transplant recipients on prednisone (5–10 mg) undergoing gingival surgery, randomized to hydrocortisone 100 mg IV or placebo preoperatively during their first surgery and then then received the opposite for the second surgery, similarly observed no symptoms consistent with AI in any patients despite several cases of abnormal ACTH stimulation testing [27]. Despite obvious sample size limitations, these studies suggest that stress-doses of corticosteroids are not required even with biochemical evidence of AI, and advanced the concept that steroid-treated patients may be continued on their preoperative-dose of corticosteroids during the perioperative period despite abnormal ACTH stimulation testing without risk of clinically significant adrenal insufficiency. Multiple meta-analysis have reported safety continuing basal glucocorticoids in minor to moderate surgeries, citing a low incidence of adrenal insufficiency secondary to exogenous corticosteroid use [28, 29].

Despite increasing evidence against stress-dose steroids during the perioperative period for steroid-treated patients, colorectal surgeons managing perioperative IBD patients on high doses of preoperative steroids remained reluctant to change their practices [3, 13, 30]. Amidst a paucity of colorectal surgery-specific data, our group performed several studies comparing low-dose steroids (LDS) to high-dose steroids (HDS) in steroid-treated IBD patients undergoing major colorectal surgery. Our LDS protocol consisted of one-third of the daily preoperative steroid dose in hydrocortisone intravenous equivalents (IVED) given at the time of surgical incision followed by one-third IVED every 8 h postoperatively, followed by a taper. For patients off steroids at the time of surgery, no perioperative steroids were given. HDS entailed hydrocortisone 100 mg IV administered preoperatively followed by 100 mg IV every 8 hours postoperatively for 24 hours, then a taper to oral prednisone over 3 days. On hospital discharge, steroids were either discontinued or tapered.

In 2012, we performed a retrospective pilot study evaluating 32 steroid-treated IBD patients (10 patients on steroids up until surgery and 22 patients treated with steroids within the past year) managed with LDS [31]. Hypotension occurred in 16% of patients, but all cases resolved spontaneously with no patients requiring fluid bolus, blood transfusion, vasopressors, or high-dose corticosteroid rescue for

AI. We later compared LDS (n = 54) versus HDS (n = 43) in IBD patients who were actively receiving steroid treatment (n = 48) or who had previously received steroid treatment (n = 49) undergoing major colorectal surgery [32, 33]. For patients previously treated with steroids, median duration since last steroid dose was 4 months (range: 0.1–12 months) and median maximum steroid dose in the past year was equivalent to prednisone 25 mg/day (range: 5–60 mg/day). Aside from a higher incidence of tachycardia in patients previously treated with steroids managed with HDS [33], we found no significant difference in hemodynamic instability between the 2 patient groups and no patients required high-dose steroid rescue for AI.

Aytac and colleagues performed a large volume IBD-specific retrospective analysis of IBD patients on steroids (n = 48) compared to IBD patients off steroids (n = 187) at the time of proctocolectomy [34]. Eighty-nine patients were treated with stress-dose steroids and 146 without. There was a higher incidence of sinus tachycardia in patients managed with stress-dose steroids. While no episodes of adrenal crisis occurred, one patient in the stress-dose group was readmitted with hypotension, fatigue and bloating and diagnosed with AI. Another patient in the stress-dose group died on postoperative day 25 due to an anastomotic leak. Further underscoring the dangers of postoperative steroids, another retrospective series of IBD patients undergoing IPAA reported that compared to stress dosing with rapid IV taper, prolonged oral taper associated with an increased rate of pelvic sepsis [35].

In 2014, our group performed a prospective, randomized non-inferiority study evaluating 92 steroid-treated IBD patients undergoing major colorectal surgery randomized to HDS or LDS [36]. LDS was non-inferior to HDS with respect to our primary outcome, absence of postural hypotension on postoperative day 1, which occurred in 95% of patients randomized to HDS versus 96% of patients assigned to LDS, p = 0.007. This study included 41 patients previously treated with steroids (median duration since last steroid dose of 4 months; interquartile range: 2–6 months), of which 25 were randomized to LDS (no perioperative steroids given). There was no difference in hemodynamic instability between the 2 patient groups and no patients were treated with rescue HDS for AI. There was, however, an insignificant trend toward more infectious complications in HDS (16%) versus LDS-treated patients (4%); p = 0.11.

While current anesthesia guidelines reference the growing body of evidence against perioperative stress-dose steroid administration for patients at low-risk for HPA axis suppression, they remain conservative and continue to recommend stress-doses of up to 100 mg hydrocortisone IV for patients with documented HPA axis dysfunction by ACTH stimulation test or those at high-risk despite evidence stating otherwise [6, 37]. These recommendations reflect the 2016 Endocrine Society Clinical Practice Guidelines [38] prioritizing adrenal crisis prevention over the potential adverse effects of short-term overtreatment with stress-dose steroids. Although both societies advocate for ACTH testing, a study by Khoo provided evidence that the threshold for diagnosis of HPA axis dysfunction may be too low [39]. They trended total serum cortisol and cortisol binding protein using modern and specific immunoassays of 93 euadrenal patients undergoing surgeries of varying severity. They concluded that (1) endogenous stress cortisol responses correlated with surgery severity, (2) a downregulation of cortisol binding protein correlated with surgery, effectively increasing free and active cortisol, and (3) their minimum peak stress cortisol response was 375 nmol/L suggesting that the previous lower limit of 580 nmol/L for diagnosis hypoadrenalism needed redefinition. A recent review article and practice recommendations summarizing perioperative optimization strategies in IBD surgery, however, recommended a gradual wean off steroids in patients undergoing IBD surgery with a goal to have patients off steroids for one week before surgery [12]. If this is not possible, the authors recommended continuing the preoperative daily dose without the need for additional steroids.

Recommendations Based on Data

Based on various retrospective and observational studies and few randomized prospective studies, stress-dose steroids appear to be unnecessary and potentially harmful in IBD patients undergoing major colorectal surgery. Several studies in both IBD and non-IBD patients have suggested that steroid-treated patients can be maintained on their usual preoperative steroid dose in the perioperative period. For patients previously treated with steroids within the past year, perioperative steroids may be avoided altogether. While preoperative ACTH stimulation and perioperative plasma cortisol levels may be evaluated, these tests tend to overestimate adrenal insufficiency with a majority of patients not exhibiting clinically significant hemodynamic instability even when perioperative steroids are held altogether. Thus, a low-dose perioperative steroid protocol consisting of the patient's preoperative dose appears to not only be sufficient but may avoid complications associated with high-dose steroids. **Based on the available data, we recommend that steroid-treated IBD patients undergoing major colorectal surgery be managed with low-dose perioperative steroids equivalent to their preoperative steroid dose in the perioperative period (*evidence quality high; strong recommendation*).**

Personal View of the Data

In our view, high-dose perioperative steroids are unnecessary and likely increase perioperative risk. In our practice we maintain patients on their preoperative steroid dose in the perioperative period. Our perioperative protocol entails hydrocortisone one-third IVED given at the time of surgical incision, followed postoperatively by oral prednisone equivalent to the patient's preoperative steroid dose or in patients unable to tolerate perioperative oral medications, hydrocortisone equivalent to the preoperative steroid dose is administered followed by a taper. Preoperative HPA axis testing is likely oversensitive, does not correlate with practical physiology, and does not need to be pursued. For patients off steroids at the time of surgery, no perioperative steroids are given.

Patients are monitored closely in the perioperative period and any unexplained hemodynamic instability is followed by ACTH stimulation testing. Patients are initially managed conservatively, and high-dose steroids are added only if the patient remains unresponsive to conservative measures and ACTH stimulation testing is positive. However, in our experience no patients have required additional high-dose steroids for AI with this protocol.

References

1. Fraser CG, Preuss FS, Bigford WD. Adrenal atrophy and irreversible shock associated with cortisone therapy. J Am Med Assoc. 1952;149(17):1542–3. https://doi.org/10.1001/jama.1952.72930340001009.
2. Lewis L, Robinson RF, Yee J, Hacker LA, Eisen G. Fatal adrenal cortical insufficiency precipitated by surgery during prolonged continuous cortisone treatment. Ann Intern Med. 1953;39(1):116. https://doi.org/10.7326/0003-4819-39-1-116.
3. Hammond K, Margolin DA, Beck DE, Timmcke AE, Hicks TC, Whitlow CB. Variations in perioperative steroid management among surgical subspecialists. Am Surg. 2010;76(12):1363–7. http://www.ncbi.nlm.nih.gov/pubmed/21265350
4. Strong S, Steele SR, Boutrous M, et al. Clinical practice guideline for the surgical management of Crohn's disease. Dis Colon Rectum. 2015;58(11):1021–36. https://doi.org/10.1097/DCR.0000000000000450.
5. Bemelman WA, Warusavitarne J, Sampietro GM, et al. ECCO-ESCP consensus on surgery for Crohn's disease. J Crohns Colitis. 2018;12(1):1–16. https://doi.org/10.1093/ecco-jcc/jjx061.
6. Woodcock T, Barker P, Daniel S, et al. Guidelines for the management of glucocorticoids during the peri-operative period for patients with adrenal insufficiency: guidelines from the Association of Anaesthetists, the Royal College of Physicians and the Society for Endocrinology UK. Anaesthesia. 2020;75(5):654–63. https://doi.org/10.1111/anae.14963.
7. Stewart PM. The adrenal cortex. In: Kronenberg HM, Melmed S, Polonsky KS, Larsen PR, editors. Williams textbook of endocrinology. 11th ed; 2008. p. 445–505. https://doi.org/1841-0987, ISBN 1843-066X.
8. Coursin DB, Wood KE. Corticosteroid supplementation for adrenal insufficiency. JAMA. 2002;287(2):236–40. https://doi.org/10.1001/jama.287.2.236.
9. Lamberts SW, Bruining HA, de Jong FH. Corticosteroid therapy in severe illness. N Engl J Med. 1997;337(18):1285–92. https://doi.org/10.1056/NEJM199710303371807.
10. Beddy D, Dozois EJ, Pemberton JH. Perioperative complications in inflammatory bowel disease. Inflamm Bowel Dis. 2011;17(7):1610–9. https://doi.org/10.1002/ibd.21504.
11. Bilavsky E, Dagan A, Yarden-Bilavsky H, et al. Adrenal insufficiency during physiological stress in children after kidney or liver transplantation. Pediatr Transplant. 2011;15(3):314–20. https://doi.org/10.1111/j.1399-3046.2010.01466.x.
12. Zangenberg MS, Horesh N, Kopylov U, El-Hussuna A. Preoperative optimization of patients with inflammatory bowel disease undergoing gastrointestinal surgery: a systematic review. Int J Color Dis. 2017;32(12):1663–76. https://doi.org/10.1007/s00384-017-2915-4.
13. Lamore RF, Hechenbleikner EM, Ha C, et al. Perioperative glucocorticoid prescribing habits in patients with inflammatory bowel disease: a call for standardization. JAMA Surg. 2014;149(5):459–66. https://doi.org/10.1001/jamasurg.2013.5278.
14. Solem JH, Lund I. Prophylaxis with corticosteroids in surgical patients receiving cortisone or other steroid therapy. Acta Anaesthesiol Scand. 1962;6:99–105. https://doi.org/10.1111/j.1399-6576.1962.tb00108.x.
15. Jasani MK, Freeman PA, Boyle JA, Reid AM, Diver MJ, Buchanan WW. Studies of the rise in plasma 11-hydroxycorticosteroids (11-OHCS) in corticosteroid-treated patients with rheumatoid arthritis during surgery: correlations with the functional integrity of the hypothalamo-pituitary-adrenal axis. QJM An Int J Med. 1968;37(3):407–21. https://doi.org/10.1093/oxfordjournals.qjmed.a067151.

16. Kehlet H, Binder C. Adrenocortical function and clinical course during and after surgery in unsupplemented glucocorticoid-treated patients. Br J Anaesth. 1973;45(10):1043–8. https://doi.org/10.1093/bja/45.10.1043.
17. Kehlet H, Binder C. Value of an ACTH test in assessing hypothalamic-pituitary-adrenocortical function in glucocorticoid-treated patients. Br Med J. 1973;2(5859):147–9. https://doi.org/10.1136/bmj.2.5859.147.
18. Knudsen L, Christiansen LA, Lorentzen JE. Hypotension during and after operation in glucocorticoid-treated patients. Br J Anaesth. 1981;53(3):295–301. https://doi.org/10.1093/bja/53.3.295.
19. Lloyd EL. A rational regimen for perioperative steroid supplements and a clinical assessment of the requirement. Ann R Coll Surg Engl. 1981;63(1):54–7. http://www.ncbi.nlm.nih.gov/pubmed/7247263
20. Symreng T, Karlberg BE, Kågedal B, Schildt B. Physiological cortisol substitution of long-term steroid-treated patients undergoing major surgery. Br J Anaesth. 1981;53(9):949–54. https://doi.org/10.1093/bja/53.9.949.
21. Shapiro R, Carroll PB, Tzakis AG, Cemaj S, Lopatin WB, Nakazato P. Adrenal reserve in renal transplant recipients with cyclosporine, azathioprine, and prednisone immunosuppression. Transplantation. 1990;49(5):1011–3. https://doi.org/10.1097/00007890-199005000-00039.
22. Bromberg JS, Alfrey EJ, Barker CF, et al. Adrenal suppression and steroid supplementation in renal transplant recipients. Transplantation. 1991;51(2):385–90. https://doi.org/10.1097/00007890-199102000-00023.
23. Bromberg JS, Baliga P, Cofer JB, Rajagopalan PR, Friedman RJ. Stress steroids are not required for patients receiving a renal allograft and undergoing operation. J Am Coll Surg. 1995;180(5):532–6. http://www.ncbi.nlm.nih.gov/pubmed/7749527
24. Friedman RJ, Schiff CF, Bromberg JS. Use of supplemental steroids in patients having orthopaedic operations. J Bone Joint Surg Am. 1995;77(12):1801–6. https://doi.org/10.2106/00004623-199512000-00002.
25. Mathis AS, Shah NK, Mulgaonkar S. Stress dose steroids in renal transplant patients undergoing lymphocele surgery. Transplant Proc. 2004;36(10):3042–5. https://doi.org/10.1016/j.transproceed.2004.10.068.
26. Glowniak JV, Loriaux DL. A double-blind study of perioperative steroid requirements in secondary adrenal insufficiency. Surgery. 1997;121(2):123–9. https://doi.org/10.1016/s0039-6060(97)90280-4.
27. Thomason JM, Girdler NM, Kendall-Taylor P, Wastell H, Weddel A, Seymour RA. An investigation into the need for supplementary steroids in organ transplant patients undergoing gingival surgery. A double-blind, split-mouth, cross-over study. J Clin Periodontol. 1999;26(9):577–82. https://doi.org/10.1034/j.1600-051x.1999.260903.x.
28. de Lange DW, Kars M. Perioperative glucocorticosteroid supplementation is not supported by evidence. Eur J Intern Med. 2008;19(6):461–7. https://doi.org/10.1016/j.ejim.2007.12.004.
29. Khazen BF, El-Hussuna A. The use of a perioperative supra-physiological dose of glucocorticoid is not supported by evidence – a systematic review. Dan Med J. 2018;65(6):1–5.
30. Zaghiyan K (@KarenZaghiyanMD). How do you manage periop steroids in IBD? 29 F with UC on 20 mg prednisone for 5 months having IPAA:#colorectalsurgery #ibd. Tweet.
31. Zaghiyan K, Melmed G, Murrell Z, Fleshner P. Safety and feasibility of using low-dose perioperative intravenous steroids in inflammatory bowel disease patients undergoing major colorectal surgery: a pilot study. Surgery. 2012;152(2):158–63. https://doi.org/10.1016/j.surg.2012.02.019.
32. Zaghiyan KN, Murrell Z, Melmed GY, Fleshner PR. High-dose perioperative corticosteroids in steroid-treated patients undergoing major colorectal surgery: necessary or overkill? Am J Surg. 2012;204(4):481–6. https://doi.org/10.1016/j.amjsurg.2011.09.036.
33. Zaghiyan K, Melmed G, Murrell Z, Fleshner P. Are high-dose perioperative steroids necessary in patients undergoing colorectal surgery treated with steroid therapy within the past 12 months? Am Surg. 2011;77(10):1295–9. http://www.ncbi.nlm.nih.gov/pubmed/22127073

34. Aytac E, Londono JMR, Erem HH, Vogel JD, Costedio MM. Impact of stress dose steroids on the outcomes of restorative proctocolectomy in patients with ulcerative colitis. Dis Colon Rectum. 2013;56(11):1253–8. https://doi.org/10.1097/DCR.0b013e3182a180b7.
35. Ritter KA, Burke JP, Stocchi L, et al. Postoperative steroid taper is associated with pelvic sepsis after ileal pouch-anal anastomosis. Inflamm Bowel Dis. 2019;25(8):1383–9. https://doi.org/10.1093/ibd/izy388.
36. Zaghiyan K, Melmed GY, Berel D, Ovsepyan G, Murrell Z, Fleshner P. A prospective, randomized, noninferiority trial of steroid dosing after major colorectal surgery. Ann Surg. 2014;259(1):32–7. https://doi.org/10.1097/SLA.0b013e318297adca.
37. Liu MM, Reidy AB, Saatee S, Collard CD. Perioperative steroid management: approaches based on current evidence. Anesthesiology. 2017;127(1):166–72. https://doi.org/10.1097/ALN.0000000000001659.
38. Bornstein SR, Allolio B, Arlt W, et al. Diagnosis and treatment of primary adrenal insufficiency: an endocrine society clinical practice guideline. J Clin Endocrinol Metab. 2016;101(2):364–89. https://doi.org/10.1210/jc.2015-1710.
39. Khoo B, Boshier PR, Freethy A, et al. Redefining the stress cortisol response to surgery. Clin Endocrinol. 2017;87(5):451–8. https://doi.org/10.1111/cen.13439.

Colonic Dysplasia in Patients with Ulcerative Colitis: Endoscopic or Surgical Management?

10

Linda Ferrari and Alessandro Fichera

Introduction

Colectomy rates for acute indications in ulcerative colitis (UC) have been decreasing during the last two decades [1–4]. This is due in part to more effective medical therapy, resulting in higher remission rates. On the other hand, operative management of ulcerative colitis appears to be slowly increasing for oncological indications, as a consequence of a more chronic course of the disease [5]. Risks factors for CRC development in patients with UC are extent and duration of the disease especially with early age at diagnosis [6, 7]. As a consequence, with improved medical therapy resulting in a prolonged duration of chronic disease, the incidence of dysplasia and malignancy in UC is expected to increase [5].

Historically, the treatment UC dysplasia has been surgical. Proctocolectomy has been the traditional approach, due to the high risk of multifocality. However, in the last decade, endoscopic management has been shown to be a treatment option for early and limited dysplasia in high volume centres [8, 9]. The aim of this chapter is to present the scientific evidence in support of endoscopic and surgical approaches for UC associated colonic dysplasia.

L. Ferrari
Guy's and St Thomas' NHS Foundation Trust, London, UK

A. Fichera (✉)
Division of Colon and Rectal Surgery, Baylor University Medical Center, Dallas, TX, USA
e-mail: alessandro.fichera@bswhealth.org

K. Umanskiy, N. Hyman (eds.), *Difficult Decisions in Colorectal Surgery*, Difficult Decisions in Surgery: An Evidence-Based Approach,
https://doi.org/10.1007/978-3-031-42303-1_10

Search Strategy (PICO Table)

A comprehensive literature search of all English-language publications was done on PubMed using the following terms "dysplasia, ulcerative colitis, neoplasia, dysplasia associated mass lesion (DALM), adenoma like lesion (ALM), endoscopic submucosal dissection, inflammatory bowel disease (IBD)". The search was limited to manuscripts published between January 1st, 1980 and December 31st, 2022. All references in each manuscript identified from the PubMed search were then individually reviewed and examined for potential inclusion if appropriate.

PICO Table

Patients	Intervention	Comparator	Outcome of interest
Patients with UC and mucosal dysplasia	Endoscopic resection	Colectomy	Progression to malignancy. Disease-free and overall survival

Results

Risk Factors for Dysplasia and Cancer in Patients with Ulcerative Colitis

In contrast with sporadic colorectal cancer, colitis associated CRCs do not follow the adenoma-carcinoma sequence. Chronic inflammation is the main driver of tumorigenesis [10]. Histologic inflammation, extent and duration of disease, presence of inflammatory polyps and colonic strictures are well-known independent risk factors for colorectal dysplasia and cancer [11, 12]. Furthermore, primary sclerosing cholangitis (PSC) is a very strong risk factor for high grade dysplasia and CRC [13] in patients with UC.

Surveillance Strategies and Techniques

Surveillance colonoscopy should be routinely performed in patients with UC. European and British guidelines stratify patients in one of three risk categories (high, intermediate, or low risk group) with surveillance intervals ranging from annually to every five years [14, 15] (Fig. 10.1). American guidelines recommend surveillance every 1–3 years considering the presence of risk factors when planning the next surveillance interval [16]. Across the board all guidelines recommend annual surveillance in patients with PSC, due to the high neoplastic risk [14–16].

Current guidelines [14–16] advocate the use of chromoendoscopy for surveillance. Superiority of high-definition chromoendoscopy to high-definition white-light endoscopy has been reported in a recent randomised controlled trial from Sweden [17]. However, high definition endoscopy is considered a less time

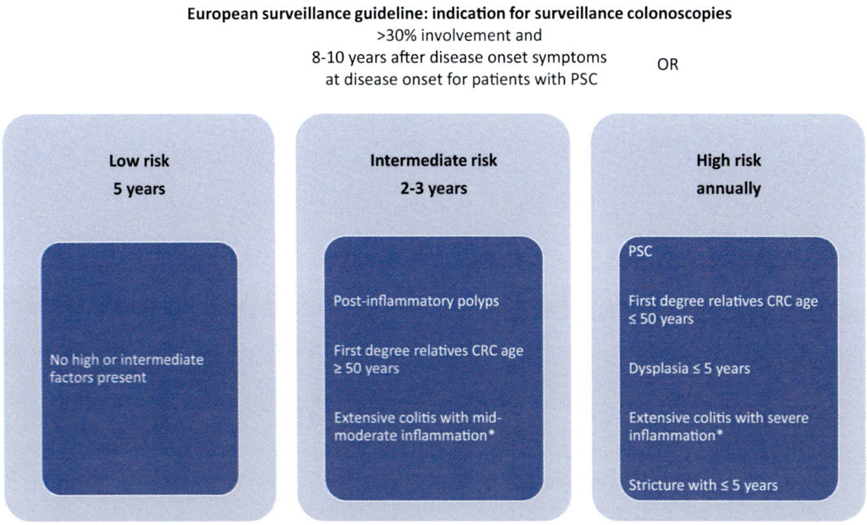

Fig. 10.1 Surveillance strategy adapted from of the European Crohn's and Colitis Organisation (ECCO) [14]. *Presence of inflammation is based on endoscopic or histologic inflammation. *CRC* Colorectal cancer, *PSC* Primary sclerosing cholangitis

consuming and a good alternative to chromoendoscopy [16] with similar dysplasia detection rates. As a consequence, the utility of random biopsies, four quadrant every ten centimetres, has been questioned with the use of high definition endoscopy systems [8]. Non-inferiority in neoplastic detection was reported for surveillance using only targeted biopsies vs targeted and random biopsies in a randomised controlled trail [18]. The added value of random biopsies is higher in patients with concomitant PSC (3.7% per colonoscopy and 0.3% per biopsy) [17–19], previous dysplasia or tubular appearing colon [19].

Classification of UC Associated Dysplasia

Diagnosis of colorectal dysplasia and cancer in patients with UC should be confirmed by two pathologists, with expertise in the field of inflammatory bowel disease [8, 14–16] due to the high level of interobserver variability for low grade dysplasia and indefinite dysplasia, especially when inflammation is present.

Dysplasia, in patients with UC, can be visible or invisible. Invisible is detected on random biopsies. According to the Scenic Consensus statement [8], visible dysplasia can be polypoid (pedunculated or sessile), non polypoid (superficial elevated, flat or depressed). Other general descriptors are presence of ulceration and assessment of borders (distinct or indistinct) [8]. Microscopically, dysplasia is also graded and ranges between mild or low grade dysplasia (LGD) to high grade dysplasia (HGD) based on the cellular and nuclear orientation changes.

According to SCENIC consensus, and endoscopically resectable lesion indicates that (1) distinct margins of the lesion could be identified, (2) the lesion appears to be completely removed on visual inspection after endoscopic resection, (3) histologic examination of the resected specimen is consistent with complete removal, and (4) biopsy specimens taken from mucosa immediately adjacent to the resection site are free of dysplasia on histologic examination.

Management of Colonic Dysplasia

Until recently, international guidelines recommended total proctocolectomy for UC patients with colorectal dysplasia [8, 14–16]. Reason behind this is the possible risk of synchronous dysplasia in the setting of long-standing extensive disease. However, there is increased evidence supporting the use of endoscopic treatment of these lesions [21–28].

For invisible dysplasia detected in random biopsies, current guidelines recommend strict surveillance by IBD endoscopists [8]. For visible dysplasia, different endoscopic and surgical options are currently available, and final decision should be made weighting grade of dysplasia, unifocal or multifocal lesions and also patient characteristics (age, comorbidities, etc.) and preferences. If visible lesions are considered suitable for endoscopic resection, first decision to be made is which technique to used. This depends on several factors: lesion size, shape, site, surface and surrounding area (known as Five "s"), risk of invasion and endoscopic accessibility [8, 29].

Small polypoid or flat lesions can be removed with simple endoscopic snare technique. For larger lesions, endoscopic mucosal resection (EMR) should be considered. This involves lifting the lesion from the muscularis propria using submucosal injection with saline to perform complete excision of the lesion. Furthermore, endoscopic submucosal dissection (ESD) should be considered for lesions larger than 20 mm, especially if they are non-polypoid or if high grade dysplasia is present. ESD allows the lesion to be lifted deeper, at the level of muscularis propria, where the lesion can be dissected. ESD has several advantages: high en block resection rate and radical (R0) resections with a relatively low risk of adverse events such as bleeding or perforation [27].

Endoscopic Submucosal Dissection (ESD)

UC patients are at increased risk of developing colorectal cancer (CRC) through the inflammation-dysplasia-carcinoma sequence. For this reason, early identification and treatment of dysplastic lesions can potentially reduce the risk of CRC. Data to support the use of endoscopic submucosal dissection (ESD) for UC associated dysplastic lesions have been collected mainly during the last eight years [22–28] (Table 10.1). Manta et al. [27] pulled together data from seven independent international research collaborations [21–27]. By cumulative analysis, there were a total of

Table 10.1 ESD to treat dysplasia in patients with ulcerative colitis

Study, year and country	UC patients	Outcomes	Dysplasia during follow-up assessment	Quality of evidence
Smith LA (2008) [21] UK	69 UC patients	En bloc resection 78%. R0 resection 94% after en bloc resection.	Median follow-up 18 months. 0 metachronous lesions or cancer. 98% cure for ESD-assisted EMR	Moderate
Iacopini F (2015) [22] Italy/Japan	9 UC patients	En block resection 80%. R0 resection 70%.	Median follow-up 24 months. 0 local recurrence 0 metachronous dysplasia.	Moderate
Suzuki N (2017) [23] UK/Japan	32 UC patients	En bloc resection 91%. R0 resection 72%.	Median follow-up 33 months. 4% local recurrence. 9% metachronous dysplasia.	Moderate
Kinoshita S (2018) [24] Japan	25 UC patients in clinical remission (Mayo total score < 2)	En block resection 100%. R0 resection 76%.	Median follow-up 21 months. 0 local recurrence. 4% metachronous HGD. Patient underwent a proctocolectomy. No cancer progression.	Moderate
Yang DH et al. (2019) [25] Korea	15 UC patients.	En block resection 93.3%. R0 resection 80%.	Median follow-up 24.7 months. 14% local recurrence. 14% metachronous recurrence. No cancer progression.	Moderate
Matsumoto K (2019) [26] Japan	17 UC patients. 7 underwent ESD and 10 total proctocolectomy.	En block resection 100%. R0 resection 86%	Median follow-up 21 months. 0 local recurrence. 71% metachronous recurrence	Moderate
Manta R et al. (2021) [27] Italy	53 UC patients	En block resection 100%. R0 resection 96.2%.	Median follow-up 27 months. 0 local recurrence. 3.7% metachronous recurrence. Both patients underwent surgery. No cancer progression.	Moderate
Kasuga K (2021) [28] Japan	17 UC patients. 9 underwent ESD. 8 subtotal colectomy.	En bloc resection 91%. R0 resections 82%.	Median follow-up 25 months. 0 local recurrence. 22% metachronous recurrence. Both patients underwent definitive ESD.	Moderate

208 patients with 216 treated lesions. There was a slight prevalence of males [M/F = 1.39] with a median age of >60 years, and there was a 59.6% prevalence of extensive colitis. The median duration disease ranged from 7 to 20 years [27].

In total, en bloc resection was successfully performed in 191 ESD procedures, corresponding to 88.4% of 216 lesions and 91.8% of 208 patients. R0 resection was achieved in 169 ESDs, equivalent to a 78.2% of lesions and 81.3% of patients. According to the operator, en bloc resection and R0, respectively, were achieved in 113 (86.9%) and 107 (82.3%) of 130 lesions treated by European endoscopists, and in 78 (92.9%) and 62 (73.8%) of 84 lesions treated by Asian endoscopists, without a statistically significant difference between groups. The median diameter of removed lesions in the different studies varied from 15 to 35 mm (range: 8–73). Submucosal fibrosis was detected in 104 (77.1%) of 135 lesions. The overall rate of complications was 9.6%, including 6.7% bleedings and 2.9% perforations, all managed endoscopically. At follow-up, recurrence was observed in only eight (3.8%) patients, and a metachronous lesion developed in 13 (6.2%) cases.

Data from the above studies [21–28] shows that ESD is a safe technique to remove non-invasive lesions in UC patients. It should be performed in selected high-volume centers, where appropriate long-term follow-up can be offered.

Surgical management of Colonic Dysplasia

Historically, surgery has been the treatment of choice for low and high grade dysplasia in patients with UC [20, 31–44]. Several series have been published, most of them retrospective, single institution and with limited numbers. Summary of the existing evidence from the literature is presented in Table 10.2.

With the recent data on ESD, surgery should be reserved for endoscopically unresectable lesions, invisible high grade dysplasia and high-risk colons, when strictures are present and surveillance might be difficult [8, 30]. When surgery is indicated, a total proctocolectomy is indicated in case of HGD or CRC to reduce overall risk of dysplasia and cancer.

Although patients with LGD have been considered at limited risk for cancer development, there are evidence that certain endoscopic characteristics are associated with increased risk of progression. Choi et al. [44] looked at risk factors for progression of LGD to HGD or CRC. In 172 patients that were followed for a median of 48 months, 21 had immediate colectomy and 152 only surveillance endoscopy. On multivariate analysis, factors associated with significant risk of HGD and CRC were: macroscopically non-polypoid dysplasia ($P < 0.001$) or invisible dysplasia ($P = 0.02$), dysplastic lesions ≥1 cm in size ($P = 0.01$), and a previous history of "indefinite for dysplasia" ($P = 0.01$). The cumulative incidence of HGD or CRC at 1 and 5 years after detection of LGD was 0% and 1.8% in patients with no risk factors, 9.6% and 17.7% with one risk factor and 29.0% and 53.4% for two risk factors. For those with three risk factors, cumulative risk of HGD or CRC development was 61.6% and 80.7% at 1 and 2 years, respectively. This important study identified endoscopic findings as prognostic factors that should be considered

Table 10.2 Surgical management for colonic dysplasia

Study and year of publication	Sample size	Dysplasia during FU	Quality of evidence
Blackstone MO (1981) [20]	112 long-standing UC patients FU: 4 years	Dysplasia in 12 patients. 7 developed CRC. Only 2 patients with CRC had HGD	Low
Woolrich AJ (1992) [31]	121 UC patients FU >7 years	Dysplasia or CRC in 27 patients (22%) Mean FU: 16 years.	Moderate
Provenzale D (1995) [32]	Computer generated population of 10,000, 30 year old UC patients with pancolitis for over 10 years	Prophylactic colectomy increased life expectancy by 2–10 months vs surveillance and 1.1–1.4 years vs no surveillance. Yearly surveillance for LGD increased life expectancy by up to 1.2 years vs no surveillance.	Poor
Befrits R (2002) [33]	60 UC patients with flat LGD FU: 10 years	LGD at index colonoscopy in 16 (26%) patients. 73% had LGD in subsequent colonoscopies.	Moderate
Ulmann T (2002) [34]	18 UC patients with flat LGD Median FU:32 months	50% developed advanced neoplasia. Incidences of progression was 13% at 1 year, 26% at 2 years and 33% at 5 years.	Mod-low
Ullman T (2003) [35]	46 UC patients with flat LGD Median FU: 15 months. 11 colectomy. 21 surveillance	19 had LGD and 2 HGD at study end 14 of the 46 progressed to advanced neoplasia (median time progression 25 months)	High-mod
Jess T (2006) [36]	29 IBD patients including Crohn's disease. Median FU:17.8 years	Among 6 patients with flat LGD, who did not undergo colectomy, none progressed to CRC. Median FU:17.8 years.	Mod-low
Lim CH (2003) [37]	128 UC patients >8 years	29 patients had LGD, and 97 no dysplasia (controls). FU: 10 years. HGD or CRC in 3/29 (10%) LGD patients vs 4/97 controls (4.0%).	Low
Rutter MD (2006) [38]	600 UC patients. Median FU: 8.5 years	74 patients (12.3%) developed neoplasia, including 30 CRC. Incidence of CRC was 2.5% at 20 years, 7.6% at 30 years, and 10.8% at 40 years.	Moderate
Pekow JR (2010) [39]	28 UC patients with LGD Median FU: 50 months	1 flat LGD progressed to HGD and 1 polypoid LGD progressed to CRC	Moderate
Goldstone R (2011) [40]	121 UC patients with extensive disease >7 years and LGH Median FU: 37 months	In total, 7 patients who progressed to CRC and 6 of 8 who progressed to HGD had distal LGD initially. Interval for progression was shorter for patients with distal vs proximal LGD.	Moderate

(continued)

Table 10.2 (continued)

Study and year of publication	Sample size	Dysplasia during FU	Quality of evidence
Stolwijk JA (2013) [41]	293 UC patients with UC >8 years. FU at 10 and 15 years	FU 10 years. Incidence of any dysplasia was 23.5%, and of CRC 4.0%. FU 15 years. 33.3% and 6.8% respectively.	Moderate
Zisman TL (2012) [42]	42 UC patients with pancolitis ≥8 years and LGD Mean FU: 3.9 years	19% (8/42) of patients progressed to advanced neoplasia (two cancer, six HGD) while 17% (7/42) had persistent LGD and 64% (27/42) indefinite dysplasia or no dysplasia	High-moderate
Wanders LK (2014) [43]	Meta-analysis 376 UC patients with polypoid dysplasia, FU: 1000 years	Pooled CRC and HGD rates were 6.7 and 9 per thousand years of patient follow-up. Longer study duration did not correlate with advanced neoplasia rates.	High
Choi CH (2015) [44] UK	172 UC patients with extensive disease and LGD 21 colectomy 152 surveillance	FU: 48 months 13% and 8.6% of patients developed HGD and CRC respectively.	High-moderate
Fumery M (2017) [45]	Meta-analysis. 671 UC patients with LGD	Annual incidence of advanced neoplasia 1.8%. Annual incidence of CRC 0.8%. High risk features associated with dysplasia progression: PSC, invisible dysplasia, distal location, and multifocal LGD.	High

UC ulcerative colitis, *FU* follow up, *LGD* low grade dysplasia, *CRC* colorectal cancer, *HGD* high grade dysplasia

to properly select patients for surgical intervention rather than just using the degree for dysplasia.

A meta-analysis including 14 surveillance cohort studies collected data on 671 patients with UC-LGD (52 developed CRC) [45]. The pooled annual incidence of CRC was 0.8% (95% CI, 0.4–1.3); the pooled annual incidence of advanced neoplasia was 1.8% (95% CI, 0.9–2.7). Factors significantly associated with dysplasia progression were concomitant primary sclerosing cholangitis (OR, 3.4; 95% CI, 1.5–7.8), invisible dysplasia (vs visible dysplasia; OR, 1.9; 95% CI, 1.0–3.4), distal location (vs proximal location; OR, 2.0; 95% CI, 1.1–3.7) and multifocal dysplasia (vs unifocal dysplasia; OR, 3.5; 95% CI, 1.5–8.5). In 12 surgical cohort studies of 450 patients who underwent colectomy for UC-LGD, 34 patients had synchronous CRC (pooled prevalence, 17%; 95% CI, 8–33) [45].

Although LGD has been considered not an absolute indications for surgical management, different endoscopic parameters should be considered to identify individual risk of progression in UC patients. Long term outcomes data on endoscopic vs surgical management of dysplasia in UC are needed to understand when to perform endoscopic treatment versus radical surgical treatment. While surgery is definitive treatment for patients with UC with oncologic implications, total proctocolectomy is associated with 1% risk of perioperative mortality and long term changes in urinary, sexual and defecatory function with significant impact on quality of life [46].

Recommendations Based on the Data

UC patients with dysplasia should be managed in a multi-disciplinary setting, including IBD gastroenterologist, advanced endoscopist, pathologist and an IBD surgeon.

Most visible dysplastic lesions are amenable to endoscopic resection which should be performed by advanced endoscopists with expertise in EMR and ESD [47], with the aim to achieve an en bloc resection with negative margins to reduce the risks of recurrence [48]. For lesions larger than 20 mm, or where EMR is unlikely to be successful in achieving an en bloc resection, ESD is a valid alternative [47]. However, ESD of dysplastic lesions has additional procedural risks quantified as 6.7% major bleeding rate and 2.9% perforation rate [27], that are usually managed successfully at the time of endoscopy.

If endoscopic resection of the all dysplastic lesions present is successful, and there is no dysplastic change in the flat mucosa surrounding the lesion(s), these patients should undergo regular endoscopic surveillance, due to low risk of CRC after complete endoscopic resection of dysplasia [49–50]. If histology confirms <1 cm polypoid LGD lesions, the next surveillance colonoscopy can be performed at 1 year. For HGD lesions, endoscopic resection is efficacious, although their presence is associated with risk of synchronous CRC of 15% [51] and for this reason a re-examination of the resection site for dysplastic recurrence should be undertaken after 3–6 months.

If the resected lesions have features of submucosal invasion, or contain significant submucosal fibrosis limiting endoscopic resection (including irregular surface architecture, mucosal depression, radiating folds or failure to lift with submucosal injection) en block resection is difficult to be achieved and these patients should be considered for a colectomy. Figure 10.2 summarises our current clinical approach to the management of visible colitis-associated dysplasia.

If invisible dysplasia is detected, then a repeat high-definition chromoendoscopy in an optimally-prepared patient should be performed by an experienced endoscopist. Invisible LGD is an independent predictor of long-term progression to advanced neoplasia in multivariate analyses (two to three-fold increased risk) [45, 50]. Invisible HGD is an indication for colectomy due to the high associated CRC risk [52].

When surgery is advocated, total proctocolectomy is the preferred surgical approach, due to multifocal risk of cancer. The role of segmental colectomy or

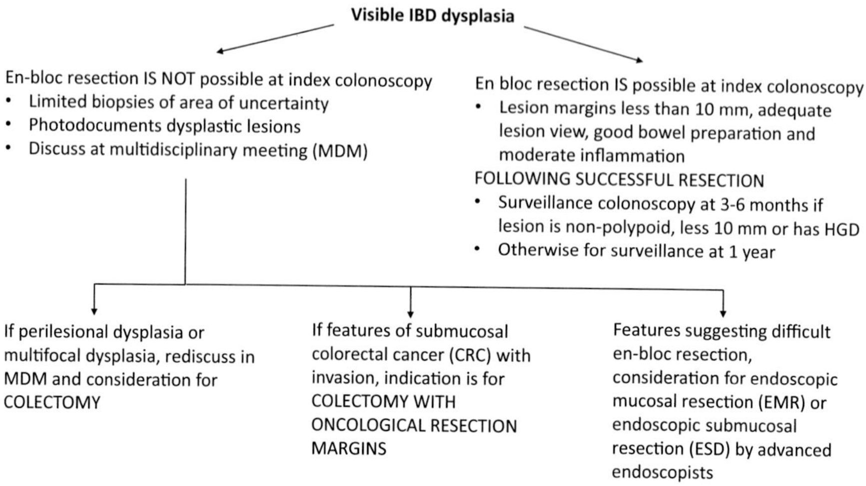

Fig. 10.2 Flowchart of the management of visible colitis-associated dysplastic lesions

rectum sparing surgery in patients with UC and dysplasia remains controversial due to the high rates of synchronous and metachronous neoplasia.

A Personal View of the Data

Colorectal cancer progression remains an area of concern in patient with UC and it is considered the most feared complication in patients with long standing colitis. Combining the aging population of UC patients with improved endoscopic techniques and increased use of medical treatment, dysplasia detection rates by experienced endoscopist can exceed 10% [53].

As previously mentioned, a multidisciplinary approach to LGD and HGD is advocated with involvement of expert IBD gastroenterologist, interventional endoscopist, IBD pathologist and IBD surgeon. Patients should be counselled about risk of metachronous neoplasia despite continuous surveillance and successful endoscopic resection. Patients should receive information about lesion-specific and patient- specific risk factors.

Dysplasia features associated with higher rates of progression to CRC comprise histologically-confirmed HGD, multifocality, invisible dysplasia, large (≥10 mm) lesion size, and non-polypoid morphology [44, 45, 54]. Patient-specific risk factors include presence of PSC, previous dysplasia, significant uncontrolled mucosal inflammation, limitations to adequate mucosal assessment (e.g. colonic stricturing or pseudopolyposis) and a family history of CRC [54]. Fumery et al. [45],in their systematic review, found that among patients with UC associated LGD under surveillance, the annual incidence of progression to CRC was 0.8%/ Concomitant primary sclerosing cholangitis, invisible dysplasia, distal location, and multifocal LGD are high-risk features associated with dysplasia progression [45]. All these risks factors should be discussed with the patient who is enrolled in a surveillance program, considering that for UC, total proctocolectomy is curative, making the patient in a position to avoid future medical treatment and their side effects. This is even more relevant in patients with more than one risk factor considering that neoplasia risk increases cumulatively in the presence of multiple risk factors [44].

Patients with well controlled disease might be reluctant to accept risks of prophylactic total proctocolectomy, with the associated changes in the quality of life. After multidisciplinary discussion and patient education a share decision approach should be applied to finalize recommendations.

References

1. Manetti N, Bagnoli S, Rogai F, Bonanomi AG, Vannozzi G, Giannotta M, Annese V. Disease course and colectomy rate of ulcerative colitis: a follow-up cohort study of a referral center in Tuscany. Inflamm Bowel Dis. 2016;22(8):1945–53.
2. Kaplan GG, Seow CH, Ghosh S, Molodecky N, Rezaie A, Moran GW, Proulx MC, Hubbard J, MacLean A, Buie D, Panaccione R. Decreasing colectomy rates for ulcerative colitis: a population based time trend study. Am J Gastroenterol. 2012;107(12):1879–87.
3. Parragi L, Fournier N, Zeitz J, Scharl M, Greuter T, Schreiner P, Misselwitz B, Safroneeva E, Schoepfer AM, Vavricka SR, Rogler G, Biedermann L, Swiss IBD Cohort Study Group. Colectomy rates in ulcerative colitis are low and decreasing: 10-year followup data from the Swiss IBD cohort study. J Crohn's Colitis. 2018;12(7):811–8.
4. Barnes EL, Jiang Y, Kappelman MD, Long MD, Sandler RS, Kinlaw AC, Herfarth HH (in press). Decreasing Colectomy Rate for Ulcerative Colitis in the United States Between 2007 and 2016: a time trend analysis. Inflamm Bowel Dis 2019; https://doi.org/10.1093/ibd/izz247.
5. Ni A, Al-Qahtani M, Salama E, Marinescu D, Khalil MA, Faria J, Morin N, Ghitulescu G, Vasilevsky CA, Boutros M. Trends in colectomies for colorectal neoplasms in ulcerative colitis: a National Inpatient Sample Database Analysis over two decades. J Gastrointest Surg. 2020 Aug;24(8):1721–8.
6. Dulai PS, Sandborn WJ, Gupta S. Colorectal cancer and dysplasia in inflammatory bowel disease: a review of disease epidemiology, pathophysiology, and management. Cancer Prev Res. 2016;9(12):887–94.
7. Fumery M, Singh S, Dulai PS, Gower-Rousseau C, Peyrin-Biroulet L, Sandborn WJ. Natural history of adult ulcerative colitis in population-based cohorts: a systematic review. Clin Gastroenterol Hepatol. 2018;16(3):343–56.
8. Laine L, Kaltenbach T, Barkun A, McQuaid KR, Subramanian V, Soetikno R. SCENIC Guideline Development Panel. SCENIC international consensus statement on surveillance and management of dysplasia in inflammatory bowel disease. Gastroenterology. 2015;148(3):639–51.
9. Wijnands AM, Mahmoud R, Lutgens MWMD, Oldenburg B. Surveillance and management of colorectal dysplasia and cancer in inflammatory bowel disease: current practice and future perspectives. Eur J Intern Med. 2021 Nov;93:35–41.
10. Itzkowitz SH. Molecular biology of dysplasia and cancer in inflammatory bowel disease. Gastroenterol Clin N Am. 2006;35:553–71.
11. Choi CR, Al Bakir I, Ding NJ, et al. Cumulative burden of inflammation predicts colorectal neoplasia risk in ulcerative colitis: a large single-centre study. Gut. 2019;68:414–22.
12. Wijnands AM, de Jong ME, Lutgens M, et al. Prognostic factors for advanced colorectal neoplasia in inflammatory bowel disease: systematic review and meta-analysis. Gastroenterology. 2021;160:1584–98.
13. Lazaridis KN, LaRusso NF. Primary sclerosing cholangitis. N Engl J Med. 2016;375:1161–70.
14. Maaser C, Sturm A, Vavricka SR, et al. ECCO-ESGAR guideline for diagnostic assessment in IBD Part 1: initial diagnosis, monitoring of known IBD, detection of complications. J Crohns Colitis. 2019;13:144–64.

15. Lamb CA, Kennedy NA, Raine T, et al. British Society of Gastroenterology consensus guidelines on the management of inflammatory bowel disease in adults. Gut. 2019;68:s1–106.
16. Rubin DT, Ananthakrishnan AN, Siegel CA, et al. ACG clinical guideline: ulcerative colitis in adults. Am J Gastroenterol. 2019;114:384–413.
17. Alexandersson B, Hamad Y, Andreasson A, et al. High-definition chromoendoscopy superior to high-definition white-light endoscopy in surveillance of inflammatory bowel diseases in a randomized trial. Clin Gastroenterol Hepatol. 2020;18:2101–7.
18. Watanabe T, Ajioka Y, Mitsuyama K, et al. Comparison of targeted vs random biopsies for surveillance of ulcerative colitis-associated colorectal cancer. Gastroenterology. 2016;151:1122–30.
19. Moussata D, Allez M, Cazals-Hatem D, et al. Are random biopsies still useful for the detection of neoplasia in patients with IBD undergoing surveillance colonoscopy with chromoendoscopy? Gut 2018;67:616–624.
20. Blackstone MO, Riddell RH, Rogers BHG, Levin B. Dysplasia-associated lesion or mass (DALM) detected by colonoscopy in long-standing ulcerative-colitis – an indication for colectomy. Gastroenterology. 1981;80:366–74.
21. Smith LA, Baraza W, Tiffin N, Cross SS, Hurlstone DP. Endoscopic resection of adenoma-like mass in chronic ulcerative colitis using a combined endoscopic mucosal resection and cap assisted submucosal dissection technique. Inflamm Bowel Dis. 2008;14:1380–6.
22. Iacopini F, Saito Y, Yamada M, et al. Curative endoscopic submucosal dissection of large nonpolypoid superficial neoplasms in ulcerative colitis (with videos). Gastrointest Endosc. 2015;82:734–8.
23. Suzuki N, Toyonaga T, East JE. Endoscopic submucosal dissection of colitis-related dysplasia. Endoscopy. 2017;49:1237–42.
24. Kinoshita S, Uraoka T, Nishizawa T, Naganuma M, Iwao Y, Ochiai Y, Fujimoto A, Goto O, Shimoda M, Ogata H, Kanai T, Yahagi N. The role of colorectal endoscopic submucosal dissection in patients with ulcerative colitis. Gastrointest Endosc. 2018 Apr;87(4):1079–84.
25. Yang DH, Kim J, Song EM, Chang K, Lee SH, Hwang SW, Park SH, Ye BD, Byeon JS, Myung SJ, Yang SK. Outcomes of ulcerative colitis-associated dysplasia patients referred for potential endoscopic submucosal dissection. J Gastroenterol Hepatol. 2019 Sep;34(9):1581–9.
26. Matsumoto K, Oka S, Tanaka S, et al. Long-term outcomes after endoscopic submucosal dissection for ulcerative colitis-associated dysplasia. Digestion. 2021;102(2):205–15.
27. Manta R, Zullo A, Telesca DA, Castellani D, Germani U, Reggiani Bonetti L, Conigliaro R, Galloro G. Endoscopic submucosal dissection for visible dysplasia treatment in ulcerative colitis patients: cases series and systematic review of literature. J Crohns Colitis. 2021 Jan 13;15(1):165–8.
28. Kasuga K, Yamada M, Shida D, Tagawa T, Takamaru H, Sekiguchi M, Sakamoto T, Uraoka T, Sekine S, Kanemitsu Y, Saito Y, Kasuga K, et al. United European. Gastroenterol J. 2021 Oct;9(8):964–72. https://doi.org/10.1002/ueg2.12118.
29. Adamina M, Feakins R, Iacucci M, et al. ECCO topical review optimising reporting in surgery, endoscopy, and histopathology. J Crohns Colitis. 2021;15:1089.
30. Oresland T, Bemelman WA, Sampietro GM, et al. European evidence based consensus on surgery for ulcerative colitis. J Crohns Colitis. 2015;9:4–25.
31. Woolrich AJ, DaSilva MD, Korelitz BI. Surveillance in the routine management of ulcerative colitis: the predictive value of low-grade dysplasia. Gastroenterology. 1992;103:431–8.
32. Provenzale D, Kowdley KV, Arora S, Wong JB. Prophylactic colectomy or surveillance for chronic ulcerative colitis? A decision analysis. Gastroenterology. 1995;109:1188–96.
33. Befrits R, Ljung T, Jaramillo E, Rubio C. Low-grade dysplasia in extensive, long-standing inflammatory bowel disease: a follow-up study. Dis Colon Rectum. 2002;45:615–20.
34. Ullman TA, Loftus EV Jr, Kakar S, Burgart LJ, Sandborn WJ, Tremaine WJ. The fate of low grade dysplasia in ulcerative colitis. Am J Gastroenterol. 2002;97:922–7.
35. Ullman T, Croog V, Harpaz N, Sachar D, Itzkowitz S. Progression of flat low-grade dysplasia to advanced neoplasia in patients with ulcerative colitis. Gastroenterology. 2003;125:1311–9.
36. Jess T, Loftus EV Jr, Velayos FS, et al. Incidence and prognosis of colorectal dysplasia in inflammatory bowel disease: a population-based study from Olmsted County, Minnesota. Inflamm Bowel Dis. 2006;12:669–76.

37. Lim CH, Dixon MF, Vail A, Forman D, Lynch DA, Axon AT. Ten year follow up of ulcerative colitis patients with and without low grade dysplasia. Gut. 2003;52:1127–32.
38. Rutter MD, Saunders BP, Wilkinson KH, et al. Thirty-year analysis of a colonoscopic surveillance program for neoplasia in ulcerative colitis. Gastroenterology. 2006;130:1030–8.
39. Pekow JR, Hetzel JT, Rothe JA, et al. Outcome after surveillance of low-grade and indefinite dysplasia in patients with ulcerative colitis. Inflamm Bowel Dis. 2010;16:1352–6.
40. Goldstone R, Itzkowitz S, Harpaz N, Ullman T. Progression of low-grade dysplasia in ulcerative colitis: effect of colonic location. Gastrointest Endosc. 2011;74:1087–93.
41. Stolwijk JA, Langers AM, Hardwick JC, et al. A thirty-year follow-up surveillance study for neoplasia of a Dutch ulcerative colitis cohort. Sci World J. 2013;2013:274715.
42. Zisman TL, Bronner MP, Rulyak S, et al. Prospective study of the progression of low-grade dysplasia in ulcerative colitis using current cancer surveillance guidelines. Inflamm Bowel Dis. 2012;18:2240–6.
43. Wanders LK, Dekker E, Pullens B, Bassett P, Travis SP, East JE. Cancer risk after resection of polypoid dysplasia in patients with longstanding ulcerative colitis: a meta-analysis. Clin Gastroenterol Hepatol. 2014;12:756–64.
44. Choi CH, Ignjatovic-Wilson A, Askari A, et al. Low-grade dysplasia in ulcerative colitis: risk factors for developing high-grade dysplasia or colorectal cancer. Am J Gastroenterol. 2015;110:1461–71.
45. Fumery M, Dulai PS, Gupta S, Prokop LJ, Ramamoorthy S, Sandborn WJ, et al. Incidence, risk factors, and outcomes of colorectal cancer in patients with ulcerative colitis with low-grade dysplasia: a systematic review and meta-analysis. Clin Gastroenterol Hepatol. 2017;15(5):665–74.e5.
46. Peyrin-Biroulet L, Germain A, Patel AS, et al. Systematic review: outcomes and post-operative complications following colectomy for ulcerative colitis. Aliment Pharmacol Ther. 2016;44:807–16.
47. Soetikno R, East J, Suzuki N, Uedo N, Matsumoto T, Watanabe K, et al. Endoscopic submucosal dissection for nonpolypoid colorectal dysplasia in patients with inflammatory bowel disease: in medias res. Gastrointest Endosc. 2018;87(4):1085–94.
48. Alkandari A, Thayalasekaran S, Bhandari M, Przybysz A, Bugajski M, Bassett P, et al. Endoscopic resections in inflammatory bowel disease: a multicentre European outcomes study. J Crohns Colitis. 2019;13(11):1394–400.
49. Cremer A, Demetter P, De Vos M, Rahier JF, Baert F, Moreels T, et al. Risk of development of more-advanced lesions in patients with inflammatory bowel diseases and dysplasia. Clin Gastroenterol Hepatol. 2020;18(7):1528–36.e5.
50. Curtius K, Kabir M, Al Bakir I, Choi CHR, Hartono JL, Johnson M, et al. Multicentre derivation and validation of a colitis-associated colorectal cancer risk prediction web tool. Gut. 2022;71(4):705–15.
51. Kabir M, Fofaria R, Arebi N, Bassett P, Tozer PJ, Hart AL, et al. Systematic review with meta-analysis: IBD-associated colonic dysplasia prognosis in the videoendoscopic era (1990 to present). Aliment Pharmacol Ther. 2020;52(1):5–19.
52. Lightner AL, Vogler S, McMichael J, Jia X, Regueiro M, Qazi T, et al. Dysplastic progression to adenocarcinoma is equivalent in ulcerative colitis and Crohn's disease. J Crohns Colitis. 2021;15(1):24–34.
53. Dekker E, Houwen BBSL, Puig I, Bustamante-Balén M, Coron E, Dobru DE, et al. Curriculum for optical diagnosis training in Europe: European Society of Gastrointestinal Endoscopy (ESGE) position statement. Endoscopy. 2020;52(10):899–923.
54. Yalchin M, Baker AM, Graham TA, Hart A. Predicting colorectal cancer occurrence in IBD. Cancers. 2021;13(12):2908.

11 Which Patients Benefit from Biologic Agents to Prevent Disease Recurrence After Resection in Crohn's Disease?

Yusuke Miyatani and Atsushi Sakuraba

Introduction

Crohn's disease is a chronic inflammatory condition that affects the entire digestive tract, resulting in bowel damage such as stricture, fistula, and perforation [3]. Up to 80% of patients experience surgery in their lifetime, of which approximately one-quarter require a second surgery, often within 5 years of their previous surgery [4]. Endoscopic recurrence occurred in about 70% of patients within one year after surgery, which precedes clinical recurrence [5].

On the other hand, the introduction of novel immunosuppressive therapies had dramatically changed treatment strategies for Crohn's disease. Biologics are also deemed effective in preventing recurrence following surgery [1], which has reduced the rate of reoperation in a cohort study [2]. However, biologics carry risks of adverse effects and can be of financial burden both on patients and health care economics. Therefore, individualized evaluations and treatment plans organized by multidisciplinary team between surgeons and gastroenterologists are imperative to reduce the risk of postoperative recurrence.

In this chapter, we describe the evidence focusing on risk factors for postoperative recurrence of Crohn's disease, and treatment options to clarify which patients benefit from biologics to prevent disease recurrence after resection.

Y. Miyatani
Inflammatory Bowel Disease Center, The University of Chicago Medicine, Chicago, IL, USA
e-mail: Yusuke.Miyatani@uchospitals.edu

A. Sakuraba (✉)
RUSH Center for Crohn's and Colitis, RUSH University Medical Center, Chicago, USA
e-mail: atsushi_sakuraba@rush.edu

K. Umanskiy, N. Hyman (eds.), *Difficult Decisions in Colorectal Surgery*, Difficult Decisions in Surgery: An Evidence-Based Approach,
https://doi.org/10.1007/978-3-031-42303-1_11

Table 11.1 PICO table

P (Patients)	I (Intervention)	C (comparator)	O (Outcomes)
Patients with Crohn's disease after resection	Prophylaxis with biologics	Other medications or no therapy	Postoperative recurrence

Search Strategy

Table 11.1 demonstrates the PICO process relevant to our research question. We searched the PubMed database in the English language between 1966 to 2022 with the following keywords "Crohn's disease" and "postoperative recurrence". Each clinically relevant article was checked as a full-article.

Results

Definition of Recurrence

Recurrence as an outcome can be mainly divided into three categories: endoscopic, symptomatic, and surgical recurrence. The definitions of endoscopic and clinical recurrence can vary in each study as follows:

Endoscopic Recurrence

Rutgeerts score has been most commonly used as a postoperative endoscopic score of neoterminal ileum which is defined as follows: i0 indicates no lesions; i1 indicates <5 aphthous lesions; i2 indicates >5 aphthous lesions with normal mucosa between the lesions, or skip areas of larger lesions or lesions confined to the ileocolonic anastomosis; i3 indicates diffuse aphthous ileitis with diffusely inflamed mucosa; i4 indicates diffuse inflammation with already larger ulcers, nodules, and/or narrowing [5]. In most clinical trials, Rutgeerts score ≥i2 was most commonly defined as endoscopic recurrence, which has been reported to predict future clinical recurrence [6]. Since the location of inflammation (e.g. at the anastomosis or at the terminal ileum) may influence the recurrence risk, a recent study analyzed clinical recurrence by dividing Rutgeerts score of i2 into i2a and i2b in accordance to the location of inflammation. However, this modified Rutgeerts score did not show a significant difference regarding the subsequent clinical recurrence and the need for endoscopic or surgical intervention [7].

Clinical Recurrence

Clinical recurrence is commonly defined as follows: symptoms of active Crohn's disease such as diarrhea and abdominal pain, Crohn's Disease Activity Index (CDAI) indicated ≥150 or 200, and Harvey-Bradshaw index (HBI) indicates ≥8, which are occasionally used as a composite outcome [1, 8, 9].

Surgical Recurrence

A new surgery including resection or stricturoplasty of the ileocolic anastomosis is homogeneously defined as surgical recurrence and reliable [10].

Risk Factors of Recurrence After Resection

The emergence of biologics has made a positive impact on the reoperation rate of Crohn's disease [2]. On the other hand, over-treatment should be avoided with regard to adverse effects and financial burden both on patients and society. Therefore, identifying high-risk patients that truly benefit from prophylactic biological treatment should be essential (Table 11.2). Here we described the risk factors of postoperative recurrence in Crohn's disease.

Table 11.2 Established risk factors associated with postoperative Crohn's disease recurrence

Risk factor
Smoking
Penetrating disease > inflammatory or fibrostenosing disease
Prior bowel resection, especially extensive resection
Multiple surgeries
Prior biologics, especially multiple failure
Short duration of disease since diagnosis or between prior surgery
Perianal disease

Biographic Feature

Smoking has been consistently reported to increase postoperative recurrence in many studies [11, 12]. A meta-analysis showed a two-fold increase in the odds of clinical recurrence in smokers compared to that in non-smokers, and a 2.5-fold increase in the risk of further surgical resection within 10 years [13]. Interestingly, current smokers have a higher odds ratio than ex-smokers which suggests smoking cessation may reduce postoperative disease recurrence [14]. Therefore, patient education for smoking cessation by a multidisciplinary approach should be conducted for smokers.

Complicated disease phenotypes such as perforation, penetrating, and perianal disease are regarded as postoperative risk factors [9, 12, 15]. Although those factors were widely used as patient selection criteria in clinical trials, they have not been fully validated.

Shorter disease duration before first surgery was reported as a risk factor for surgical recurrence [16, 17]. Another study demonstrated that a shorter interval between first and second surgery was associated with higher risk for a third surgery [18]. Although these studies utilized different definitions in terms of duration, a shorter timing of the need for surgery may suggest a more progressive phenotype.

Age and gender are controversial in regards to postoperative recurrence of Crohn's disease [11].

Gut microbiota is considered to affect pathogenesis in Crohn's disease. Dysbiosis in the mucosa such as reduction of alpha diversity and increase in pro-inflammatory pathogenic bacteria may be associated with postoperative recurrence [19]. Several bacteria (e.g. Proteobacteria phylum and the Firmicutes phylum) were reported to predict endoscopic recurrence, but further study is needed to clarify the role of microbiome [20].

Genetic factors also may contribute to postoperative recurrence. There is a variety of single-nucleotide polymorphism (SNP) that predispose the individual to recurrence of Crohn's disease. NOD2 has been shown to be associated with not only disease development and progressive phenotype but with postoperative surgical recurrence [21, 22]. SNPs in CARD15, SMAD3, and CARD8 were also found as risk factors for postoperative recurrence, but further validation is required [14, 23].

Preoperative Treatment

Whereas tumor necrosis factor inhibitors (TNFi) brought a paradigm shift in the treatment of Crohn's disease, a significant proportion of patients still require surgery. Previous TNFi exposure as the risk of recurrence is understandable considering the general efficacy of TNFi [9, 24]. Whereas ileocecal resection in uncomplicated ileitis may be a more beneficial treatment option in regards to patient's quality of life and long-term surgical recurrence compared with continued TNFi use or intensification without surgical resection, patients with a previous history of resection have been considered to have a higher risk of clinical recurrence [9, 11, 25, 26].

Surgery

Surgical strategy can influence the rate of postoperative recurrence. A meta-analysis comparing laparoscopic resection with open ileocolic resection indicated that the surgical recurrence rate is not significantly different between the two groups [27], while laparoscopic surgery is beneficial in that it is less invasive than open surgery with possibly less postoperative complications [28, 27].

Stapled ileocolonic side-to-side anastomosis is associated with lower surgical recurrence than end-to-end anastomosis, which might suggest the importance of a wide diameter of anastomosis [29, 30].

An antimesenteric functional end-to-end handsewn anastomosis (Kono-S anastomosis) has recently been designed to maintain a wide anastomotic lumen and shape [31]. A recent RCT comparing Kono-S anastomosis and stapled ileocolonic side-to-side showed that Kono-S anastomosis significantly decreased the rate of postoperative endoscopic recurrence at 6 months and presented a longer recurrence-free duration [32].

Severe inflammation of ileocolonic Crohn's disease develops mesenteric thickening and fat wrapping. Some evidence showed ileocolic resection with the mesentery may reduce the rate of surgical recurrence since the removal of mesentery could reduce immunological input and recruitment of fibroblast precursors [29, 33].

Positive resection margins, granuloma, and plexitis are associated with risk of postoperative recurrence [34, 35, 36]. However, an expanded resection margin was not preventative reoperation [37] and recent guidelines do not recommend extended resection [38, 39].

Postoperative Preventive Therapy

TNFi

TNFi have been a mainstream treatment for high-risk postoperative patients with Crohn's disease. The first placebo-controlled RCT which evaluated the efficacy of postoperative infliximab demonstrated that the infliximab group had a significantly lower rate of endoscopic recurrence than the placebo group at one year [40]. Covering the limitation of small number of participants, the largest RCT which enrolled higher-risk populations with at least one of the following factors defined as short disease duration (<10 years), penetrating phenotype, history of perianal fistulae, or smoking history, revealed significantly lower postoperative endoscopic recurrence at week 76 in infliximab treated patients [9].

While combination therapy with infliximab and thiopurine is associated with a favorable outcome in Crohn's disease, there is no RCT assessing the superiority of combination therapy in postoperative Crohn's disease [41]. A nationwide study using propensity-matched analysis showed the superiority of combination therapy to infliximab monotherapy with regard to postoperative endoscopic recurrence [42]. Considering the fact that patients with a preoperative history of multiple TNFi exposures were associated with postoperative recurrence, these refractory patients with high-risk features may be considered as candidates for combination therapy [24].

On the other hand, adalimumab has also been used as prophylaxis after operation in Crohn's disease. The first RCT compared adalimumab with thioprine and mesalamine group showed that the adalimumab group had a much lower endoscopic and clinical recurrence 2 years after surgery [43]. Each group was not stratified according to well-known recurrence risks in this study. Notably, only 6% of patients demonstrated endoscopic recurrence at the 2-year follow-up after surgery, though the adalimumab group included more patients who were active smokers [44].

In addition, a sub-analysis of the POCER study which enrolled patients with high-risk recurrence factors defined as smokers, penetrating disease, or history of at least one resection, demonstrated that adalimumab was more likely to maintain complete endoscopic remission than azathioprine combined with 3 months metronidazole [45]. Although this study was not designed to directly compare the efficacy of adalimumab with that of azathioprine in that all patients who were intolerant to thioprine were assigned to the adalimumab group, it may show feasible evidence of the superiority of adalimumab to thiopurine in postoperative Crohn's disease.

Meta-analysis of postoperative prophylaxis with TNFi which included six RCTs with infliximab and two with adalimumab indicated that the relative risk of endoscopic and clinical recurrence was 0.34[95% CI 0.22–0.53] and 0.60[0.36–1.02], respectively [1]. Furthermore, no difference between infliximab and adalimumab was indicated by other meta-analyses [10, 46].

On the other hand, real-world data shows that the same TNFi was often used as postoperative treatment partially due to a lack of alternative options as maintenance therapy [47]. Is it effective to use the same drug following surgery even though it failed before surgery? A retrospective study indicated that patients treated with the same TNFi as a preoperative treatment showed similar efficacy as TNFi naïve patients who used TNFi after surgery. In addition, the study also analyzed pharmacokinetics data of drug levels and antidrug antibodies of TNFi before and after surgery, which showed that patients with preoperative primary failure or secondary loss of response to TNFi despite therapeutic serum drug levels without antidrug antibodies responded adequately to TNFi after surgery. This data may suggest that removal of the disease burden of TNF-α in the tissue of severely inflamed areas led to improvement of TNFi pharmacokinetics [48].

Other Biologics

There is scarce evidence regarding the effect of other biologics for postoperative Crohn's disease.

The first study which compared ustekinumab to azathioprine in postoperative Crohn's disease using propensity score analysis of data from RCT indicated that ustekinumab treated patients were significantly less likely to develop endoscopic recurrence at 6 months after resection than azathioprine treated patients. Notably, ustekinumab was effective even though approximately 90% of patients had a history of TNFi before surgery [49].

While vedolizumab improved the endoscopic inflammation even detected at postoperative follow-up endoscopy, [50] postoperative prophylaxis with vedolizumab demonstrated a significantly higher rate of endoscopic recurrence within one year compared to that with infliximab [47].

The latest retrospective multicenter study was conducted to compare the rate of endoscopic recurrence with TNFi with those with vedolizumab and ustekinumab in a real-world setting. Although patients treated with ustekinumab had the highest rate of endoscopic recurrence at one year (ustekinumab 61% vs. TNFi 40.2% vs. vedolizumab 33%), there was no statistical difference after adjusted by the numbers of pre-biologics and surgical histories with inverse probability of treatment weighting. Past history of infliximab and adalimumab is associated with postoperative endoscopic recurrence factor at one year adjusted by multivariable logistic regression analysis [51].

Conclusion

The emergence of novel therapies will provide us with more prophylaxis options in postoperative Crohn's disease. Further head-to-head RCTs between biologics are warranted to assess postoperative prophylaxis. Based on available evidence, it is proposed that patients with multiple risk factors of postoperative recurrence should be treated with TNFi and followed up with a colonoscopy 6 months after surgery for step-up treatment for recurrence (Fig. 11.1). Fecal calprotectin may be used in between colonoscopies for early detection of endoscopic recurrence [52]. Individualized risk stratification and approach with a multidisciplinary team are indispensable to prevent disease recurrence after resection in Crohn's disease.

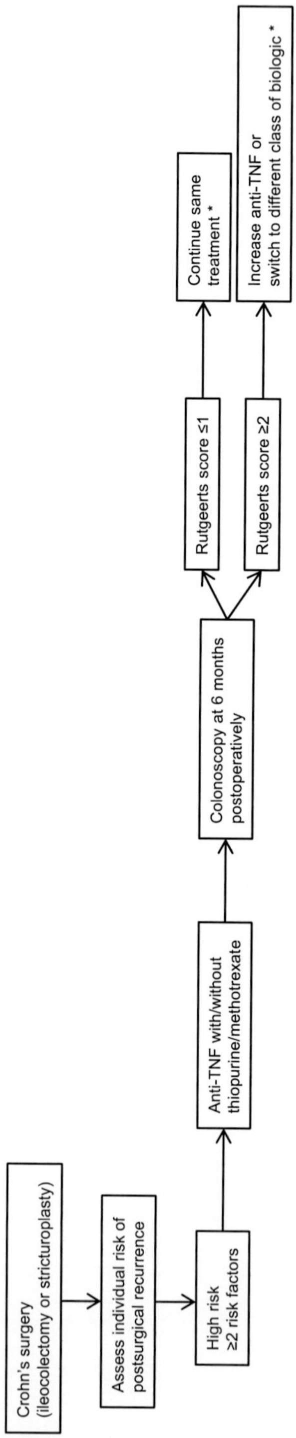

Fig. 11.1 Recommended strategy for postoperative Crohn's disease with high-risk features. *Fecal calprotectin measurement in between colonoscopies may be useful

References

1. Uchino M, Ikeuchi H, Hata K, Minagawa T, Horio Y, Kuwahara R, et al. Does anti-tumor necrosis factor alpha prevent the recurrence of Crohn's disease? Systematic review and meta-analysis. J Gastroenterol Hepatol. 2021;36(4):864–72.
2. Shinagawa T, Hata K, Ikeuchi H, Fukushima K, Futami K, Sugita A, et al. Rate of reoperation decreased significantly after year 2002 in patients with Crohn's disease. Clin Gastroenterol Hepatol. 2020;18(4):898–907.e5.
3. Torres J, Mehandru S, Colombel JF, Peyrin-Biroulet L. Crohn's disease. Lancet. 2017;389(10080):1741–55.
4. Pascua M, Su C, Lewis JD, Brensinger C, Lichtenstein GR. Meta-analysis: factors predicting post-operative recurrence with placebo therapy in patients with Crohn's disease. Aliment Pharmacol Ther. 2008;28(5):545–56.
5. Rutgeerts P, Geboes K, Vantrappen G, Beyls J, Kerremans R, Hiele M. Predictability of the postoperative course of Crohn's disease. Gastroenterology. 1990;99(4):956–63.
6. Khanna R, Ma C, Jairath V, Vande Casteele N, Zou G, Feagan BG. Endoscopic assessment of inflammatory bowel disease activity in clinical trials. Clin Gastroenterol Hepatol. 2022;20(4):727–36.e2.
7. Rivière P, Vermeire S, Irles-Depe M, Van Assche G, Rutgeerts P, de Buck van Overstraeten A, et al. No change in determining Crohn's disease recurrence or need for endoscopic or surgical intervention with modification of the Rutgeerts' scoring system. Clin Gastroenterol Hepatol. 2019;17(8):1643–5.
8. Ble A, Renzulli C, Cenci F, Grimaldi M, Barone M, Sedano R, et al. The relationship between endoscopic and clinical recurrence in postoperative Crohn's disease: a systematic review and meta-analysis. J Crohns Colitis. 2022;16(3):490–9.
9. Regueiro M, Feagan BG, Zou B, Johanns J, Blank MA, Chevrier M, et al. Infliximab reduces endoscopic, but not clinical, recurrence of Crohn's disease after ileocolonic resection. Gastroenterology. 2016;150(7):1568–78.
10. Jain SR, Ow ZGW, Chin YH, Lim WH, Kong G, Tham HY, et al. Quantifying the rate of recurrence of postoperative Crohn's disease with biological therapy. A meta-analysis. J Dig Dis. 2021;22(7):399–407.
11. Auzolle C, Nancey S, Tran-Minh ML, Buisson A, Pariente B, Stefanescu C, et al. Male gender, active smoking and previous intestinal resection are risk factors for post-operative endoscopic recurrence in Crohn's disease: results from a prospective cohort study. Aliment Pharmacol Ther. 2018;48(9):924–32.
12. De Cruz P, Kamm MA, Hamilton AL, Ritchie KJ, Krejany EO, Gorelik A, et al. Crohn's disease management after intestinal resection: a randomised trial. Lancet. 2015;385(9976):1406–17.
13. Reese GE, Nanidis T, Borysiewicz C, Yamamoto T, Orchard T, Tekkis PP. The effect of smoking after surgery for Crohn's disease: a meta-analysis of observational studies. Int J Colorectal Dis. 2008;23(12):1213–21.
14. Fowler SA, Ananthakrishnan AN, Gardet A, Stevens CR, Korzenik JR, Sands BE, et al. SMAD3 gene variant is a risk factor for recurrent surgery in patients with Crohn's disease. J Crohns Colitis. 2014;8(8):845–51.
15. Bernell O, Lapidus A, Hellers G. Risk factors for surgery and recurrence in 907 patients with primary ileocaecal Crohn's disease. Br J Surg. 2000;87(12):1697–701.
16. Poggioli G, Laureti S, Selleri S, Brignola C, Grazi GL, Stocchi L, et al. Factors affecting recurrence in Crohn's disease. Results of a prospective audit. Int J Colorectal Dis. 1996;11(6):294–8.
17. Chardavoyne R, Flint GW, Pollack S, Wise L. Factors affecting recurrence following resection for Crohn's disease. Dis Colon Rectum. 1986;29(8):495–502.
18. Watanabe T, Sasaki I, Sugita A, Fukushima K, Futami K, Hibi T, et al. Interval of less than 5 years between the first and second operation is a risk factor for a third operation for Crohn's disease. Inflamm Bowel Dis. 2012;18(1):17–24.

19. Zhuang X, Tian Z, Li N, Mao R, Li X, Zhao M, et al. Gut microbiota profiles and microbial-based therapies in post-operative Crohn's disease: a systematic review. Front Med (Lausanne). 2020;7:615858.
20. Sokol H, Brot L, Stefanescu C, Auzolle C, Barnich N, Buisson A, et al. Prominence of ileal mucosa-associated microbiota to predict postoperative endoscopic recurrence in Crohn's disease. Gut. 2020;69(3):462–72.
21. Adler J, Rangwalla SC, Dwamena BA, Higgins PD. The prognostic power of the NOD2 genotype for complicated Crohn's disease: a meta-analysis. Am J Gastroenterol. 2011;106(4):699–712.
22. Kline BP, Weaver T, Brinton DL Jr, Harris L, Yochum GS, Berg AS, et al. Clinical and genetic factors impact time to surgical recurrence after ileocolectomy for Crohn's disease. Ann Surg. 2021;274(2):346–51.
23. Germain A, Guéant RM, Chamaillard M, Bresler L, Guéant JL, Peyrin-Biroulet L. CARD8 gene variant is a risk factor for recurrent surgery in patients with Crohn's disease. Dig Liver Dis. 2015;47(11):938–42.
24. Collins M, Sarter H, Gower-Rousseau C, Koriche D, Libier L, Nachury M, et al. Previous exposure to multiple Anti-TNF is associated with decreased efficiency in preventing postoperative Crohn's disease recurrence. J Crohns Colitis. 2017;11(3):281–8.
25. Ponsioen CY, de Groof EJ, Eshuis EJ, Gardenbroek TJ, Bossuyt PMM, Hart A, et al. Laparoscopic ileocaecal resection versus infliximab for terminal ileitis in Crohn's disease: a randomised controlled, open-label, multicentre trial. Lancet Gastroenterol Hepatol. 2017;2(11):785–92.
26. Stevens TW, Haasnoot ML, D'Haens GR, Buskens CJ, de Groof EJ, Eshuis EJ, et al. Laparoscopic ileocaecal resection versus infliximab for terminal ileitis in Crohn's disease: retrospective long-term follow-up of the LIR!C trial. Lancet Gastroenterol Hepatol. 2020;5(10):900–7.
27. Patel SV, Patel SV, Ramagopalan SV, Ott MC. Laparoscopic surgery for Crohn's disease: a meta-analysis of perioperative complications and long term outcomes compared with open surgery. BMC Surg. 2013;13:14.
28. Stocchi L, Milsom JW, Fazio VW. Long-term outcomes of laparoscopic versus open ileocolic resection for Crohn's disease: follow-up of a prospective randomized trial. Surgery. 2008;144(4):622–7; discussion 7-8.
29. Reynolds IS, Doogan KL, Ryan ÉJ, Hechtl D, Lecot FP, Arya S, et al. Surgical strategies to reduce postoperative recurrence of Crohn's disease after ileocolic resection. Front Surg. 2021;8:804137.
30. Adamina M, Bonovas S, Raine T, Spinelli A, Warusavitarne J, Armuzzi A, et al. ECCO guidelines on therapeutics in Crohn's disease: surgical treatment. J Crohns Colitis. 2020;14(2):155–68.
31. Kono T, Ashida T, Ebisawa Y, Chisato N, Okamoto K, Katsuno H, et al. A new antimesenteric functional end-to-end handsewn anastomosis: surgical prevention of anastomotic recurrence in Crohn's disease. Dis Colon Rectum. 2011;54(5):586–92.
32. Luglio G, Rispo A, Imperatore N, Giglio MC, Amendola A, Tropeano FP, et al. Surgical prevention of anastomotic recurrence by excluding mesentery in Crohn's disease: the SuPREMe-CD Study – a randomized clinical trial. Ann Surg. 2020;272(2):210–7.
33. Coffey CJ, Kiernan MG, Sahebally SM, Jarrar A, Burke JP, Kiely PA, et al. Inclusion of the mesentery in ileocolic resection for Crohn's disease is associated with reduced surgical recurrence. J Crohns Colitis. 2018;12(10):1139–50.
34. Poredska K, Kunovsky L, Marek F, Kala Z, Prochazka V, Dolina J, et al. The influence of microscopic inflammation at resection margins on early postoperative endoscopic recurrence after ileocaecal resection for Crohn's disease. J Crohns Colitis. 2020;14(3):361–8.
35. Tandon P, Malhi G, Abdali D, Pogue E, Marshall JK, de Buck van Overstraeten A, et al. Active margins, plexitis, and granulomas increase postoperative Crohn's recurrence: systematic review and meta-analysis. Clin Gastroenterol Hepatol. 2021;19(3):451–62.
36. Lemmens B, de Buck van Overstraeten A, Arijs I, Sagaert X, Van Assche G, Vermeire S, et al. Submucosal plexitis as a predictive factor for postoperative endoscopic recurrence in patients

with Crohn's disease undergoing a resection with ileocolonic anastomosis: results from a prospective single-centre study. J Crohns Colitis. 2017;11(2):212–20.
37. Fazio VW, Marchetti F, Church M, Goldblum JR, Lavery C, Hull TL, et al. Effect of resection margins on the recurrence of Crohn's disease in the small bowel. A randomized controlled trial. Ann Surg. 1996;224(4):563–71; discussion 71-3
38. Bemelman WA, Warusavitarne J, Sampietro GM, Serclova Z, Zmora O, Luglio G, et al. ECCO-ESCP consensus on surgery for Crohn's disease. J Crohns Colitis. 2018;12(1):1–16.
39. Adamina M, Feakins R, Iacucci M, Spinelli A, Cannatelli R, D'Hoore A, et al. ECCO topical review optimising reporting in surgery, endoscopy, and histopathology. J Crohns Colitis. 2021;15(7):1089–105.
40. Regueiro M, Schraut W, Baidoo L, Kip KE, Sepulveda AR, Pesci M, et al. Infliximab prevents Crohn's disease recurrence after ileal resection. Gastroenterology. 2009;136(2):441–50.e1; quiz 716
41. Burr NE, Hall B, Hamlin PJ, Selinger CP, Ford AC, O'Connor A. Systematic review and network meta-analysis of medical therapies to prevent recurrence of post-operative Crohn's disease. J Crohns Colitis. 2019;13(6):693–701.
42. Cañete F, Mañosa M, Pérez-Martínez I, Barreiro-de Acosta M, González-Sueyro RC, Nos P, et al. Antitumor necrosis factor agents to treat endoscopic postoperative recurrence of Crohn's disease: a nationwide study with propensity-matched score analysis. Clin Transl Gastroenterol. 2020;11(8):e00218.
43. Hanauer SB, Korelitz BI, Rutgeerts P, Peppercorn MA, Thisted RA, Cohen RD, et al. Postoperative maintenance of Crohn's disease remission with 6-mercaptopurine, mesalamine, or placebo: a 2-year trial. Gastroenterology. 2004;127(3):723–9.
44. Savarino E, Bodini G, Dulbecco P, Assandri L, Bruzzone L, Mazza F, et al. Adalimumab is more effective than azathioprine and mesalamine at preventing postoperative recurrence of Crohn's disease: a randomized controlled trial. Am J Gastroenterol. 2013;108(11):1731–42.
45. De Cruz P, Kamm MA, Hamilton AL, Ritchie KJ, Krejany EO, Gorelik A, et al. Efficacy of thiopurines and adalimumab in preventing Crohn's disease recurrence in high-risk patients – a POCER study analysis. Aliment Pharmacol Ther. 2015;42(7):867–79.
46. Erős A, Farkas N, Hegyi P, Szabó A, Balaskó M, Veres G, et al. Anti-TNFα agents are the best choice in preventing postoperative Crohn's disease: a meta-analysis. Dig Liver Dis. 2019;51(8):1086–95.
47. Yamada A, Komaki Y, Patel N, Komaki F, Pekow J, Dalal S, et al. The use of Vedolizumab in preventing postoperative recurrence of Crohn's disease. Inflamm Bowel Dis. 2018;24(3):502–9.
48. Assa A, Bronsky J, Kolho KL, Zarubova K, de Meij T, Ledder O, et al. Anti-TNFα treatment after surgical resection for Crohn's disease is effective despite previous pharmacodynamic failure. Inflamm Bowel Dis. 2017;23(5):791–7.
49. Buisson A, Nancey S, Manlay L, Rubin DT, Hebuterne X, Pariente B, et al. Ustekinumab is more effective than azathioprine to prevent endoscopic postoperative recurrence in Crohn's disease. United European Gastroenterol J. 2021;9(5):552–60.
50. Macaluso FS, Cappello M, Crispino F, Grova M, Privitera AC, Piccillo G, et al. Vedolizumab may be an effective option for the treatment of postoperative recurrence of Crohn's disease. Dig Liver Dis. 2022;54(5):629–34.
51. Yanai H, Kagramanova A, Knyazev O, Sabino J, Haenen S, Mantzaris GJ, et al. Endoscopic postoperative recurrence in Crohn's disease after curative ileocecal resection with early Prophylaxis by Anti-Tnf, Vedolizumab Or Ustekinumab: a real-world multicenter European Study. J Crohns Colitis. 2022;16(12):1882–92.
52. Wright EK, Kamm MA, De Cruz P, Hamilton AL, Ritchie KJ, Krejany EO, et al. Measurement of fecal calprotectin improves monitoring and detection of recurrence of Crohn's disease after surgery. Gastroenterology. 2015;148(5):938–47.e1.

Part II

Colon Cancer

12 Is Intensive Surveillance Necessary After Curative Resection for Colon Cancer?

Terrah J. Paul Olson

Introduction

Colorectal cancer is consistently in the top three cancer diagnoses both in the United States and worldwide. According to the American Cancer Society, estimated incidence of colorectal cancer in 2020 was 147,950, with 53,200 estimated deaths attributable to colorectal cancer [1]. About 40% of new CRC diagnoses are stage I or II (local disease), 36% are stage III (locoregional disease), and 20% at stage IV (metastatic disease) [2]. Local and locoregional disease is often able to be treated with curative surgery. Following treatment, patients embark on a period of surveillance as there is a definite risk of recurrence even after appropriate therapy. Risk of recurrence ranges from 30% to 50%, with a yearly incidence of 9.9% at one year, increasing to 26.2% by 3 years, and 31.5% at 5 years when grouping various stages together [3]. There are different rates based on stage and clinicopathologic characteristics.

While there is consensus that surveillance needs to be provided to patients after definite treatment, the exact timing and nature of that surveillance has been a contentious topic, with more or less intensive strategies being adopted. More frequent surveillance would hopefully find recurrences sooner, thereby allowing salvage treatment, but at the expense of increased interactions with the medical system, potentially leading to mental, physical, and financial costs to both patients and medical systems. This chapter will review the data for more versus less intensive surveillance following curative surgery for colorectal cancer. Surveillance modalities include blood tests, imaging studies, and colonoscopy.

T. J. Paul Olson (✉)
Division of Colorectal Surgery, Department of Surgery, Emory University, Atlanta, GA, USA
e-mail: tpaulol@emory.edu

K. Umanskiy, N. Hyman (eds.), *Difficult Decisions in Colorectal Surgery*, Difficult Decisions in Surgery: An Evidence-Based Approach,
https://doi.org/10.1007/978-3-031-42303-1_12

Table 12.1 PICO table

Population	Intervention	Comparison	Outcome
Patients with non-metastatic colon cancer who underwent curative resection, +/– adjuvant therapy	Intensive surveillance with routine labs, imaging, and endoscopy	Less intensive surveillance	Overall survival Cancer specific survival Recurrence treated with surgery

Search Strategy

Table 12.1 summarized the PICO question used to design this search strategy. A comprehensive search of PubMed, EMBASE, and Cochrane Library was performed. Search strategies employed search engine-appropriate combinations of terms including: "colon cancer surveillance", "intensive surveillance", "surveillance", "overall survival", "disease free survival", and "colon cancer surgery". Articles from 2004–July 2022 were included. Search limits included human studies, articles and/or conference reviews/abstracts, and English language. The references of included articles were reviewed to identify additional relevant articles.

Results

A total of 4326 titles were retrieved with this search strategy. There were three duplicate titles. After reviewing titles and abstracts, 48 articles underwent full text review for data extraction and summary of recommendations. Four randomized controlled trials and three meta-analyses were selected for detailed discussion. Of note, most studies combined colon and rectal cancer outcomes, making it difficult to tease out the exact role of different surveillance programs for these two malignancies.

Tjandra et al. [4] performed a meta-analysis of randomized trials examining this issue available up to 2007. This included a total of eight trials with a cumulative patient population of 2923. These were patients who had undergone curative resection for colorectal cancer. They were randomized to intensive follow up (n = 1474) or less intensive/minimal follow up (n = 1449). Criteria for follow up intensity were variable between trials, but typically included serum carcinoembryonic antigen (CEA) levels, chest radiographs (CXR), and colonoscopy or flexible sigmoidoscopy, with variable liver imaging. Less intensive follow up ranged from only written instructions to the same surveillance modalities but at less frequent intervals. Overall mortality was reduced with intensive surveillance (21.8% vs 25.7%, OR 0.74, $p = 0.01$), with serum CEA levels ($p = 0.0002$) and colonoscopy ($p = 0.04$) contributing to this effect. Cancer-related mortality was not significantly different between groups (11.5% vs 12.5%; OR 0.91, $p = 0.52$). Recurrences were found 5.91 months earlier ($p < 0.0001$) and more frequently while asymptomatic with intensive surveillance (odds ration [OR] 3.42, $p < 0.0001$). When recurrences happened, they were more amenable to re-resection (10.7% vs 5.7%, p = 0.0002) and had higher rates of curative surgery in the intensive surveillance group (24.3% vs 9.9%, p = 0.0001) [4].

The GILDA trial was an international randomized clinical trial based out of Italy examining outcomes after curative treatment for Dukes B2 or C colorectal cancer [5]. Subjects were randomized to high intensity surveillance with CEA, complete blood count, Ca 19-9, colonoscopy, CXR, and liver ultrasound or low intensity with CEA, colonoscopy, and liver ultrasonography at less frequent intervals. From 1998 until 2006, 1228 subjects were randomized from three countries, with median follow up of 62 months in both arms, and 90% of subjects completing surveillance as planned. By calculating the difference between the disease-free survival curves, intensive surveillance was shown to detect recurrences 5.9 months earlier (95% confidence interval [CI] 2.71–9.11). However, this did not translate to a difference in overall survival (hazard ratio [HR] 1.14, 95% CI 0.87–1.48, p = 0.34) or disease free survival (HR 1.22, 95% CI 0.95–1.57, p = 0.11). Health related quality of life was similar between groups [5].

The FACS (Follow-up After Colorectal Surgery) trial was a randomized clinical trial with four arms evaluating different strategies using CEA and CT imaging for surveillance after curative surgical treatment for stage I-III colorectal cancer [6]. This multisite trial in the UK enrolled 1202 subjects between 2003 and 2009 who were randomized to minimal follow up with a single CT chest/abdomen/pelvis; CEA surveillance; CT scan surveillance; or combined CEA and CT scan surveillance. Subjects were followed for a mean of 4.4 years, and surveillance with either CEA monitoring or CT scans had higher rates of surgical treatment of recurrence with curative intent. Specifically, rate of surgery with curative intent for recurrence was 2.3% in the minimum follow up group, whereas rates were 6.7% in CEA group (adjusted OR 3.00, 95% CI 1.23–7.33), 8% in CT group (adjusted OR 3.63, 95% CI 1.51–8.69), and 6.6% in CEA and CT group (adjusted OR 3.10, 95% CI 1.10–8.71). The combination of CEA and CT scans did not significantly increase the yield of surveillance, and there were not differences in overall or cancer specific deaths between the minimal follow up group and the intensive surveillance groups (15.9% vs 18.2%, difference 2.3%, 95% CI −2.6% to 7.1%). While intensive surveillance again had a higher rate of surgically treatable recurrences, no survival benefit was demonstrated [6].

The COLOFOL trial was an international randomized clinical trial of subjects with stage II or III colorectal cancer after curative surgery [7]. This study randomized 2509 subjects looking specifically at overall and colorectal cancer-specific mortality rates, and time to colorectal cancer specific recurrence in subjects undergoing more frequent vs less frequent surveillance with CEA and CT scans of the abdomen. Overall 5-year mortality rate was 13.0% in the high frequency group vs 14.1% in the low frequency group (risk difference 1.1%, 95% CI −1.6% to 3.8%, p = 0.43). Likewise, there was no significant difference in 5-year colorectal cancer specific mortality between groups – 10.6% vs 11.4% (risk difference 0.8%, 95% CI −1.7 to 3.3%, p = 0.52). Detection rates of colorectal cancer recurrence was also similar between groups – 21.6% vs 19.4% (risk difference 2.2%, 95% CI −1.0% to 5.4%, p = 0.15) [7].

The CEAwatch multicenter randomized trial examined different frequencies of CEA serum testing after curative surgery for colorectal cancer, and if CEA rose twice consecutively, used this to trigger cross-sectional imaging. From 2010 to 2012, 3223 patients were included. More frequent CEA testing found recurrences sooner (HR 1.45, 95% CI 1.08–1.95, $p = 0.013$); this also led to higher rates of curative treatment (OR 3.12, 95% CI 1.25–6.02, $p = 0.0145$) [8]. However, there were no differences in overall survival or cancer specific survival with the intensive surveillance regimen (HR 0.73, 95% CI 0.46–1.17; HR 0.78, 95% CI 0.48–1.28, respectively). The more intensive regimen tended to find recurrences before they were symptomatic, and this was associated with better survival than when subjects developed symptoms from their recurrence (HR 0.39, 95% CI 0.25–0.63) [9]. Patients did not report adverse psychological effects associated with more intense follow up [10].

An updated Cochrane review published in 2019 collated data on surveillance strategies for non-metastatic colorectal cancer [11]. There were 19 studies with 13,216 subjects included, and meta-analysis was performed using data from 16 of the studies. As seen with the individual trial discussed above, there was no difference in overall survival or colorectal cancer specific survival with intensive follow up regimen. Symptomatic recurrences were less frequent with intensive surveillance, and salvage surgery for recurrence was more frequent as well. When colonoscopy is part of surveillance, this can lead to more complications from bleeding or perforation. Intensive surveillance did not have a measurable effect on quality of life, anxiety, or depression. Cost may be increased with more intensive follow up [11]. Table 12.2 summarizes the results of these trials and meta-analyses.

An updated Cochrane review examined the role of serum CEA levels in detecting colorectal cancer [12]. This review focused on the pooled sensitivity and sensitivity of different cutoff values for CEA for detecting colorectal cancer recurrence. They concluded that CEA was insufficiently sensitive or specific to be used alone, even with low cutoff values, for surveillance. Additionally, 20% of recurrences showed no increase in CEA [12].

Table 12.2 Randomized controlled trials and meta-analyses included

Study	Study type	Years of accrual	N	Intensive regimen	Control regimen	Outcomes of intensive regimen	Quality of evidence
Tjandra 2007	Meta-analysis	1966–2007	2923	Variable, including: labs CEA CXR FOBT liver u/s CT colonoscopy	Variable	-reduced overall mortality -no difference in cancer specific mortality -early detection -more asymptomatic recurrence detection -more amenable to surgery -better chance of curative resection	Moderate
GILDA 2016	RCT	1998–2006	1228	Office visit, CEA, CBC, CA 19–9 q 4mo CXR and colonoscopy yearly Liver u/s q 4 mo × 4, then yearly	Office visit and CEA q 4 mo Colonoscopy at year 1 and 2 -liver u/s at 4 months and 16 months	Recurrence found 5.9 mo earlier No difference in overall or disease free survival Similar HQoL	Moderate
FACS 2014	RCT	2003–2009	1202	Either: CT c/a/p q6 mo × 2 years, then yearly CEA and CT c/a/p q6 mo × 2 years, then yearly CEA q3 mo × 2 years, then q6 mo × 3 years, with single CT c/a/p at 12–18 months if requested	No scheduled follow up except CT c/a/p at 12–18 months if requested	Similar OS and CSS Higher rates of surgery with curative intent for recurrence CT and CEA combined did not have higher yield than either alone	Moderate

(continued)

Table 12.2 (continued)

Study	Study type	Years of accrual	N	Intensive regimen	Control regimen	Outcomes of intensive regimen	Quality of evidence
COLOFOL 2018	RCT	2006–2010	2509	CT c/a and CEA at 6, 12, 18, 24, and 36 mo Endoscopy and pelvic CT at discretion of treating MD	CT c/a and CEA at 12 and 36 mo Endoscopy and pelvic CT at discretion of treating MD	No difference in OS and CSS No difference in CRC recurrence	Moderate
CEAWatch 2017	RCT	2010–2012	3223	CEA q 8 weeks Year 1–3: Annual CT and, output clinic visit Year 4–5: Annual output clinic visit	Year 1–3: CEA q 3mo, output clinic visit, u/s liver, CXR q6 mo Year 4–5: CEA q6 mo, annual clinic visit, u/s liver, CXR	More recurrences detected More surgically treatable More definitive surgical tx No difference in OS, CSS No difference in adverse psych events	Moderate
Jeffrey 2019	Meta-analysis	1966–2019	13,216	Variable	Variable	No difference in OS and CSS Recurrence found while asymptomatic More frequent salvage surgery for recurrence No difference in QoL, anxiety, depression	Strong

Abbreviations: *CEA* carcinoembryonic antigen, *CXR* chest xray, *FOBT* fecal occult blood test, *u/s* ultrasound, *RCT* randomized clinical trial, *mo* month, *HQoL/QoL* health-care related/quality of life, *OS* overall survival, *CSS* cancer specific survival, *CRC* colorectal cancer

Recommendations Based on Data

There are no compelling results to link any particular intensive surveillance regimen compared with minimal to less frequent surveillance to improved overall or cancer-specific survival. However, high quality studies have consistently shown that more intensive surveillance is correlated with earlier detection of recurrences, detection of recurrence while asymptomatic which associated with improved outcomes [13], and increased rates of both surgically treatable recurrences and successfully resected recurrences. (Evidence: moderate; recommendation: strong).

The trials and meta-analyses presented here used a variety of different blood tests, imaging modalities, and timing of surveillance, making it difficult to recommend an exact unified surveillance regimen. Additionally, colonoscopy is an important part of post-resection surveillance for colorectal cancer, but this modality was inconsistently included in the trials reviewed in this chapter. That being said, the value of colonoscopy is established for detection of luminal recurrence [14]. Finally, given the variety of ways colorectal cancer can recur, any modality in isolation is unlikely to be adequate for meaningful surveillance.

Personal View of the Data

The data examining the role of more intensive vs less intensive surveillance after curative resection for non-metastatic colorectal cancer is vexing. Despite the fact that numerous well-designed studies, as well as a multitude of case series and cohort studies, show that more frequent surveillance by whichever regimen is being studied correlates with earlier detection of recurrence, detection before recurrence becomes symptomatic, and at a point when recurrences are more likely to be surgically salvageable, this has not translated to improvements in overall survival or cancer specific mortality. How to make sense of this discrepancy?

One reason may be the evolving landscape of cancer treatments. While these trials were appropriately powered based on older rates of recurrence seen with colorectal cancer, there were decreases in recurrence with concurrent changes in adjuvant and neoadjuvant therapy. As Popp et al. discuss in their analysis of the combined results of the GILDA, FACS, and COLOFOL trials, between lower than expected accrual rates to these studies as well as possibly decreased recurrence rates than were included in power calculations, these studies may not have been adequately powered to detect a small survival benefit from curative surgery when recurrences happened [15]. As there is evidence to suggest that treatment of recurrences, whether with surgery or palliative chemotherapy, can provide benefit, intensive surveillance regimens that allow detection of recurrences before they become symptomatic make it more likely that patients can receive these treatments [13]. The consistent signal in the trials and meta-analyses that more subjects were able to receive salvage surgery of recurrences is encouraging and a reason to continue close monitoring of colorectal cancer patients despite the lack of obvious survival benefit. Additionally, better outcomes associated with asymptomatic detection of recurrences support the practice of close monitoring in colorectal cancer patients after curative surgery [13, 16].

The most efficacious combination of surveillance tests is also not entirely settled. Colorectal cancer can follow several patterns of recurrence. There can be luminal, anastomotic recurrences. Local recurrences are also seen in surrounding lymphatic tissue and nodal basins. Common sites of distant metastases include lung or liver lesions. Additionally, while some tumors produce carcinoembryonic enzymes, elevations in this tumor marker are not universally seen. Because of these myriad presentations, a panel of complementary surveillance tests are needed to monitor colorectal cancer patients. This is demonstrated by the various modalities included in the trials discussed here, and reflect the ongoing attempts to find the most accurate, most effective surveillance strategy. In particular, the move from chest radiographs and liver ultrasonography to CT imaging is seen in the trials reported here. Other imaging modalities are also being studied to see if there is any role in colorectal cancer surveillance, such as PET-CT. There is not currently data to support incorporation of this into surveillance, but this may continue to evolve [17, 18]. Likewise, ongoing studies working to determine better use of serum CEA to maximize the sensitivity and specificity of this testing could prove beneficial for improved surveillance [12, 19, 20].

Another area to potentially improve the granularity of surveillance could be to incorporate specific pathologic or histologic features into risk estimates for recurrence. A number of groups have been correlating factors such as perineural invasion, number of lymph nodes retrieved, lymphovascular invasion, and novel classification of log odds of positive lymph nodes to clarify risk of recurrence and better tailor surveillance regimens [21–24]. While large randomized trials are useful in providing an aggregate view of a population, some of the finer details can be obscured in the process. Likewise, the practice of combining colon and rectal cancers in these studies may obscure divergence in outcomes, as the treatments for these malignancies are evolving differently.

Two of the three large trials discussed here included only stage II and III subjects. How to appropriately surveil stage I patients as well as resected stage IV patients are ongoing questions that are likely not appropriate for extrapolation from current trial data. Regarding stage I patients, while there is a low risk of recurrence, certainly pathologic markers may warrant closer surveillance [22, 25, 26]. Attempts are also being made to clarify surveillance protocols for resected stage IV patients as well, as there is little data to guide this management [27].

One important consideration is how the data on surveillance after resection for colorectal cancer is actually being used. Multiple studies surveying practitioners internationally show that there is hesitancy or difficulty in arranging the degree of surveillance that is recommended by current guidelines [28–31]. This could reflect lack of buy-in by practitioners to high intensity surveillance, logistical difficulties in arranging follow up for patients, lack of robust systems for tracking patients, or some combination of these and other elements. If controlled studies with high rates of retention and adherence to surveillance protocols could demonstrate only indirect improvements and benefits, this degree of low engagement in "real world" settings suggests that implementation of high intensity surveillance programs will have a hard time demonstrating noticeable benefits.

As a final point, while I do think there is benefit in close and careful surveillance with complementary modalities in patients after surgery for colorectal cancer, there is certainly room for improvement of current recommended protocols. It will be interesting to see what changes might arise from improved incorporation of pathologic data or more targeted use of different imaging modalities, as well as diverging treatment strategies for colon and rectal cancer. Another promising modality is circulating tumor cell technology; the role of this as part of surveillance regimens is still very much a work in progress, and it will be intriguing to see if this becomes incorporated in surveillance going forward.

References

1. Society AC. Colorectal Cancer Facts & Figures 2020–2022. 2020.
2. El-Shami K, Oeffinger KC, Erb NL, Willis A, Bretsch JK, Pratt-Chapman ML, et al. American Cancer Society colorectal cancer survivorship care guidelines. CA Cancer J Clin. 2015;65(6):428–55.
3. Guraya SY. Pattern, stage, and time of recurrent colorectal cancer after curative surgery. Clin Colorectal Cancer. 2019;18(2):e223–e8.
4. Tjandra JJ, Chan MK. Follow-up after curative resection of colorectal cancer: a meta-analysis. Dis Colon Rectum. 2007;50(11):1783–99.
5. Rosati G, Ambrosini G, Barni S, Andreoni B, Corradini G, Luchena G, et al. A randomized trial of intensive versus minimal surveillance of patients with resected Dukes B2-C colorectal carcinoma. Ann Oncol. 2016;27(2):274–80.
6. Primrose JN, Perera R, Gray A, Rose P, Fuller A, Corkhill A, et al. Effect of 3 to 5 years of scheduled CEA and CT follow-up to detect recurrence of colorectal cancer: the FACS randomized clinical trial. JAMA. 2014;311(3):263–70.
7. Wille-Jørgensen P, Syk I, Smedh K, Laurberg S, Nielsen DT, Petersen SH, et al. Effect of more vs less frequent follow-up testing on overall and colorectal cancer-specific mortality in patients with stage II or III colorectal cancer: the COLOFOL randomized clinical trial. JAMA. 2018;319(20):2095–103.
8. Verberne CJ, Zhan Z, van den Heuvel E, Grossmann I, Doornbos PM, Havenga K, et al. Intensified follow-up in colorectal cancer patients using frequent Carcino-Embryonic Antigen (CEA) measurements and CEA-triggered imaging: results of the randomized "CEAwatch" trial. Eur J Surg Oncol. 2015;41(9):1188–96.
9. Verberne CJ, Zhan Z, van den Heuvel ER, Oppers F, de Jong AM, Grossmann I, et al. Survival analysis of the CEAwatch multicentre clustered randomized trial. Br J Surg. 2017;104(8):1069–77.
10. Zhan Z, Verberne CJ, van den Heuvel ER, Grossmann I, Ranchor AV, Wiggers T, et al. Psychological effects of the intensified follow-up of the CEAwatch trial after treatment for colorectal cancer. PLoS One. 2017;12(9):e0184740.
11. Jeffery M, Hickey BE, Hider PN. Follow-up strategies for patients treated for non-metastatic colorectal cancer. Cochrane Database Syst Rev. 2019;9:CD002200.
12. Nicholson BD, Shinkins B, Pathiraja I, Roberts NW, James TJ, Mallett S, et al. Blood CEA levels for detecting recurrent colorectal cancer. Cochrane Database Syst Rev. 2015;2015(12):Cd011134.
13. Smoragiewicz M, Lim H, Peixoto RD. Surveillance for asymptomatic recurrence in resected stage III colon cancer: does it result in a more favorable outcome? J Gastrointest Oncol. 2015;6(3):268–73.

14. Liu SL, Cheung WY. Role of surveillance imaging and endoscopy in colorectal cancer follow-up: quality over quantity? World J Gastroenterol. 2019;25(1):59–68.
15. Popp JWD, Enns E, Nyman JA, Beck JR, Kuntz KM. Reevaluating the evidence for intensive postoperative extracolonic surveillance for nonmetastatic colorectal cancer. Value Health. 2022;25(1):36–46.
16. Leijssen LGJ, Dinaux AM, Kunitake H, Bordeianou LG, Berger DL. Detrimental impact of symptom-detected colorectal cancer. Surg Endosc. 2020;34(2):569–79.
17. Jiménez Londoño GA, García Vicente AM, Sánchez Pérez V, Jiménez Aragón F, León Martin A, Cano Cano JM, Domínguez Ferreras E, Gómez López OV, Espinosa Arranz J, Soriano Castrejón ÁM. ^{18}F-FDG PET/contrast enhanced CT in the standard surveillance of high risk colorectal cancer patients. Eur J Radiol. 2014;83(12):2224–30.
18. Monteil J, Le Brun-Ly V, Cachin F, Zasadny X, Seitz JF, Mundler O, et al. Comparison of 18FDG-PET/CT and conventional follow-up methods in colorectal cancer: a randomised prospective study. Dig Liver Dis. 2021;53(2):231–7.
19. Saito GSS, Kamata H, Miyakita H, Okada K, Tanaka A, Suzuki T. Monitoring of serum carcinoembryonic antigen levels after curative resection of colon cancer: cutoff values determined according to preoperative levels enhance the diagnostic accuracy for recurrence. Oncology. 2017;92(5):276–82.
20. Huang CS, Chen CY, Huang LK, Wang WS, Yang SH. Prognostic value of postoperative serum carcinoembryonic antigen levels in colorectal cancer patients who smoke. PLoS One. 2020;15(6):e0233687.
21. Maeda HKK, Aoyama T, Oba K, Honda M, Mayanagi S, Kanda M, Hamada C, Sadahiro S, Sakamoto J, Saji S, Yoshikawa T. Hazard rate of tumor recurrence over time in patients with colon cancer: implications for postoperative surveillance from three Japanese Foundation for Multidisciplinary Treatment of Cancer (JFMC) clinical trials. J Cancer. 2017;8(19):4057–64.
22. Lee SY, Lee J, Park HM, Kim CH, Kim HR. Perineural invasion and number of retrieved lymph nodes are prognostic factors for T2N0 colon cancer. Langenbeck's Arch Surg. 2021;406(6):1979–85.
23. Lin Y, Liu S, Hong L, Shao L, Wu J. Postoperative locoregional recurrence pattern and treatment management of stage pT4 sigmoid colon cancer: a retrospective cohort study. Radiat Oncol. 2022;17(1):95.
24. Pei JP, Zhao ZM, Sun Z, Gu WJ, Zhu J, Zhu J, et al. Development and validation of a novel classification scheme for combining pathological T stage and log odds of positive lymph nodes for colon cancer. Eur J Surg Oncol. 2022;48(1):228–36.
25. Gilardoni E, Bernasconi DP, Poli S, Garancini M, Luperto M, Zucchini N, et al. Surveillance for early stages of colon cancer: potentials for optimizing follow-up protocols. World J Surg Oncol. 2015;13:260.
26. Leijssen LGJ, Dinaux AM, Kinutake H, Bordeianou LG, Berger DL. Do stage I colorectal cancers with lymphatic invasion require a different postoperative approach? J Gastrointest Surg. 2019;23(9):1884–92.
27. Kishiki T, Lapin B, Matsuoka H, Watanabe T, Takayasu K, Kojima K, et al. Optimal surveillance protocols after curative resection in patients with stage IV colorectal cancer: a multicenter retrospective study. Dis Colon Rectum. 2018;61(1):51–7.
28. Sisler JJ, Seo B, Katz A, Shu E, Chateau D, Czaykowski P, et al. Concordance with ASCO guidelines for surveillance after colorectal cancer treatment: a population-based analysis. J Oncol Pract. 2012;8(4):e69–79.
29. Paulson EC, Veenstra CM, Vachani A, Ciunci CA, Epstein AJ. Trends in surveillance for resected colorectal cancer, 2001–2009. Cancer. 2015;121(19):3525–33.
30. Moritani K, Shida D, Kanemitsu Y, Shunsuke T, Hamaguchi T, Shimada Y. Surveillance of patients with stage I or II colorectal cancer in Japan: a JCOG study group questionnaire survey. Jpn J Clin Oncol. 2021;51(12):1761–4.
31. Viehl CT, Ochsner A, von Holzen U, Cecini R, Langer I, Guller U, et al. Inadequate quality of surveillance after curative surgery for colon cancer. Ann Surg Oncol. 2010;17(10):2663–9.

13 Surgical Versus Endoscopic Options for Management of Malignant Large Bowel Obstruction

Marco Bertucci Zoccali and Athanasios Angistriotis

Introduction

The incidence of colorectal cancer (CRC) has been steadily increasing overtime, representing the fourth most common malignancy and the third leading cause of cancer related death worldwide [1]. With advances in early diagnosis and treatment strategies, CRC mortality has progressively decreased, with a reported 64% 5-year relative survival rate for all colon cancer stages combined in the US [2]. Elective colon resection remains the mainstay of treatment for locoregional disease, with low morbidity and mortality rates, particularly after the widespread adoption of minimally invasive techniques [3]. Despite the intensification of screening, large bowel obstruction (LBO) is still the initial presentation of up to 30% of colon cancers [4]. Emergency surgery (ES) has traditionally represented the treatment of choice for these patients, with reported higher complication rates and worse oncologic outcomes compared to elective operations [5, 6]. In an effort to avoid the morbidity associated with emergency surgery, the use of endoscopically placed self-expanding metal stents (SEMS) has been proposed and implemented over the last 3 decades for the restoration of intestinal flow in patients presenting with malignant LBO [7]. While initially proposed as definitive palliation for unresectable tumors or in patients unfit for surgery, overtime SEMS have been commonly used as a bridge to surgery (BTS), with the aim of converting a surgical emergency into a condition amenable to a safer elective procedure [8]. Despite some concerns related to potentially worse oncologic outcomes in the event of an iatrogenic perforation during stent placement, this approach has gained popularity, as data regarding its safety and efficacy, particularly in avoiding the need for a stoma, has accumulated in the

M. Bertucci Zoccali (✉) · A. Angistriotis
Division of Colorectal Surgery, Columbia University Irving Medical Center-New York Presbyterian Hospital, New York, NY, USA

K. Umanskiy, N. Hyman (eds.), *Difficult Decisions in Colorectal Surgery*, Difficult Decisions in Surgery: An Evidence-Based Approach,
https://doi.org/10.1007/978-3-031-42303-1_13

Table 13.1 PICO table

P (patients)	I (intervention)	C (comparator)	O (outcomes)
Patients with malignant LBO	ES (colectomy, diversion)	SEMS placement	Short term (morbidity, mortality), long term (oncologic outcomes), quality of life.

literature [9, 10]. This chapter provides a critical review of the current literature on the topic, discussing advantages and disadvantages of the use of SEMS over emergency surgeries in the setting of malignant LBO, with some special considerations for right sided and rectal cancers as well as extracolonic malignancies (ECMs) (Table 13.1).

Search Strategy

For the purposes of this chapter, a literature search was performed on the management of malignant SBO to identify all the English language publications on the Cochrane Database of Collected Research, EMBASE, MEDLINE, and PubMed from inception to 2021, with particular focus on those published after 2015. Key words used for the search included: "colon cancer", "rectal cancer", "obstruction", "stent", "stenting", "surgery", "emergency", "stoma", "colostomy", "diversion". Randomized controlled trials (RCT), systematic reviews and large retrospective studies were reviewed in details and findings were summarized in table form in the results section (Table 13.2). Small retrospective series were also assessed and referenced as appropriate.

Table 13.2 Summary of the most notable studies published in the literature to date

	Study	Intent	N	Design	Technical success of stenting	Outcome	SEMS	Emergent surgery	Quality of evidence
1	Hill 2016	BTS	246	RCT	82%	30-day mortality	5.3%	4.4%	High
						Hospital stay	15.5 days	16 days	
						Stoma rate[a]	45%	69%	
2	Arezzo 2017	BTS	56 BTS 59 surgery	RCT	87.5%	60-day complication rate	51.8%	57.6%	High
						1-year complication rate	60.7%	69.4%	
						Stoma rate[a]	19.6%	39%	
						Hospital stay[a]	15 days	11 days	
3	Siddiqui 2017	Palliative	69 SEMS 36 surgery	Retrospective cohort	89.9%	30-day morbidity[a]	7.2%	30.5%	Moderate
						30-day mortality	0	5.5%	
						Hospital stay[a]	4 days	8 days	
						Maintenance of decompression until death[a]	73.9%	94.4%	
						Long-term morbidity	21%	11%	
4	Ribeiro 2018	Palliative	4 RCT (125 total)	Meta-analysis	87.3%	30-day Morbidity	36.5%	24.2%	High
						30-day mortality	6.3%	6.4%	
						Stoma rate[a]	14.3%	84%	
						Mean survival	279 days	244 days	
5	Fiori 2019	Palliative	16 SEMS 17 surgery	RCT	–	30-day Karnofsky[a]	65	56	Moderate
						180-day Karnofsky	58	52	
						Hospital stay[a]	4 days	9.8 days	
						1-year survival	25%	29%	

(continued)

Table 13.2 (continued)

	Study	Intent	N	Design	Technical success of stenting	Outcome	SEMS	Emergent surgery	Quality of evidence
6	Foo 2019	BTS	7 RCT (222 SEMS 226 surgery)	Meta-analysis	–	Morbidity[a]	RR 0.605		High
						30-day mortality	RR 0.963		
						Overall recurrence[a]	37%	25.9%	
						Systemic recurrence[a]	25.3%	15%	
						3-year disease-free survival	OR 1.429		
						3-year overall survival	OR 1.659		
7	Amelung 2019	BTS	222 SEMS 444 surgery	Propensity-matched retrospective	87.4%	Primary anastomosis[a]	74.3%	39.9%	Moderate
						Stoma rate[a]	28.4%	65.3%	
						Morbidity	42.8%	41.9%	
						90-day mortality	5.4%	6.3%	
						Need for adjuvant chemo	37.8%	37.2%	
						Time to adj chemo	6 weeks	9 weeks	
						Distant metastases	21.6%	26.6%	
						3-year locoregional recurrence	11.4%	13.6%	
						3-year disease-free survival	58.8%	52.6%	
						3-year overall survival	74%	68.3%	
8	Tomita 2019	BTS/ palliative	426 BTS 288 palliative (only BTS were included in the analysis)	Prospective observational	98.1%	30-day complication	8.5%		Moderate
						Perforation	1.9%		
						Stent migration	1.2%		
						Primary anastomosis	91.8%		
						Stoma rate	10.6%		
						Morbidity	16.9%		
						Mortality	0.5%		

9	Veld 2020	Palliative	3 RCT/ 2 prospective observational / 13 retrospective (758 SEMS 540 surgery 220 decompressing stoma)	Meta-analysis	–	Early complication[a]	13.6%	25.5	High
						30-day mortality[a]	3.9%	9.4%	
						Stoma rate[a]	14.3%	51.4%	
						Hospital stay	8 days	15 days	
						Need for adjuvant chemo	70.4%	69.5%	
						Time to start adj chemo[a]	19 days	37 days	
						Late complication[a]	23.2%	9.8%	
						Mean survival	259 days	287 days	
10	Spannenburg 2020	BTS/ palliative	14 RCTs/ 13 NRCTs (18 BTS, 7 palliative, 2 both) 1266 BTS 2628 surgery	Meta-analysis	–	3-year disease-free survival	HR 1.15		High
						5-year disease-free survival	HR 1.08		
						3-year overall survival	HR 0.93		
						5-year overall survival	HR 0.93		
						30-day mortality[a]	6.5%	8.1%	
						Morbidity[a]	26.1%	41.4%	
						Tumor recurrence	RR 1.32		
						Hospital stay[a]	Mean difference -7.2		
						Primary anastomosis[a]	73.8%	50.8%	
						Stoma rate[a]	40.3%	82.9%	
11	Jain 2020	BTS	8 RCT/ 25 observational (11,596 surgery 1928 SEMS)	Meta-analysis	90%	Primary anastomosis[a]	OR 3.179		High
						Stoma rate[a]	OR 0.385		
						Anastomotic leak[a]	OR 0.589		
						Post-op ileus[a]	OR 0.557		
						90-day mortality[a]	OR 0.687		
						Hospital stay[a]	Difference 2.5 days		

(continued)

Table 13.2 (continued)

	Study	Intent	N	Design	Technical success of stenting	Outcome	SEMS	Emergent surgery	Quality of evidence
12	Cirocchi 2021	BTS	387 SEMS 386 surgery	Meta-analysis	89.3%	Primary anastomosis[a]	69.8%	55.1%	High
						Overall morbidity[a]	32.7%	48.2%	
						Overall recurrence	35.1%	24.7%	
						3-year overall survival	67.8%	73.5%	
						3-year disease-free survival	58.7%	63.5%	
13	Cao 2021	BTS	49 SEMS 49 surgery	Propensity matched retrospective observational	44/49 (89.8)	3-year OS[a]	53%	77.2%	Moderate
						5-year OS[a]	30.6%	55%	
						Median OS[a]	41 months	65 months	
						Total recurrence rate[a]	51%	26.5%	
						Regional recurrence	20.4%	8.2%	
						Distant metastasis	30.6%	18.4%	
14	Mahfouz 2022	Palliative	35 SEMS 29 surgery	Prospective observational	100%	Hospital stay[a]	3.5 days	7.7 days	Moderate
						Morbidity	20%	20.7%	

BTS bridge to surgery, *RCT* randomized controlled trial, *RR* relative risk, *OR* odds ratio
[a]Indicates statistically significant difference in the outcome

Results

Emergency Surgery

In the face of an overall increase in early diagnosis, it is estimated that up to one third of CRC patients would require an emergency intervention upon initial presentation [11]. Malignancy represents the leading cause of LBO in adults, and over two thirds of the obstructing tumors occur in the left side of the colon, the majority of which are distal to the splenic flexure [12, 13]. Due to the smaller diameter of the bowel, more distal tumors (occurring in the left and sigmoid colon) are more likely to present as an obstruction compared to more proximal cancers. Surgical options in this setting include simple diversion with loop colostomy versus resection with or without primary anastomosis. The creation of a diverting or blowhole colostomy proximal to the tumor presents several advantages: (1) it can be performed quickly, with minimal surgical trauma, potentially even under local anesthesia in particularly frail patients; (2) it is an effective temporizing measure allowing completion of staging and definition of the most appropriate multidisciplinary treatment strategy, while avoiding a resection in the setting of an unprepped colon; (3) it represents an effective treatment when a radical resection is not feasible due to the extent of the disease or the tenuous conditions of the patient [4, 14]. However, colostomies are associated with non-trivial complication rates, including prolapse, herniation, necrosis, and infection, and the risk is demonstrably higher when performed in the emergent setting [15]. A loop colostomy negatively affects overall quality of life (QoL) when meant as definitive palliation, and imposes the need for additional operations when used as a bridge to elective resection [16]. The safety of an emergency colectomy, when technically feasible, is suggested by several studies in the literature, with reported equal morbidity, mortality and oncologic outcomes compared to loop colostomy, and shorter overall length of stay [17, 18]. A segmental resection is the preferred operation, while a subtotal colectomy – reportedly associated with worse functional outcomes - is reserved for those cases where bowel ischemia or serosal tear/perforation occurs in the proximal colon, or in the presence of synchronous tumors [19]. In a RCT published in 2014, 75 patient with obstructing rectosigmoid cancer were randomized to either loop colostomy or resection with end colostomy (Hartmann's procedure); after stratifying patients by age and comorbidities, the two approaches had comparable surgical and non-surgical complication rates, blood transfusion requirement, length of stay, and mortality [20]. Additionally, although the quality of the data is limited, there seems to be a survival benefit in resecting the primary tumor even in the presence of synchronous metastases [21]. The feasibility of an oncologically sound resection in the emergent setting was assessed in a retrospective study by Teixeira et al.; 87 patient had an ES (77% of which for bowel obstruction); while the complication rates were higher than those reported for elective procedures (34% morbidity and 20% mortality), the vast majority of the specimens were adequate in terms of surgical margins and lymph node harvest [22]. While a Hartmann's procedure leaves open the possibility of restoration of bowel continuity, actual colostomy reversal rates are much lower than generally thought, with 95% of patients still having a stoma at 18 months in the UK National Bowel Cancer Audit published in 2015 [23]. Furthermore, Hartmann's reversal is a morbid procedure, as reported in a series of 103 patients from University of Vermont, where nearly one third of the patients experienced a postoperative complication; interestingly, during the study period, the number of Hartmann procedures exceeded by fivefold the take downs, once again suggesting that most of these end colostomies will, in reality, become permanent [24]. Over the last two decades, several retrospective and prospective studies have been conducted asserting the feasibility and safety of resection with primary anastomosis in the emergent setting for appropriately selected cases [25]. Bearing in mind the potential for bias inherent to the non-randomized design of the studies, primary anastomosis seems to have more favorable outcomes over a staged approach (14% vs 35% mortality, respectively, in a historical series), with leak rates reported between 2% and 12%, not dissimilar to the leak rates reported for elective left sided resections [25–29]. Recognized risk factors for poor outcomes after primary anastomosis are age, comorbidities, advanced cancer stage, and surgeon's expertise [30, 31]. In a recent international audit on nearly 600 patients, those who received a primary anastomosis experienced a similar major complication rate compared to those managed with end colostomy; interestingly, in the anastomosis group, while a diverting stoma did not decrease the leak rate (12% vs 13% for diverted versus not diverted, respectively), it did decrease the rate of severe complications (75% vs 87%), need for reoperation (50% vs 75%), and postoperative mortality (0% vs 20%) [32].

SEMS as Bridge to Surgery

For patients with resectable disease who are fit for surgery, SEMSs have been used to avoid ES and allow for definitive treatment in a more controlled environment with a one-step resection, thus acting as a bridge to surgery (BTS). This section of the chapter summarizes the current literature by reported outcomes.

Success Rate Overall, the reported clinical and technical success rates for SEMSs are excellent. Atukorale et al., in their systematic review, defined technical success as satisfactory placement and deployment of the SEMS, and clinical success as improvement of obstructive symptoms within 48 h and resumption of bowel function and oral intake. Over the 6 studies included in their review (2 RCTs and 4 non-randomized comparative studies), technical and clinical success were observed in 91% and 89% of the patients, respectively. The need for reintervention due to recurrent obstruction was reported in 4 studies, and this occurred in 17% of the patients [33]. The CReST study (246 patients with left-sided colonic obstruction randomized to either endoluminal stenting as a bridge to surgery or surgical decompression, 92% of which treated with curative intent), reported a success rate of 82% after stenting [34]. In a more recent pooled analysis from 2 prospective multicenter trials (426 patients total), technical and clinical success rates were found to be 98% and 94% respectively [35]. Lastly, in a meta-analysis that included 8 RTC and 25 observational studies (15,224 patients total), SEMSs had technical and clinical success rates of 90% (1426 patients) and 81% (860 patients), respectively [36].

Morbidity and Mortality The safety aspect of the use of SEMS has been extensively scrutinized in the literature. Arezzo et al., in a meta-analysis of 8 RCTs, reported an overall 60-day morbidity rate of 34%, not statistically different compared to ES [37]. The ESCO RTC published in 2017 reported 8 cases of stent-related complications in the 56 patients treated with SEMS, the most common being perforation at the tumor site (9%) [38]. Perforation remains the most feared stent-related complication, with a reported incidence ranging from 2% to 10%, followed by stent migration (reported rates 1–10%) [35, 36, 39]. In a meta-analysis by Van Halsema et al., chemotherapy regimen including bevacizumab was an independent risk factor for perforation following SEMS placement (incidence 12% vs 7% for non-bevacizumab based regimens) [40]. Many studies have been published investigating whether the use of SEMSs improves surgical outcomes at the time of resection when compared to emergent operations. A recent updated meta-analysis comparing the two approaches demonstrated significantly lower overall postoperative complications rates in the SEMS group (33%) than in the ES group (48%), along with a higher rate of successful primary anastomosis formation (70% vs 55%, respectively) [41]. In a meta-analysis of seven RCTs by Huang et al., patients managed with SEMS achieved significantly better rates of primary anastomoses (OR 2.01, p = 0.007), wound infection (OR 0.31, p = 0.004)] and overall complication (OR 0.30, p = 0.03); no difference was demonstrated in anastomotic leak rate following curative resection (OR 0.74, p = 0.47), mortality (OR 0.88, p = 0.76), or organ space infections (OR 0.62, p = 0.57)] [42]. Similar findings were reported in a propensity matching study by Harvey et al. based on NHS data, where the rate of anastomotic leak, wound dehisce and sepsis were comparable between stenting and ES [43]. Across the most recent literature, the reported rates of successful primary anastomosis and overall post-operative complications are consistently more favorable in patients treated with SEMS [10, 37, 41, 42]. Procedure-related mortality is more difficult to assess, as many studies do not distinguish between procedure- and disease-related mortality, making survival a more reliable indicator, which will be discussed later in the chapter. Nonetheless, Amelung et al. reported a procedure-related mortality of 1.6%, most commonly secondary to bowel perforation [44]. While an earlier meta-analysis failed to demonstrate a difference in overall 60-day-mortality,[37] subsequent studies have shown significant lower 30-day, 90-day and 1-year mortality in subjects undergoing stenting prior to surgery [10, 36, 43].

Permanent Stoma Rate In the ESCO RCT, the stoma formation rate was 22.2% vs 39% (P = .031) for SEMS and ES, respectively; at the time the study was published, the overall stoma reversal rate was 30% [38]. Similar results were reported by Amelung in a propensity score-matched analysis from the Netherlands (stoma rate 24% for SEMS vs 45% for ES; p < 0·001) [45]. This finding was confirmed in 2 recent meta-analyses of RTCs, thus minimizing the possibility that the observed difference is affected by selection bias [37, 41].

Recurrence Rates Since the introduction of stents for the management of malignant colonic obstruction, oncologic safety has represented the primary concern [46, 47]. Amelung et al., both in their propensity score-matched retrospective study and in their meta-analysis, showed comparable local (11% vs 14%) and overall (27% vs 26%) recurrence rates between SEMS and ES, respectively [44, 45]. Similarly, no difference in recurrence rates was observed in the ESCO RCT (17% vs 20%, median follow-up of 36 months) and a more recent meta-analysis (25 vs 35%) [38, 41]. Conversely, Cao et al., in their propensity-matched study published in 2021, showed higher rates of perineural invasion (51% vs 26%, p = 0.013) and worse overall recurrence rates for the SEMS group (51% vs 26%, p = 0.013) [9]. Along the same lines, in a 2019 meta-analysis of 7 RCTs, the overall recurrence rate was higher in the stent group (37% vs 26%; p = 0.049), although this did not translate into a significant difference in 3-year disease-free and overall survival [48]. In terms of risk factors for recurrence, a 2020 meta-analysis specifically looking at the negative effects of procedural complications, stent-related perforation (reported incidence 9%) was significantly associated with higher locoregional (27% vs 12%; p = 0.004) and global recurrence rates (41 vs. 31%; p = 0.04), although 3- and 5-year survival was not affected [49].

Long Term Survival and Quality Of Life Notwithstanding the considerations regarding the previously discussed outcomes, the literature is rather consistent in reporting comparable long-term survival between the two approaches. Huang et al. observed no difference in 3- (65 vs 75%; p = 0.25) and 5-year overall survival (48 vs. 58%, p = 0.38), in keeping with the results from the ESCO trial and the meta-analysis by Cirocchi et al.[38, 41, 42]. It is worth reporting that a handful of retrospective studies have observed worse long-term outcomes associated with SEMS [46, 50]. Particularly, in the propensity-matched study by Cao, 3-year overall survival (53% vs 77%, p = 0.039) and 5-year overall survival (31 vs 55%, p = 0.025) were significantly worse in the stent group; stenting was an independent predictor of poorer survival on multivariable analysis (hazard ratio = 2.309, p = 0.037) [9]. Lastly, the CReST trial is one of the few studies looking at quality of life metrics and did not demonstrate significant differences at the 3 and 12 months between the patients treated with SEMS when compared to ES [34].

SEMS as Definitive Palliation

Owing to a lesser concern regarding oncologic safety, the use of SEMSs in the palliative setting has been more rapidly and broadly accepted; however, the volume and quality of the data is limited when compared to that available for patients treated with curative intent.

Success Rates Overall, SEMSs are very effective in the symptomatic management of malignant LBO, with clinical success rates reported above 90% across the literature [51–53]. In a 2020 meta-analysis by Veld et al., pooled clinical success rate from 10 studies including 406 SEMS procedures was 94% [54]. Lower success rates (86%) were reported in a meta-analysis by Ribeiro et al., however the inclusion of rectal cancer patients might have represented a confounding factor, since this tumor location appears to be associated with worse outcomes, as discussed later in this chapter [55].

Morbidity Depending on the studies and definitions, overall stent-related complication rates are reported between 23% and 36%, with the most common adverse events being restenosis/migration (15–21%), perforation (5–16%), and bleeding (3%) [51, 55, 56]. Several studies, some of which randomized, have compared adverse event rates between SEMSs and ES for palliation, without demonstrating any statistically significant differences [51, 55, 57]. The use of SEMS for palliation is consistently associated with shorter hospital stay and earlier resumption of oral nutrition [51, 55, 57, 58]. When looking at long-term morbidity, Siddiqui et al. reported stent occlusion (10%), stent migration (5%), and colonic ulcer (6%) as the most common occurrences in the SEMS group, at a median follow up of 26 weeks [58]. In this RCT, patients managed with stenting experienced worse long term maintenance of decompression (until death or latest follow-up) compared to surgical patients (74% vs 97%; respectively, $p = 0.003$), while overall long-term complication rate was higher (21% vs 11%, respectively; $p = 0.27$) [58].

Similarly, a retrospective series on 114 patients described shorter patency duration after SEMS compared to surgery (163 vs 349 days; $p < 0.001$), even after additional intervention (202 vs 349 days; $p < .001$); the presence of carcinomatosis has been significantly associated with long term stent failure and need of re-intervention [59, 60].

In a recent retrospective population based study, Abelson et al. showed that, compared to those palliated surgically, patients undergoing SEMS had similar or fewer complications (major events: OR 0.81; $p = 0.68$; procedural complications: OR 0.57; $p = 0.10$) with no significant difference between the groups in terms of 90-day and 1-year hospital readmission (OR 0.93; $p = .83$; OR 0.72; $p = .30$ respectively); SEMS patient had a higher risk of requiring an additional intervention at 1 year (OR 2.93; $p = 0.03$), most commonly re-stenting [61].

Long Term Survival and Quality of Life Most of the published studies suggest no significant difference in long-term survival between SEMS and ES [55, 56, 62]. One retrospective study, however, showed that surgery was an independent predictor of better survival in patients with good performance status (ECOG 0-1), emphasizing the importance of patient selection in the treatment decision making [59]. Quality of life is arguably the most important outcome of treatment in the palliative setting. Data is scarce, however, Fiori et al,. in their 2019 RCT, observed a bimodal distribution of outcomes; at one month, QoL was significantly better in patients treated with stenting, whereas, at 6 months, patients who had surgical treatment reported higher scores [57]. The authors speculated that this may be due to stent-related late side effects such as tenesmus and minor rectal bleeding, in line with the evidence available in the literature demonstrating higher long term morbidity associated with stenting as compared to ES [59, 62, 63]. Lastly, in an RCT published in 2017, Young et al., while unable to demonstrate any significant difference in QoL at 4 weeks, found stenting significantly more cost effective compared to surgery, with an estimated incremental cost-effectiveness ratio of about $22.000 [64].

Special Considerations

Proximal Tumors Because of the larger caliber of the proximal colon, right sided malignant obstructions are less common. Even in those uncommon instances, emergency resections tend to be less challenging compared to left sided procedures and, except for the frailest patients, a primary anastomosis can be safely performed, in spite of a more advanced age and stage at presentation [65]. Anastomotic leak rates after emergency right colectomy for obstruction are reported in the range of 1–5%, significantly lower compared to emergent distal colocolonic and colorectal anastomoses, and not far off from the rates commonly reported for ileocolostomies performed in the elective setting (~1%) [4]. In order to minimize metabolic derangements and improve quality of life, a surgical ileocolonic bypass is the preferred palliation in patients with unresectable right sided tumors, with surgical/percutaneous cecostomy reserved for extremely unfit patients [66]. The use of SEMS in the right colon is technically more challenging, which, along with the favorable outcomes after ES, have hampered the diffusion of endoscopic stenting for obstructing proximal tumors. A 2016 retrospective multicenter retrospective study from South Korea comparing ES versus stenting as bridge to surgery for obstructing right colon cancer suggests the safety of the latter approach, with comparable short- and long-term results for all the assessed outcomes [67]. An earlier metanalysis on 14 studies showed better outcomes when resection was performed after initial stent placement, with statistically significant less major morbidity (1% vs 24%) and mortality (0% vs 11%), and a trend towards less anastomotic leaks (0% vs 9%); these results must be interpreted with caution due to the limited quality and the high heterogeneity of the included studies (mostly retrospective) [44]. In a more recent retrospective multicenter trial where SEMSs were used both for definitive palliation (15%) and as bridge to surgery (85%), stenting achieved clinical success in 78% of the cases and long term maintenance of patency in 74%, with 21% long term complication rate (compared to 11% for patients undergoing ES upon presentation) [58]. Lastly, in a retrospective study from China, the use of SEMSs in the acute setting not only provided better short-term outcomes compared to emergent colectomy (intensive care admission 11.4% vs. 34.7%, $p = 0.011$; overall complications 11.4% vs. 29.2%, $P = 0.042$; length of stay 8.23 ± 6.50 vs. 11.18 ± 6.71 days, $p = 0.033$) but, in the stage IV subgroup, patients treated with stent were 3 times more likely to undergo a synchronous liver metastasis resection at the time of surgery (85.7% vs 14.3%, $p = 0.029$; HR = 3.26, $p = 0.041$) [68].

Extraperitoneal Rectal Cancer Tumors involving the mid and distal rectum present some distinctive features that call for a different approach compared to more proximal CRCs. A distal rectal cancer causing an obstruction is almost always locally advanced at presentation, hence best managed with neoadjuvant chemoradiation [69]. A diverting colostomy represents the treatment modality of choice in the acute setting, as it reliably manages the obstruction with minimal trauma, allowing from prompt initiation and minimal interruptions of oncologic treatments. While a loop ileostomy is the preferred diversion modality after low anterior resection, it should be used with caution in the emergent setting, as it does not represent a suitable option in the presence of complete obstruction or of a competent ileocecal valve [70]. The choice of type and placement of the colostomy should be based on the anticipated definitive surgery. Vermeer et al., in a paper from 2016, suggested to perform a right sided transverse colostomy or very distal loop sigmoid colostomy if an eventual lower anterior resection (LAR) is anticipated, while an end sigmoid colostomy is preferred in those cases where an abdominoperineal resection will be required; left sided colostomies should be avoided as they could compromise the future conduit in case of an LAR [71]. The use of SEMSs for lower rectal cancers (<5 cm from the anal verge) is limited by the potential for pain, tenesmus and incontinence, ultimately worsening patients' quality of life; additionally, stent migration and bleeding are common complications during neoadjuvant treatment [72]. In a meta-analysis including 32 articles, technical success was reported in 97% of the cases, however, the clinical success rate was only 69%, with a considerable rate of complications (28%) [73].

Extracolonic Malignancies Conflicting results have been reported in the literature on the safety and efficacy SEMs for the management of LBO cause by advanced ECM, with earlier series documenting higher morbidity as well as lower success rates when compared to primary CRC [72, 74]. More recent reports have mitigated those concerns, with comparable technical and clinical success rates as well as complications, irrespective of the underlying malignancy, when used both as definitive palliation or BTS; one study reported significant shorter long term patency for extracolonic primaries in the palliative setting, however, this was not of clinical relevance given the shorter life expectancy of this cohort [75–77]. Because of the rarity of this presentation, high quality data is lacking, nonetheless, based on the current evidence, SEMSs are a viable option for the treatment of LBO secondary to ECM.

Recommendations Based on the Data

The recommendations summarized below are based on the data presented in this chapter and are in keeping with those put forward by the American Society of Colon and Rectal Surgeons in the current Clinical Practice Guidelines Management of Rectal Cancer (2020) and Colon Cancer (2022), as well as the ones formulated by the World Society of Emergency Surgery [4, 69, 78].

In patients with malignant large bowel obstruction secondary to potentially curable left sided disease, stenting as a bridge to surgery is associated with high rates of technical (>90%) and clinical success (>80%), improved short term outcomes at the time of surgical resection (particularly in terms of overall complications and primary anastomosis rates), and lower permanent stoma rates [33, 36, 37, 41, 42]. Concerns remain regarding the reported perforation rates (2–10%) and worse overall recurrence rates with the use of SEMS, while the majority of the literature suggests comparable long term survival rates [35, 36, 38, 39, 41, 42, 48]. Therefore, patients with obstructing left-sided colon cancer and curable disease, particularly if averse to diversion, can be management with stenting as bridge to surgery, if properly counselled about the risks (strong recommendation based on high-quality evidence).

Surgical options in this setting include simple diversion (loop colostomy) versus resection with or without primary anastomosis and loop ileostomy. Colostomies are associated with detrimental effects on QoL and, while technically reversible, they tend to become permanent in the majority of the patients [16, 23]. Evidence has accumulated in the literature supporting the feasibility of an oncologically sound emergency colectomy, as well as the safety of primary anastomosis in the acute setting [22, 25, 32]. Hence, in patients undergoing emergency surgery for left sided malignant obstruction, an oncologic resection (with or without diverting ileostomy) should be preferred over simple diversion or Hartmann's procedure, when technically feasible (strong recommendation based on moderate-quality evidence).

For patients with incurable disease, stenting represents an appealing option for the treatment of obstructing colon cancer, associated with shorter length of stay and quicker resumption of diet compared to emergent surgery [51, 55, 57]. Surgery, however, seems to provide longer lasting decompression with less need for repeated procedures [59, 61]. Based on these considerations, stenting should be considered the treatment modality of choice for obstructing colon cancer in the palliative setting, especially in patients with poor overall prognosis and performance status (strong recommendation based on moderate-quality evidence).

Obstructing right sided tumors are generally amenable to primary resection and anastomosis with acceptable complication rates [4]. While some data exists suggesting a role for stenting as bridge to surgery in this setting to improve surgical outcomes, more evidence is needed prior to recommending the widespread adoption of this strategy [44, 68]. Currently, patients with right sided malignant LBO who are fit for surgery should be preferentially managed with primary resection and anastomosis; stenting can be considered as an option for palliation or, in selected cases, as a bridge to elective surgery (weak recommendation based on low-quality evidence).

The use of stents for extraperitoneal obstructing rectal cancer or extracolonic malignancies remains controversial with only low-quality data available in the literature [72–74]. Particularly for rectal cancer, the treatment strategy should prioritize the reliable delivery of optimal oncologic care. Patients with obstructing extraperitoneal rectal cancer and extracolonic malignancies are best managed with surgical diversion; stenting can be considered in patients who are poor surgical candidates or with short life expectancy (strong recommendation based on low-quality evidence).

Personal View of the Data

Due to the intrinsically different nature of the associated complications, comparing the outcomes of endoscopic and surgical treatments is challenging. In particular, adverse events after stenting might become immediately apparent (for example in the event of a perforation), while those related to a surgical procedure tend to extend far beyond the immediate postoperative period, particularly when a diversion is involved. Additionally, differences in technique, patient selection as well as definition of complications and outcomes can contribute to the inconsistency of the findings across studies. Lastly, the variability of the clinical presentation, especially in the emergent setting, along with the varying degree of expertise - a crucial determinant of outcomes - across centers makes any comparison even more challenging.

Currently, a trial is enrolling patients in Goteborg, Sweden comparing emergency surgery versus stenting or stoma prior to elective resection for malignant LBO, while 2 trials are being conducted in Beijing, China looking at the role of neoadjuvant chemotherapy after stent placement as a bridge to surgery (www.clinicaltrials.gov).

These considerations further emphasize the importance of a tailored approach based on disease stage and presentation, the patient's overall conditions and goals of care. When a patient presents with malignant LBO, after appropriate resuscitation and staging imaging, overall goals of treatment should be clarified. Most patients with right sided tumors are best treated with right colectomy and primary anastomosis. For left sided tumors, granted that the necessary expertise is locally available, stenting is a valuable treatment to relieve the obstruction and allow for a subsequent elective resection, particularly in patients who are reluctant to the idea of a stoma; proper discussion regarding the potential benefits as well as the risks associated with this approach (including iatrogenic perforation and the potential for suboptimal oncologic outcomes) is crucial. In patients with metastatic disease, stenting is becoming the treatment modality of choice, both for palliation in patients with overall poor prognosis, and for those who are good surgical candidates and could become resectable after systemic treatment. It is worth involving a medical oncologist in the treatment planning early on, as the use of medications such as anti-VEGF agents (Bevacizumab) has been associated with higher rates of stent related complications. For obstructing tumors of the mid and distal rectum, optimal oncologic treatment almost invariably involves neoadjuvant treatments, hence the acute management should be aimed at achieving reliable, long-lasting resolution of the obstruction thus minimizing interruptions in the administration of systemic therapy, and this is usually best accomplished with a proximal diversion.

Summary of Recommendations

1. Patients with obstructing left-sided colon cancer and curable disease, particularly if averse to diversion, can be managed with stenting as bridge to surgery, if properly counselled about the risks (strong recommendation based on high-quality evidence).
2. In patients undergoing emergent surgery for left sided malignant obstruction, an oncologic resection (with or without diverting ileostomy) should be preferred over simple diversion or Hartmann's procedure, when technically feasible (strong recommendation based on moderate-quality evidence)
3. Stenting should be considered the treatment modality of choice for obstructing colon cancer in the palliative setting, especially in patients with poor overall prognosis and performance status (strong recommendation based on moderate-quality evidence).
4. Patients with right sided malignant LBO who are fit for surgery should be preferentially managed with primary resection and anastomosis; stenting can be considered as an option for palliation or, in selected cases, as a bridge to elective surgery (weak recommendation based on low-quality evidence).
5. Patients with obstructing extraperitoneal rectal cancer and extracolonic malignancies are best managed with surgical diversion; stenting can be considered in patients who are poor surgical candidates or with short life expectancy (strong recommendation based on low-quality evidence).

References

1. Rawla P, Sunkara T, Barsouk A. Epidemiology of colorectal cancer: incidence, mortality, survival, and risk factors. Prz Gastroenterol. 2019;14:89.
2. Cancer Statistics Review, 1975–2016 - SEER Statistics. https://seer.cancer.gov/archive/csr/1975_2016/. Accessed 24 Jun 2022.
3. Song XJ, Liu ZL, Zeng R, Ye W, Liu CW. A meta-analysis of laparoscopic surgery versus conventional open surgery in the treatment of colorectal cancer. Medicine. 2019; https://doi.org/10.1097/MD.0000000000015347.
4. Pisano M, Zorcolo L, Merli C, et al. 2017 WSES guidelines on colon and rectal cancer emergencies: obstruction and perforation. BioMed. 2018;13:1–27.
5. Chen TM, Huang YT, Wang GC. Outcome of colon cancer initially presenting as colon perforation and obstruction. World J Surg Oncol. 2017;15:1–7.
6. Bakker IS, Snijders HS, Grossmann I, Karsten TM, Havenga K, Wiggers T. High mortality rates after nonelective colon cancer resection: results of a national audit. Color Dis. 2016;18:612–21.

7. Dohmoto M. New method endoscopic implantation of rectal stent in palliative treatment of malignant stenosis. Endoscopia Digestiva. 1991;3:1507–12.
8. Cheung HYS, Chung CC, Tsang WWC, Wong JCH, Yau KKK, Li MKW. Endolaparoscopic approach vs conventional open surgery in the treatment of obstructing left-sided colon cancer: a randomized controlled trial. Arch Surg. 2009;144:1127–32.
9. Cao Y, Chen Q, Ni Z, Wu F, Huang C, Zhou J, Zhang S, Ge B, Huang Q. Propensity score-matched comparison of stenting as a bridge to surgery and emergency surgery for acute malignant left-sided colonic obstruction. BMC Surg. 2021; https://doi.org/10.1186/S12893-021-01144-Z.
10. Spannenburg L, Sanchez Gonzalez M, Brooks A, Wei S, Li X, Liang X, Gao W, Wang H. Surgical outcomes of colonic stents as a bridge to surgery versus emergency surgery for malignant colorectal obstruction: a systematic review and meta-analysis of high quality prospective and randomised controlled trials. Eur J Surg Oncol. 2020;46:1404–14.
11. Baer C, Menon R, Bastawrous S, Bastawrous A. Emergency presentations of colorectal cancer. Surg Clin North Am. 2017;97:529–45.
12. Webster PJ, Aldoori J, Burke DA. Optimal management of malignant left-sided large bowel obstruction: do international guidelines agree? World J Emerg Surg. 2019;14:1–8.
13. Aslar AK, Özdemir S, Mahmoudi H, Kuzu MA. Analysis of 230 cases of emergent surgery for obstructing colon cancer–lessons learned. J Gastrointest Surg. 2011;15:110–9.
14. DiGiacomo JC, Lehman M. The colostomy of Duret for the high risk patient. J Investig Surg. 2021;34:257–61.
15. Krishnamurty DM, Blatnik J, Mutch M. Intestinal stoma: stoma complications. Clin Colon Rectal Surg. 2017;30:193.
16. Stavropoulou A, Vlamakis D, Kaba E, Kalemikerakis I, Polikandrioti M, Fasoi G, Vasilopoulos G, Kelesi M. "Living with a stoma": exploring the lived experience of patients with permanent colostomy. Int J Environ Res Public Health. 2021;18:8512.
17. Kronborg O. Acute obstruction from tumour in the left colon without spread. Int J Colorectal Dis. 1995;1(10):1–5.
18. de Salvo GL, Gava C, Lise M, Pucciarelli S. Curative surgery for obstruction from primary left colorectal carcinoma: primary or staged resection? Cochrane Database Syst Rev. 2004; https://doi.org/10.1002/14651858.CD002101.PUB2/INFORMATION/EN.
19. Ross S, Krukowski ZH, Munro A, Russell IT. Single-stage treatment for malignant left-sided colonic obstruction: a prospective randomized clinical trial comparing subtotal colectomy with segmental resection following intraoperative irrigation. Br J Surg. 2005;82:1622–7.
20. Krstic S, Resanovic V, Alempijevic T, Resanovic A, Sijacki A, Djukic V, Loncar Z, Karamarkovic A. Hartmann's procedure vs loop colostomy in the treatment of obstructive rectosigmoid cancer. World J Emerg Surg. 2014;9:1–6.
21. van Rooijen KL, Shi Q, Goey KKH, et al. Prognostic value of primary tumour resection in synchronous metastatic colorectal cancer: individual patient data analysis of first-line randomised trials from the ARCAD database. Eur J Cancer. 2018;91:99–106.
22. Teixeira F, Akaishi EH, Ushinohama AZ, Dutra TC, Netto SD do C, Utiyama EM, Bernini CO, Rasslan S. Can we respect the principles of oncologic resection in an emergency surgery to treat colon cancer? World J Emerg Surg. 2015;10:1–5.
23. National Bowel Cancer Audit Report – 2015 – NHS Digital. https://digital.nhs.uk/data-and-information/publications/statistical/national-bowel-cancer-audit/national-bowel-cancer-audit-report-2015. Accessed 1 Jul 2022.
24. Garber A, Hyman N, Osler T. Complications of Hartmann takedown in a decade of preferred primary anastomosis. Am J Surg. 2014;207:60–4.
25. Zorcolo L, Covotta L, Carlomango N, Bartolo DCC. Safety of primary anastomosis in emergency colo-rectal surgery. Colorectal Dis. 2003;5:262–9.
26. Fielding LP, Stewart-Brown S, Blesovsky L. Large-bowel obstruction caused by cancer: a prospective study. Br Med J. 1979;2:515.

27. Meyer F, Marusch F, Koch A, Meyer L, Führer S, Köckerling F, Lippert H, Gastinger I. Emergency operation in carcinomas of the left colon: value of Hartmann's procedure. Tech Coloproctol. 2004; https://doi.org/10.1007/S10151-004-0164-3.
28. Tekkis PP, Kinsman R, Thompson MR, Stamatakis JD. The Association of Coloproctology of Great Britain and Ireland study of large bowel obstruction caused by colorectal cancer. Ann Surg. 2004;240:76.
29. McKenna NP, Bews KA, Cima RR, Crowson CS, Habermann EB. Validation of a left-sided colectomy anastomotic leak risk score and assessment of diversion practices. Am J Surg. 2022; https://doi.org/10.1016/J.AMJSURG.2022.04.018.
30. Zorcolo L, Covotta L, Carlomagno N, Bartolo DCC, O'Connell PR. Toward lowering morbidity, mortality, and stoma formation in emergency colorectal surgery: the role of specialization. Dis Colon Rectum. 2003;46:1461–7.
31. Biondo S, Parés D, Frago R, Martí-Ragué J, Kreisler E, de Oca J, Jaurrieta E. Large bowel obstruction: predictive factors for postoperative mortality. Dis Colon Rectum. 2004;47:1889–97.
32. Sánchez-Guillén L, Nepogodiev D, Sivrikoz E, et al. Safety of primary anastomosis following emergency left sided colorectal resection: an international, multi-centre prospective audit. Color Dis. 2018;20:47–57.
33. Atukorale YN, Church JL, Hoggan BL, Lambert RS, Gurgacz SL, Goodall S, Maddern GJ. Self-expanding metallic stents for the management of emergency malignant large bowel obstruction: a systematic review. J Gastrointest Surg. 2016;20:455–62.
34. Hill J, Kay C, Morton D, Magill L, Handley K, Gray RG. CREST: Randomised phase III study of stenting as a bridge to surgery in obstructing colorectal cancer—Results of the UK ColoRectal Endoscopic Stenting Trial (CREST). J Clin Oncol. 2016;34:3507. https://doi.org/10.1200/JCO20163415_suppl3507.
35. Tomita M, Saito S, Makimoto S, et al. Self-expandable metallic stenting as a bridge to surgery for malignant colorectal obstruction: pooled analysis of 426 patients from two prospective multicenter series. Surg Endosc. 2019;33:499–509.
36. Jain SR, Yaow CYL, Ng CH, Neo VSQ, Lim F, Foo FJ, Wong NW, Chong CS. Comparison of colonic stents, stomas and resection for obstructive left colon cancer: a meta-analysis. Tech Coloproctol. 2020;24:1121–36.
37. Arezzo A, Passera R, lo Secco G, Verra M, Bonino MA, Targarona E, Morino M. Stent as bridge to surgery for left-sided malignant colonic obstruction reduces adverse events and stoma rate compared with emergency surgery: results of a systematic review and meta-analysis of randomized controlled trials. Gastrointest Endosc. 2017;86:416–26.
38. Arezzo A, Balague C, Targarona E, et al. Colonic stenting as a bridge to surgery versus emergency surgery for malignant colonic obstruction: results of a multicentre randomised controlled trial (ESCO trial). Surg Endosc. 2017;31:3297–305.
39. Padwick RT, Chauhan V, Newman M, et al. Endoscopic stenting of acutely obstructing colorectal cancer: a 10-year review from a tertiary referral Centre. ANZ J Surg. 2016;86:778–81.
40. van Halsema EE, van Hooft JE, Small AJ, et al. Perforation in colorectal stenting: a meta-analysis and a search for risk factors. Gastrointest Endosc. 2014; https://doi.org/10.1016/J.GIE.2013.11.038.
41. Cirocchi R, Arezzo A, Sapienza P, Crocetti D, Cavaliere D, Solaini L, Ercolani G, Sterpetti AV, Mingoli A, Fiori E. Current status of the self-expandable metal stent as a bridge to surgery versus emergency surgery in colorectal cancer: results from an updated systematic review and meta-analysis of the literature. Medicina (Kaunas). 2021; https://doi.org/10.3390/MEDICINA57030268.
42. Huang X, Lv B, Zhang S, Meng L. Preoperative colonic stents versus emergency surgery for acute left-sided malignant colonic obstruction: a meta-analysis. J Gastrointest Surg. 2014;18:584–91.
43. Harvey PR, Rees J, Baldwin S, Waheed H, Tanner JR, Evison F, Patel P, Trudgill NJ. Outcomes of colorectal stents when used as a bridge to curative resection in obstruction secondary to colorectal cancer. Int J Color Dis. 2019; https://doi.org/10.1007/S00384-019-03302-5.

44. Amelung FJ, de Beaufort HWL, Siersema PD, Verheijen PM, Consten ECJ. Emergency resection versus bridge to surgery with stenting in patients with acute right-sided colonic obstruction: a systematic review focusing on mortality and morbidity rates. Int J Color Dis. 2015;30:1147–55.
45. Amelung FJ, Borstlap WAA, Consten ECJ, et al. Propensity score-matched analysis of oncological outcome between stent as bridge to surgery and emergency resection in patients with malignant left-sided colonic obstruction. Br J Surg. 2019;106:1075–86.
46. Sabbagh C, Browet F, Diouf M, et al. Is stenting as "a bridge to surgery" an oncologically safe strategy for the management of acute, left-sided, malignant, colonic obstruction? A comparative study with a propensity score analysis. Ann Surg. 2013;258:107–15.
47. Kim HJ, Choi GS, Park JS, Park SY, Jun SH. Higher rate of perineural invasion in stent-laparoscopic approach in comparison to emergent open resection for obstructing left-sided colon cancer. Int J Color Dis. 2013;28:407–14.
48. Foo CC, Poon SHT, Chiu RHY, Lam WY, Cheung LC, Law WL. Is bridge to surgery stenting a safe alternative to emergency surgery in malignant colonic obstruction: a meta-analysis of randomized control trials. Surg Endosc. 2019;33:293–302.
49. Balciscueta I, Balciscueta Z, Uribe N, García-Granero E. Long-term outcomes of stent-related perforation in malignant colon obstruction: a systematic review and meta-analysis. Int J Color Dis. 2020;35:1439–51.
50. Kim JS, Hur H, Min BS, Sohn SK, Cho CH, Kim NK. Oncologic outcomes of self-expanding metallic stent insertion as a bridge to surgery in the management of left-sided colon cancer obstruction: comparison with nonobstructing elective surgery. World J Surg. 2009;33:1281–6.
51. Mahfouz MF, Saeid Salama TM, Afifi AH, Dabous HMK. Effectiveness and early postoperative outcomes of palliative endoluminal stenting versus Hartmann's procedure in acute malignant bowel obstruction in high-risk patients. Ann Coloproctol. 2022;38:141–5.
52. Sousa M, Pinho R, Proença L, Silva J, Ponte A, Rodrigues J, Carvalho J. Predictors of complications and mortality in patients with self-expanding metallic stents for the palliation of malignant colonic obstruction. GE Port J Gastroenterol. 2017;24:122–8.
53. Naruse N, Miyahara K, Sakata Y, et al. Utility and safety of the self-expandable metallic colonic stent in Japanese patients who received systemic chemotherapy or palliative treatment for obstructive primary advanced colorectal cancer: a retrospective single-center medical chart evaluation. JGH Open. 2022;6:324–9.
54. Veld J, Umans D, van Halsema E, et al. Self-expandable metal stent (SEMS) placement or emergency surgery as palliative treatment for obstructive colorectal cancer: a systematic review and meta-analysis. Crit Rev Oncol Hematol. 2020; https://doi.org/10.1016/J.CRITREVONC.2020.103110.
55. Ribeiro I, Bernardo W, Martins B, et al. Colonic stent versus emergency surgery as treatment of malignant colonic obstruction in the palliative setting: a systematic review and meta-analysis. Endosc Int Open. 2018;6:E558–67.
56. Finlayson A, Hulme-Moir M. Palliative colonic stenting: a safe alternative to surgery in stage IV colorectal cancer. ANZ J Surg. 2016;86:773–7.
57. Fiori E, Lamazza A, Sterpetti AV, Crocetti D, de Felice F, di Muzio M, Mingoli A, Sapienza P, de Toma G. Quality of life for patients with incurable stage IV colorectal cancer: randomized controlled trial comparing resection versus endoscopic stenting. In Vivo. 2019;33:2065–70.
58. Siddiqui A, Cosgrove N, Yan LH, et al. Long-term outcomes of palliative colonic stenting versus emergency surgery for acute proximal malignant colonic obstruction: a multicenter trial. Endosc Int Open. 2017;5:E232.
59. Ahn HJ, Kim SW, Lee SW, Lee SW, Lim CH, Kim JS, Cho YK, Park JM, Lee IS, Choi MG. Long-term outcomes of palliation for unresectable colorectal cancer obstruction in patients with good performance status: endoscopic stent versus surgery. Surg Endosc. 2016;30:4765–75.
60. Kwon SJ, Yoon J, Oh EH, et al. Factors associated with clinical outcomes of palliative stenting for malignant colonic obstruction. Gut Liver. 2021;15:579–87.

61. Abelson JS, Yeo HL, Mao J, Milsom JW, Sedrakyan A. Long-term postprocedural outcomes of palliative emergency stenting vs stoma in malignant large-bowel obstruction. JAMA Surg. 2017;152:429–35.
62. Zhao XD, Cai BB, Cao RS, Shi RH. Palliative treatment for incurable malignant colorectal obstructions: a meta-analysis. World J Gastroenterol. 2013;19:5565–74.
63. Takahashi H, Okabayashi K, Tsuruta M, Hasegawa H, Yahagi M, Kitagawa Y. Self-expanding metallic stents versus surgical intervention as palliative therapy for obstructive colorectal cancer: a meta-analysis. World J Surg. 2015;39:2037–44.
64. Young CJ, Zahid A. Randomized controlled trial of colonic stent insertion in non-curable large bowel obstruction: a post hoc cost analysis. Color Dis. 2018;20:288–95.
65. Faucheron JL, Paquette B, Trilling B, Heyd B, Koch S, Mantion G. Emergency surgery for obstructing colonic cancer: a comparison between right-sided and left-sided lesions. Eur J Trauma Emerg Surg. 2018;44:71–7.
66. Tewari SO, Getrajdman GI, Petre EN, Sofocleous CT, Siegelbaum RH, Erinjeri JP, Weiser MR, Thornton RH. Safety and efficacy of percutaneous cecostomy/colostomy for treatment of large bowel obstruction in adults with cancer. J Vasc Interv Radiol. 2015;26:182–8.
67. Kye BH, Lee YS, Cho HM, et al. Comparison of long-term outcomes between emergency surgery and bridge to surgery for malignant obstruction in right-sided colon cancer: a multicenter retrospective study. Ann Surg Oncol. 2016;23:1867–74.
68. Li B, Cai SL, Lv ZT, et al. Self-expandable metallic stenting as a bridge to elective surgery versus emergency surgery for acute malignant right-sided colorectal obstruction. BMC Surg. 2020; https://doi.org/10.1186/S12893-020-00993-4.
69. You YN, Hardiman KM, Bafford A, Poylin V, Francone TD, Davis K, Paquette IM, Steele SR, Feingold DL. The American Society of colon and rectal surgeons clinical practice guidelines for the management of rectal cancer. Dis Colon Rectum. 2020;63:1191–222.
70. Geng HZ, Nasier D, Liu B, Gao H, Xu YK. Meta-analysis of elective surgical complications related to defunctioning loop ileostomy compared with loop colostomy after low anterior resection for rectal carcinoma. Ann R Coll Surg Engl. 2015;97:494–501.
71. Vermeer TA, Orsini RG, Nieuwenhuijzen GAP, Rutten HJT, Daams F. Stoma placement in obstructive rectal cancer prior to neo-adjuvant treatment and definitive surgery: a practical guideline. Eur J Surg Oncol (EJSO). 2016;42:273–80.
72. Lee HJ, Hong SP, Cheon JH, Kim TI, Kim WH, Park SJ. Clinical outcomes of self-expandable metal stents for malignant rectal obstruction. Dis Colon Rectum. 2018;61:43–50.
73. Trabulsi N, Halawani H, Alshahrani E, et al. Short-term outcomes of stents in obstructive rectal cancer: a systematic review and meta-analysis. Saudi J Gastroenterol. 2021;27:127–35.
74. Keswani RN, Azar RR, Edmundowicz SA, Zhang Q, Ammar T, Banerjee B, Early DS, Jonnalagadda SS. Stenting for malignant colonic obstruction: a comparison of efficacy and complications in colonic versus extracolonic malignancy. Gastrointest Endosc. 2009;69:675–80.
75. Moon SJ, Kim SW, Lee BI, Lim CH, Kim JS, Cho YK, Park JM, Lee IS, Choi MG, Choi KY. Palliative stent for malignant colonic obstruction by extracolonic malignancy: a comparison with colorectal cancer. Dig Dis Sci. 2014;59:1891–7.
76. Kim JY, Kim SG, Im JP, Kim JS, Jung HC. Comparison of treatment outcomes of endoscopic stenting for colonic and extracolonic malignant obstruction. Surg Endosc. 2013;27:272–7.
77. Kim EJ, Han SH, Kim KO, Chung JW, Park DK, Kwon KA, Kim JH. Stenting as a bridge to surgery for extra-colonic malignancy induced colorectal obstruction: preliminary experience. BMC Gastroenterol. 2020;20:1–7.
78. Vogel JD, Felder SI, Bhama AR, et al. The American Society of colon and rectal surgeons clinical practice guidelines for the management of colon cancer. Dis Colon Rectum. 2022;65:148–77.

14 Metastatic Colorectal Cancer in the Asymptomatic Patient: Is There a Benefit in Resection of Primary Tumor?

Paolo Goffredo and Martin R. Weiser

Approximately 25% of patients with colorectal cancer present with synchronous metastatic disease at diagnosis, and the primary treatment is chemotherapy [1]. For patients with limited metastases, complete resection of the primary tumor and distant metastases is associated with a 30–50% increase in the likelihood of 5-year overall survival, depending on patient and tumor characteristics [2–4]. Primary tumor resection in medically fit patients with resectable metastases, either before or after chemotherapy, is therefore optimal [5]. Likewise, there is no debate regarding the need to resect the primary tumor in the setting of metastases if the tumor causes abdominal pain, gastrointestinal bleeding, or bowel obstruction. For patients with an asymptomatic primary tumor and unresectable metastases, however, the role of surgery has been debated. One of the main goals of care for such patients is to maximize survival while maintaining the highest quality of life possible [6–8].

Data from some retrospective studies suggest that in patients with unresectable metastases, resection of the primary tumor in combination with chemotherapy may provide a survival benefit [9, 10]. However, the benefit observed may be associated with a selection bias in those studies toward younger, healthier patients with good performance status and low disease burden. Another suggested benefit of upfront resection of an asymptomatic primary tumor is prevention of subsequent development of symptoms, such as bleeding, obstruction, or perforation, which occur in

P. Goffredo
Division of Colon & Rectal Surgery, University of Minnesota, Minneapolis, MN, USA
e-mail: goffr002@umn.edu

M. R. Weiser (✉)
Stuart Quan Chair in Colorectal Surgery, Memorial Sloan Kettering Cancer Center, New York, NY, USA

Weill Cornell Medical College, New York, NY, USA
e-mail: weiser1@mskcc.org

K. Umanskiy, N. Hyman (eds.), *Difficult Decisions in Colorectal Surgery*, Difficult Decisions in Surgery: An Evidence-Based Approach,
https://doi.org/10.1007/978-3-031-42303-1_14

10–20% of patients [11, 12]. Over the past decade, these considerations led to randomized controlled trials aimed at determining whether resection of an asymptomatic primary tumor in patients with unresectable metastases provides an oncologic or quality-of-life benefit.

Search Strategy

A detailed search of the PubMed, Embase, Medline, and Cochrane databases was conducted for medical literature published between 2010 and 2022. The following search terms were employed to identify relevant articles: ("colon" OR "colorectal" OR "rectal") AND ("cancer" OR "carcinoma" OR "adenocarcinoma") AND ("metastatic" OR "Stage IV" OR "Stage 4") AND "asymptomatic" AND ("surgery" OR "colectomy" OR "resection") (Table 14.1). The titles and abstracts of English language articles were assessed for relevance. Reasons for exclusion were as follows: duplicate, not relevant, lack of comparator group (trend analysis), review or opinion article without primary data, and systematic review or meta-analysis. We sought to focus our review on the highest-quality evidence, with emphasis on level 1 and level 2 data.

Table 14.1 PICO table

Patients	Intervention	Comparator	Outcomes
Patients with asymptomatic metastatic colorectal cancer	Primary tumor resection (colectomy, proctectomy)	Chemotherapy alone	Overall survival, morbidity

Table 14.2 Results from clinical trials[a]

Trial	No. of patients		% Survival[b]		% Morbidity grade ≥ 3		% Mortality[c]		% CTX patients who had palliative surgery
	PTR	CTX	PTR	CTX	PTR	CTX	PTR	CTX	
PTR [13]	26	22	70	45	20	23	4	0	18
CAIRO4 [15]	97	99	NA	NA	23	30	11	3[d]	NA
iPACS [14]	81	84	33	33	21	NA	4	0	13

[a]PTR, primary tumor resection; CTX, chemotherapy; NA, not available
[b]Overall survival at 2 years (PTR trial) or 3 years (iPACS trial)
[c]Within 60 days after randomization (CAIRO4 trial) or within 30 days after surgery (PTR trial and iPACS trial)
[d]$P = 0.03$

Results

Our literature search identified three published multicenter randomized controlled trials aimed at comparing patients with metastatic colorectal cancer who underwent primary tumor resection followed by chemotherapy and patients who underwent chemotherapy alone: the PTR trial (n = 48), the iPACS trial (n = 165), and the CAIRO4 trial (n = 196) (Table 14.2) [13–15]. Four ongoing trials have not yet reported relevant results: SYNCHRONOUS (ISRCTN 30964555), GRECCAR-8 (NCT 02314182), CLIMAT (NCT 02363049), and the China multicenter study (NCT 02149784).

Overall Survival

The PTR trial and the iPACS trial found no significant difference in overall survival rates between primary tumor resection and chemotherapy alone. The 2-year rates in the PTR trial were 70 and 45%, respectively ($P = 0.06$) [13]. In the iPACS trial, the 3-year rate was 33% in both groups, with median overall survival of approximately 26 months in each (hazard ratio, 1.10; 95% confidence interval, 0.76–1.59; $P = 0.69$) [14, 16]. These results were consistent with the findings of an analysis of data from the National Cancer Database [17].

With no level 1 data in favor of primary tumor resection, some relatively weak evidence supporting primary tumor resection has been reported by retrospective analyses—a single-institution series from Japan and two population-based cohort studies from Canada and the United States—which were limited by selection biases and lack of details on possible confounders [18–20]. A 2018 meta-analysis of ARCAD database data from eight randomized controlled trials that included patients with metastatic colorectal cancer found a moderate benefit in overall survival: 22.2 months for patients who underwent resection of the primary tumor vs.

16.4 months for patients who underwent chemotherapy alone (hazard ratio, 1.60; 95% confidence interval, 1.43–1.78) [21]. The authors acknowledged the potential for bias, since the reasons for resection and nonresection were not available. Moreover, data from patients who did not meet the inclusion criteria for the trials, such as morbidity or mortality after primary tumor resection, were not available.

Morbidity and Mortality

Resection of the primary tumor is associated with high morbidity. In the iPACS trial, grade ≥ 2 complications occurred in 38% of the patients and grade ≥ 3 complications occurred in 21% [14]. The rates of anastomotic leak and 30-day mortality were 4%. Additionally, both grade ≥ 2 and grade ≥ 3 nonhematological adverse events were more frequent than after chemotherapy alone (87% vs. 77% and 48% vs. 34%, respectively). Similarly, the PTR trial found higher morbidity in patients who underwent resection, with postoperative complications in 19% of the patients, including 1 death, and a 30-day readmission rate of 12% [13]. There were no cases of anastomotic leakage. The rate of chemotherapy-related toxicities was approximately 27% in both groups. The CAIRO4 trial reported comparable rates of grade ≥ 3 toxicity in the two groups (23% for resection vs. 30% for chemotherapy alone, $P = 0.25$) [15]. However, within 60 days from randomization, mortality was 11% in the resection group vs. 3% in the chemotherapy group ($P = 0.03$).

Postoperative recovery and morbidity can significantly delay or sometimes prevent initiation of chemotherapy. This has frequently been considered a drawback to resection of the primary tumor in patients with metastasis. In the iPACS trial, the median time to initiation of systemic chemotherapy after surgery was 34 days, compared with 9 days after enrollment for patients who did not undergo resection [14]. In the PTR trial, the median interval from surgery to initiation of systemic chemotherapy was 25 days [13]. In the CAIRO4 trial, the median interval from randomization to initiation of systemic chemotherapy was 7 days for patients who did not undergo resection and 46 days for patients who did [15].

Conversion to Resectability

The guidelines of the American Society of Colon and Rectal Surgeons advise against primary tumor resection in patients with asymptomatic unresectable stage IV disease and strongly recommend neoadjuvant chemotherapy as a means of facilitating conversion to resectability [22]. This recommendation is based in part on a 2020 systematic review of 20 trials, which found that neoadjuvant treatment with oxaliplatin- or irinotecan-based chemotherapy plus bevacizumab or cetuximab produced a response in 55–85% of patients and conversion to resectability in 10–61% of patients, with R0 resection rates as high as 54% [23]. The PTR and iPACS trials reported conversion to resectability in 18 and 6% of patients randomized to chemotherapy alone, respectively [13, 14].

Natural History of Nonresected Primary Disease

One argument for resecting the primary tumor electively is potential prevention of obstruction, perforation, severe bleeding, or another cancer-related complication. However, these events are relatively rare. In the multicenter prospective phase II trial NSABP C-10, in which patients with an asymptomatic primary tumor and unresectable metastases received oxaliplatin-based chemotherapy and bevacizumab, with median follow-up of 21 months, 14% of the patients had major morbidity related to the primary tumor and 12% required an operation, mostly for obstruction [12]. A 2019 population-based SEER study of 4692 patients with stage IV colorectal cancer (74% of the patients had colon cancer and 26% had rectal cancer) obtained similar results, with unplanned operations required in only 12% of the patients [24]. In the PTR trial, 4 (18%) of the 22 patients assigned to chemotherapy alone underwent surgery during chemotherapy and 5 (23%) of the 22 patients required interventional therapy (colonic stent placement or salvage radiotherapy) [13]. The rate of palliative surgery in patients assigned to chemotherapy alone was 13% in the iPACS trial and 6% in the CAIRO4 trial [14, 15]. These data indicate that if upfront resection was performed routinely in order to prevent possible acute surgery during chemotherapy, approximately 5 to 10 patients would undergo an unnecessary intervention in order to prevent an emergency intervention in 1 patient. Resection of an asymptomatic primary tumor, therefore, does not provide a significant prophylactic benefit for most patients.

It is important to note that complications associated with an untreated primary tumor may be more common for rectal cancer than for colon cancer. In a recent single-institution series from Memorial Sloan Kettering Cancer Center, of 190 patients who did not undergo an upfront or elective intervention for the primary tumor, 68 (36%) experienced complications; 42 (62%) of the 68 patients ended up with a diverting ostomy [25]. These data suggest that closer follow-up may be needed for metastatic rectal cancer than for metastatic colon cancer.

Recommendations Based on the Data

Asymptomatic patients with unresectable metastatic colorectal cancer should proceed with systemic therapy and not undergo resection of the primary tumor (evidence quality high; strong recommendation).

Personal View of the Data

Until recently, the value of resecting an asymptomatic primary tumor in patients with incurable metastatic colon cancer was debatable, based on biased retrospective series. We now have data from randomized controlled trials demonstrating the futility of resection for most patients. Immediate surgery is associated with morbidity and is not associated with longer survival, and it can delay initiation of systemic chemotherapy. Timely intervention can rescue patients who develop complications related to the primary lesion.

Clinical judgment should guide the decision-making process, with the goal of optimizing survival and balancing the quality of life. Our current practice is to administer chemotherapy first, based on the fact that in a subset of patients, current multimodal therapies substantially prolong life and facilitate the possibility of a curative resection.

When developing a treatment plan, patients' symptoms, colonoscopy reports, and cross-sectional images should be carefully reviewed. In patients who present with anemia, the symptoms can be managed medically, with improvement within two to four cycles of chemotherapy. Similarly, upfront chemotherapy with close observation may be safely employed in patients with mild obstructive symptoms, which generally improve with systemic treatment. However, when patients present with significant symptoms or evidence of proximal dilation on CT, surgical intervention in the form of a diverting ostomy or tumor resection should be considered, keeping in mind the significant risk of complications and potential delay in chemotherapy.

Future investigations may identify clinicopathologic or molecular factors that can be used to predict which patients may indeed benefit form upfront surgery. Currently, based on the evidence, the standard of care should be upfront chemotherapy, evaluation of response, estimation of prognosis, and further discussion in a multidisciplinary setting.

References

1. U.S. Cancer Statistics Working Group. U.S. Cancer Statistics Data Visualizations Tool, based on 2020 submission data (1999–2018) www.cdc.gov/cancer/dataviz: U.S. Department of Health and Human Services, Centers for Disease Control and Prevention and National Cancer Institute; 2021.
2. Corsini EM, Mitchell KG, Correa A, Morris VK, Antonoff MB. Effect of primary colorectal cancer tumor location on survival after pulmonary metastasectomy. J Thorac Cardiovasc Surg. 2021;162(1):296–305.
3. Tomlinson JS, Jarnagin WR, DeMatteo RP, Fong Y, Kornprat P, Gonen M, et al. Actual 10-year survival after resection of colorectal liver metastases defines cure. J Clin Oncol. 2007;25(29):4575–80.
4. Engstrand J, Nilsson H, Strömberg C, Jonas E, Freedman J. Colorectal cancer liver metastases – a population-based study on incidence, management and survival. BMC Cancer. 2018;18(1):78.
5. National Comprehensive Cancer Network. NCCN clinical practical guidelines in oncology: colon cancer: NCCN; (updated Version 1.2019 – March 15, 20192019). Available from: https://www.nccn.org/professionals/physician_gls/pdf/colon.pdf.
6. Weiser MR. Primum non nocere: a word of caution regarding prophylactic colectomy in the setting of incurable metastatic disease. Ann Surg Oncol. 2011;18(12):3229–31.
7. Yamada Y, Takahari D, Matsumoto H, Baba H, Nakamura M, Yoshida K, et al. Leucovorin, fluorouracil, and oxaliplatin plus bevacizumab versus S-1 and oxaliplatin plus bevacizumab in patients with metastatic colorectal cancer (SOFT): an open-label, non-inferiority, randomised phase 3 trial. Lancet Oncol. 2013;14(13):1278–86.
8. Yamazaki K, Nagase M, Tamagawa H, Ueda S, Tamura T, Murata K, et al. Randomized phase III study of bevacizumab plus FOLFIRI and bevacizumab plus mFOLFOX6 as first-line treatment for patients with metastatic colorectal cancer (WJOG4407G). Ann Oncol. 2016;27(8):1539–46.
9. Ahmed S, Leis A, Fields A, Chandra-Kanthan S, Haider K, Alvi R, et al. Survival impact of surgical resection of primary tumor in patients with stage IV colorectal cancer: results from a large population-based cohort study. Cancer. 2014;120(5):683–91.

10. Ishihara S, Hayama T, Yamada H, Nozawa K, Matsuda K, Miyata H, et al. Prognostic impact of primary tumor resection and lymph node dissection in stage IV colorectal cancer with unresectable metastasis: a propensity score analysis in a multicenter retrospective study. Ann Surg Oncol. 2014;21(9):2949–55.
11. Poultsides GA, Servais EL, Saltz LB, Patil S, Kemeny NE, Guillem JG, et al. Outcome of primary tumor in patients with synchronous stage IV colorectal cancer receiving combination chemotherapy without surgery as initial treatment. J Clin Oncol. 2009;27(20):3379–84.
12. McCahill LE, Yothers G, Sharif S, Petrelli NJ, Lai LL, Bechar N, et al. Primary mFOLFOX6 plus bevacizumab without resection of the primary tumor for patients presenting with surgically unresectable metastatic colon cancer and an intact asymptomatic colon cancer: definitive analysis of NSABP trial C-10. J Clin Oncol. 2012;30(26):3223–8.
13. Park EJ, Baek JH, Choi GS, Park WC, Yu CS, Kang SB, et al. The role of primary tumor resection in colorectal cancer patients with asymptomatic, synchronous, unresectable metastasis: a multicenter randomized controlled trial. Cancers (Basel). 2020;12(8):2306.
14. Kanemitsu Y, Shitara K, Mizusawa J, Hamaguchi T, Shida D, Komori K, et al. Primary tumor resection plus chemotherapy versus chemotherapy alone for colorectal cancer patients with asymptomatic, synchronous unresectable metastases (JCOG1007; iPACS): a randomized clinical trial. J Clin Oncol. 2021;39(10):1098–107.
15. van der Kruijssen DEW, Elias SG, Vink GR, van Rooijen KL, t Lam-Boer J, Mol L, et al. Sixty-day mortality of patients with metastatic colorectal cancer randomized to systemic treatment vs primary tumor resection followed by systemic treatment: the CAIRO4 phase 3 randomized clinical trial. JAMA Surg. 2021;156(12):1093–101.
16. Moritani K, Kanemitsu Y, Shida D, Shitara K, Mizusawa J, Katayama H, et al. A randomized controlled trial comparing primary tumour resection plus chemotherapy with chemotherapy alone in incurable stage IV colorectal cancer: JCOG1007 (iPACS study). Jpn J Clin Oncol. 2020;50(1):89–93.
17. Alawadi Z, Phatak UR, Hu CY, Bailey CE, You YN, Kao LS, et al. Comparative effectiveness of primary tumor resection in patients with stage IV colon cancer. Cancer. 2017;123(7):1124–33.
18. Ahmed S, Fields A, Pahwa P, Chandra-Kanthan S, Zaidi A, Le D, et al. Surgical resection of primary tumor in asymptomatic or minimally symptomatic patients with stage IV colorectal cancer: a Canadian province experience. Clin Colorectal Cancer. 2015;14(4):e41–7.
19. Shida D, Hamaguchi T, Ochiai H, Tsukamoto S, Takashima A, Boku N, et al. Prognostic impact of palliative primary tumor resection for unresectable stage 4 colorectal cancer: using a propensity score analysis. Ann Surg Oncol. 2016;23(11):3602–8.
20. Tarantino I, Warschkow R, Worni M, Cerny T, Ulrich A, Schmied BM, et al. Prognostic relevance of palliative primary tumor removal in 37,793 metastatic colorectal cancer patients: a population-based, propensity score-adjusted trend analysis. Ann Surg. 2015;262(1):112–20.
21. van Rooijen KL, Shi Q, Goey KKH, Meyers J, Heinemann V, Diaz-Rubio E, et al. Prognostic value of primary tumour resection in synchronous metastatic colorectal cancer: individual patient data analysis of first-line randomised trials from the ARCAD database. Eur J Cancer. 2018;91:99–106.
22. Vogel JD, Felder SI, Bhama AR, Hawkins AT, Langenfeld SJ, Shaffer VO, et al. The American Society of Colon and Rectal Surgeons clinical practice guidelines for the Management of Colon Cancer. Dis Colon Rectum. 2022;65(2):148–77.
23. Bolhuis K, Kos M, van Oijen MGH, Swijnenburg RJ, Punt CJA. Conversion strategies with chemotherapy plus targeted agents for colorectal cancer liver-only metastases: a systematic review. Eur J Cancer. 2020;141:225–38.
24. Lorimer PD, Motz BM, Kirks RC, Han Y, Symanowski JT, Hwang JJ, et al. Frequency of unplanned surgery in patients with stage IV colorectal cancer receiving palliative chemotherapy with an intact primary: an analysis of SEER-Medicare. J Surg Oncol. 2019;120(3):407–14.
25. Tan WJ, Patil S, Guillem JG, Paty PB, Weiser MR, Nash GM, et al. Primary tumor-related complications and salvage outcomes in patients with metastatic rectal cancer and an untreated primary tumor. Dis Colon Rectum. 2021;64(1):45–52.

What Are the Options for Management of Large Colonic Polyps?

15

Sumeyye Yilmaz and Emre Gorgun

Introduction

Colorectal cancer is the third most commonly diagnosed cancer and second leading cause of cancer-related mortality globally [1, 2]. Based on adenoma-carcinoma sequence theory, early detection and removal of colorectal neoplasms is essential for improving cancer incidence and mortality [3]. Ideally, a neoplastic lesion should be resected in one-piece (en-bloc) with histologically negative margins (R0). Fortunately, 80–90% of polyps are ≤1 cm and can effectively be managed by conventional polypectomy [4]. However, management of large colorectal polyps (≥2 cm) require more advanced resection techniques, as conventional snare-based techniques might result in piecemeal resection, which precludes proper histopathological evaluation and increases the risk for recurrence [5]. Given that large polyps may have an increased risk for harboring malignancy [6], adequate treatment is of the utmost importance. Further, risks of different procedures should be considered.

Search Strategy

A comprehensive literature search of Cochrane Database of Collected Research, EMBASE, and MEDLINE was performed. The search strategy included different combinations of the following terms: "colon or colorectal", "large polyp or polyp ≥2 cm", "polypectomy", "endoscopic mucosal resection (EMR)", "endoscopic submucosal dissection (ESD)", "surgery or colectomy", "en-bloc resection",

S. Yilmaz · E. Gorgun (✉)
Department of Colorectal Surgery, Digestive Disease and Surgery Institute, Cleveland, OH, USA
e-mail: gorgune@ccf.org

K. Umanskiy, N. Hyman (eds.), *Difficult Decisions in Colorectal Surgery*, Difficult Decisions in Surgery: An Evidence-Based Approach,
https://doi.org/10.1007/978-3-031-42303-1_15

Table 15.1 PICO table

Patients	Intervention groups	Comparator groups	Outcomes
Patients with large (≥2 cm) colorectal polyps	ESD	Conventional polypectomy EMR U-EMR Hybrid ESD Surgery	Primary: • Postoperative/procedural complications • En-bloc and R0 resection • Local recurrence
	EMR	Conventional polypectomy U-EMR Hybrid ESD Surgery	Secondary: • Procedure time • Length of hospital stay • Cost

ESD Endoscopic Submucosal Dissection, *EMR* Endoscopic Mucosal Resection, *U-EMR* Underwater EMR

En-bloc resection: Resection of a neoplasm in one piece. R0 resection: En-bloc resection of a lesion with histologically proven negative margins

"perforation", "bleeding", "recurrence" in "All fields", and the related Mesh terms to identify all English-language publications from 1999 (the year ESD was first described [7]) to 2022. Since guidelines' recommendation is to use ESD for resection of polyps larger than 2 cm [5, 8], ESD is identified as the intervention group, and studies comparing ESD with any of the following were included: conventional polypectomy (CP), EMR, Underwater EMR (U-EMR), Hybrid ESD, and surgery. However, while conducting the search, studies comparing EMR with different techniques (other than ESD) were found. They were also included to give a more comprehensive information about efficacy and safety of different resection techniques. Primary outcomes were: postoperative/procedural complications (mainly bleeding and perforation), en-bloc resection, R0 resection, and tumor recurrence. Secondary outcomes were: procedure time, length of hospital stay, and cost (Table 15.1). Studies were excluded according to the following criteria: (a) Articles without a control group (non-comparative studies); (b) Articles including patients with polyps ≤2 cm without a subgroup analysis for patients with large polyps; (c) Conference abstracts (since evaluation for quality of evidence would not be possible), systematic reviews, meta-analyses, guidelines, book chapters, editorials. Only the most recent study was included in the presence of multiple articles reporting data from the same study population. The references of the included studies were reviewed to identify additional studies that were incorporated as appropriate.

Results

Colorectal ESD was first described in 1999 [7]. Since then, literature on the outcomes of different management techniques for colorectal polyps has been expanding. Guidelines recommend CP and/or EMR for most superficial colorectal lesions and ESD for lesions larger than 2 cm and/or lesions with suspicion of submucosal invasion [5, 8]. However, reports published in this area are mostly case series (non-comparative) and/or include polyps regardless of their size without a subgroup analysis for large polyps.

12 studies comparing ESD with: CP&EMR [9], EMR [10–15], U-EMR [16], Hybrid ESD [12, 17–19], and surgery [20] were identified and summarized in Table 15.2. 5 studies comparing EMR with: CP [21], U-EMR [22, 23], Hybrid ESD [12], and surgery [24] were identified and summarized in Table 15.3. 1 study [12] was included in both tables, as it compared the outcomes of EMR, Hybrid ESD, and ESD. Reports included: 2 randomized controlled trials (RCTs) [21, 22], 2 prospective cohort [9, 18] and 12 retrospective cohort studies [10–17, 19, 20, 23, 24].

En-Bloc, R0 and Complete Resection

In terms of efficacy of different techniques, most studies [9–14, 16–19, 22, 23] reported en-bloc resection (resection of a neoplasm in one-piece) with some [10, 12, 14, 16–19] reporting R0 resection (en-bloc resection of a lesion with histologically proven negative margins) rates. Oka et al. [9] combined CP with EMR and compared the en-bloc resection rate with ESD, and reported that ESD achieved significantly higher en-bloc resection rates. Studies comparing ESD with EMR reported significantly higher en-bloc [11–14] and R0 [12, 14] resection rates with ESD. Iizuka et al. [10] compared 38 ESDs with 83 EMRs and found no significant difference between en-bloc resection rates. However, R0 resection rate was significantly higher for ESD. Hybrid ESD achieved similar en-bloc and R0 resection rates with ESD in 2 studies [18, 19]; whereas in other 2 studies [12, 17], ESD achieved significantly higher en-bloc and R0 resection rates.

Chien et al. [23] compared EMR with U-EMR, and reported that there was no statistically significant difference in en-bloc resection rates. Lee et al. [12] reported that Hybrid ESD achieved higher en-bloc and R0 resection rates when compared with EMR.

2 studies [15, 21] reported complete resection as resection of a lesion with histologically proven negative margins (instead of resection of a lesion in one-piece with negative margins). ESD achieved significantly higher complete resection rate when compared with EMR [15], as EMR with CP [21]. When EMR was compared with U-EMR, there was no significant difference in incomplete resection rates [22].

Postoperative/Procedural Complications

Regarding safety of different techniques, most commonly reported complications were bleeding [9, 11–19, 22, 23] and perforation [9–19]. 5 studies [12, 14, 20, 22, 24] reported total complication rates. Surgery was associated with higher complication rates compared to EMR [24] and ESD [20]. Bleeding (either early or delayed) rates were not different between different techniques in the majority of the studies [9, 11–19, 22]. Oka et al. [9] reported no significant differences between perforation rates of

Table 15.2 Studies comparing ESD with other techniques

Study	Study Design	Intervention group	Control Group	Outcome measures	Results	Significance	Quality of evidence
Oka 2015 [9]	Prospective Cohort	ESD *dissection* (816)	CP & EMR (1,029)	Delayed bleeding Perforation En bloc resection Recurrence	2.5% vs. 1.4% 1.1% vs. 0.9% 95.0% vs. 53.2% 1.4% vs. 6.8%	NS NS p<0.00001 p<0.01	Moderate
Iizuka 2009 [10]	Retrospective Cohort	ESD (38)	EMR (83)	Perforation En bloc resection R0 resection	8% vs. 1% 61% vs. 54% 58% vs. 37%	p=0.056 NS p<0.05	Low
Saito 2009 [11]	Retrospective Cohort	ESD (145)	EMR (228)	Delayed bleeding Perforation En bloc resection Recurrence Procedure time, min	1.4% vs. 3.1% 6.2% vs. 1.3% 84% vs. 33% 2% vs. 14% 108±71 vs. 29±25	NS NS p<0.0001 p<0.0001 p<0.0001	Moderate
Lee 2011 [12]	Retrospective Cohort	ESD (314)	EMR (140)	Complication (any) Bleeding Perforation En bloc resection R0 resection Recurrence	11.5% vs. 5.7% 0.6% vs. 0% 8% vs. 0% 92.7% vs. 42.9% 87.6% vs. 32.9% 0.8% vs. 25.7%	p=0.024 NS p<0.001 p<0.001 p<0.001 p<0.001	Low
		ESD (314)	Hybrid ESD (69)	Complication (any) Bleeding PerforationEn bloc resection R0 resection Recurrence	11.5% vs. 15.9% 0.6% vs. 2.9% 8% vs. 2.9% 92.7% vs. 65.2% 87.6% vs. 59.4% 0.8% vs. 3.1%	NS NS p=0.048 p=0.004 p=0.006 NS	
Tajika 2011 [13]	Retrospective Cohort	ESD (85)	EMR (104)	Bleeding Perforation En bloc resection Recurrence Procedure time, min	2.4% vs. 2.9% 5.9% vs. 0% 83.5% vs. 48.1% 1.2% vs. 15.4% 87.2±49.7 vs. 29.4±26.1	NS p=0.04 p<0.001 p=0.002 p<0.001	Low

Study	Study Design	Intervention group	Control Group	Outcome measures	Results	Significance	Quality of evidence
Soliman 2018 [14]	Retrospective Cohort	ESD (157)	EMR (217)	Complication (any) Bleeding Perforation En bloc resection R0 resection Recurrence Length of stay, days	9.5% vs. 6.4% 3.8% vs. 4.1% 5.7% vs. 2.3% 87.3% vs. 26.3% 83.4% vs. 26.3% 7.6% vs. 15.2% 2.2±1.79 vs. 0.97±1.32	NS NS NS p<0.0001 p<0.0001 p=0.026 p<0.0001	Low
Ham 2019 [15]	Retrospective Cohort	ESD (429)	EMR – piecemeal (115)	Intraprocedural bleeding Delayed bleeding Perforation Complete resection Recurrence Procedure time, min Length of stay, days Cost (initial resection), p<0.001 Cost (cumulative), p<0.001	19.1% vs. 12.4% 6.1% vs. 3.3% 2.6% vs. 4.9% 83.9% vs. 32.2% 0.5% vs. 7.1% 55.4±47.0 vs. 25.6±32.7 2.4±1.1 vs. 2.5±1.4 1480.0±728.0 vs. 729.8±299.7 847.6±823.0 vs. 871.9±994.4	NS NS NS p<0.001 p<0.001 p<0.001 NS p<0.001 NS	Low
Inoue 2021 [16][a]	Retrospective Cohort	ESD (74)	U-EMR (74)	Delayed bleeding Perforation En bloc resection R0 resection Recurrence Procedure time, min	2.7% vs. 5.4% 5.4% vs. 0% 99% vs. 61% 89% vs. 34% 0% vs 0% 64.8 vs. 6.7	NS Significant N/A N/A NS Significant	Low

(continued)

Table 15.2 (continued)

Study	Study Design	Intervention group	Control Group	Outcome measures	Results	Significance	Quality of evidence
Byeon 2011 [17]	Retrospective Cohort	ESD (141)	Hybrid ESD (47)	Immediate bleeding Delayed bleeding Perforation En bloc resection R0 resection Procedure time, min	1% vs. 0% 1% vs. 4% 6% vs. 2% 85% vs. 49% 73% vs. 43% 52±37 vs. 40±25	NS NS NS p<0.01 p<0.01 p=0.05	Low
Bae 2016 [18]	Prospective Cohort	ESD (36)	Hybrid ESD (34)	Bleeding Perforation En bloc resection R0 resection Procedure time, min	3.2% vs. 2.9% 6.5% vs. 8.8% 100% vs. 94.1% 93.5% vs. 91.2% 40.6±22.1 vs. 27.4±12.7	NS NS NS NS p=0.005	Low
Yang 2017 [19]	Retrospective Cohort	ESD (102)	Hybrid ESD (34)	Bleeding Perforation En bloc resection R0 resection Procedure time, min	1.0% vs. 2.9% 2.9% vs. 5.9% 100% vs. 94.1% 90.2% vs. 76.5% 45.6±30.1 vs. 12.7±7.0	NS NS NS NS p<0.001	Low
Gamaleldin 2017 [20]	Retrospective Cohort	ESD (48)	Surgery (48)	Complication (any) Procedure time, min Length of stay, days Cost	13% vs. 15% 133±72.7 vs. 136±45 1.5±1.4 vs. 5.2±2.4 ESD/surgery: 60%	p<0.001 NS NS p<0.001	Low

CP Conventional polypectomy, *EMR* Endoscopic mucosal resection, *ESD* Endoscopic submucosal dissection, *NS* Non-significant, *U-EMR* Underwater EMR En bloc resection: resection of a polyp in one-piece. R0 resection: resection of a polyp in one-piece with histologically proven negative margins. Complete resection: resection of a polyp with histologically proven negative margins (not necessarily in one-piece)

[a] No information regarding the significance level for perforation, en bloc and R0 resection rates, and procedure time

Table 15.3 Summary of studies comparing EMR with other techniques

Study	Study Design	Intervention group	Control group	Outcome measures	Results	Significance	Quality of evidence
Horiuchi 2015 [21]	RCT	EMR (12)	CP (11)	Complete resection	75% vs. 18%	p=0.006	High
Yen et al. [22][a]	RCT	EMR (16)	U-EMR (16)	Immediate bleeding Complication (other) En bloc resection Incomplete resection Procedure time, min	12.5% vs. 18.8% 0% vs. 0% 43.8% vs. 25% 0% vs. 6.3% 9.5±0.7 vs. 7.3±0.6	N/A N/A N/A NS p=0.015	High
Chien et al. [23][b]	Retrospective Cohort	EMR (42)	U-EMR (42)	Bleeding En bloc resection Procedure time, min	28.6% vs. 4.8% 52.4% vs. 69.1% 17.7±9.3 vs. 12±7.4	Significant NS Significant	Moderate
Lee 2011 [14]	Retrospective Cohort	EMR (140)	Hybrid ESD (69)	Complication (any) Bleeding Perforation En bloc resection R0 resection Recurrence	5.7% vs. 15.9% 0% vs. 2.9% 0% vs. 2.9% 42.9% vs. 65.2% 32.9% vs. 59.4% 25.7% vs. 3.1%	p=0.038 NS NS p<0.001 p<0.001 p<0.001	Low
Patel 2019 [24]	Retrospective Cohort	EMR (310)	Surgery (81)	Complication (any)	0.6% vs. 22.2%	p=0.00001	Low

CP Conventional Polypectomy, *EMT* Endoscopic Mucosal Resection, *ESD* Endoscopic Submucosal Dissection, *NS* Non-significant, *RCT* Randomized Controlled Trial, *U-EMR* Underwater EMR

En bloc resection: resection of a polyp in one-piece. R0 resection: resection of a polyp in one-piece with histologically proven negative margins. Complete resection: resection of a polyp with histologically proven negative margins (not necessarily in one-piece). Incomplete resection: histologically proven margin positivity

[a] Model failed to converge to assess the significance level for immediate bleeding, complications, and en bloc resection

[b] Difference (%95 CI) levels for bleeding and procedure time are -23.8 ([-38.9]-[-8.7]) and -5.2 ([-8.9]-[-1.6]), respectively

ESD vs. CP + EMR. Studies comparing ESD with EMR reported conflicting results on perforation rates [10–16]. Some studies reported significantly higher perforation rates with ESD (when compared with EMR) [12, 13, 16], whereas some [10, 11, 14, 15] reported no significant difference. When Hybrid ESD was compared to EMR [12] and ESD [17–19], there was no significant difference in perforation rates, with the exception of 1 study, in which ESD was associated with higher perforation rates [12].

Tumor Recurrence

7 studies reported tumor recurrence rates [9, 11–16]. Compared with CP + EMR [9] and EMR [11–15], ESD was associated with significantly lower local recurrence rates. No significant difference was observed when ESD and U-EMR were compared with each other [16]. Compared to EMR, Hybrid ESD was associated with lower recurrence rates [12].

Secondary Outcomes

[10] [11, 13, 15–20, 22, 23], studies evaluated the procedure time. ESD, when compared with EMR and Hybrid ESD, was associated with significantly higher procedure time [11, 13, 15–19]. Gamaleldin et al. [20] compared procedure times between ESD and surgery (laparoscopic resection) and found no significant difference. U-EMR achieved significantly shorter procedure times than EMR [22, 23].

[3] [14, 15, 20], studies assessed the length of hospital stay. Among 2 studies comparing EMR and ESD [14, 15], Soliman et al. [14] reported significantly higher length of hospital stay associated with ESD, whereas Ham et al. [15] reported no significant difference. Compared to surgery, ESD was associated with shorter length of hospital stay in one study [20], but the result was not statistically significant.

Ham et al. [15] compared the cost of initial resection between ESD and EMR (piecemeal), and reported that ESD was associated with significantly higher cost. However, patients undergoing EMR needed significantly higher number of follow-up colonoscopies, which in turn evened up the cumulative costs associated with two procedures. Gamaleldin et al. [20] compared the technical costs associated with ESD vs. surgery and reported that the cost of ESD was 60% of the cost of surgery. This result was statistically significant.

Recommendation

Management of large colonic polyps (≥2 cm) require more invasive techniques than CP (Evidence: moderate; Recommendation: strong). ESD is associated with higher en-bloc and R0 resection, and lower recurrence rates than EMR. Therefore, for the management of colonic polyps ≥2 cm, ESD should be considered (Evidence: low-moderate; Recommendation: strong).

Compared to surgery, EMR and ESD are associated with lower complication rates and cost. Furthermore, some patients might be poor surgical candidates (*e.g.*, patients with severe comorbidities). Therefore, when possible, EMR and ESD should be preferred rather than surgery (Evidence: low, Recommendation: strong).

Hybrid ESD is an alternative option for the management of large colonic polyps, providing shorter procedure times than ESD with equal or lower complication rates. However, it can be associated with lower en-bloc and R0 resection rates. Therefore, it can be an option in the treatment of large colonic polyps in certain situations (Evidence: low, Recommendation: weak).

Personal View

Early detection and removal of colorectal neoplasms with colonoscopic polypectomy is a well-established means of decreasing colorectal cancer incidence and mortality [25, 26]. In general, majority of colorectal neoplasms are ≤1 cm and can safely and effectively be removed with standard polypectomy [4]. However, 2–15% of polyps are not amenable for conventional colonoscopic removal due to a variety of reasons such as large size, difficult location, previous resection attempts etc [27, 28]

Traditionally, treatment of endoscopically unresectable tumors has required surgical resection / colectomy due to limited availability of management options and concerns for malignancy. However, we have previously reported that only 8.4% of these specimens harbor malignancy [28]. Moreover, colectomy for endoscopically unresectable tumors is associated with 17–25.3% morbidity and 0.8–1.5% mortality risk [29, 30].

Advanced endoscopic resection techniques such as EMR, ESD and Hybrid ESD have been introduced for removal of these complex lesions while allowing patients to avoid the morbidity and mortality of surgical resection [31, 32]. EMR is highly effective in the treatment of colorectal lesions <2 cm, achieving 86–97.5% en-bloc and 76.6–95.5% R0 resection rates [33, 34]. When EMR is used to resect large lesions, en-bloc and R0 resection rates range 26.3–54% [10–14, 35] and 26.3–37% [10, 12, 14], respectively. Luigiano et al. [35] reported their outcomes with 174 EMRs performed for lesions larger than 2 cm, and mentioned that en-bloc resection was possible only for lesions <3 cm. Iizuka et al. [10] reported that tumor size ≥2 cm is an independent risk factor for piecemeal resection following EMR. Piecemeal resection reduces the reliability of the histopathological assessment, and is associated with higher local recurrence rates [15, 36]. Given that increased polyp size is a predictor for malignancy [6, 37], en-bloc resection is preferred to allow accurate histopathological assessment and curative resection [5]. U-EMR uses floating effect of water submersion instead of submucosal injection. Water submersion helps mucosa and submucosa to be separated from the muscularis layer, hence enables snaring of the polyp [38]. A meta-analysis published in 2020 [39] showed that U-EMR is associated with higher en-bloc resection and lower recurrence rates, and shorter procedure time without any difference in complication rates when compared with conventional EMR.

Colorectal ESD is an endoscopic resection technique which allows for en-bloc resection of a neoplasm regardless of its size [8]. For treatment of polyps larger than 2 cm, several case series and comparative studies reported 83.5–100% [9, 11–19, 40, 41] en-bloc and 73–94.9% [12, 14–19, 40, 41] R0 resection rates with ESD. Consequently, tumor recurrence rates following ESD range from 0.5% to 7.6% [9, 11, 13–15], which is significantly lower compared to EMR [11, 12, 14, 16] and CP [9]. Despite these advantages, colorectal ESD has not been widely accepted in clinical practice because it is a technically challenging procedure given the troublesome anatomy of the colon with its folds, flexures, thinner wall and narrower lumen. In fact, perforation rates following ESD can be as high as 10.7% [42].

Colorectal ESD requires a high level of skill. In 2011, Nakajima et al. [43] evaluated the learning curve for ESD in trainees who are experienced in gastric ESD. They reported that after experience with ≥30 cases, trainees were able to perform colorectal ESD without significant complications. In their systematic review, Rajendran et al. [44] assessed learning curves for colorectal polyp resection techniques. They concluded that to achieve en-bloc resection rate of 80% and R0 resection rate of 70%, a trainee must perform 20–40 cases. Competency in safety was achieved at 20–200 cases. Compared to other techniques, ESD requires a longer procedure time [11, 13, 16–19]. Rajendran et al. [44] also reported that procedural speed increases after 30 cases. Nevertheless, for lesions >4 cm, ESDmust be performed by experienced endoscopists, due to the longer procedure time [9]. In our experience and based on our unpublished data, proficiency in performing ESD was achieved after completing around 100 cases.

Hybrid ESD involves circumferential mucosal incision followed by submucosal dissection to a certain degree and snare resection of the polyp. Since it is a technique that can use the advantages of both ESD and snaring, it is an attractive method to achieve safe, rapid, en-bloc resection of colorectal neoplasms [18]. While studies agree on Hybrid ESD being performed faster [17–19] than ESD, it might be inferior in terms of achieving en-bloc & R0 resection of large polyps [12, 17].

In conclusion, large polyps are not amenable to be resected with CP. EMR is an attractive option for the management of polyps that are unsuitable for CP, however, its efficacy is limited for lesions larger than 2 cm [5]. ESD achieves higher en-bloc and R0 resection and lower tumor recurrence rates. However, it is a technically challenging procedure and might be associated with higher perforation rates. Nevertheless, it remains to be safer and more cost-effective than surgery [20].

References

1. World Health Organization. Cancer. https://www.who.int/news-room/fact-sheets/detail/cancer. Published February 2022. Accessed Dec 2022.
2. Xi Y, Xu P. Global colorectal cancer burden in 2020 and projections to 2040. Transl Oncol. 2021;14(10):101174.
3. Muto T, Bussey HJ, Morson BC. The evolution of cancer of the colon and rectum. Cancer. 1975;36(6):2251–70.

4. Ma MX, Bourke MJ. Complications of endoscopic polypectomy, endoscopic mucosal resection and endoscopic submucosal dissection in the colon. Best Pract Res Clin Gastroenterol. 2016;30(5):749–67.
5. Pimentel-Nunes P, Dinis-Ribeiro M, Ponchon T, et al. Endoscopic submucosal dissection: European Society of Gastrointestinal Endoscopy (ESGE) guideline. Endoscopy. 2015;47(9):829–54.
6. He X, Wu K, Ogino S, Giovannucci EL, Chan AT, Song M. Association between risk factors for colorectal cancer and risk of serrated polyps and conventional adenomas. Gastroenterology. 2018;155(2):355–373.e18.
7. Gotoda T, Kondo H, Ono H, et al. A new endoscopic mucosal resection procedure using an insulation-tipped electrosurgical knife for rectal flat lesions: report of two cases. Gastrointest Endosc. 1999;50(4):560–3.
8. Hashiguchi Y, Muro K, Saito Y, et al. Japanese Society for Cancer of the colon and Rectum (JSCCR) guidelines 2019 for the treatment of colorectal cancer. Int J Clin Oncol. 2020;25(1):1–42.
9. Oka S, Tanaka S, Saito Y, et al. Local recurrence after endoscopic resection for large colorectal neoplasia: a multicenter prospective study in Japan. Am J Gastroenterol. 2015;110(5):697–707.
10. Iizuka H, Okamura S, Onozato Y, Ishihara H, Kakizaki S, Mori M. Endoscopic submucosal dissection for colorectal tumors. Gastroenterol Clin Biol. 2009;33(10–11):1004–11.
11. Saito Y, Fukuzawa M, Matsuda T, et al. Clinical outcome of endoscopic submucosal dissection versus endoscopic mucosal resection of large colorectal tumors as determined by curative resection. Surg Endosc. 2010;24(2):343–52.
12. Lee EJ, Lee JB, Lee SH, Youk EG. Endoscopic treatment of large colorectal tumors: comparison of endoscopic mucosal resection, endoscopic mucosal resection-precutting, and endoscopic submucosal dissection. Surg Endosc. 2012;26(8):2220–30.
13. Tajika M, Niwa Y, Bhatia V, et al. Comparison of endoscopic submucosal dissection and endoscopic mucosal resection for large colorectal tumors. Eur J Gastroenterol Hepatol. 2011;23(11):1042–9.
14. Soliman H, Brieau B, Guillaumot MA, et al. Invasive pit pattern, macronodule and depression are predictive factors of submucosal invasion in colorectal laterally spreading tumours from a Western population. United European Gastroenterol J. 2018;6(10):1569–77.
15. Ham NS, Kim J, Oh EH, et al. Cost of endoscopic submucosal dissection versus endoscopic piecemeal mucosal resection in the Colorectum. Dig Dis Sci. 2020;65(4):969–77.
16. Inoue T, Nakagawa K, Yamasaki Y, et al. Underwater endoscopic mucosal resection versus endoscopic submucosal dissection for 20-30 mm colorectal polyps. J Gastroenterol Hepatol. 2021;36(9):2549–57.
17. Byeon JS, Yang DH, Kim KJ, et al. Endoscopic submucosal dissection with or without snaring for colorectal neoplasms. Gastrointest Endosc. 2011;74(5):1075–83.
18. Bae JH, Yang DH, Lee S, et al. Optimized hybrid endoscopic submucosal dissection for colorectal tumors: a randomized controlled trial. Gastrointest Endosc. 2016;83(3):584–92.
19. Yang DH, Kwak MS, Park SH, et al. Endoscopic mucosal resection with circumferential mucosal incision for colorectal neoplasms: comparison with endoscopic submucosal dissection and between two Endoscopists with different experiences. Clin Endosc. 2017;50(4):379–87.
20. Gamaleldin M, Benlice C, Delaney CP, Steele S, Gorgun E. Management of the colorectal polyp referred for resection: a case-matched comparison of advanced endoscopic surgery and laparoscopic colectomy. Surgery. 2018;163(3):522–7.
21. Horiuchi A, Makino T, Kajiyama M, Tanaka N, Sano K, Graham DY. Comparison between endoscopic mucosal resection and hot snare resection of large nonpedunculated colorectal polyps: a randomized trial. Endoscopy. 2016;48(7):646–51.
22. Yen AW, Leung JW, Wilson MD, Leung FW. Underwater versus conventional endoscopic resection of nondiminutive nonpedunculated colorectal lesions: a prospective randomized controlled trial (with video). Gastrointest Endosc. 2020 Mar;91(3):643–654.e2.

23. Chien HC, Uedo N, Hsieh PH. Comparison of underwater and conventional endoscopic mucosal resection for removing sessile colorectal polyps: a propensity-score matched cohort study. Endosc Int Open. 2019;7(11):E1528–36.
24. Patel M, Haque M, Kohli D, et al. Endoscopic resection reduces morbidity when compared to surgery in veterans with large and complex colorectal polyps. Surg Endosc. 2021;35(3):1164–70.
25. Winawer SJ, Zauber AG, Ho MN, et al. Prevention of colorectal cancer by colonoscopic polypectomy. The National Polyp Study Workgroup. N Engl J Med. 1993;329(27):1977–81.
26. Lin JS, Perdue LA, Henrikson NB, Bean SI, Blasi PR. Screening for colorectal cancer: updated evidence report and systematic review for the US preventive services task force [published correction appears in JAMA. 2021 Jul 20;326(3):279]. JAMA. 2021;325(19):1978–98.
27. Zhang M, Shin EJ. Successful endoscopic strategies for difficult polypectomy. Curr Opin Gastroenterol. 2013;29(5):489–894.
28. Gorgun E, Benlice C, Church JM. Does cancer risk in colonic polyps unsuitable for polypectomy support the need for advanced endoscopic resections? J Am Coll Surg. 2016;223(3):478–84.
29. Vu JV, Sheetz KH, De Roo AC, Hiatt T, Hendren S. Variation in colectomy rates for benign polyp and colorectal cancer. Surg Endosc. 2021;35(2):802–8.
30. Ma C, Teriaky A, Sheh S, et al. Morbidity and mortality after surgery for nonmalignant colorectal polyps: a 10-year Nationwide analysis. Am J Gastroenterol. 2019;114(11):1802–10.
31. Shirai M, Nakamura T, Matsuura A, Ito Y, Kobayashi S. Safer colonoscopic polypectomy with local submucosal injection of hypertonic saline-epinephrine solution. Am J Gastroenterol. 1994;89(3):334–8.
32. Yamamoto H, Kawata H, Sunada K, et al. Successful en-bloc resection of large superficial tumors in the stomach and colon using sodium hyaluronate and small-caliber-tip transparent hood. Endoscopy. 2003;35(8):690–4.
33. Zhang XQ, Sang JZ, Xu L, et al. Endoscopic mucosal resection-precutting vs conventional endoscopic mucosal resection for sessile colorectal polyps sized 10-20 mm. World J Gastroenterol. 2022;28(45):6397–409.
34. Li D, Wang W, Xie J, et al. Efficacy and safety of three different endoscopic methods in treatment of 6-20 mm colorectal polyps. Scand J Gastroenterol. 2020;55(3):362–70.
35. Luigiano C, Consolo P, Scaffidi MG, et al. Endoscopic mucosal resection for large and giant sessile and flat colorectal polyps: a single-center experience with long-term follow-up. Endoscopy. 2009;41(10):829–35.
36. Mandic O, Jovanovic I, Cvetkovic M, et al. Factors predicting malignant occurrence and polyp recurrence after the endoscopic resection of large colorectal polyps: a single center experience. Medicina (Kaunas). 2022;58(10):1440.
37. Bujanda L, Cosme A, Gil I, Arenas-Mirave JI. Malignant colorectal polyps. World J Gastroenterol. 2010;16(25):3103–11.
38. Nett A, Binmoeller K. Underwater endoscopic mucosal resection. Gastrointest Endosc Clin N Am. 2019;29(4):659–73.
39. Choi AY, Moosvi Z, Shah S, et al. Underwater versus conventional EMR for colorectal polyps: systematic review and meta-analysis. Gastrointest Endosc. 2021;93(2):378–89.
40. Xu MD, Wang XY, Li QL, et al. Colorectal lateral spreading tumor subtypes: clinicopathology and outcome of endoscopic submucosal dissection. Int J Color Dis. 2013;28(1):63–72.
41. Draganov PV, Aihara H, Karasik MS, et al. Endoscopic submucosal dissection in North America: a large prospective multicenter study. Gastroenterology. 2021;160(7):2317–2327.e2.
42. Tanaka S, Oka S, Chayama K. Colorectal endoscopic submucosal dissection: present status and future perspective, including its differentiation from endoscopic mucosal resection. J Gastroenterol. 2008;43(9):641–51.
43. Sakamoto T, Saito Y, Fukunaga S, Nakajima T, Matsuda T. Learning curve associated with colorectal endoscopic submucosal dissection for endoscopists experienced in gastric endoscopic submucosal dissection. Dis Colon Rectum. 2011;54(10):1307–12.
44. Rajendran A, Pannick S, Thomas-Gibson S, et al. Systematic literature review of learning curves for colorectal polyp resection techniques in lower gastrointestinal endoscopy. Color Dis. 2020;22(9):1085–100.

16 Management of the Malignant Colon Polyp: Resection or Surveillance?

Ahmed A. Eltahir and Radhika K. Smith

Introduction

Malignant polyps are defined as polyps containing cancer cells that invade into but not through the submucosa of the colon [1]. Malignant polyps make up to 11% of colorectal polyps [2–4]. Over the last 20 years, participation in age appropriate colonoscopy screening has more than doubled leading to a 60% increase in the detection of malignant polyps [5]. With the adoption of advanced endoscopic techniques such as endoscopic mucosal resection (EMR) and, more recently, endoscopic submucosal dissection (ESD), complete polypectomy at the time of endoscopy is becoming more commonplace. When these polyps are completely removed at the time of endoscopy it questions the need for an oncologic resection at these very early stages of malignancy. Complete endoscopic removal could potentially avoid the morbidity and mortality associated with subsegmental colectomies and lymphadenectomy.

When weighing the risks and benefits of surgical resection versus ongoing surveillance after polypectomy, the main clinical dilemma to consider is the potential for regoinal spread to the lymph nodes. It is assumed that malignant polyps are all very early cancers but our current locoregional staging relies on lymphadenectomy. The submucosal plane houses the lymphatics and vasculature, and invasive cells in this layer allow for the potential for regional lymph node metastasis [6]. There are also certain histological characteristics such as positive margins, poor differentiation, lymphovascular invasion, tumor budding, and deep submucosal invasion which are associated with lymph node spread and worse outcomes [7, 8]. The

A. A. Eltahir (✉) · R. K. Smith (✉)
Washington University St. Louis, St. Louis, MO, USA
e-mail: a.a.eltahir@wustl.edu; radhikasmith@wustl.edu

K. Umanskiy, N. Hyman (eds.), *Difficult Decisions in Colorectal Surgery*, Difficult Decisions in Surgery: An Evidence-Based Approach,
https://doi.org/10.1007/978-3-031-42303-1_16

consideration of these factors, in addition to patients' underlying health and preferences, should drive the conversation for management of malignant polyps.

Search Strategy

A comprehensive search of PUBMED, Cochrane Library, and the Embase database was completed to identify cohort studies, reviews, meta-analysis, and other articles pertaining to malignant colon polyps. The search was limited to articles published in English between 2002 and 2022. The following keywords were used: malignant, colon, polyp, carcinoma, pT1, endoscopic resection, and surveillance.

Studies were included if they examined histological characteristics and their association with mortality, lymph node spread, residual disease, recurrence, or adverse outcomes. Studies which had incomplete histological evaluations of specimen were excluded. Studies which included benign polyps or advanced carcinomas in their analysis were also excluded. If articles were published using the same data, only the most recent article was included.

Results

Malignant polyps account for up to 11% of colorectal polyps [2–4]. Their lymph node metastatic potential ranges from 6.6 to 16% [9–12]. A variety of retrospective and prospective studies were conducted to better prognosticate the risks of these early malignancies to spread to the regional lymph nodes. These data could better inform clinicians on how to best manage these polyps and potentially avoid overtreatment with surgical resection. Studies published over the last several decades have reported on the metastatic risk to the lymph node of malignant polyps, differentiating them into low and high risk features [13].

Depth of Invasion

Polyp morphology has been linked to risk for nodal invasion with sessile polyps having a higher likelihood of lymph node spread when compared to pedunculated polyps. Different classifications are used to grade the level of invasion of pedunculated and sessile polyps. The Haggitt classification is used for pedunculated polyps as seen in Fig. 16.1. Overall incidence of lymph node spread in pedunculated polyps is approximately 6%. Many studies have shown that risk of lymph node spread is <1% of polyps with Haggitt level 1,2, and 3 invasion when the polyp is completely removed. Level four invasion, however, is associated with a lymph node metastasis risk of up to 27% [14, 15]. Depth of submucosal invasion in sessile polyps on the other hand are divided into thirds according to the Kikuchi classification as seen in Fig. 16.2, which can also be seen in the histology slides in Figs. 16.3, 16.4 and 16.5. SM1 polyps carry a risk of lymph node spread of 1–3%, SM2 have an 8% risk, and

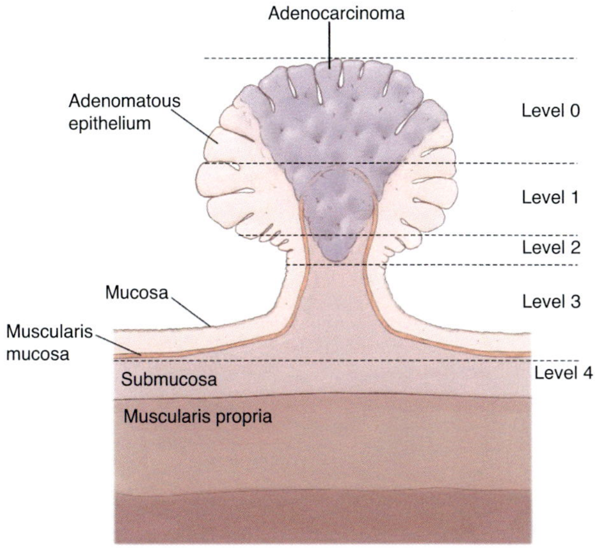

Fig. 16.1 Haggitt classification of pedunculated polyp. (This figure was illustrated by Shawna Duan)

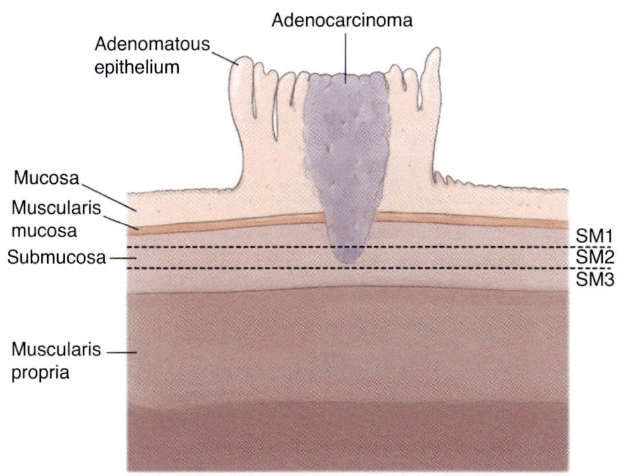

Fig. 16.2 Kikuchi classification of sessile polyp. (This figure was illustrated by Shawna Duan)

SM3 have a risk of 23–27% [16, 17]. It is hard to measure relative invasion of endoscopically resected polyps as the whole submucosa is usually not resected. Therefore, studies have looked at the degree of invasion with invasion of more than 1 mm associated with a higher risk of lymph node spread [7].

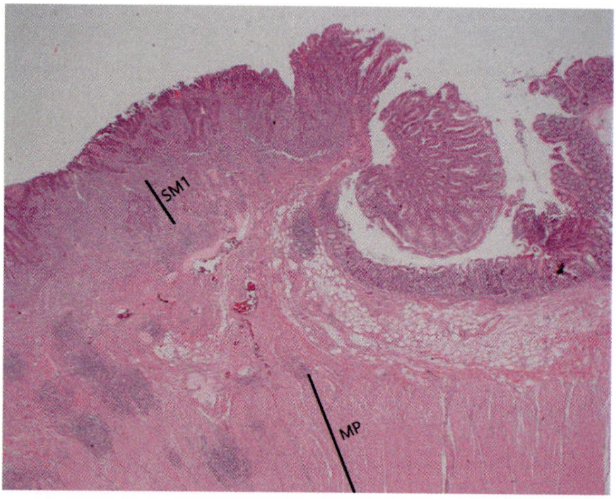

Fig. 16.3 Kikuchi SM 1. (This figure produced thanks to Dr. Kathleen Byrnes and Washington University in St. Louis Pathology Department)

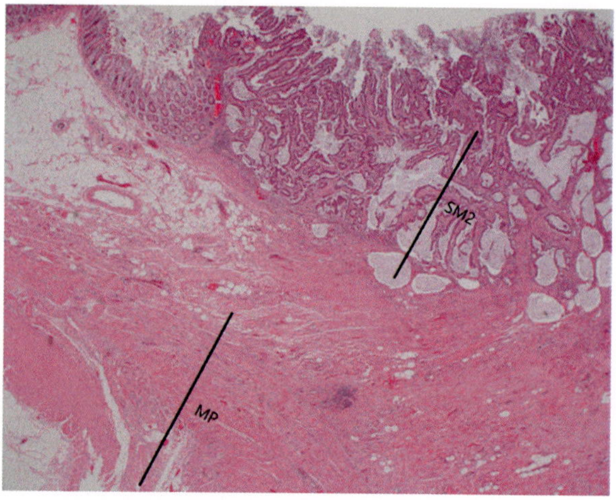

Fig. 16.4 Kikuchi SM 2. (This figure produced thanks to Dr. Kathleen Byrnes and Washington University in St. Louis Pathology Department)

Margin Positivity

Histologically incomplete resection of malignant polyps is associated with both lymph node metastasis and residual disease. Boenicke et al. retrospectively studied 105 patients with malignant polyps. They found that histologically incomplete removal was significantly associated with lymph node spread with an odds ratio of 10.2 [18]. A meta-analysis encompassing 815 patients found that tumors with lymph node spread had a 2.36 odds of having positive margins [19]. Butte et al. found that 16% of patients with less than 1 mm margins had residual disease while no patients with a margin 1 mm or greater had residual disease [20]. Kim et al. also found that positive margins were twice as likely to have residual disease [21].

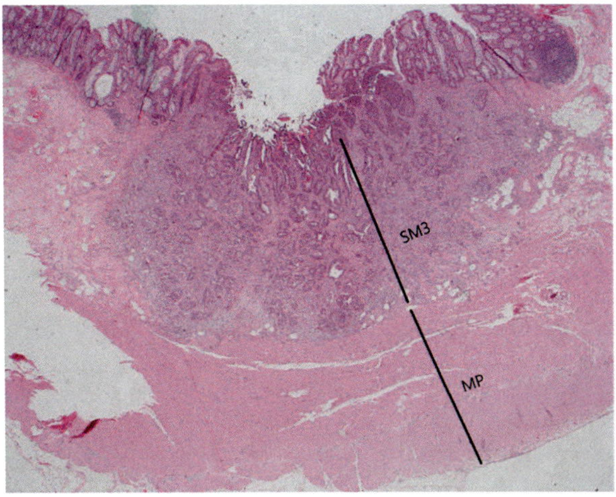

Fig. 16.5 Kikuchi SM 3. (This figure produced thanks to Dr. Kathleen Byrnes and Washington University in St. Louis Pathology Department)

Lymphovascular Invasion

The presence of lymphatics and blood vessels in the submucosa is the reason malignant cells in this layer are able to spread. The majority of published literature on the risks of lymph node spread have demonstrated that lymphovascular invasion is a risk factor. Samuolis et al., a recently retrospective study, found that half of specimens with positive lymph nodes had lymphovascular invasion [22]. Butte et al. demonstrated odds of 5.3 of lymphovascular invasion when lymph nodes are positive [20].

Poor Differentiation

Poor differentiation is another risk factor associated with lymph node spread. The 2014 meta-analysis demonstrated that specimens with positive lymph nodes were associated with positive margins with an odds ratio 3.52. It was also significantly associated with disease-specific mortality [19]. Kim et al. showed that poor differentiation was 7.5 times as likely to have residual disease [21].

Tumor Budding

Tumor budding which is defined as a single cancer cell or a cluster of up to 4 cells at the advancing edge of the tumor, is not as well studied as the other features. Nevertheless, more recent studies have demonstrated an association with lymph node spread. Two studies, Choi et al. and Kye et al. found that tumor budding was independently associated with 16 and 7.7 increased odds of having lymph node metastasis respectively [12, 23]. A large meta-analysis encompassing 4510 patients published in 2013 also found that tumor budding was independently associated with lymph node metastasis (OR 7.74) [7].

Recommendations

Patients who present with malignant colon polyps with no high-risk features can undergo surveillance with frequent colonoscopies instead of surgical resection with no increase in risk of adverse outcomes (Recommendation: Strong; Evidence: Moderate).

The decision to manage malignant colon polyps should be a collaborative approach between the physician and patient, taking into account the patient's fitness, preference, and ability to adhere to a surveillance schedule. After expert pathology review demonstrates no high-risk features such as positive margins, poor differentiation, lymphovascular invasion, deep submucosal invasion, or tumor budding in the colonic polyp, patients can opt for surveillance with a low risk of lymph node spread or recurrent disease. However, if high-risk features are identified, patients should consider surgical resection if medically fit.

Personal View

Treating colorectal cancer is largely dependent on its potential to metastasize. Given the scarcity of lymphatic vessels in the colonic mucosa, truly intramucosal carcinomas have no risk of metastasizing to the lymph node [24]. Numerous studies have demonstrated that endoscopic management of these polyps is cost effective and associated with lower morbidity and mortality [25, 26]. The potential for morbidity and mortality of surgery should prompt physicians and patients to avoid surgery if it does not offer any clinical benefits.

With more widespread adoption of colorectal cancer screening, more carcinomas are detected at an earlier state. Over the last several decades, dozens of articles have been published to better understand the risk of lymph node metastasis in malignant polyps allowing for more informed consent and shared decision making. The known literature points to certain histological features that are known to increase the risk of spread such as positive margins, lymphovascular invasion, poor differentiation, deep submucosal invasion and, to some degree, tumor budding. In order to best evaluate these features, the first step is an en-bloc resection of the polyp allowing pathologists to best evaluate the margins and architecture of the specimen. Realistically, many of these features are surprisingly difficult to differentiate and can have poor inter-operator reliability. Given that the decision to forgo surgery will largely depend on the lack of high-risk features on histological evaluation, expert pathologic assessment is paramount however this is often times limited by the specimen itself. The original endoscopist must make every effort to resect the polyp completely and in one piece. In almost every study, positive margins were associated with residual disease or lymph node spread. Piecemeal dissection makes it difficult for the pathologist to evaluate the specimen and can lead to inaccurate or incomplete interpretation. One study demonstrated there was an increase in recurrence for polyps removed in a piecemeal fashion [27]. Regardless, piecemeal dissection in and of itself is not an indication for surgical resection but it should prompt the conversation between the patient and physician even if there are no other high-risk features.

Another issue to consider is that the alternative to surgical resection is surveillance with frequent colonoscopies. There are no exact guidelines on the frequency of these colonoscopies, and they are institution and physician dependent. The patient and physician must consider the feasibility of patient adherence to the surveillance schedule. If there is a serious risk of not following up with medical care either due to logistical issues or lack of insurance, then surgical resection should be weighed more favorably. Ultimately, risks of nodal disease, the patient's preference, and their fitness for surgery must be clearly considered in the treatment of malignant polyps.

PICO table

Patients	Intervention	Comparator	Outcome
Patients with pT1 malignant colon polyps	Colectomy	Surveillance	Lymph node metastasis, mortality, recurrent disease

Data summary

Study	Patients	Intervention	Outcome	Result	Quality of evidence
Choi [12]	87	Surgery vs surveillance	Lymph node spread	20% vs 0%	Strong
Pizarro [28]	42	Surgery	Residual disease	22%	Moderate
Di Gregorio [19]	105	Surgery vs surveillance	Cancer related mortality	6% vs 0%	Moderate
Butte [20]	143	Surgery	Lymph node spread	7%	Moderate
Boenicke [18]	105	Surgery vs surveillance	Lymph node spread	Odd ratio (OR) 9.2	Weak
Samuolis [22]	40	Surgery	Lymph node spread	12.5%	Moderate
Kim [21]	148	Surgery	Residual disease	10.9%	Weak
Okabe [29]	428	Surgery	Lymph node spread	10%	Moderate
Kye [23]	55	Surgery	Lymph node spread	14.5%	Moderate

References

1. Aarons CB, Shanmugan S, Bleier JI. Management of malignant colon polyps: current status and controversies. World J Gastroenterol WJG. 2014;20(43):16178–83. https://doi.org/10.3748/wjg.v20.i43.16178.
2. Netzer P, Forster C, Biral R, et al. Risk factor assessment of endoscopically removed malignant colorectal polyps. Gut. 1998;43(5):669–74. https://doi.org/10.1136/gut.43.5.669.
3. Hackelsberger A, Frühmorgen P, Weiler H, Heller T, Seeliger H, Junghanns K. Endoscopic polypectomy and management of colorectal adenomas with invasive carcinoma. Endoscopy. 1995;27(2):153–8. https://doi.org/10.1055/s-2007-1005654.
4. Bujanda L, Cosme A, Gil I, Arenas-Mirave JI. Malignant colorectal polyps. World J Gastroenterol WJG. 2010;16(25):3103–11. https://doi.org/10.3748/wjg.v16.i25.3103.
5. Colorectal Cancer Screening | Cancer Trends Progress Report. Accessed 28 Sept 2022. https://progressreport.cancer.gov/detection/colorectal_cancer
6. Rex DK, Shaukat A, Wallace MB. Optimal Management of Malignant Polyps, from endoscopic assessment and resection to decisions about surgery. Clin Gastroenterol Hepatol. 2019;17(8):1428–37. https://doi.org/10.1016/j.cgh.2018.09.040.
7. Beaton C, Twine CP, Williams GL, Radcliffe AG. Systematic review and meta-analysis of histopathological factors influencing the risk of lymph node metastasis in early colorectal cancer. Colorectal Dis Off J Assoc Coloproctology G B Irel. 2013;15(7):788–97. https://doi.org/10.1111/codi.12129.
8. Choi JY, Jung SA, Shim KN, et al. Meta-analysis of predictive clinicopathologic factors for lymph node metastasis in patients with early colorectal carcinoma. J Korean Med Sci. 2015;30(4):398–406. https://doi.org/10.3346/jkms.2015.30.4.398.
9. Tateishi Y, Nakanishi Y, Taniguchi H, Shimoda T, Umemura S. Pathological prognostic factors predicting lymph node metastasis in submucosal invasive (T1) colorectal carcinoma. Mod Pathol Off J U S Can Acad Pathol Inc. 2010;23(8):1068–72. https://doi.org/10.1038/modpathol.2010.88.
10. Kikuchi R, Takano M, Takagi K, et al. Management of early invasive colorectal cancer. Risk of recurrence and clinical guidelines. Dis Colon Rectum. 1995;38(12):1286–95. https://doi.org/10.1007/BF02049154.
11. Risio M, Fiocca R. Malignant adenoma: diagnosis, staging, risk factors, lymph node involvement and problems of sampling. Tech Coloproctol. 2004;8(Suppl 2):s253–6. https://doi.org/10.1007/s10151-004-0171-4.
12. Choi DH, Kyung Sohn D, Jin Chang H, Lim SB, Seong Choi H, Jeong SY. Indications for subsequent surgery after endoscopic resection of Submucosally invasive colorectal carcinomas: a prospective cohort study. Dis Colon Rectum. 2009;52(3):438–45. https://doi.org/10.1007/DCR.0b013e318197e37f.
13. Coverlizza S, Risio M, Ferrari A, Fenoglio-Preiser CM, Rossini FP. Colorectal adenomas containing invasive carcinoma. Pathologic assessment of lymph node metastatic potential. Cancer. 1989;64(9):1937–47. https://doi.org/10.1002/1097-0142(19891101)64:9<1937::aid-cncr2820640929>3.0.co;2-x.
14. Nivatvongs S, Rojanasakul A, Reiman HM, et al. The risk of lymph node metastasis in colorectal polyps with invasive adenocarcinoma. Dis Colon Rectum. 1991;34(4):323–8. https://doi.org/10.1007/BF02050592.
15. Ramirez M, Schierling S, Papaconstantinou HT, Scott TJ. Management of the Malignant Polyp. Clin Colon Rectal Surg. 2008;21(4):286–90. https://doi.org/10.1055/s-0028-1089944.
16. Nascimbeni R, Burgart LJ, Nivatvongs S, Larson DR. Risk of lymph node metastasis in T1 carcinoma of the colon and rectum. Dis Colon Rectum. 2002;45(2):200–6. https://doi.org/10.1007/s10350-004-6147-7.
17. Tytherleigh MG, Warren BF, Mortensen NJM. Management of early rectal cancer. Br J Surg. 2008;95(4):409–23. https://doi.org/10.1002/bjs.6127.

18. Boenicke L, Fein M, Sailer M, Isbert C, Germer CT, Thalheimer A. The concurrence of histologically positive resection margins and sessile morphology is an important risk factor for lymph node metastasis after complete endoscopic removal of malignant colorectal polyps. Int J Color Dis. 2010;25(4):433–8. https://doi.org/10.1007/s00384-009-0836-6.
19. Di Gregorio C, Bonetti LR, de Gaetani C, Pedroni M, Kaleci S. Ponz de Leon M. clinical outcome of low- and high-risk malignant colorectal polyps: results of a population-based study and meta-analysis of the available literature. Intern Emerg Med. 2014;9(2):151–60. https://doi.org/10.1007/s11739-012-0772-2.
20. Butte JM, Tang P, Gonen M, et al. Rate of residual disease after complete endoscopic resection of malignant colonic polyp. Dis Colon Rectum. 2012;55(2):122–7. https://doi.org/10.1097/DCR.0b013e3182336c38.
21. Kim KJ, Lee HS, Jeon SW, Jin S, Lee SW. Association of Poor Differentiation or positive vertical margin with residual disease in patients with subsequent colectomy after complete macroscopic endoscopic resection of early colorectal cancer. Gastroenterol Res Pract. 2017;2017:7129626. https://doi.org/10.1155/2017/7129626.
22. Samuolis N, Samalavicius NE, Dulskas A, et al. Surgical or endoscopic management of malignant colon polyps. ANZ J Surg. 2018;88(12):E824–8. https://doi.org/10.1111/ans.14846.
23. Kye BH, Jung JH, Kim HJ, Kang SG, Cho HM, Kim JG. Tumor budding as a risk factor of lymph node metastasis in submucosal invasive T1 colorectal carcinoma: a retrospective study. BMC Surg. 2012;12:16. https://doi.org/10.1186/1471-2482-12-16.
24. Risio M. The natural history of pT1 colorectal cancer. Front Oncol 2012;2. Accessed 21 Aug 2022. https://www.frontiersin.org/articles/10.3389/fonc.2012.00022
25. Ma C, Teriaky A, Sheh S, et al. Morbidity and Mortality After Surgery for Nonmalignant Colorectal Polyps: A 10-Year Nationwide Analysis. Am J Gastroenterol. 2019;114(11):1802–10. https://doi.org/10.14309/ajg.0000000000000407.
26. Jayanna M, Burgess NG, Singh R, et al. Cost analysis of endoscopic mucosal resection vs surgery for large laterally spreading colorectal lesions. Clin Gastroenterol Hepatol Off Clin Pract J Am Gastroenterol Assoc. 2016;14(2):271–278.e1-2. https://doi.org/10.1016/j.cgh.2015.08.037.
27. Hassan C, Repici A, Sharma P, et al. Efficacy and safety of endoscopic resection of large colorectal polyps: a systematic review and meta-analysis. Gut. 2016;65(5):806–20. https://doi.org/10.1136/gutjnl-2014-308481.
28. Pizarro-Moreno A, Cordero-Fernández C, Garzón-Benavides M, et al. Malignant colonic adenomas. Therapeutic criteria. Long-term results of therapy in a series of 42 patients in our healthcare area. Rev Espanola Enfermedades Dig Organo Of Soc Espanola Patol Dig. 2009;101(12):830–6. https://doi.org/10.4321/s1130-01082009001200002.
29. Okabe S, Shia J, Nash G, et al. Lymph node metastasis in T1 adenocarcinoma of the colon and rectum. J Gastrointest Surg. 2004;8(8):1032–40. https://doi.org/10.1016/j.gassur.2004.09.038.

Stage II Colon Cancer: Towards an Individualized Treatment Approach

17

Gideon Dosunmu and Chih-Yi Liao

Introduction

The decision on whether to administer adjuvant chemotherapy in stage II colon cancer continues to be an ongoing debate. There are no clear-cut guidelines or data on the majority of cases. Ultimately, every patient is different, and that decision will vary from patient to patient depending on their unique characteristics and tumor biology. The problem is that stage II colon cancer is so heterogeneous biologically with SEER 5-year survival rates ranging from 66% in stage IIA cancers to 37% for stage IIC disease [1]. In this chapter, we will present the current state of the science for stage II colon cancer with the hopes of allowing the practitioner to better risk-stratify patients and thereby select those who are most likely to benefit from adjuvant chemotherapy. We will conclude with our recommendations for specific cases with the strength of that recommendation based on the evidence.

Patient population	Intervention	Comparators	Outcomes studied
Patients with stage II colon cancer	Chemotherapy	Observation	Disease free survival, overall survival

G. Dosunmu (✉) · C.-Y. Liao
Section of Hematology/Oncology, Department of Medicine, University of Chicago, Chicago, IL, USA
e-mail: gideon.dosunmu@uchicagomedicine.org; andyliao@medicine.bsd.uchicago.edu

K. Umanskiy, N. Hyman (eds.), *Difficult Decisions in Colorectal Surgery*, Difficult Decisions in Surgery: An Evidence-Based Approach,
https://doi.org/10.1007/978-3-031-42303-1_17

Results

Non-Risk-Stratified Patients

In attempting to answer the questions as to whether chemotherapy is important in stage II colorectal cancer, we will explore available studies. A comprehensive list of the relevant studies is listed in Table 17.1. A noteworthy trial is the QUASAR trial [2] which explored the use of adjuvant 5-FU based therapy in stage II colon cancer. Although not a perfect study, with the study power and randomization, it reasonably answers our question of chemotherapy benefit. In the QUASAR trial, 5-FU chemotherapy resulted in a statistically significant improvement in overall survival and disease-free survival. The absolute magnitude of the survival benefit was 3.6% (95% CI: 1–6%), and number needed to treat was 28. No other study confirms this survival advantage statistically, but most suggest a magnitude of benefit that is not inconsistent with the QUASAR results either for overall survival (OS) or at least for disease-free survival (DFS) [3–10].

A limitation of most of the studies aimed at addressing our question is that they are either underpowered or are pooled subset analyses of randomized trials which subjects them to biases inherent in pooled analysis, including a meta-analysis done by the Cochrane group [3]. MOSAIC and NSABP C-07 are two trials that incorporated oxaliplatin-based chemotherapy. They however did not appear to have shown a significant improvement over 5-FU alone for stage II colon cancer patients [5, 10]. Even the 10-year MOSAIC update failed to show an overall survival advantage of one chemotherapy over the other (78.4% vs. 79.5%) [11]. The limitation of these studies is that they are underpowered to answer our question with any certainty.

Looking at some registry data which are weaker study types in our table, such as the BCCA and SEER-Medicare. They showed no advantage to chemotherapy in stage II colon cancer and even suggest it may be detrimental [12, 13]. However, data from the National Cancer Database consisting of 153,110 stage II colon cancer patients showed increased OS in those who received adjuvant chemotherapy compared to those who did not 51% vs 35% [14]. The limitation of these registry studies is uncontrolled threats to internal validity.

Risk-Stratification: Clinical and Pathologic Factors

To better understand risk stratification, let's clarify the basic terminology surrounding risk stratification, namely the distinction between a prognostic versus a predictive factor. Prognostic factors are features of a disease that tells us about the natural course and outcomes of the disease. This can help guide in deciding whether to treat cancer. Predictive factors give information as to whether a patient will benefit from an intervention or not. It is important to note that prognostic is not equal to predictive. A common fallacy to which we are all susceptible is that patients with the worst prognosis are the ones most likely to benefit from aggressive treatment. It is sometimes the case but often it is not.

Table 17.1 Role of chemotherapy for stage II colon cancer

Study	Trial type	Stage II cancer Pts	Therapies	RFS (95% CI)	OS (95% CI)	Strength
QUASAR [2]	RCT	2146	5-FU vs surgery alone	0.78 (0.66–0.93)	0.82 (95% CI: 0.7–0.95)	High
NACCP [9]	RCT (subset)	468	5-Fu vs surgery alone	71% vs. 65% (OR crosses 1)	5 year: 78% vs 70% (OR crosses 1)	Moderate
INT-0035 [8]	RCT	318	5-Fu vs surgery alone	7 years: 79% vs 71% (p = 0.1)	7 year: 72% vs 72% (p = 0.83)	Moderate
Nordic [7]	Pooled RCT	812	5-FU vs surgery alone	NR	79% vs 79% (p = 0.81)	Moderate
IMPACT-B2 [4]	Pooled RCT	1016	5-FU vs surgery alone	5 year: 76% vs 73% (p = 0.061)	Year: 82% vs. 80% (p = 0.057)	Moderate
Gill et al. [6]	Pooled RCT (IMPACT-B2 + 2 Additional trials)	1440	5-FU vs surgery alone	5 year: 76% vs. 72% (p = 0.049)	5 year: 81% vs 80% (p = 0.1127)	Moderate
MOSAIC [5], 18	RCT (subset)	899	FOLFOX vs 5-FU	5 year: 83.7% vs 79.9% (p = 0.258)	6 year OS: 86.9 vs 86.8 (0.986) 10 year OS: 79.5% 78.4% (0.980)	Moderate
NSABP C-07 [10]	RCT (subset)	699	FLOX vs 5-FU	5 year: 82.1% vs. 80.1%	89.7 vs 89.6	Moderate
Cochrane [3]	Meta-analysis	7097	Chemo vs. surgery alone	HR 0.83 (0.77–0.92)	HR 0.96 (0.91–1.02)	Moderate
SEER-Medicare [13]	Registry	6234	Chemo vs. surgery alone	NR	5 year: 70% vs. 69.5%	Moderate
BCCA data base [11]	Registry	1697a	Chemo vs. surgery alone	5 year: 87.1% vs. 92% (p = 0.18)	5 year: 82.9 vs 83.3 (p = 0.561)	Moderate

NR not reported
a = Stage II with no poor prognostic feature (obstruction/perf, T4, poor/undiff histology, >12 LN, emergent surgery)

The most commonly recognized prognostic factors in stage II colon cancer are as follows: T4 disease, inadequate lymph node sampling (<12 lymph nodes), poorly differentiated histology (in MSI-L/S patients), perforation, obstruction, lymphovascular invasion, perineural invasion, and positive resection margins [15]. It is very important that the reader pays special attention to the high-grade tumor histology and the importance of interpreting this in the context of the mismatch repair (MMR) or microsatellite instability (MSI) status of the tumor. As we will go into detail below, tumors with MMR deficiency or MSI-H phenotype are often high grade yet have an excellent prognosis. Whether these adverse risk factors are predictive of the benefit of chemotherapy is less clear. The strongest data to suggest a benefit of chemotherapy in high-risk groups comes from the British Columbia Cancer Agency (BCCA) registry which found a significant survival advantage for patients with T4 tumors who received 5-FU chemotherapy (HR 0.5 95% CI: 0.33–0.77) [12]. The National Cancer Database also showed that the high-risk group benefited from adjuvant chemotherapy at 57% vs 76% ($P < 0.001$) [14]. A study of the California cancer registry Showed that patients with T4 disease as the single highest risk factor had improved OS with chemotherapy (HR 0.51, 95% CI 0.34–0.78) [16]. In contrast, the SEER registry study could discern any differential chemotherapy advantage for high versus low-risk groups [6, 13].

The MOSAIC study utilizing oxaliplatin-based therapy suggested a disease-free survival advantage in the high-risk stage II group only with 5-year DFS of 82.3% versus 74.6% (HR 0.72; 95% CI: 0.5–1.02) for FOLFOX versus infusional 5-FU [5]. 10-year OS was 79.5% versus 78.4% in 5-FU/LV versus FOLFOX arms [11]. Although there was a statistically significant improvement in DFS and OS, the benefit of FOLFOX was less pronounced with only a small absolute improvement in DFS and OS. Overall, the MOSAIC study provides some evidence supporting the use of an oxaliplatin-based regimen in patients with stage II colon cancer with high-risk features. The benefit is however less clear than in stage III colon cancer patients. Therefore, treatment and chemotherapy decisions should be individualized based on patient and disease characteristics.

Risk-Stratification: Molecular Factors

The strongest data for both a prognostic and predictive factor exists for a deficiency in the mismatch repair pathway. It is beyond the scope of this chapter to explain the nuances of MMR deficiency and testing for it; but in brief, patients with defective MMR tumors either have a germline loss of one of the MMR proteins (MLH1, MSH2, MSH6, PMS2) or epigenetic silencing of the MLH1 promoter [17]. The former is associated with Lynch syndrome and the latter is often in the setting of a CpG Island methylator phenotype (CIMP). Defective MMR tumors can either be tested for using a PCR panel of 5 reference microsatellite sites; if at least 2 show instability then the tumor is characterized as MSI-H. More often in the clinical setting, immunohistochemistry testing (IHC) is used to stain for the presence or absence of one of the MMR proteins. By convention in the literature, we call a tumor as defective MMR.

(dMMR) if they are either MSI-H or have an absence of an MMR protein by IHC. Table 17.2 lists the major studies which have explored the prognostic and Predictive value of MMR testing in stage II colon cancer. The majority of these studies clearly show that those with dMMR stage II tumors have a superior prognosis compared to those with pMMR with hazards of recurrence or death often 50% lower [18–22]. In the study by Sargent, et al. [21] patients with dMMR tumors who received chemotherapy had a hazard of death which was nearly three times those who were on observation (HR 2.95; 95% CI: 1.02–8.54). The reason why this may be the case is speculative, but we know patients with dMMR often have an intense immune response to their tumors and are in fact the only colon cancer cohort to date where immune checkpoint inhibitors appear to be effective in the metastatic setting [23]. It is suggested that chemotherapy may blunt this immune response. This hypothesis is further corroborated by recent data suggesting that if there is a chemotherapy benefit for these patients, it is only for those with germline tumors which tend not to express the hyper-mutated phenotype [24]. These findings of a detrimental impact have not been corroborated by the other studies listed in Table 17.2. However, no study has found a clearly beneficial impact of chemotherapy for this cohort, who have an otherwise excellent prognosis. It is important to note that all of

Table 17.2 Role of dMMR as prognostic and predictive marker for stage II colon cancer

Study	dMMR colon patients	Therapies	DFS (vs pMMR)	OS (vs pMMR)	OS w/chemo vs w/o chemo
Sargent et al. [21]	102 (stage II)	5-FU vs surgery alone	0.51 (95% CI: 0.29–0.89)a	0.47 (0.26–0.83)[a]	2.95 (95% CI:1.02–8.54)
Jover et al. [27]	76 (38 stage II)	5-FU vs surgery Alone	6 year: 71% vs 63% (p = 0.3)	6 year: 57.7% vs 67.6% (p = 0.6)[b]	69.2% vs 73.5% (p = 0.8)b
Kim et al. (NSABP c01-c04) [28]	98 (II and III)	5-FU vs surgery alone	HR 0.77 (95% CI: 0.4–1.48)[a]	Interaction p = 0.68[b]	Interaction p = 0.62b
Klingbiel et al. (PETACC-3) [20]	86 (stage II)	FOLFIRI vs 5FU	HR 0.26 (95% CI: 0.1–0.65)	HR 1.27 (0.65–2.49)	HR 1.47 (0.65–3.36)
Hutchings et al. (QUASAR) [19]	167 (stage II)	5-Fu vs surgery alone	RR 0.44 (95% CI: 0.29–0.67)	2 year: 2.2% vs 5.1% Interaction p = 0.55	NR
Gavin et al (NSABP C07-C08) [18]	207 (93 stage II)	FOLFOX	HR 0.48 (95% CI: 0.3–0.7)	Interaction 0.97	Interaction p = 0.848

dMMR defective DNA mismatch repair, *pMMR* proficient mismatch repair, *NR* not reported

[a] Includes only patients not treated with chemotherapy

[b] Includes stage II and III

these studies are severely limited by the power to test for the interaction between dMMR status and chemotherapy effect. Several studies have also looked at other molecular mutations in the BRAF and KRAS genes including interactions of these factors with dMMR status as well as those with CpG Island methylator phenotype [18, 19, 25, 26]. No clear consensus has emerged with one study suggesting a BRAF mutation is prognostic for poorer overall survival in all stage II patients [18] and another in only those with pMMR status [25]. An additional study suggested a poorer survival for KRAS mutant tumors but not BRAF [19]. In none of the studies were KRAS, BRAF, or CIMP predictive of benefit from chemotherapy and as such have not found their way into our treatment algorithms.

Risk-Stratification: ctDNA and Minimal Residual Disease

Circulating tumor DNA (ctDNA) are DNA fragments that are released by neoplastic cells [29]. Its positivity after curative surgery provides evidence of micrometastases and minimal residual disease. It offers to be a promising noninvasive tool for personalizing treatment and deciding which patients will receive adjuvant chemotherapy, and which regimen to use.

A phase II study evaluated whether ctDNA guided approach could reduce the use of adjuvant therapy while reducing the risk of recurrence. This study enrolled patients based on either ctDNA or clinicopathologic features. ctDNA-negative patients were not treated. 15% in ctDNA guided group received chemotherapy compared to 28% in the standard management group. The primary endpoint, recurrence-free survival (RFS) at 2 years, was non-inferior to the standard group (93.5% vs 92.4%; 95% CI: 1.25–2.65%). At 3 years, RFS was 91.7% vs. 92.4%. Essentially, fewer patients received chemotherapy when the ctDNA-based approach was employed without sacrificing the risk of recurrence, suggesting that potential role of ctDNA in guiding adjuvant therapy decisions [30]. While this study offered prognostic information, it did not provide evidence about the effect of chemotherapy treatment, and larger validation studies are needed. A major limitation of ctDNA is its sensitivity which can range from 50 to 60% [31], especially in early-stage tumors with few DNA fragments [29].

The CIRCULATE-US study (NCT05174169) is a prospective study to evaluate the role of ctDNA to guide adjuvant therapy decisions in high-risk stage II and III colon cancer. This phase II/III clinical trial stratified patients with resected colon cancer based on their ctDNA status, and randomized them to different adjuvant therapy regimens, with the primary objective of measuring DFS (Fig. 17.1). Patients with negative baseline ctDNA (cohort A) will get randomized to receive adjuvant FOLFOX/CAPOX, or no adjuvant chemotherapy. Patients with baseline positive ctDNA (cohort B) will get randomized to receive adjuvant FOLFOX/CAPOX or FOLFOXIRI. Both cohorts will involve serial ctDNA monitoring. Patients from cohort A with detectable ctDNA at any point will be switched to cohort B. The CIRCULATE-US study will hopefully better enlighten practitioners on the potential use of ctDNA as a monitoring, prognostic, and treatment decision tool. If

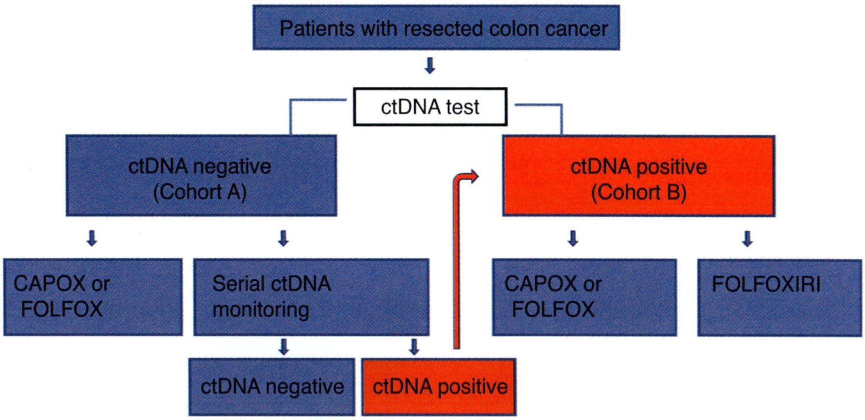

Fig. 17.1 Circulate-US study (NCT05174169)

successful, the trial may lead to the development of new treatment paradigms for stage II colon cancer, including MRD-directed adjuvant therapy.

Duration of Adjuvant Therapy

The International Duration Evaluation of Adjuvant Chemotherapy (IDEA) was a collaboration of four to six phase III studies involving 3273 high-risk stage II colon cancer patients, that attempted to answer the question of the optimal duration of adjuvant chemotherapy in stage II colorectal cancer. Patients were randomly assigned to receive 3 months vs. 6 months of adjuvant chemotherapy. Adjuvant therapy regimen was up to investigator discretion, and included FOLFOX (5-fluorouracil, leucovorin, and oxaliplatin) or CAPOX (capecitabine and oxaliplatin). The primary endpoint was 5-year disease-free survival. In the overall population, noninferiority was not demonstrated for 3 months of adjuvant therapy vs. 6 months of adjuvant therapy (DFS 80.7% vs 83.9%, HR, 1.17; 80% CI, 1.05 to 1.31; P [for noninferiority] .39). However, preplanned subgroup comparisons showed a statistically significant difference in patients receiving CAPOX vs. FOLFOX regimens. The 5-year DFS of 3 months adjuvant CAPOX vs 6 months was 81.7 vs 82%. (HR 1.02; 95% CI, 0.82 to 1.27) with fewer grade 3–5 toxicities in the 3 months cohort. The 5-year DFS was higher with 6 months of FOLFOX compared to 3 months of FOLFOX (79.2% vs 86.5%, HR 1.41; 95% CI, 1.08 to 1.84), though 6 months of FOLFOX was associated with more toxicities. Essentially, 3 months of FOLFOX was inferior to 6 months of FOLFOX, while 3 months of CAPOX was comparable to 6 months of CAPOX with a HR closer to 1. This suggests a potential use of 3 months of CAPOX in high-risk stage II patients, especially when taking into consideration the cost and toxicity profile. 6 months of FOLFOX was superior to 3 months of FOLFOX but had more toxicities [32]. A limitation of the IDEA study was that OS was not yet evaluated due to the short follow-up; longer follow-up is needed to fully evaluate the long-term outcomes of patients receiving 3 months of CAPOX. The sample size was also not sufficiently large to accurately detect small differences in DFS.

Overall, 3 months CAPOX or 6 months single-agent 5FU can be considered in high-risk stage II colon cancer patients taking into account the patient's specific risk profile, comorbidities, side effects, and preferences. We reserve 6-months of oxaliplatin based adjuvant therapy for patients with multiple high-risk features.

Recommendations Based on the Data

1. All stage II colon cancer patients should be tested for dMMR either by IHC or PCR and those with dMMR should not receive chemotherapy (evidence quality high, strong recommendation).
2. Patients with T4 tumors, high grade (pMMR), <12 LN sampled, or with perforation should receive adjuvant chemotherapy (evidence quality moderate, moderate recommendation).
3. Adjuvant therapy with 3 months CAPOX or 6 months single-agent 5FU can be considered in high-risk stage II colon cancer patients taking into account the patient's specific risk profile, comorbidities, side effects, and preferences. Patients with multiple high-risk features may be considered for 6-months of oxaliplatin-based adjuvant therapy (evidence quality moderate, moderate recommendation).
4. Patients with T4b tumors should receive oxaliplatin-based adjuvant therapy (evidence quality weak, moderate recommendation).
5. ctDNA should be considered for surveillance and risk-stratification, and studies are underway to investigate its role in guiding adjuvant therapy regimen. (evidence quality moderate, moderate recommendation).

References

1. Edge SB, Byrd DR, Compton CC, Fritz AG, Greene FL, Trotti A, editors. AJCC cancer staging manual. 7th ed. New York: Springer; 2010.
2. Quasar Collaborative G, Gray R, Barnwell J, McConkey C, Hills RK, Williams NS, et al. Adjuvant chemotherapy versus observation in patients with colorectal cancer: a randomised study. Lancet. 2007;370(9604):2020–9. https://doi.org/10.1016/S0140-6736(07)61866-2.
3. Figueredo A, Coombes ME, Mukherjee S. Adjuvant therapy for completely resected stage II colon cancer. Cochrane Database Syst Rev. 2008;2010(3):CD005390. https://doi.org/10.1002/14651858.CD005390.pub2.
4. Erlichman C. Efficacy of adjuvant fluorouracil and folinic acid in B2 colon cancer. International multicentre pooled analysis of B2 colon cancer trials (IMPACT B2) investigators. J Clin Oncol Off J Am Soc Clin Oncol. 1999;17(5):1356–63.
5. Andre T, Boni C, Navarro M, Tabernero J, Hickish T, Topham C, et al. Improved overall survival with oxaliplatin, fluorouracil, and leucovorin as adjuvant treatment in stage II or III colon

cancer in the MOSAIC trial. J Clin Oncol Off J Am Soc Clin Oncol. 2009;27(19):3109–16. https://doi.org/10.1200/JCO.2008.20.6771.

6. Gill S, Loprinzi CL, Sargent DJ, Thome SD, Alberts SR, Haller DG, et al. Pooled analysis of fluorouracil-based adjuvant therapy for stage II and III colon cancer: who benefits and by how much? J Clin Off J Am Soc Clin Oncol. 2004;22(10):1797–806. https://doi.org/10.1200/JCO.2004.09.059.
7. Glimelius B, Dahl O, Cedermark B, Jakobsen A, Bentzen SM, Starkhammar H, et al. Adjuvant chemotherapy in colorectal cancer: a joint analysis of randomised trials by the Nordic gastrointestinal tumour adjuvant therapy group. Acta Oncol. 2005;44(8):904–12. https://doi.org/10.1080/02841860500355900.
8. Moertel CG, Fleming TR, Macdonald JS, Haller DG, Laurie JA, Tangen CM, et al. Intergroup study of fluorouracil plus levamisole as adjuvant therapy for stage II/dukes' B2 colon cancer. J Clin Oncol Off J Am Soc Clin Oncol. 1995;13(12):2936–43.
9. Taal BG, Van Tinteren H, Zoetmulder FA. Group N. Adjuvant 5FU plus levamisole in colonic or rectal cancer: improved survival in stage II and III. Br J Cancer. 2001;85(10):1437–43. https://doi.org/10.1054/bjoc.2001.2117.
10. Yothers G, O'Connell MJ, Allegra CJ, Kuebler JP, Colangelo LH, Petrelli NJ, et al. Oxaliplatin as adjuvant therapy for colon cancer: updated results of NSABP C-07 trial, including survival and subset analyses. J Clin. Oncol Off J Am Soc Clin Oncol. 2011;29(28):3768–74. https://doi.org/10.1200/JCO.2011.36.4539.
11. André T, de Gramont A, Vernerey D, et al. Adjuvant fluorouracil, Leucovorin, and Oxaliplatin in stage II to III colon cancer: updated 10-year survival and outcomes according to BRAF mutation and mismatch repair status of the MOSAIC study. J Clin Oncol. 2015;33(35):4176–87. https://doi.org/10.1200/JCO.2015.63.4238.
12. Kumar A, Kennecke HF, Renouf DJ, Lim HJ, Gill S, Woods R, et al. Adjuvant chemotherapy use and outcomes of patients with high-risk versus low-risk stage II colon cancer. Cancer. 2015;121(4):527–34. https://doi.org/10.1002/cncr.29072.
13. O'Connor ES, Greenblatt DY, LoConte NK, Gangnon RE, Liou JI, Heise CP, et al. Adjuvant chemotherapy for stage II colon cancer with poor prognostic features. J Clin Oncol Off J Am Soc Clin Oncol. 2011;29(25):3381–8. https://doi.org/10.1200/JCO.2010.34.3426.
14. Casadaban L, Rauscher G, Aklilu M, Villenes D, Freels S, Maker AV. Adjuvant chemotherapy is associated with improved survival in patients with stage II colon cancer. Cancer. 2016;122(21):3277–87. https://doi.org/10.1002/cncr.30181.
15. NCCN Guidelines. Colon Cancer Version 3.2022. NCCN.org.
16. Babcock BD, Aljehani MA, Jabo B, et al. High-risk stage II colon cancer: not all risks are created equal. Ann Surg Oncol. 2018;25:1980–5. https://doi.org/10.1245/s10434-018-6484-8.
17. Sinicrope FA. DNA mismatch repair and adjuvant chemotherapy in sporadic colon cancer. Nat Rev Clin Oncol. 2010;7(3):174–7. https://doi.org/10.1038/nrclinonc.2009.235.
18. Gavin PG, Colangelo LH, Fumagalli D, Tanaka N, Remillard MY, Yothers G, et al. Mutation profiling and microsatellite instability in stage II and III colon cancer: an assessment of their prognostic and oxaliplatin predictive value. Clin Cancer Res Off J Am Assoc Cancer Res. 2012;18(23):6531–41. https://doi.org/10.1158/1078-0432.CCR-12-0605.
19. Hutchins G, Southward K, Handley K, Magill L, Beaumont C, Stahlschmidt J, et al. Value of mismatch repair, KRAS, and BRAF mutations in predicting recurrence and benefits from chemotherapy in colorectal cancer. J Clin. Oncol Off J Am Soc. 2011;29(10):1261–70. https://doi.org/10.1200/JCO.2010.30.1366.
20. Klingbiel D, Saridaki Z, Roth AD, Bosman FT, Delorenzi M, Tejpar S. Prognosis of stage II and III colon cancer treated with adjuvant 5-fluorouracil or FOLFIRI in relation to microsatellite status: results of the PETACC-3 trial. Ann Oncol Off J Eur Soc Med Oncol/ESMO. 2015;26(1):126–32. https://doi.org/10.1093/annonc/mdu499.
21. Sargent DJ, Marsoni S, Monges G, Thibodeau SN, Labianca R, Hamilton SR, et al. Defective mismatch repair as a predictive marker for lack of efficacy of fluorouracil-based adjuvant therapy in colon cancer. J Clin Oncol Off J Am Soc Clin Oncol. 2010;28(20):3219–26. https://doi.org/10.1200/JCO.2009.27.1825.

22. Gray RG, Quirke P, Handley K, Lopatin M, Magill L, Baehner FL, et al. Validation study of a quantitative multigene reverse transcriptase-polymerase chain reaction assay for assessment of recurrence risk in patients with stage II colon cancer. J Clin Oncol Off J Am Soc Clin Oncol. 2011;29(35):4611–9. https://doi.org/10.1200/JCO.2010.32.8732.
23. Le DT, Uram JN, Wang H, Bartlett BR, Kemberling H, Eyring AD, et al. PD-1 blockade in tumors with mismatch-repair deficiency. N Engl J Med. 2015;372(26):2509–20. https://doi.org/10.1056/NEJMoa1500596.
24. Sinicrope FA, Foster NR, Thibodeau SN, Marsoni S, Monges G, Labianca R, et al. DNA mismatch repair status and colon cancer recurrence and survival in clinical trials of 5-fluorouracil-based adjuvant therapy. J Natl Cancer Inst. 2011;103(11):863–75. https://doi.org/10.1093/jnci/djr153.
25. Roth AD, Tejpar S, Delorenzi M, Yan P, Fiocca R, Klingbiel D, et al. Prognostic role of KRAS and BRAF in stage II and III resected colon cancer: results of the translational study on the PETACC-3, EORTC 40993, SAKK 60-00 trial. J Clin Oncol Off J Am Soc Clin Oncol. 2010;28(3):466–74. https://doi.org/10.1200/JCO.2009.23.3452.
26. Watanabe T, Kobunai T, Yamamoto Y, Matsuda K, Ishihara S, Nozawa K, et al. Chromosomal instability (CIN) phenotype, CIN high or CIN low, predicts survival for colorectal cancer. J Clin Oncol Off J Am Soc Clin Oncol. 2012;30(18):2256–64. https://doi.org/10.1200/JCO.2011.38.6490.
27. Jover R, Zapater P, Castells A, Llor X, Andreu M, Cubiella J, et al. The efficacy of adjuvant chemotherapy with 5-fluorouracil in colorectal cancer depends on the mismatch repair status. Eur J Cancer. 2009;45(3):365–73. https://doi.org/10.1016/j.ejca.2008.07.016.
28. Kim GP, Colangelo LH, Wieand HS, Paik S, Kirsch IR, Wolmark N, et al. Prognostic and predictive roles of high-degree microsatellite instability in colon cancer: a National Cancer Institute-National Surgical Adjuvant Breast and bowel project Collaborative study. J Clin Oncol Off J Am Soc Clin Oncol. 2007;25(7):767–72. https://doi.org/10.1200/JCO.2006.05.8172.
29. Sun X, Huang T, Cheng F, Huang K, Liu M, He W, Li M, Zhang X, Xu M, Chen S, Xia L. Monitoring colorectal cancer following surgery using plasma circulating tumor DNA. Oncol Lett. 2018;15(4):4365–75.
30. Tie J, Cohen JD, Lahouel K, et al. Circulating tumor DNA analysis guiding adjuvant therapy in stage II colon cancer. N Engl J Med. 2022;386(24):2261–72. https://doi.org/10.1056/NEJMoa2200075.
31. Dasari A, Grothey A, Kopetz S. Circulating tumor DNA-defined minimal residual disease in solid tumors: opportunities to accelerate the development of adjuvant therapies [published online ahead of print, 2018 Oct 30]. J Clin Oncol. 2018;36(35):JCO2018789032. https://doi.org/10.1200/JCO.2018.78.9032.
32. Iveson TJ, Sobrero AF, Yoshino T, et al. Duration of Adjuvant Doublet Chemotherapy (3 or 6 months) in Patients With High-Risk Stage II Colorectal Cancer [published correction appears in J Clin Oncol. 2021 May 20;39(15):1691]. J Clin Oncol 2021;39(6):631–641. doi:https://doi.org/10.1200/JCO.20.01330.

18 Is There a Benefit in Cytoreduction and Hyperthermic Intraperitoneal Chemotherapy in Colorectal Cancer?

Arsha Ostowari and Oliver S. Eng

Introduction

Colorectal cancer (CRC) is the third most common type of cancer with 1.9 million new cases in 2020 and second in terms of cancer deaths with 935,000 deaths in 2020 [1]. The peritoneum is a common site of metastasis for CRC that is associated with poor prognosis. It is estimated that around 5% of patients with CRC are synchronously diagnosed with peritoneal carcinomatosis (PC) and a greater proportion ranging from 5–20% of CRC patients will develop metachronous PC later in their disease course [2–4]. Additionally, this is likely an under-estimation of PC incidence as tumor deposits are small (<1 cm) and difficult to be captured on imaging alone, requiring more invasive procedures such as laparoscopy to better evaluate the abdomen [2–5]. Autopsy studies that have looked at patients who died from CRC found PC in up to 40% of patients [6]. This raises the importance of appropriately managing and treating patients with metastatic CRC, which has evolved over the past few decades with changes in the systemic and surgical treatment options available. Currently, cytoreductive surgery (CRS) with or without hyperthermic intraperitoneal chemotherapy (HIPEC) is a potential modality for treatment of patients with PC [7]. In the 2000s, as is summarized in Table 18.1, studies showed that CRS/

A. Ostowari (✉)
Department of Surgery, University of California, Orange, CA, USA
e-mail: ostowari@hs.uci.edu

O. S. Eng (✉)
Division of Surgical Oncology, Department of Surgery, University of California, Orange, CA, USA
e-mail: oeng@uci.edu

K. Umanskiy, N. Hyman (eds.), *Difficult Decisions in Colorectal Surgery*, Difficult Decisions in Surgery: An Evidence-Based Approach,
https://doi.org/10.1007/978-3-031-42303-1_18

Table 18.1 Summary of CRS/HIPEC studies

Study	Participants (Treatment vs. Control)	Study design	Outcome	Quality of evidence
Verwaal et al. (2003)	54 vs. 51	CRS/HIPEC vs SCT	Median OS: 22.3 vs 12.6 m Median OS (complete reduction): 48 m 45% alive at 5 years	Moderate
Verwaal et al. (2008)	54 vs. 51	CRS/HIPEC vs SCT	Median PFS: 12.6 vs 7.7 m Median disease-specific survival: 22.2 vs 12.6 m	Moderate
Glehen et al. (2004)	506	CRS/HIPEC	1y, 3y, 5y OS: 72%, 39%, 19% 1y, 3y, 5y DFS: 40%, 16%, 10% Median OS: 19.2 m Median OS: CCR-0 (32.4 m), CCR-1 (24 m), CCR-2 (8.4 m)	Moderate
Franko et al. (2010)	67 vs. 38	CRS/HIPEC vs SCT	Median OS: 34.7 vs 16.8 m	Moderate
Goéré et al. (2013)	107	CRS/IPC	OS: 5 year (35%), 10 year (15%) 16% cure rate PCI (cure vs noncured): 4 vs 12	Moderate
Esquivel et al. ASPSM (PSDSS) (2014)	1013	CRS/HIPEC vs SCT	Median OS: 41 vs 10 m 3y OS: 66% vs 25% 5y OS: 58% vs 19% Median OS (PSDSS I/II/III/IV): 86 vs 49 m, 43 vs 19 m, 29 vs 8 m, 28 vs 6 m Median OS (CC-0/CC≥1): 51 vs 28 m	Moderate
Prada-Villaverde et al. ASPSM (2014)	539	CRS/HIPEC (Oxaliplatin) vs CRS/HIPEC (Mitomycin)	Median OS: 32.6 m Median OS (PSDSS I/II): 28.2 vs 54.3 m No OS difference between mitomycin and oxaliplatin	Moderate

(continued)

Table 18.1 (continued)

Study	Participants (Treatment vs. Control)	Study design	Outcome	Quality of evidence
Cashin et al. (2016)	24 vs. 24	CRS/IPC vs SCT	OS (2 years): 54% vs 38% Median OS: 25 vs 18 m Survival at 5 years: 33% vs 4%	Low
Klaver et al. COLOPEC (2019)	100 vs. 102	Adjuvant HIPEC + SCT vs SCT	Peritoneal-free survival (18 m): 80.9% vs 76.2% DFS (18 m): 69% vs 69.3% OS (18 m): 93% vs 94.1% Time to diagnosis of PM: 9 vs 14 m	High
Goéré et al. PROPHYLOCHIP (2020)	75 vs. 71	2nd-look CRS/HIPEC vs surveillance	3y DFS: 44% vs 53% 3y peritoneal recurrence free survival: 59% vs 61% 3y OS: 79% vs 80% 5y OS: 68% vs 72% 41% in second-look group had grade 3–4 complications	High
Quénet et al. PRODIGE 7 (2021)	133 vs 132	CRS/HIPEC vs CRS	No difference in OS or RFS At 30 days, no difference in frequency of grade 3 or worse adverse events Between 30–60 days, higher rate of grade 3 or worse adverse events in CRS/HIPEC group Subset with PCI 11–15, improved OS and RFS in CRS/HIPEC	High

HIPEC provide CRC patients with a significant mortality benefit when compared to standard chemotherapy (SCT) in the setting of PC [8]. Since then, CRS/HIPEC has been studied extensively in order to optimize the treatment modality and to determine if and who would benefit most from CRS/HIPEC (Table 18.1).

Search Strategy

A literature review was performed using the MEDLINE/PubMed database to identify relevant studies after the year 2000 using the following terms: "colorectal cancer", "peritoneal carcinomatosis", "cytoreductive surgery", "Intraperitoneal chemotherapy", "Adjuvant chemotherapy", "HIPEC", "Novel therapies".

P (Patients)	I (Intervention)	C (Comparator)	O (Outcomes)
Patients with colorectal cancer and peritoneal carcinomatosis	CRS/HIPEC	Systemic therapy, CRS alone	Overall Survival (OS), Progression free survival (PFS), Disease free survival (DFS)

Results

In the 2000s, a sentinel study was carried out by Verwaal et al. that evaluated the efficacy of CRS/HIPEC versus SCT in patients with PC from CRC. 105 patients were enrolled in this study with 54 randomized to the CRS/HIPEC (Mitomycin C) arm and 51 to the control arm consisting of SCT (Fluorouracil, Leucovorin) with or without palliative surgery. At a median follow-up of 21.6 months, the CRS/HIPEC arm exhibited a longer median survival of 22.3 months compared to 12.6 months ($p = 0.032$) in the control arm [8]. Subgroup analyses of patients that underwent CRS/HIPEC showed that those with disease in 6–7 regions of the abdomen had poorer median survival compared to those patients with disease involvement of zero to five regions (5.4 months vs >29 months, $p < .0001$) [8]. Additionally, only 1/18 patients who underwent a complete resection died versus 14/21 with limited residual disease and 7/10 with extensive residual disease ($p < .0001$) [8]. Overall, those whom underwent complete cytoreduction had a median OS of 48 months with a 5-year survival of 45% [9]. The subgroup analyses within the experimental arm brought up two important concepts regarding CRS/HIPEC with improved survival in those with lower burden of disease, reported as the peritoneal carcinomatosis index (PCI), and the importance in achieving a complete cytoreduction. These results were additionally demonstrated in an 8-year follow up of the initial study by Verwaal et al. This study illustrated a durable survival benefit when comparing CRS/HIPEC to SCT in the treatment of CRC patients with PC. This follow-up study showed an increased median progression-free survival in CRS/HIPEC of 12.6 months vs 7.7 months and an improved median disease-specific survival of 22.2 months vs 12.6 months [9]. Two limitations in this study were related to the systemic chemotherapy and patient population, which can impact its generalizability to present day treatment of CRC patients. 5-FU/Leucovorin was used as the SCT, which is not the optimal first-line therapy today and 17% of the patient cohort had a diagnosis of primary appendiceal malignancies [8]. Appendiceal cancer is a distinct malignancy from CRC with heterogeneous long-term oncologic outcomes that therefore may have affected the results of the study.

In subsequent follow-up studies, Glehen et al. carried out a large retrospective multicenter study that further evaluated the efficiency of CRS/HIPEC and additional prognostic indicators. This study included 506 patients from 28 institutions between May 1987 and December 2002 that underwent CRS and perioperative intraperitoneal chemotherapy. The overall morbidity and mortality rate in the patient cohort was 22.9% and 4% with a median OS of 19.2 months [10]. When the patient cohort was sub-divided based on the completeness of cytoreduction, a significantly improved survival benefit was seen. Patients that underwent a complete cytoreduction (CCR-0) had a median OS of 32.4 months versus 24 months in CCR-1 patients and 8.4 months ($p < 0.001$) in those with an incomplete cytoreduction (CCR-2) [10]. Multivariate analysis showed that positive independent prognostic indicators included complete cytoreduction, treatment with a second procedure, limited PC, age < 65 and use of adjuvant therapy, while negative prognostic indicators were the use of neoadjuvant chemotherapy, lymph node involvement, presence of liver metastasis and poor histologic differentiation. The completeness of cytoreduction was the principal independent prognostic indicator ($p < 0.0001$) [10]. When subgroup analysis was performed based on the extent of PC, the OS of those with limited PC (PCI < 13 and stage I and II from the Gilly's classification) was higher than extended PC (PCI ≥ 13 and stage III and IV from the Gilly's classification) with 1-year, 3-year and 5-year OS of 92%, 50%, and 33% versus 62%, 22%, and 11%, respectively ($p < 0.0001$) [10]. These findings reaffirmed some of the existing concepts introduced in the previous study regarding the prognostic benefit of lower PC burden and improved survival with complete cytoreduction. In addition, this study addressed a limitation of the previous study by excluding all malignancies of appendiceal origin. However, in addition to the retrospective nature this study, authors acknowledged treatment variability, for example, in HIPEC technique regarding exposure, drugs, drug doses, duration, temperature, type of perfusate and flow rates [10]. Following this, a study carried out by Goéré et al. evaluated the long-term outcomes of CRS and intraperitoneal chemotherapy (IPC). This study looked at 107 patients from 1995 to 2006 who underwent complete CRS followed by IPC [11]. At a median follow up of 77 months, the 5-year and 10-year OS was 35% and 15% and 16% of patients ($n = 17$) were considered cured, defined as having a disease-free interval of at least 5 years. Comparing patients that were considered cured to the rest of the cohort, a significantly lower PCI was noted (4 vs 12, $p = .0002$). Additionally, after multivariate analysis, a PCI ≤ 10 was the only independent factor predictive of a cure in the patient population [11].

Franko et al. performed a single-institution retrospective case study that compared patients undergoing CRS/HIPEC versus modern SCT alone. 105 patients were included from 2001 to 2007 with 67 patients in the CRS/HIPEC (Mitomycin) arm and 38 patients in the SCT alone group. Median OS favored the CRS/HIPEC group at 34.7 months compared to 16.8 months in the SCT alone group ($p < 0.001$) [12]. In addition, this study found that the presence of a liver metastasis was a significant negative predictor of survival with a HR of 2.13 [12]. Following this, Cashin et al. designed a prospective, randomized control trial that compared patients undergoing CRS/IPC versus patients undergoing SCT alone. Unfortunately, this study closed after 7 years due to poor patient accrual with only 48 patients enrolled (24/arm) [13]. Median OS favored the CRS/IPC arm at 25 months versus 18 months in the SCT only arm (p = .04) with a 2-year OS of 54% in the experimental arm versus 38% in the SCT arm (p = .04). There was no significant difference in PFS, but at 5 years 33% of the experimental arm versus 4% of the control arm were still alive (p = .02) [13]. Therefore, these studies demonstrated some survival benefit to the implementation of CRS with IPC over SCT alone.

The American Society of Peritoneal Surface Malignancies Multi-Institution (ASPSM) sought to improve patient selection by identifying who would likely benefit most from CRS/HIPEC by establishing the Peritoneal Surface Disease Severity Score (PSDSS). This score was based off of three criteria prior to surgery, which included the patient's symptoms, PCI score, and primary tumor histological grade [14]. A retrospective review of 1013 CRC patients with PC between 1985 and 2012 was performed, comparing survival data from patients who underwent CRS/HIPEC versus SCT alone. 884 patients had PSDSS scores calculated for, of which 609 patients underwent CRS/HIPEC and 275 patients underwent systemic treatment alone [14]. Overall median survival favored the CRS/HIPEC group at 41 months versus 10 months (p < 0.001) and 3-year/5-year survival also favored the CRS/HIPEC group at 66%/58% versus 25%/19%. After multivariate analysis, two factors identified as independent prognostic factors for survival were the PSDSS and CC score (P < 0.001) [14]. The median survival of patients who underwent CRS/HIPEC based on their PSDSS (I, II, III, IV) was 86, 43, 29, and 28 months, respectively versus 45, 19, 8, and 6 months in patients with systemic therapy alone (P < 0.001). Subgroup analysis of patients that underwent CRS/HIPEC showed improved median survival in patients undergoing complete cytoreduction (CC-0) versus an incomplete cytoreduction (51 vs 28 months, p < 0.001) [14]. This confirmed the importance of achieving a complete cytoreduction during CRS for patient survival and provided data on the use of the PSDSS as a tool to define CRC patients with PC with the highest likelihood of long-term survival after undergoing CRS/HIPEC. Following this, the ASPSM looked further into survival differences based on the type of HIPEC performed while stratifying patients based on PSDSS. 539 patients were included in this study and underwent complete CRS and HIPEC with either oxaliplatin or mitomycin C. Median OS was not significantly different between the two types of utilized chemoperfusion agents [15]. However, when patients were stratified by their PSDSS, there was a significant difference in median OS in patients with a PSDSS of I or II that favored mitomycin C (54.3 vs 28.2 months, p = 0.012). On the other hand, patients with a PSDSS of III or IV showed no significant difference in median OS between the two agents [15]. This demonstrated that mitomycin C might be more effective than oxaliplatin in the treatment of patients with better tumor histology and lower disease burden.

More recently, several studies have been carried out that have looked at the effectiveness of HIPEC in CRC patients with PC or at high risk of developing PC. The COLOPEC study was a multicenter, open-label, randomized control trial that looked at the efficacy of adjuvant HIPEC in patients with locally advanced colon cancer amongst 9 HIPEC specialty hospitals in the Netherlands [16]. Between April

1, 2015 and February 20, 2017, 204 patients were enrolled in a 1:1 fashion to adjuvant HIPEC followed by routine SCT (n = 100, 2 patients dropped out) versus SCT alone (n = 102). Patients with primary clinical or pathological stage T4N0-2 M0 or perforated colon cancer were included, while those with metastatic disease were excluded. Adjuvant HIPEC consisted of a combination of IV fluorouracil and leucovorin with intraperitoneal oxaliplatin delivered either simultaneously at the time of resection or 5–8 weeks after resection [16]. All patients received 6 months of adjuvant SCT consisting of capecitabine and oxaliplatin or fluorouracil and oxaliplatin ideally started within 6–8 weeks of resection, but no later than 12 weeks. After 18 months, every patient without radiographic evidence of recurrence underwent a diagnostic laparoscopy [16]. At 18 months, there was no significant difference seen between the groups in terms of peritoneal metastasis-free survival, overall survival, and disease-free survival. 14% (n = 12) of patients in the adjuvant HIPEC group developed postoperative complications and 1% (n = 1) developed a long-term morbidity (encapsulating peritoneal sclerosis) requiring a surgical intervention [16]. The median time to diagnosis of peritoneal metastasis was 9 months in the experimental group versus 14 months in the control group (p = .059). Of those with peritoneal metastases, 68% (13/19) of patients in the experimental group underwent CRS/HIPEC and 65% (15/23) in the control group. Overall, there was a 21% peritoneal recurrence amongst all patients in this study [16]. This study showed no benefit in peritoneal metastasis-free survival, overall survival, or disease-free survival at 18 months in patients undergoing adjuvant HIPEC after resection even though we did see a trend of earlier diagnosis of peritoneal metastasis. Some of the limitations of this study included later administration of adjuvant chemotherapy in the experimental group versus the control group though this still occurred within 12 weeks. Furthermore, 37% (n = 74) of patients did not agree to undergo diagnostic laparoscopy at 18 months, possibly due to the invasiveness of undergoing a second procedure [16].

After the COLOPEC trial, the PROPHYLOCHIP study evaluated survival benefits in undergoing a second-look surgery and HIPEC versus standard surveillance in CRC patients with high risk of developing PC. This was an open-label, phase 3 study among 23 hospitals in France. 150 patients were enrolled from June 11, 2010 to March 31, 2015 in a 1:1 fashion to a second-look surgery and HIPEC group (n = 75) versus a standard surveillance group (n = 75) [17]. Patients included in this study had CRC with either synchronous/localized PC removed during the operation, resection of ovarian metastasis or a perforated tumor and underwent 6 months of adjuvant chemotherapy following resection without evidence of tumor recurrence, while patients with cancer other than CRC, and detectable recurrence or metastasis other than to the peritoneum or ovaries were excluded from the study [17]. Chemoperfusion agents consisted of oxaliplatin, oxaliplatin/irinotecan or mitomycin C. Every patient in this study received adjuvant SCT and those in the experimental group without signs of disease recurrence underwent second-look surgery/HIPEC 6 months afterwards [17]. At a median follow up of 50.8 months, 47% (n = 35) of patients in the experimental group and 48% (n = 36) in the control group experienced recurrence. There was no significant difference seen in 3-year disease-free survival or peritoneal recurrence-free survival between the two groups [17]. In addition, there were no treatment related deaths reported, but 41% (n = 29) of patients in the experimental group had grade 3–4 complications most commonly being an intra-abdominal event such as hemorrhage or GI leak followed by a hematologic adverse event. 3-year OS was 79% in the experimental group and 80% in the control group, while 5-year OS was 68% in the experimental group and 72% in the control group [17]. Similar to the COLOPEC trial, this study showed that a second-look surgery and HIPEC does not improve disease-free or overall survival compared to standard surveillance. However, this study brought up the importance of identifying CRC patients with high risk of developing PC to potentially diagnose and treat them at an earlier stage [17].

The HIPECT4 study is a multicenter, randomized control trial among 15 Spanish HIPEC specialty centers that looked at the effectiveness and safety of adjuvant HIPEC in preventing PC development in CRC patients with high risk of PC recurrence. Between November 2015 and January 2021, 184 patients with locally advanced colon cancer were enrolled and randomly assigned to an adjuvant HIPEC group followed by SCT (n = 89) versus SCT alone (n = 95) [18]. Adjuvant HIPEC consisted of mitomycin and was performed simultaneously with tumor resection. At a median follow-up of 36 months, there was no difference seen in DFS, OS, or morbidity between the two groups, but loco-regional control was improved in the experimental arm (35.3 versus 33.2 months) with a 3-year loco-regional rate of 97% versus 87% (p = 0.025). Additionally, subgroup analysis showed a clear benefit in loco-regional control in the adjuvant HIPEC arm among patients with T4 disease [18]. This study showed that while the addition of mitomycin HIPEC to surgical resection did not lead to improved DFS and OS in patients with locally advanced colon cancer, it does improve loco-regional control rate especially in patients with T4 colon cancer.

More recently, the PRODIGE 7 trial has brought into question whether the addition of HIPEC to CRS adds survival benefit compared to CRS alone. This was a phase 3, randomized control trial across 17 centers in France. Between February 11, 2008 and January 6, 2014, 265 patients were enrolled and randomized into the CRS/HIPEC arm (n = 133) and CRS only arm (n = 132) [19]. The HIPEC component included intravenous 5-FU/Leucovorin with 30 minutes of intraperitoneal oxaliplatin, and all patients either received neoadjuvant and/or adjuvant systemic chemotherapy. After a median follow-up period of 63.8 months, no significant difference was seen in median OS and RFS between the two groups. However, a post-hoc subgroup analysis of patients with a PCI of 11–15 did show a significant improvement in OS and RFS in the CRS/HIPEC arm versus CRS alone [19]. When looking at the frequency of grade 3 or worse adverse events, there was no significant difference at 30 days, but between 30 and 60 days there was a higher rate in the CRS/HIPEC group versus CRS alone group at 26% versus 15% [19]. This study showed that there was no survival benefit with the addition of HIPEC to CRS aside from possibly a small subset of patients with a PCI of 11–15 [19].

As more data emerges on the efficacy and survival benefits of CRS and HIPEC in the management of CRC patients with PC or high risk of developing PC, we continue to optimize this treatment modality for our patients. Factors associated with survival along with patient selection criteria have been described and give us insight on which population of patients might benefit the most from CRS and HIPEC. The Chicago Consensus Working Group currently provides us with multidisciplinary recommendations incorporating all of those factors on the management of CRC with both synchronous and metachronous peritoneal metastasis. [20] Novel approaches are always being studied, which include modified/improved techniques of administering intraperitoneal or system chemotherapy, immunotherapy, monoclonal antibodies, and others [4]. As the treatment paradigm to CRC with PM continues to evolve over time, the management of these patients should always be a multidisciplinary collaboration to provide patients with the best treatments available to them.

Expert Opinion

Based on the data presented, we would strongly recommend the practice of CRS alone in patients with CRC and PC in the context of multidisciplinary evaluation at an expert center. We would provide a moderate to strong recommendation for the practice of CRS/HIPEC in CRC patients with PC under certain clinical scenarios (PSDSSI/II with mitomycin C and PCI 11–15 with Oxaliplatin) in the context of multidisciplinary evaluation at an expert center. Based on the results of recent studies, we would not recommend the prophylactic or adjuvant use of HIPEC at this time for patients with CRC and high risk of PC.

Personal View

Colorectal cancer with peritoneal carcinomatosis was at one time a diagnosis without surgical treatment options and consisted of systemic palliative chemotherapy as the mainstay in management. Over time, the management of CRC with PC has evolved with now established cytoreductive surgery techniques along with intraperitoneal chemotherapy, to supplement the practice of systemic chemotherapy. As described above, various studies have shown survival benefits with the use of CRS and HIPEC in the management of CRC patients with PC resulting in this becoming an increasingly accepted treatment modality in this patient population. However, many questions remain, including whether certain HIPEC regimens add survival benefit versus CRS alone and their use as an adjuvant/prophylactic option in patients with high risk to develop PC. Yet given the vast heterogeneity of disease processes and clinical practice patterns, some open questions may remain as such, thus emphasizing the importance of coordinated multidisciplinary decision-making. What appears most apparent though is that survival is consistently related to achieving a complete cytoreduction and having a lower burden of disease. Our ability to intervene during times of lower disease burdens may perhaps be better informed by improvement in detection and surveillance in the future. In addition, the ever-evolving landscape of novel therapeutics likewise provides the prospect of future treatments such as targeted therapies and/or enhanced drug delivery systems which may be utilized in these patients. While CRC with PC is undoubtedly a challenging disease process, the increasing momentum in improving outcomes is apparent and has been a long time coming.

Abstract Recommendations

- Patients with CRC and PC should undergo CRS alone after multidisciplinary evaluation at an expert center (evidence quality moderate to high; strong recommendation)
- Patients with CRC and PC under certain clinical scenarios (PSDSSI/II with mitomycin C and PCI 11–15 with Oxaliplatin) should undergo CRS/HIPEC after multidisciplinary evaluation at an expert center (evidence quality moderate to high; moderate to strong recommendation)
- Patients with CRC and high risk of PC should not undergo prophylactic or adjuvant HIPEC (evidence quality moderate to high; strong recommendation)

References

1. Sung H, Ferlay J, Siegel RL, et al. Global Cancer Statistics 2020: GLOBOCAN estimates of incidence and mortality worldwide for 36 cancers in 185 countries. CA Cancer J Clin. 2021;71(3):209–49. https://doi.org/10.3322/caac.21660.
2. Klaver YLB, Lemmens VEPP, Nienhuijs SW, Luyer MDP, de Hingh IHJT. Peritoneal carcinomatosis of colorectal origin: Incidence, prognosis and treatment options. World J Gastroenterol: WJG. 2012;18(39):5489–94. https://doi.org/10.3748/wjg.v18.i39.5489.
3. Lenos KJ, Bach S, Ferreira Moreno L, et al. Molecular characterization of colorectal cancer related peritoneal metastatic disease. Nat Commun. 2022;13(1):4443. https://doi.org/10.1038/s41467-022-32198-z.
4. Vierra MA, Morgan RB, Eng OS. Advances in therapeutics for peritoneal metastases from colorectal cancer: a narrative review. Dig Med Res. 2022;5(0) https://doi.org/10.21037/dmr-21-88.
5. Behrenbruch C, Hollande F, Thomson B, et al. Treatment of peritoneal carcinomatosis with hyperthermic intraperitoneal chemotherapy in colorectal cancer. ANZ J Surg. 2017;87(9):665–70. https://doi.org/10.1111/ans.14077.
6. Koppe MJ, Boerman OC, Oyen WJG, Bleichrodt RP. Peritoneal Carcinomatosis of Colorectal Origin. Ann Surg. 2006;243(2):212–22. https://doi.org/10.1097/01.sla.0000197702.46394.16.
7. Bakkers C, Simkens GAAM, De Hingh IHJT. Systemic therapy in addition to cytoreduction and hyperthermic intraperitoneal chemotherapy for colorectal peritoneal metastases: recent insights from clinical studies and translational research. J Gastrointest Oncol. 2021;12(Suppl 1):S206–13. https://doi.org/10.21037/jgo-20-133.
8. Verwaal VJ, van Ruth S, de Bree E, et al. Randomized trial of cytoreduction and hyperthermic intraperitoneal chemotherapy versus systemic chemotherapy and palliative surgery in patients with peritoneal carcinomatosis of colorectal cancer. J Clin Oncol Off J Am Soc Clin Oncol. 2003;21(20):3737–43. https://doi.org/10.1200/JCO.2003.04.187.

9. Verwaal VJ, Bruin S, Boot H, van Slooten G, van Tinteren H. 8-year follow-up of randomized trial: cytoreduction and hyperthermic intraperitoneal chemotherapy versus systemic chemotherapy in patients with peritoneal carcinomatosis of colorectal cancer. Ann Surg Oncol. 2008;15(9):2426–32. https://doi.org/10.1245/s10434-008-9966-2.
10. Glehen O, Kwiatkowski F, Sugarbaker PH, et al. Cytoreductive surgery combined with perioperative intraperitoneal chemotherapy for the management of peritoneal carcinomatosis from colorectal cancer: a multi-institutional study. J Clin Oncol Off J Am Soc Clin Oncol. 2004;22(16):3284–92. https://doi.org/10.1200/JCO.2004.10.012.
11. Goéré D, Malka D, Tzanis D, et al. Is there a possibility of a cure in patients with colorectal peritoneal carcinomatosis amenable to complete cytoreductive surgery and intraperitoneal chemotherapy? Ann Surg. 2013;257(6):1065–71. https://doi.org/10.1097/SLA.0b013e31827e9289.
12. Franko J, Ibrahim Z, Gusani NJ, Holtzman MP, Bartlett DL, Zeh Iii HJ. Cytoreductive surgery and hyperthermic intraperitoneal chemoperfusion versus systemic chemotherapy alone for colorectal peritoneal carcinomatosis. Cancer. 2010;116(16):3756–62. https://doi.org/10.1002/cncr.25116.
13. Cashin PH, Mahteme H, Spång N, et al. Cytoreductive surgery and intraperitoneal chemotherapy versus systemic chemotherapy for colorectal peritoneal metastases: A randomised trial. Eur J Cancer (Oxford, England: 1990). 2016;53:155–62. https://doi.org/10.1016/j.ejca.2015.09.017.
14. Esquivel J, Lowy AM, Markman M, et al. The American Society of Peritoneal Surface Malignancies (ASPSM) Multiinstitution Evaluation of the Peritoneal Surface Disease Severity Score (PSDSS) in 1,013 Patients with colorectal cancer with peritoneal carcinomatosis. Ann Surg Oncol. 2014;21(13):4195–201. https://doi.org/10.1245/s10434-014-3798-z.
15. Prada-Villaverde A, Esquivel J, Lowy AM, et al. The American Society of Peritoneal Surface Malignancies evaluation of HIPEC with Mitomycin C versus Oxaliplatin in 539 patients with colon cancer undergoing a complete cytoreductive surgery. J Surg Oncol. 2014;110(7):779–85. https://doi.org/10.1002/jso.23728.
16. Klaver CEL, Wisselink DD, Punt CJA, et al. Adjuvant hyperthermic intraperitoneal chemotherapy in patients with locally advanced colon cancer (COLOPEC): a multicentre, open-label, randomised trial. Lancet Gastroenterol Hepatol. 2019;4(10):761–70. https://doi.org/10.1016/S2468-1253(19)30239-0.
17. Goéré D, Glehen O, Quenet F, et al. Second-look surgery plus hyperthermic intraperitoneal chemotherapy versus surveillance in patients at high risk of developing colorectal peritoneal metastases (PROPHYLOCHIP-PRODIGE 15): a randomised, phase 3 study. Lancet Oncol. 2020;21(9):1147–54. https://doi.org/10.1016/S1470-2045(20)30322-3.
18. Arjona-Sánchez A, Barrios P, Boldo-Roda E, et al. HIPECT4: multicentre, randomized clinical trial to evaluate safety and efficacy of Hyperthermic intra-peritoneal chemotherapy (HIPEC) with Mitomycin C used during surgery for treatment of locally advanced colorectal carcinoma. BMC Cancer. 2018;18:183. https://doi.org/10.1186/s12885-018-4096-0.
19. Quénet F, Elias D, Roca L, et al. Cytoreductive surgery plus hyperthermic intraperitoneal chemotherapy versus cytoreductive surgery alone for colorectal peritoneal metastases (PRODIGE 7): a multicentre, randomised, open-label, phase 3 trial. Lancet Oncol. 2021;22(2):256–66. https://doi.org/10.1016/S1470-2045(20)30599-4.
20. Group CCW. The Chicago Consensus on peritoneal surface malignancies: management of colorectal metastases. Cancer. 2020;126(11):2534–40. https://doi.org/10.1002/cncr.32874.

Colorectal Cancer Management in Older Adults: Use of Geriatric Assessment to Guide Patient-Centered Care

19

Jeffrey L. Roberson and Nicole M. Saur

Introduction

Age and/or physician-perceived frailty have historically been inappropriately used as relative contraindications to abdominal surgery in geriatric patients. Specific to colorectal cancer, 56% of new diagnoses in the United States occur in patients over 65 years of age [1]. Currently, a 75-year-old American man in good health has a life expectancy of 18 years with his 82-year-old counterpart has a 10-year life expectancy. However, the presence of any severe comorbidity decreases their expectancies to 6 and 2 years respectively [2, 3]. While the definition and cutoff age for geriatrics remains debated, it is generally agreed upon that patients should not be treated solely on chronological age [4]. Despite this, however, many elderly colorectal cancer patients are either undertreated based on age or over-treated despite their frailty [5, 6]. Therefore, the approach to elderly patients with colorectal cancer should include comprehensive evaluation for and optimization of frailty with a focus on patient-centered outcomes.
PICO Table

Formatted for: Difficult Decisions in Colorectal Surgery

J. L. Roberson
Department of Surgery, Hospital of the University of Pennsylvania, Philadelphia, PA, USA
e-mail: jeffrey.roberson@pennmedicine.upenn.edu

N. M. Saur (✉)
Division of Colon and Rectal Surgery, Department of Surgery, Hospital of the University of Pennsylvania, Philadelphia, PA, USA
e-mail: Nicole.Saur@uphs.upenn.edu

K. Umanskiy, N. Hyman (eds.), *Difficult Decisions in Colorectal Surgery*, Difficult Decisions in Surgery: An Evidence-Based Approach,
https://doi.org/10.1007/978-3-031-42303-1_19

Patient	Intervention	Comparator	Outcome
Elderly patients with colorectal cancer	Prehabilitation or geriatric assessment prior to surgical or chemotherapeutic intervention	Patients without prehabilitation or assessment	Perioperative and/or chemotherapeutic outcomes

Search Strategy

Comprehensive literature searches of the Cochrane Database, EMBASE, MEDLINE, and PubMed was performed to identify all of the English-language publications related to geriatric colorectal cancer patients with or without geriatric assessments and prehabilitation and their subsequent perioperative/chemotherapeutic outcomes from 1985 to 2022. Key search terms included "geriatric," "colorectal cancer," "prehabilitation," "perioperative," "perioperative outcomes," "outcomes," and "elderly." Studies were excluded if they did not focus on geriatric patients with colorectal cancer and/or discuss prehabilitation or if the full texts were not available in English. Only the most recent study was included if similar studies from the same institution were encountered. All references of the included studies were subsequently reviewed to identify any additional studies that were appropriate for inclusion.

Results

Of the 145 potential studies, seven independent studies were identified for inclusion. To date, a variety of methods have been utilized to attempt to quantify frailty and influence perioperative management in colorectal cancer. Of the seven studies, three utilized scoring systems, three performed comprehensive geriatric assessments (CGA), and one was intervention-based with respect to patients' frailty assessments.

A variety of scoring systems were utilized to investigate patients' frailty. Li et al. [8] performed a subgroup analysis of patients enrolled in a multicenter study for gastrointestinal malignancy prior to chemotherapy initiation. They utilized serial measures of the Cooperative Oncology Group score, Barthel's ADL scale, Lawton's IADL scale, the G-8 questionnaire, and the QLQ-C30 questionnaire. Of the 20 analyzed patients, most were receiving palliative chemotherapy. Patients with unstable ADL and IADL scores had significantly shorter overall survival (OS) than those without changes in their scores. However, there was no difference in progression-free survival. IADL instability was also correlated with QoL deterioration. Bessems et al. [11], however, was a retrospective study comparing G8 and 4MGST scores with postoperative complications. Of the 132 patients screened for frailty, a higher complication rate was seen in patients with G8 less than or equal to 14 and/or 4MGST under 1 m/s. Pneumonia and cardiac complications were most prevalent among these patients. Souwer et al. [10] utilized a geriatric sumscore comprised of undernutrition, physical impairment, risk for delirium, and fall risk to retrospectively investigate an association between score and perioperative morbidity of 555 patients undergoing elective CRC surgery. One point was awarded per criteria with intermediate being

1–2 and high being 3–4. Ultimately, intermediate and high scores were associated with lower OS and presence of a postoperative complication.

A comprehensive geriatric assessment (CGA) was performed in three of the studies. The aim of CGA is to assess comorbidity, polypharmacy, functional status, geriatric syndromes, mood, cognition, and social support. CGA typically classifies patients into three groups: fit, medium-fit, or unfit. Antonio et al. [7] prospectively enrolled 195 patients with stage II and stage III colorectal cancer. 43% were deemed fit, 29% medium-fit, and 28% unfit with 5-year survival rates of 74%, 52%, and 27% respectively. Fit and medium-fit patients were more likely to die due to cancer progression, and unfit patients were at a significantly greater risk of a non-cancer related cause of death. Decoster et al. [9] performed CGA in 193 patients with colorectal cancer, identifying at least one abnormality or area for improvement in 75%. Treatment was modified in 37% of patients based on this assessment. Baseline IADL, depression, fatigue, and cognition were all predictors for ADL decline. Verweij et al. [11] analyzed 168 geriatric consultations for patients with colorectal cancer. 93% of these patients were found to have some sort of geriatric impairment with the main recommendation for improvement being addressing nutritional status. In regards to oncologic treatment, the geriatrician ultimately recommended the "more intensive treatment" in 69% and "less intensive" in 31%, 63% of whom were recommended for "supportive care" alone.

Finally, the GERICO study [13] is a randomized phase 3 trial of 142 patients receiving adjuvant or first-line palliative chemotherapy for colorectal cancer. Prior to study initiation, a G8 questionnaire was performed with vulnerability being defined as a score less than or equal to 14. These patients were subsequently randomized to CGA-based interventions or standard care, along with guideline based chemotherapy. Of the enrolled patients, 58% were receiving adjuvant therapy and 42% first-line palliative chemotherapy. In the intervention group, 62% of patients had medication changes, 51% received nutritional therapy, and 39% engaged in physical therapy. There was no difference in severe treatment toxicity; however, significantly more interventional patients completed their full chemotherapy (45% vs. 28%, $p = 0.0366$) than the standard care patients. Additionally, the interventional patients had significantly improved QoL compared to standard care patients, most notably with decreased burden of illness ($p = 0.048$ and improved mobility ($p = 0.008$).

Recommendations

Depending upon the clinical encounter and the resources available, frailty can be assessed in a variety of ways in older adults with colorectal cancer. In regions without readily accessible geriatric consultation, the G8 and 4MGST scales can provide important insight about expected perioperative and/or chemotherapeutic morbidity. However, if the resource is available, a CGA referral to a geriatric specialist should be pursued as it provides much more information about a patients' overall functional status and can influence treatment plans, ultimately enhancing outcomes of older adults with colorectal cancer (strong recommendation, moderate evidence).

Study	Study design	Patients	Measure	Results	Conclusion	Quality of evidence
Antonio [7]	Prospective cohort	195 patients over age 74 with high-risk stage II and III CRC	Comprehensive geriatric Assessment (CGA)	–43% classified as fit; 74% 5-year survival –29% classified as medium-fit; 52% 5-year survival –27% as unfit; 27% 5-year survival –31% died due to cancer progression	CGA can predict survival and assist in the decision-making process of elderly CRC management.	Moderate
Li [8]	Subgroup analysis, prospective multicenter	20 patients over 74 years of age with gastrointestinal(GI) malignancy	-eastern cooperative oncology group score -Barthel's ADL scale -Lawton's IADL scale -G8 questionnaire -QLQ-C30 questionnaire	-Most patients received palliative chemotherapy -unstable ADL and IADL had shorter OS	-deterioration of functional status during chemotherapy negatively impacted overall survival and quality of life	Low
Decoster [9]	Prospective cohort	193 patients over age 69 with colorectal cancer	-geriatric assessment	–75% had an abnormal GA -unknown problems were discovered in 40% -GA led to intervention in 5% -baseline IADL, depression, fatigue, and cognition predict ADL decline	-GA identifies previously unknown problems but has limited impact on interventions and treatment decisions	Moderate

Souwer [10]	Retrospective	550 patients over age 70 undergoing elective colorectal cancer surgery	-geriatric risk factor assessment	-intermediate or high risk scores were associated with lower perioperative OS -sum scores were associated with postoperative complications	-geriatric sum score is associated with long-term outcome and perioperative morbidity data	Low
Bessems [11]	Retrospective	149 patients over 69 years of age undergoing elective colorectal cancer surgery	-G8 score -4MGST score	-higher complication rate with G8 under 15 and/or 4GMST less than 1 m/s	-frailty screening can identify patients at higher risk for postoperative complications	Low
Verweij [12]	Prospective cohort	168 patients over 59 years of age with colorectal cancer referred for geriatric consultation	-geriatric consultation	–93% had geriatric impairments –69% were referred for 'more intensive treatment option'	-geriatric consultation can alter the treatment plan in colorectal cancer	Moderate
Lund [13]	Randomized phase III trial	–142 patients receiving adjuvant or first-line palliative chemotherapy -patients with G8 score under 14 were randomized to CGA-based interventions or standard care	-CGA-based intervention	-Most common interventions included medication changes, nutritional therapy, and physiotherapy -more interventional patients completed chemotherapy than control -QoL and morbidity improved in interventional patients -burden of disease decreased in interventional patients	-geriatric interventions increase the number of older CRC patients completing adjuvant chemotherapy and can improve mobility and illness burden.	High

Personal View

The multidimensional CGA, typically performed by geriatricians, is the gold standard for assessing frailty and can provide important insight and treatment guidance in the perioperative setting in patients with colorectal cancer. However, as a limited resource, only a minority of surgeons are able to collaborate with geriatricians [14, 15]. Therefore, it is imperative that surgeons familiarized themselves with the components of a CGA and collaborate with geriatricians whenever possible. The main domains of a CGA, for surgeons' reference, are functional assessment, cognitive assessment, evaluation of comorbidities, and nutrition assessment.

At the crux of creating a treatment plan for an older adult with colorectal cancer, however, is aligning patient goals with possible outcomes. While maintaining independence and a desire to die at home are common health priorities among seniors, both medical and surgical interventions can result in complications requiring further invasive procedures, ICU admissions, or hasten an in-hospital death [16]. Therefore, in the elective, outpatient setting, the provider should elicit a patient's goals of care and identify factors that influence their quality of life through the process of shared decision making [17]. A variety of communication aids have been developed for elective surgery that help with information exchange and mutual decision making. Specifically, one question prompt list (QPL) encourages discussions to cover three main areas: (1) Should I have surgery? (2) What should I expect if everything goals well? And (3) What happens if things go wrong? [18] These types of questions change the focus of the office visits from specific technical details to instead patient goals and possible outcomes and, combined with the overall clinical assessment, can help guide towards treatment for oncologic cure versus palliation.

To assist surgeons in this endeavor, the American College of Surgeons (ACS) Geriatric Surgery Task Force has launched the Geriatric Surgery Verification Program. The goal of this program is to support all hospitals, regardless of size and/or resources, in caring for older adults with surgical diagnoses. The ACS has identified four phases of care of special importance, acknowledging that the ultimate goal is to preserve functional independence and prioritize quality of life: (1) goals of care and decision making, (2) cognitive function and prevention of delirium, (3) maintenance of function and mobility, and (4) nutrition and hydration optimization [19].

Looking forward and outside of the outpatient encounter, inpatient geriatric comanagement for surgical patients has been shown to decrease perioperative complications. Specifically, within vascular surgery, prospectively enrolled patients with an inpatient surgical procedure were compared in a pre-post fashion following implementation of formal comanagement. The post-group saw a significant reduction in hospital-acquired geriatric syndromes such as delirium as well as cardiac and infective complications [20].

With an aging population, it is the responsibility of the surgeon to be comfortable caring for older adults, crafting care plans congruent with a patient's goals, and consulting with geriatricians. If proceeding with surgery, there are a variety of assessments and interventions that can ultimately improve perioperative outcomes and assist the patient in achieving their health goals.

References

1. Siegel RL, Miller KD, Fedewa SA, et al. Colorectal cancer statistics, 2017. CA Cancer J Clin. 2017;67:177–93.
2. Walter LC, Covinsky KE. Cancer screening in elderly patients: a framework for individualized decision making. JAMA. 2001;285:2750–6.
3. Saur NM, Montroni I, Shahrokni A, Kunitake H, Potenti FM, Goodacre RC, Davis BR, Carli F. Care of the geriatric colorectal surgical patient and framework for creating a geriatric program: a compendium from the 2019 American society of colon and rectal surgeons annual meeting. Dis Colon Rectum. 2020;63(11):1489–95. https://doi.org/10.1097/DCR.0000000000001793. PMID: 32947418; PMCID: PMC7547896
4. Shahrokni A, Alexander K. The age of talking about age alone is over. Ann Surg Oncol. 2019;26:12–4.
5. Lawler M, Selby P, Aapro MS, Duffy S. Ageism in cancer care. BMJ. 2014;348:g1614.
6. Aparicio T, Canouï-Poitrine F, Caillet P, François E, Cudennec T, Carola E, Albrand G, Bouvier AM, Petri C, Couturier B, Phelip JM, Bengrine-Lefevre L, Paillaud E. Treatment guidelines of metastatic colorectal cancer in older patients from the French Society of Geriatric Oncology (SoFOG). Dig Liver Dis. 2020;52(5):493–505. https://doi.org/10.1016/j.dld.2019.12.145. Epub 2020 Feb 3
7. Antonio M, Saldaña J, Carmona-Bayonas A, Navarro V, Tebé C, Nadal M, Formiga F, Salazar R, Borràs JM. Geriatric assessment predicts survival and competing mortality in elderly patients with early colorectal cancer: can it help in adjuvant therapy decision-making? Oncologist. 2017;22(8):934–43. https://doi.org/10.1634/theoncologist.2016-0462. Epub 2017 May 9. PMID: 28487465; PMCID: PMC5553962
8. Li M, Schulte N, Elting F, Winkler EC, Hetjens S, Berger AK, Zschäbitz S, Hofmann J, Hofmann J, Hilbertz L, Kuhn M, Khakzar C, Jesenofsky R, Betge J, Zhan T, Belle S, Ebert MP, Härtel N. Sequential geriatric assessment in older patients with colorectal cancer during chemotherapy: subgroup analysis of a prospective, multicenter study EpiReal 75. Oncol Res Treat. 2022;45(11):670–80. https://doi.org/10.1159/000525101. Epub 2022 Jun 8
9. Decoster L, Vanacker L, Kenis C, Prenen H, Van Cutsem E, Van Der Auwera J, Van Eetvelde E, Van Puyvelde K, Flamaing J, Milisen K, Lobelle JP, De Grève J, Wildiers H. Relevance of geriatric assessment in older patients with colorectal cancer. Clin Colorectal Cancer. 2017;16(3):e221–9. https://doi.org/10.1016/j.clcc.2016.07.010. Epub 2016 Aug 8
10. Souwer ETD, Hultink D, Bastiaannet E, Hamaker ME, Schiphorst A, Pronk A, van der Bol JM, Steup WH, Dekker JWT, Portielje JEA, van den Bos F. The prognostic value of a geriatric risk score for older patients with colorectal cancer. Ann Surg Oncol. 2019;26(1):71–8. https://doi.org/10.1245/s10434-018-6867-x. Epub 2018 Oct 25. PMID: 30362061; PMCID: PMC6338720
11. Bessems SAM, Konsten JLM, Vogelaar JFJ, Csepán-Magyar R, Maas HAAM, van de Wouw YAJ, Janssen-Heijnen MLG. Frailty screening by Geriatric-8 and 4-meter gait speed test is feasible and predicts postoperative complications in elderly colorectal cancer patients. J Geriatr Oncol. 2021;12(4):592–8. https://doi.org/10.1016/j.jgo.2020.10.012. Epub 2020 Nov 4
12. Verweij NM, Souwer ETD, Schiphorst AHW, Maas HA, Portielje JEA, Pronk A, van den Bos F, Hamaker ME. The effect of a geriatric evaluation on treatment decisions for older patients with colorectal cancer. Int J Color Dis. 2017;32(11):1625–9. https://doi.org/10.1007/s00384-017-2883-8. Epub 2017 Sep 20
13. Lund CM, Vistisen KK, Olsen AP, Bardal P, Schultz M, Dolin TG, Rønholt F, Johansen JS, Nielsen DL. The effect of geriatric intervention in frail older patients receiving chemotherapy for colorectal cancer: a randomised trial (GERICO). Br J Cancer. 2021;124(12):1949–58. https://doi.org/10.1038/s41416-021-01367-0. Epub 2021 Apr 7. PMID: 33828260; PMCID: PMC8185087
14. Korc-Grodzicki B, Holmes HM, Shahrokni A. Geriatric assessment for oncologists. Cancer Biol Med. 2015;12:261–74.

15. Kottek A, Bates T, Spetz MJ. The roles and value of geriatricians in healthcare teams: a landscape analysis. UCSF Health Workforce Research Center on Long-Term Care; 2017. Accessed 15 Oct 2019. https://healthworkforce.ucsf.edu/sites/healthworkforce.ucsf.edu/files/REPORT_Geriatricians_Lit_FINAL.pdf.
16. Ballou JH, Brasel KJ. Palliative care and geriatric surgery. Clin Geriatr Med. 2019;35(1):35–44. https://doi.org/10.1016/j.cger.2018.08.004. Epub 2018 Sep 28
17. Kon AA, Davidson JE, Morrison W, et al. Shared decision making in ICUs: an American college of critical care medicine and American Thoracic Society policy statement. Crit Care Med. 2016;44(1):188–201.
18. Steffens NM, Tucholka JL, Nabozny MJ, Schmick AE, Brasel KJ, Schwarze ML. Engaging patients, health care professionals, and community members to improve preoperative decision making for older adults facing high-risk surgery. JAMA Surg. 2016;151(10):938–45. https://doi.org/10.1001/jamasurg.2016.1308. PMID: 27368074; PMCID: PMC5071104
19. Ma M, Zhang L, Rosenthal R, Finlayson E, Russell MM. The American College of surgeons geriatric surgery verification program and the practicing colorectal surgeon. Semin Colon Rectal Surg. 2020;31(4):100779. https://doi.org/10.1016/j.scrs.2020.100779. Epub 2020 Oct 2. PMID: 33041604; PMCID: PMC7531280
20. Thillainadesan J, Aitken SJ, Monaro SR, Cullen JS, Kerdic R, Hilmer SN, Naganathan V. Geriatric comanagement of older vascular surgery inpatients reduces hospital-acquired geriatric syndromes. J Am Med Dir Assoc. 2022;23(4):589–595.e6. https://doi.org/10.1016/j.jamda.2021.09.037. Epub 2021 Oct 29

Colon Cancer in the Splenic Flexure: Which Operation?

20

Himani Bhatt and Kellie Mathis

Introduction

Adenocarcinoma of the colon is the fourth most common cancer worldwide, and tumor location within the splenic flexure is rare, occurring in less than 10% of cases. Splenic flexure cancers (SFC) have been anatomically defined as cancers located within 10 cm in either direction from the left upper quadrant maximal bend of the colon or alternatively as a cancer located between the distal 1/3 of the transverse colon and the proximal 1/3 of the descending colon [1–3]. Embryologically, the splenic flexure is located between the final portion of the midgut and the starting portion of the hindgut, and it is supplied by both superior mesenteric and inferior mesenteric arteries. This dual vasculature and lymphatic drainage has led to uncertainty about the most appropriate extent of resection for SFCs. Understanding the complex anatomy and embryology of the splenic flexure is important to determine the optimal surgical approach for a SFC [3].

SFCs have a less favorable prognosis compared to other colon locations, often present at an advanced stage, have a high metastatic potential, have a high incidence of bowel obstruction, and are associated with a higher rate of lymph node positivity [4, 5]. The reason for these poor outcomes is not entirely understood. Multiple operations have been described for SFC including extended right hemicolectomy with an ileocolic anastomosis (and sometimes referred to as subtotal colectomy), left hemicolectomy with a colorectal anastomosis, segmental colectomy with a colocolonic anastomosis, and a total colectomy with an ileorectal anastomosis. The

H. Bhatt · K. Mathis (✉)
Department of Surgery, Mayo Clinic, Rochester, MN, USA
e-mail: Bhatt.himani@mayo.edu; Mathis.kellie@mayo.edu

K. Umanskiy, N. Hyman (eds.), *Difficult Decisions in Colorectal Surgery*, Difficult Decisions in Surgery: An Evidence-Based Approach,
https://doi.org/10.1007/978-3-031-42303-1_20

literature is limited on consensus for the best approach to treat SFCs and consists of only retrospective and heterogenous data from single institutions, making generalizable recommendations difficult. In this chapter we aim to provide a thorough literature review to collate an evidence-based optimal surgical approach for SFC resection.

Methods

An extensive literature review of several databases was conducted on May 18, 2022. The databases included: Ovid MEDLINE(R) and Epub Ahead of Print, In-Process & amp; Other Non-Indexed Citations, and Daily, Ovid EMBASE, Ovid Cochrane Central Register of Controlled Trials, Ovid Cochrane Database of Systematic Reviews, and Scopus. Controlled vocabulary supplemented with keywords like: "left colic flexure", "splenic flexure", "transverse colon", "Adenomatous polyposis", "Familial polyposis", "colorectal or bowel* or colon*", "left colic flexure", "splenic flexure", "transverse colon", "cancer* or neoplasm* or tumor* or tumour* or carcinoma* or adenocarcinoma* or carcinogenes*", "extended right colectomy*", "extended right hemicolectomy*", "extended right hemi-colectomy*", "right extended colectomy*", "right extended hemicolectomy*", "right extended hemi-colectomy*", "left colectomy*", "left hemicolectomy*", "left hemicolectomy*". Directed searches of the references from the primary articles were also performed to look for additional relevant articles. Results from observational studies and metanalyses were found. We found that all the relevant observational studies were already incorporated in the metanalyses and thus, we only included these meta-analyses in this review. Search was limited to: [1] Articles only in English, [2] Articles published in last 5 years [3] Articles related to splenic flexure cancer resection, and [4] Full text articles. See PICO information in Table 20.1. The Final 3 Metanalysis studies were reviewed in detail and their results are presented in the Table 20.2.

Table 20.1 PICO table

Patient population	Intervention	Comparators	Outcomes
Patients with splenic flexure cancer	Extended right/ subtotal colectomy	Left/segmental colectomy	Perioperative outcome, overall survival, disease free survival

Table 20.2 Summary of 3 Metanalyses Included in this Review

Author	Year	Country	Timeline	Type of study	Number of Studies	Total number of patients	ERH	LH	STC	SC	Outcomes	Study Quality
Hajibandeh et al.	2020	UK	1946 to 2020	Systematic review and meta-analysis	7 retrospective studies	956	353	361		242	No difference between ERH, LH and SC in terms of postoperative morbidity and mortality, lymph node yield and cancer survival.	Low
Wang et al.	2021	China	up to August 2020	Network meta-analysis	10 retrospective studies	2734	596	928	109	928	SC, LH, ERH and STC for the curative resection of splenic flexure tumors provide similar survival.	Low
Martınez-Perez et al.	2017	France	1990 to 2016	Systematic review and meta-analysis	12 retrospective studies (6 comparative, 6 case series)	569	132	437			No difference in ERH or LC	Low

ERH Extended right hemicolectomy *LH* Left hemicolectomy *SC* Segmental colectomy, *STC* Subtotal colectomy

Results

Extensive literature review yielded 3 meta-analysis studies that matched our search criteria. We found no prospective or randomized control trials published to date. The studies included in the meta-analysis were all retrospective in nature leaving us with low quality evidence.

This study included a total of 3264 non-overlapping subjects, but variable numbers of patients were included in each individual comparison.

Intra-Operative Outcomes

The intra-operative outcomes of interest include operative time, margin status, success of the anastomosis, the number of lymph nodes harvested, and minimally invasive surgery (MIS) use.

Extended Right Hemicolectomy vs Left Hemicolectomy

When comparing extended right hemicolectomy with left hemicolectomy, Hajibandeh et al., found no difference in operative times, rate of R0 resection, or the proportion of patients who had more than 12 LNs harvested. They did report that ERH resulted in a higher number of total lymph nodes harvested as compared to LH [fixed effects model: MD 3.52, 95% CI 2.14, 4.89; $P < 0.00001$; low heterogeneity (I2 = 43%); high GRADE certainty of evidence] [6]. Wang et al., reported a higher rate of primary anastomosis in the ERH group compared to the LH group [7].

Martinez Perez et al., found no differences in LN retrieval, R0 resection between ERH and LH [8].

Extended Right Hemicolectomy vs Segmental Colectomy

Hajibandeh et al., found no difference in rate of R0 resection, total number of LNs harvested, or the proportion of patients who had more than 12 LNs harvested. Operative times were significantly longer in the ERH group compared to segmental colectomy [6]Wang et al., found a higher rate of ileus in the ERH group compared to segmental colectomy (OR = 4.2, 95% CI 1.3–18.0, $P = 0.019$: low heterogeneity (I2 = 14.8%) [7].

Segmental Colectomy vs Left Hemicolectomy

Hajibandeh et al., found no difference in rate of R0 resection, total number of LNs harvested, or the proportion of patients who had more than 12 LNs harvested. Operative times were significantly longer in the left hemicolectomy group compared to segmental colectomy [6].

In the ACS NSQIP study, there were no differences in the proportion of patients with <12 LNs. 73% of all cases were done with an MIS technique. Patients in the segmental colectomy group had shorter operative times compared to left hemicolectomy [2].

Direct Comparison of 4 Techniques: Subtotal Colectomy, Extended Right Hemicolectomy, Left Hemicolectomy and Segmental Colectomy

Wang et al., reported no difference in rate of minimally invasive technology use or proportion of patients with >12 LNs harvested [7].

Post-Operative Outcomes/Morbidity

The postoperative outcomes reported include postoperative mortality, total complication rate, severe complication rate, anastomotic leak, ileus, need for reoperation, and length of hospital stay.

Extended Right Hemicolectomy Versus Left Hemicolectomy

Hajibandeh et al., found no statistical difference in total postoperative complications [fixed effects model: OR 1.16, 95% CI 0.83, 1.63; P = 0.37; low heterogeneity (I2 = 0%); high GRADE certainty of evidence], severe complications [fixed effects model: OR 0.69, 95% CI 0.43, 1.12; P = 0.13; low heterogeneity (I2 = 28%); high GRADE certainty of evidence], wound infection [fixed effect model: OR 0.63, 95% CI _0.14, 2.80; P = 0.55; low heterogeneity (I2 = 0%); low GRADE certainty of evidence], pancreatic fistula [fixed effects model: OR 1.00, 95% CI 0.06, 16.85; P = 1.00; very low GRADE certainty of evidence], and intra-abdominal abscess [fixed effects model: OR 2.08, 95% CI 0.18, 24.41; P = 0.56; very low GRADE certainty of evidence]. They also found no difference in anastomotic leak rates, mortality, ileus, need for reoperation and length of hospital stay [6]. Martinez Perez et al., found no differences in operative times, anastomotic leaks, postop complications [8].

Extended Right Hemicolectomy vs Segmental Colectomy

Hajibandeh et al., found no statistical difference in total postoperative complications, anastomotic leak, severe complications, mortality, need for reoperation, or length of hospital stay. They did report a higher rate of postoperative ileus in in the ERH group compared to segmental colectomy [6].

Segmental Colectomy vs Left Hemicolectomy

Hajibandeh et al., found no statistical difference in total postoperative complications, anastomotic leak, severe complications, mortality, need for reoperation, or length of hospital stay [6]. In the ACS-NSQIP study, there was no difference in major morbidity rates [2].

Direct Comparison of 4 Techniques: Subtotal Colectomy, Extended Right Hemicolectomy, Left Hemicolectomy and Segmental Colectomy

Wang, et al. reported no difference in need for reoperation, anastomotic leak, or mortality [7].

Laparoscopic Techniques (all Operations Combined) Versus Open Technique

Martinez Perez found no difference in postoperative complication rates comparing patients undergoing MIS surgery versus open surgery. The time to tolerance of an oral diet and the length of hospital stay both favored the laparoscopic group [8].

Survival Outcomes

All studies showed no differences in overall survival or disease-free survival among all comparisons. Survival outcomes were reported as 5 year outcomes in Hajibandeh et al., and Wang et al., studies [6, 7]. Wang et al., also reported no differences in local recurrence rates or distant recurrence rates [7].

Recommendation

After an in-depth review of the surgical literature for management of splenic flexure adenocarcinoma, there is no consensus for a "best" operation. All operations, including extended right hemicolectomy, left hemicolectomy, segmental colectomy, and subtotal colectomy, have similar post-operative outcomes and no differences in long-term oncologic outcomes. Two surveys about surgeons' choice regarding SFC resection approach yielded different outcomes, where one favored ERH at 63% [9] and the other favored SC for 70% [10]. Therefore, the surgical care of each patient with splenic flexure adenocarcinoma should be individualized.

A principle of colon cancer surgery is to base the extent of resection on the lymphovascular drainage of the region where the tumor is located [11]. This is where some of the uncertainty stems from with splenic flexure cancers as the lymphovascular drainage is not clear cut and predictable. Advocates of the ERH believe that lymph nodes along the middle colic proper should be removed in addition to those around the left colics while advocates of left hemicolectomy or segmental colectomy believe that left colic lymph node excision is sufficient. A clinical trial by Vasey et al., was conducted on 30 patients to assess the lymphatic drainage of SFC using scintigraphic mapping intraoperatively. It demonstrated that lymphatic flow was usually directed towards the left colic pedicle (96% of patients) followed by the left branch of the middle colic and the inferior mesenteric artery [12]. Watanabe et al., injected peritumoral indocyanine green at the time of laparoscopy for splenic flexure adenocarcinoma and found that the left colic basin was dominant in most and one patient had flow along the left branch of the middle colic [13]. Additionally, there was fluorescence along the inferior mesenteric vein in multiple patients [12, 13]. Both left hemicolectomy and segmental colectomy ligate the left branch of the middle colic and the left colic vessels, so either operation would allow sufficient lymph node resection in the vast majority.

A significant number of patients with SFCs will present with obstruction and require urgent operations. In these cases, there may be significant dilation of the proximal colon with resultant ischemia or serosal splitting, and this may necessitate an extended right colectomy [4, 6]. ERH is associated with a higher number of lymph nodes harvested in comparison to LH [7].

Lymph node resection has been a surrogate marker of quality for lymphadenectomy, but neither approach had significant difference in yielding ≥12 LNs [7]. And there was no difference in survival outcomes in any study.

The long-term function and quality of life should also be considered when choosing an operation for SFC. You et al., found measurable differences in quality of life and number of bowel motions per day when comparing segmental versus extended resections [14]. Because there is no clear oncologic benefit of ERH or STC over LH or SC, a segmental resection is preferred for SFC.

There are multiple limitations of this review. First, the definitions of each operation vary among studies, making it difficult to lump and compare, demonstrated in Table 20.3. Additionally, the three included metanalyses had several overlapping studies among themselves and in one case a single institution had publications on SFC with overlapping dates, suggesting that all patients were not unique [15, 16]. The meta-analysis by Hajibandeh et al., acknowledged this and performed sensitivity analyses which yielded no differences in outcomes [6]. All studies are retrospective from single institutions. No studies have been reported from the North American population with the exception of a recently published NSQIP study with only short-term outcomes [2].

Table 20.3 Definition of the surgical approaches used for splenic flexure cancer resection

Author	Extended right hemicolectomy definition	Left hemicolectomy definition	Subtotal colectomy definition	Segmental colectomy/ segmental left colectomy/splenic flexure colectomy definition
Hajibandeh et al.	Ligation of ileocolic (ICA), right colic (RCA), middle colic (MCA) and ascending branch of the left colic vessels (LCA).	Ligation of left colic and left branch of the middle colic vessels.		Ligation of left colic artery and left branches of the middle colic artery.
	Resection of the right and transverse colon and a part of descending colon.	Resection of the colon from the middle of the transverse colon to the recto-sigmoid junction.		Resection of the distal part of the transverse colon, the splenic flexure, and the proximal descending colon.
	Formation of an ileocolic anastomosis.	Formation of a colorectal or Colo-distal sigmoid anastomosis.		Colocolonic anastomosis.

(continued)

Table 20.3 (continued)

Author	Extended right hemicolectomy definition	Left hemicolectomy definition	Subtotal colectomy definition	Segmental colectomy/ segmental left colectomy/splenic flexure colectomy definition
Wang et al.	Ligation of the ICA, RCA, MCA and LCA.	Ligation of the left branch of the MCA and IMA.	Ligation of the ileocecal artery, right colic artery, middle colic artery and inferior mesenteric artery (IMA).	Resection of the bowel between the left branch of the MCA and the LCA at its origin from the IMA.
	Resection from the terminal ileum to the middle descending colon.	Resection of the last third of the transverse colon, descending and sigmoid colon down to the recto-sigmoid union.	Resection of the right, transverse, descending and sigmoid colon down to the rectosigmoid union.	
Martı ´nez-Pe´rez et al.	Ligation of ileocolic, right colic, middle colic, and left colic arteries.	Ligation of the inferior mesenteric artery and the left branch of the middle colic artery		The left colic and left branches of the middle colic vessels are ligated.
	Resection of the terminal ileus and the right, transverse, and proximal descending colon.	Resection of the colonic segment between the left third of the transverse colon and the colorectal juncture (ie, left half of the colon).		Resection of the distal part of the transverse colon, the splenic flexure, and the proximal descending colon.
	Formation of an ileocolostomy.	Colorectal anastomosis or a terminal colostomy		Colocolonic anastomosis is performed between the transverse and descending sigmoid colon.

Personal View of Data/ Expert Opinion

A standard operation for cancers of the splenic flexure remains elusive due at least in part to the unclear lymphovascular drainage of the splenic flexure and the relatively rare presentation of a tumor at this location. Many single institutions have reported outcomes comparing multiple operations, including extended right colectomy, left colectomy and segmental colectomy, and no significant differences in long-term outcomes been shown or even suggested. We believe the operation should be individualized to the patient rather than protocolized. For early stage, non-obstructing tumors at the splenic flexure, we perform a segmental colectomy with ligation of the left branch of the middle colic vessels and the left colic vessels as well as the IMV followed by a colocolonic anastomosis. In a patient who also has extensive diverticular disease, we may consider a left colectomy with a colorectal anastomosis. When a preoperative staging CT scan shows concern for central lymphadenopathy, we will consider an extended right colectomy or subtotal colectomy with high ligation of the ileocolic and middle colic vessels in addition to the left-sided vessels. And when the patient presents with obstruction, we will perform an extended right colectomy if there is a concern of cecal ischemia.

All elective SFC operations should be done in a minimally invasive fashion given the oncologic safety and improvements in recovery outcomes.

While it is always preferred to have randomized trial evidence to inform these decisions, it is not likely that a randomized trial will be feasible given the relative rarity of SFCs. Prospective registries among many institutions would add value as well as the public reporting of data from institutions in North America to further understand patterns and outcomes. Additionally, the intraoperative ICG pilot studies are fascinating and with some refinement may allow a real time decision to be made about extent of resection based on the fluorescence.

In the meantime, we believe that the culmination of many low-quality studies supports the use of a segmental colectomy for patients undergoing surgery for SFCs.

References

1. Ardu M, Bergamini C, Martellucci J, Prosperi P, Valeri A. Colonic splenic flexure carcinoma: is laparoscopic segmental resection a safe enough oncological approach? Surg Endosc. 2020;34(10):4436–43. https://doi.org/10.1007/s00464-019-07221-y.
2. Pang AJ, Marinescu D, Morin N, Vasilevsky CA, Boutros M. Segmental resection of splenic flexure colon cancers provides an adequate lymph node harvest and is a safe operative approach – an analysis of the ACS-NSQIP database. Surg Endosc. 2022;36(8):5652–9. https://doi.org/10.1007/s00464-021-08926-9.
3. Matsuda T, Sumi Y, Yamashita K, et al. Anatomical and embryological perspectives in laparoscopic complete mesocoloic excision of splenic flexure cancers. Surg Endosc. 2018;32(3):1202–8. https://doi.org/10.1007/s00464-017-5792-6.
4. Aldridge MC, Phillips RKS, Hittinger R, Fry JS, Fielding LP. Influence of tumour site on presentation, management and subsequent outcome in large bowel cancer. Br J Surg. 2005;73(8):663–70. https://doi.org/10.1002/bjs.1800730829.

5. Kim MJ, Kim JH, Lee YS, et al. Short- and long-term outcomes of laparoscopic segmental left colectomy for splenic flexure colon cancer: comparison with propensity score matching. Ann Surg Treat Res. 2021;101(5):274–80. https://doi.org/10.4174/astr.2021.101.5.274.
6. Hajibandeh S, Hajibandeh S, Hussain I, Zubairu A, Akbar F, Maw A. Comparison of extended right hemicolectomy, left hemicolectomy and segmental colectomy for splenic flexure colon cancer: a systematic review and meta-analysis. Color Dis. 2020;22(12):1885–907. https://doi.org/10.1111/codi.15292.
7. Wang X, Zheng Z, Chen M, et al. Subtotal colectomy, extended right hemicolectomy, left hemicolectomy, or splenic flexure colectomy for splenic flexure tumors: a network meta-analysis. Int J Color Dis. 2021;36(2):311–22. https://doi.org/10.1007/s00384-020-03763-z.
8. Martínez-Pérez A, Brunetti F, Vitali GC, Abdalla S, Ris F, de'Angelis N. Surgical treatment of colon cancer of the splenic flexure: A systematic review and meta-analysis. Surg Laparosc Endosc Percutan Tech. 2017;27(5):318–27. https://doi.org/10.1097/SLE.0000000000000419.
9. Degiuli M, Reddavid R, Ricceri F, et al. Segmental colonic resection is a safe and effective treatment option for colon cancer of the splenic flexure: a nationwide retrospective study of the Italian society of surgical oncology–colorectal cancer network collaborative group. Dis Colon Rectum. 2020;63(10):1372–82. https://doi.org/10.1097/DCR.0000000000001743.
10. Manceau G, Mori A, Bardier A, et al. Lymph node metastases in splenic flexure colon cancer: is subtotal colectomy warranted?: MANCEAU ET AL. J Surg Oncol. 2018;118(6):1027–33. https://doi.org/10.1002/jso.25169.
11. Steele SR, Hull TL, Hyman N, Maykel JA, Read TE, Whitlow CB, editors. The ASCRS textbook of colon and Rectal surgery. Springer International Publishing; 2022. https://doi.org/10.1007/978-3-030-66049-9.
12. Vasey CE, Rajaratnam S, O'Grady G, Hulme-Moir M. Lymphatic drainage of the splenic flexure defined by intraoperative Scintigraphic mapping. Dis Colon Rectum. 2018;61(4):441–6. https://doi.org/10.1097/DCR.0000000000000986.
13. Watanabe J, Ota M, Suwa Y, Ishibe A, Masui H, Nagahori K. Evaluation of lymph flow patterns in splenic flexural colon cancers using laparoscopic real-time indocyanine green fluorescence imaging. Int J Color Dis. 2017;32(2):201–7. https://doi.org/10.1007/s00384-016-2669-4.
14. You YN, Chua HK, Nelson H, Hassan I, Barnes SA, Harrington J, Segmental vs. Extended colectomy: measurable differences in morbidity, function, and quality of life. Dis Colon Rectum. 2008;51(7):1036–43. https://doi.org/10.1007/s10350-008-9325-1.
15. de'Angelis N, Hain E, Disabato M, et al. Laparoscopic extended right colectomy versus laparoscopic left colectomy for carcinoma of the splenic flexure: a matched case–control study. Int J Color Dis. 2016;31(3):623–30. https://doi.org/10.1007/s00384-015-2469-2.
16. The SFC Study Group, de'Angelis N, Martínez-Pérez A, et al. Extended right colectomy, left colectomy, or segmental left colectomy for splenic flexure carcinomas: a European multicenter propensity score matching analysis. Surg Endosc. 2021;35(2):661–72. https://doi.org/10.1007/s00464-020-07431-9.

Part III

Rectal Cancer

Management of T1 Rectal Cancer

21

Maggie L. Westfal and Matthew G. Mutch

Introduction

Colorectal cancer is the third most common cancer for both men and women and is the second leading cause of cancer-related deaths in the United States annually. In 2019, it was estimated that 145,600 new colorectal cancer cases were diagnosed in the last year and an estimated 51,020 deaths will have occurred [1]. The treatment for rectal cancer depends on the stage of disease at diagnosis. T1 cancers are defined as those that have grown into the submucosa only. The Kudo classification defines the degree of invasion into the submucosa as: upper third (sm1), middle third (sm2), and lower third (sm3) of the depth into the submucosa [2]. The depth of invasion is important as it is one of the characteristics that is used to classify lesions as low-risk or high-risk of developing locoregional disease. The management of T1 rectal tumors varies depending on the risk of locoregional disease, therefore this classification system is an important tool for surgeons.

Surgical management of rectal cancer is divided between local and radical resection. Total mesorectal excision (TME) is still considered the gold standard for the curative surgical treatment of rectal cancer. TME is believed to result in a significant decrease in local recurrence rates and increased disease-free survival for locally advanced disease, but is also associated with perioperative mortality ranging between 2–4% [3, 4] and morbidity as high as 59% [5]. In order to decrease the morbidity associated with a radical resection, several local excision techniques have been developed. Despite the success of local excision in managing the tumor at the index procedure with lower morbidity, many studies have questioned the oncologic outcomes of local excision, specifically in terms of high recurrence rates. This

M. L. Westfal (✉) · M. G. Mutch
Washington University St. Louis, Colon and Rectal Surgery, St. Louis, MO, USA
e-mail: maggiew@wustl.edu; mutchm@wustl.edu

K. Umanskiy, N. Hyman (eds.), *Difficult Decisions in Colorectal Surgery*, Difficult Decisions in Surgery: An Evidence-Based Approach,
https://doi.org/10.1007/978-3-031-42303-1_21

chapter will explore the management of T1 rectal cancer including presentation and evaluation, operative management approaches, oncologic and quality of life outcomes, as well as review the evidence-based guidelines from both the National Comprehensive Cancer Network (NCCN) and the American Society of Colon and Rectal Surgeons (ASCRS).

PICO table

Patients	Intervention	Comparator	Outcome
Patients with malignant rectal polyp (T1 rectal cancer)	Trans-anal excision	Total mesorectal excision	Recurrence-free survival, overall survival, quality of life

Presentation and Evaluation

Presentation

The widespread implementation of screening colonoscopy has led to a parallel increase in the detection of early staged rectal cancer including T1N0M0 lesions. Rectal cancers at this stage have invaded into the submucosal layer of the rectal wall without metastasis to the lymph nodes and other organs. The two most common presentations of T1 rectal cancer are those that are discovered on colonoscopy before or after endoscopic resection. Patients present with a pedunculated or sessile polyp and are subsequently diagnosed with cancer either post-endoscopic resection or post-endoscopic biopsy. A malignant rectal polyp is defined as an adenoma that harbors a focus of cancer invading through the mucosa and into the submucosa [6]. Before making a decision about formal surgical resection for an endoscopically resected pedunculated or sessile malignant polyp, surgeons should review the pathology and consult with the patient regarding their management options [7].

If the patient undergoes endoscopic resection and is found to have cancer in the polyp that is removed, it is imperative that the site be marked at the time of removal or within 2 weeks of removal in order monitor the site of removal going forward [8]. Additionally, the pathology should reviewed and mismatch repair gene (MMR) and microsatellite instability (MSI) testing should be completed. If a pedunculated poly is removed and found to have invasive cancer with favorable histologic features and clear margins then the patient can be clinically observed [7, 9]. However, if a sessile polyp is removed and found to have invasive cancer, the patient can be observed or undergo transanal local excision or transabdominal resection pending the presence of high-risk features and the status of the resection margins. If the patient undergoes fragmented resection and the margin cannot be assessed or there is evidence of unfavorable histologic features then the patient should undergo pre-operative work up for either local or radical excision [8]. Further details regarding the indications for operative intervention and pre-operative work-up will be discussed further below.

Evaluation

A cancer-specific history should be obtained eliciting disease-specific symptoms, associated symptoms, family history and perioperative medical risk. Symptoms of rectal cancer that need to be discussed are bleeding, pain, or symptoms related to obstruction. Urinary, sexual and bowel function should be reviewed, and symptoms indicative of malignant fistulas or severe radiating pain may alert the surgeon to locally advanced disease involving adjacent pelvic organs. Family history should include documentation of relevant pre-malignant lesions and cancers including details like age at diagnosis and the lineage of affected first- and second-degree relatives. Patients should be asked about known predisposing hereditary cancer syndromes, prior genetic testing, and family ancestry or ethnicity that may be relevant. Finally, a patient's medical fitness to undergo surgery should be assessed in order to plan for the appropriate operative intervention [1]. Routine lab values including preoperative chemistry, blood counts and a baseline CEA should be obtained before initiating treatment [10].

Physical exam should include documentation of the distance of the distal extent of the tumor from the anal verge and the cancer's relationship to the sphincter complex. Distance should be assessed by digital examination and endoscopy. Rigid proctoscopy may provide a more accurate measurement than flexible endoscopy. Endoscopic tattooing for purposes of anticipated intraoperative localization or to facilitate mucosal surveillance in the event of a clinical complete response in the setting of neo-adjuvant therapy may be helpful [1]. Before elective treatment, the histological diagnosis of invasive cancer should be confirmed and patients should undergo a full colonoscopy in order to rule out synchronous lesions. The incidence of synchronous colorectal cancer is low at 1–3% but the incidence of synchronous adenomas or other polyps remains as high as 30% in the literature [11–14]. If preoperative colonoscopy is not performed due to the need for urgent intervention or in the setting of an obstructing rectal cancer, then completion colonoscopy should be performed post-operatively.

In terms of staging, rectal cancer should be staged accordingly to the American Joint Committee on Cancer TNM system before initiating any treatment. A rectal cancer protocol MRI is the preferred modality for locoregional clinical staging. Endorectal ultrasound may be considered when differentiating between early T stages or when MRI is contraindicated [1, 15]. The recommendations for MRI staging of rectal cancer includes using a standardized technical protocol and reporting template that includes assessment of the depth of tumor penetration, presence of loco-regional nodal metastases, and the relationship between the lesions within the mesorectum and mesorectal fascia [16–18]. The NCCN defines a positive circumferential resection margin (CRM) as within one millimeter of the mesorectal fascia [19] and MRI can help predict surgical clearance of the CRM [16, 18, 20]. In addition to MRI, clinical staging for metastatic disease includes a CT scan of the chest, abdomen, and pelvis [1].

Finally, the management of patients with rectal cancer should utilize a multidisciplinary approach. Each case should be discussed in a tumor board that includes representatives from surgery, pathology, radiology, radiation oncology, and medical oncology. The decision of treatment modality is a balance between the presence of luminal disease, risk of nodal metastasis, functional impact and patient preference. Due to the complexity of decision making, extensive patient counseling is imperative. Additionally, if patients are going to have an ostomy as part of their surgical treatment, pre-operative education and stoma site marking should be performed by a trained ostomy educator. Pre-operative stoma marking and education has been shown to improve time to ostomy proficiency and decrease ostomy-related complications [21, 22].

Management Approach

Local Resection

Transanal local excision can be considered for patients with favorable tumors that are mobile and non-fixed, less than 30% of the circumference of the bowel, less than 3 cm in size, a margin that is clear for greater than 3 mm, within 8 cm from the anal verge, T1 depth of invasion, well to moderately differentiated without lymphovascular invasion (LVI), perineural invasion (PNI), or tumor budding [7, 8, 23]. The currently available transanal approaches to resection of T1 tumors include: transanal excision (TAE), transanal endoscopic surgery (TES), transanal endoscopic microsurgery (TEM), and transanal minimally invasive surgery (TAMIS). There is a robotic assisted TAMIS (R-TAMIS) platform that utilizes the Da Vinci robotic system that it is not yet approved for use but has been shown to be both effective and safe in small trials [24]. The use of TEM and TAMIS can allow for local excision of more proximal lesions. The benefit of a full thickness excision compared to endoscopic removal allows for a more comprehensive pathologic evaluation. Final pathologic review of a locally excised T1 rectal cancer maximizes the ability to stratify for the risk of nodal metastasis allowing for a final decision between local excision and radical resection. For patients with low-risk tumors (sm1 depth of invasion, no high risk features (LVI, PNI, tumor budding), and well or moderately differentiated) the risk of nodal metastasis is low at 1–3%. However, sm3 tumors with high-risk features can have a risk of nodal metastasis as high as 35%, thus these factors must be considered when making a decision regarding the need for radical resection [25].

There is controversy as to whether malignant colorectal polyps with a sessile configuration can be successfully treated by endoscopic removal. Per the ASCRS guidelines, the literature remains varied with some data indicating that endoscopically removed sessile malignant polyps have a significantly greater incidence of adverse outcomes (residual disease, recurrent disease, mortality, and hematogenous metastasis but not lymph node metastasis), while other data suggests that configuration by itself is not a significant variable for adverse outcomes and sessile polyps with grade I or grade II histology, negative margins, and no LVI can be successfully treated with endoscopic polypectomy alone [1]. If the lesion has low-risk features, there may still be benefit from further transanal or TEM excision to ensure there is no residual local disease.

Local excision involves full-thickness excision down to perirectal fat ideally with a greater than or equal to 10 millimeter grossly normal circumferential margin and 2-millimeter-deep margin [19]. The advantages to this approach are minimal morbidity, sphincter sparing, rapid recovery, and minimal mortality [26, 27]. The significant limitation of this approach is the inability to pathologically stage the mesorectal lymph nodes. Given this limitation and the significantly higher local recurrence rate after local excision compared to APR or LAR, some authors suspect that this is due to lymph node micrometastatic disease that is undetectable on imaging and not assessed with local excision [23, 27, 28]. Thus, highlighting the importance of a thorough pathologic evaluation and patient counseling.

Radical Resection

As mentioned previously, the gold standard for the treatment of rectal cancer remains a transabdominal resection with total mesorectal excision. In terms of operative approaches, depending on the location of the tumor, an abdominoperineal resection or low anterior resection with colorectal or coloanal anastomosis can be performed. The treating surgeon should be experienced in rectal cancer surgery and specifically with TME. Sphincter preservation and restoration of organ integrity should be achieved without compromise of oncologic resection and consideration of anticipated patient functional outcome and quality of life [1, 8]. TME involves en bloc removal of the mesorectum, including associated vascular and lymphatic structures, fatty tissue, and mesorectal fascia as a tumor package through sharp dissection that spares the autonomic nerves [29–31].

For patients with T1 malignant polyps with unfavorable histologic features (positive margins, LVI, PNI, poor differentiation or sm2 or 3 invasion into the submucosa) [25, 32] or when the specimen is fragmented and/or margins cannot be assessed, further rectal resection is warranted. A positive margin for an endoscopically removed polyp has been defined as the presence of tumor cells within the diathermy of the transected margin [7, 33–35]. Additionally, several studies have shown that tumor budding is an adverse histologic feature associated with adverse outcomes and may preclude polypectomy as an adequate treatment of endoscopically removed T1 tumors [36, 37]. These poor prognostic features carry a 10–19% risk of nodal metastasis so local excision will not provide adequate treatment. Additionally, in terms of timing of radical resection, results of immediate surgery in cases of high-risk pathology have shown superior results to those after salvage surgery at the time of local recurrence [38, 39].

Neoadjuvant and Adjuvant Therapy

Several studies have attempted to discern whether neo-adjuvant or adjuvant therapy may benefit patients undergoing local excision for T1 rectal cancer. Local excision has also been performed after neoadjuvant chemoradiation for select T1/T2 lesions and this has been studied in clinical trials but remains controversial [28, 40–42]. Taira et al. looked at the prognosis of patients with T1 rectal cancer stratified by pre-operative chemo-radiation therapy. In 86 patients there was no significant difference in relapse-free survival but they did find that in a multivariate analysis, tumor location within 5 cm from the anal verge was a significant risk factor associated with a poor relapse-free survival [43].

In terms of adjuvant therapy, Minsky et al. concluded that post-operative radiation therapy is not needed after local excision in patients with T1 tumors and negative prognostic features [44]. On the other hand, Taylor et al [45] and Lamont et al. [46] reported that adjuvant radiation therapy improved both recurrence rate and survival in their patient cohorts. Paty et al. [47] reported that local recurrence was delayed in patient that received adjuvant pelvic radiation. Finally, Borstlap et al. concluded that local recurrence rates in T1 rectal cancer between patients with local excision with adjuvant therapy and those who underwent radical surgery were comparable [48].

When patients with high-risk T1 lesions refuse radical resection or prioritize sphincter preservation, adjuvant chemoradiation in combination with local excision has been considered. A systematic review of patients with T1/T2 rectal lesions removed by local excision compared the patients who received adjuvant chemoradiation with those that underwent radical resection. The authors report a 10% recurrence rate after local excision with adjuvant therapy versus a 6% recurrence rate after radical resection of T1 tumors [49]. Oostendorp et al. performed a meta-analysis of 73 studies and showed a local recurrence rate of 6.7% for low risk T1 tumors with local excision alone and no local recurrences in patients treated with adjuvant pelvic radiation and concurrent chemotherapy. High risk T1 tumors had a local recurrence rate of 13.6% compared to 3.9% with LE alone versus adjuvant therapy, therefore the authors concluded that local excision with adjuvant chemoradiation therapy may provide an alternative approach to radical surgery for patients with high-risk features. In a small study, Balyasnikova et al. found no recurrence at a median follow-up of 4 years in 18 patients with high-risk rectal cancer after undergoing local excision with adjuvant radiotherapy [50]. Al-Sawat et al. concluded that local excision with adjuvant radiotherapy is a better treatment option to avoid complications and stoma formation compared with radical excision and is a safe alternative for patients with T1 rectal cancer with fewer than three high-risk features [51]. Finally, Swanton et al. found similar results and concluded that local excision followed by adjuvant pelvic radiation is feasible, safe and yields good locoregional control in T1 rectal cancers, thereby avoiding definitive surgery and the morbidity associated with LAR or APR. [52]

In summary, the NCCN guidelines[8] recommend that for node negative T1 rectal cancer, lesions can be treated with trans-abdominal resection or trans-anal resection as appropriate. If pathology review after local excision reveals no high-risk features, then no further treatment is required. However, if pathology shows poorly differentiated histology, positive margins, invasion into the deepest third of the submucosa (sm3), LVI or PNI, then additional treatment is required. Trans-abdominal resection is the preferred next step in management followed by adjuvant therapy based on pathologic stage. If patients instead undergo adjuvant chemoradiation therapy after local excision, additional treatment will be determined by whether there is evidence of residual disease. If there is no evidence of disease, observation or additional chemotherapy can be considered based the patient's risk factors. If there is evidence of disease, then trans-abdominal resection should be performed with or without adjuvant chemotherapy. It is imperative that the patient undergo careful surveillance if they forego trans-abdominal resection.

Surveillance

Whether or not patients with T1N0M0 rectal cancer require further surveillance remains controversial. ASCRS and NCCN guidelines both recommend surveillance for stage 1 rectal cancer with a regular history and exam, CEA, flexible sigmoidoscopy/proctoscopy and colonoscopy. There is no role for routine imaging for these patients [1, 8]. On the other hand the Cancer Care Ontario (CCO) and the American Society of Clinical Oncology (ASCO) do not recommend surveillance for stage I patients for colon or rectal cancer [53]. The decision regarding surveillance for patients with T1 rectal cancer should be made on an individual basis based on the patient's risk factors.

Outcomes

Local Recurrence

The risk of local recurrence for patients undergoing local excision remains unknown. One retrospective study by Nash et al. showed that in 282 patients undergoing either transanal local excision or radical resection for T1 rectal cancer, the respective local recurrence rates were 13.2% and 2.7% respectively [23]. A similar retrospective study by You et al. showed local recurrence rates of 12.5% for transanal excision patients and 6.9% for radical resection patients [27]. Rates of local control following local excision have been shown to be favorable in T1 sm1–2 tumors [54], while prognostic factors for increased local recurrence rates include high grade tumors, LVI, PNI, tumor budding, sm3 tumors, mucinous type tumors, and positive resection margins [36, 37, 55]. Overall, several studies have found recurrence rates of 10–30% for patients undergoing local resection for T1 rectal cancer [45, 56–58].

In high-risk patients the risk of local recurrence is higher. One meta-analysis looking at local recurrence in patients with high-risk T1 and T2 rectal cancer who did not receive additional therapy showed a substantial risk of local recurrence. Completion TME or adjuvant chemoradiation for T1 patient was found to mitigate that risk. This provides support for using full thickness local excision as a guide to definitive management. Another meta-analysis reported a substantial risk of local recurrence in patients with high-risk T1 and T2 rectal cancer who received no additional therapy following local excision. The authors conclude that neo-adjuvant chemoradiation therapy followed by local excision may be safe and effective alternative for patients with any T stage of cancer who refuse or are unfit for transabdominal resection but understand that further studies are needed to explore this management suggestion [59].

Finally, Madbouly et al [60] showed that the 5-year recurrence rate after transanal excision was 29.4%. 5-year cancer specific and overall survival were 89% and 75% respectively. Nearly all patients with a recurrence underwent salvage treatment with a 56.3% five-year survival rate. They concluded that although overall cancer survival rates might be regarded as satisfactory, the high recurrence and low salvage rate raises the issue about the role of transanal excision alone for early rectal cancer and the potential need to consider adjuvant therapy for these patients.

Metastasis

Lymph node (LN) metastasis occurs in 2–35% of T1 lesions. When looking at the depth of tumor involvement into the submucosa and LN metastasis in T1 rectal cancer, the rates of LN metastasis for sm1, sm2 and sm3 tumors was 2%, 9%, and 35% respectively [25]. Additionally, Kitajima et al. established the method for measuring submucosal invasion depth (SID) and found that lesions with SID less than 1000 micrometers had no evidence of lymph node metastasis. The clinical guidelines of the Japanese Society for Cancer of the Colon and Rectum describe the method of measuring an SID and advise additional surgical resection with lymph node dissection after endoscopic treatment for lesions with SID greater than 1000 micrometers. This "1000 micrometer rule" is recommended as a criterion for additional resection in many previous papers [34, 61, 62] and is used as a gold-standard indicator for endoscopic diagnoses, such as magnifying endoscopy or image-enhanced endoscopy [63]. As endoscopic techniques progress, endoscopic treatment is becoming more widely acceptable for lesions with SID greater than or equal to 1000 micrometers [61, 64, 65].

Disease Free and Overall Survival

Although limited, some data suggests that TEM may have similar oncologic outcomes in patients with T1N0M0 rectal cancer compared with radical resection, while additionally offering patients the benefits of local resection [66, 67]. Additionally, Lu et al. showed that although the local recurrence rate after TEM was higher than that after TME, distant metastasis, overall survival and disease-free survival rates did not differ between these groups [68]. Clancy et al. performed a meta-analysis in 2015 and found that TEM provides superior oncologic outcomes compared to transanal local excision as it had a higher rate of negative microscopic margins, reduced rate of specimen fragmentation, and reduced rate of lesion recurrence [69]. Endreseth et al. completed a prospective study from the Norwegian Rectal Cancer Project looking at 291 patients with T1 rectal cancer treated with radical resection or trans-anal excision. They found that the 5-year survival for trans-anal excision was 70% compared to 80% in the radical resection group [55]. Hyun et al. performed a retrospective review from multicenter data and used propensity score matching to form two groups of patients who underwent local excision and compared them to patients who underwent TME for T1 rectal cancer. They found that although patients who underwent local excision had higher local recurrence rates, there was no difference in disease-free survival or overall survival [70]. Several other studies found that there was not a significant difference in overall survival rate between patients undergoing local excision versus TME with T1 rectal cancer [27, 57, 71].

Quality of Life

Local excision is associated with improved quality of life secondary to overall decreased morbidity in terms of bowel function, sexual function, and micturition function. In the NSABP R-04 trial, patients who had an APR reported worse body image, worse micturition symptoms, and less sexual enjoyment at 1 year post-surgery compared to those who had sphincter-sparing surgery [8]. An extra-levator APR may have benefits over a conventional APR approach, including lower rates of intra-operative perforation, CRM involvement and local recurrence although the data remains varied [72, 73]. Further studies comparing the quality of life of patients after radical resection and local excision are needed to further delineate these outcomes in more detail.

Conclusion

In patients found to have T1 rectal cancer, a careful review of the pathology as well was local and distant staging is necessary in order to determine if a local excision or a radical resection is appropriate. All resected specimens should undergo pathologic review to assess for high-risk features because presence of these features are associated with an increased likelihood of mesorectal lymph node involvement and therefore a radical resection with TME would be warranted in this setting. If the patient has significant co-morbidities and is not a candidate for radical resection, then a local excision should be considered. Although this is the safer approach from an operative standpoint in terms of morbidity, mortality and sphincter function, there is a possible increased risk of local and distant failure. For patients that opt for a local excision, close surveillance is necessary in order to identify local recurrence quickly should it occur. The use of either neo-adjuvant and/or adjuvant chemoradiation therapy remains controversial but may provide better outcomes for patients opting to undergo local excision. A multi-disciplinary clinical team should be utilized in order to review each case on an individual basis and provide the patient with all possible options for the management of T1 rectal cancer. Overall, it is important to match the treatment plan approach to the individual patient and all risk factors must be explained to the patient in order to allow them to make an informed decision that considers short and long-term risks and benefits.

References

1. You YN, Hardiman KM, Bafford A, et al. The American Society of Colon and Rectal Surgeons clinical practice guidelines for the Management of Rectal Cancer. Dis Colon Rectum. 2020;63(9):1191–222.
2. Kudo S, Tamegai Y, Yamano H, et al. Endoscopic mucosal resection of the colon: the Japanese technique. Gastrointest Endosc Clin N Am. 2001;11(3):519–35.
3. Marijnen CA, Kapiteijn E, van de Velde CJ, et al. Acute side effects and complications after short-term preoperative radiotherapy combined with total mesorectal excision in primary rectal cancer: report of a multicenter randomized trial. J Clin Oncol. 2002;20(3):817–25.
4. Snijders HS, Wouters MW, van Leersum NJ, et al. Meta-analysis of the risk for anastomotic leakage, the postoperative mortality caused by leakage in relation to the overall postoperative mortality. Eur J Surg Oncol. 2012;38(11):1013–9.
5. Guillou PJ, Quirke P, Thorpe H, et al. Short-term endpoints of conventional versus laparoscopic-assisted surgery in patients with colorectal cancer (MRC CLASICC trial): multicentre, randomised controlled trial. Lancet. 2005;365(9472):1718–26.
6. Hamilton S. Carcinoma of the colon and rectum. Pathology and genetics of tumours of the digestive system. 2000:103–43.
7. Cooper HS, Deppisch LM, Gourley WK, et al. Endoscopically removed malignant colorectal polyps: clinicopathologic correlations. Gastroenterology. 1995;108(6):1657–65.
8. Benson AB, Venook AP, Al-Hawary MM, et al. Rectal cancer, version 2.2022, NCCN clinical practice guidelines in oncology. J Natl Compr Cancer Netw. 2022;20(10):1139–67.
9. Yoshii S, Nojima M, Nosho K, et al. Factors associated with risk for colorectal cancer recurrence after endoscopic resection of T1 tumors. Clin Gastroenterol Hepatol. 2014;12(2):292–302 e293.
10. Tarantino I, Warschkow R, Worni M, et al. Elevated preoperative CEA is associated with worse survival in stage I-III rectal cancer patients. Br J Cancer. 2012;107(2):266–74.
11. Adloff M, Arnaud JP, Bergamaschi R, Schloegel M. Synchronous carcinoma of the colon and rectum: prognostic and therapeutic implications. Am J Surg. 1989;157(3):299–302.
12. Barillari P, Ramacciato G, De Angelis R, et al. Effect of preoperative colonoscopy on the incidence of synchronous and metachronous neoplasms. Acta Chir Scand. 1990;156(2):163–6.
13. Bat L, Neumann G, Shemesh E. The association of synchronous neoplasms with occluding colorectal cancer. Dis Colon Rectum. 1985;28(3):149–51.
14. Isler JT, Brown PC, Lewis FG, Billingham RP. The role of preoperative colonoscopy in colorectal cancer. Dis Colon Rectum. 1987;30(6):435–9.
15. Beets-Tan RGH, Lambregts DMJ, Maas M, et al. Magnetic resonance imaging for clinical management of rectal cancer: updated recommendations from the 2016 European Society of Gastrointestinal and Abdominal Radiology (ESGAR) consensus meeting. Eur Radiol. 2018;28(4):1465–75.
16. Lahaye MJ, Engelen SM, Nelemans PJ, et al. Imaging for predicting the risk factors—the circumferential resection margin and nodal disease—of local recurrence in rectal cancer: a meta-analysis. Semin Ultrasound CT MR. 2005;26(4):259–68.
17. Faletti R, Gatti M, Arezzo A, et al. Preoperative staging of rectal cancer using magnetic resonance imaging: comparison with pathological staging. Minerva Chir. 2018;73(1):13–9.
18. Klessen C, Rogalla P, Taupitz M. Local staging of rectal cancer: the current role of MRI. Eur Radiol. 2007;17(2):379–89.
19. Benson AB, Venook AP, Al-Hawary MM, et al. Rectal cancer, version 2.2018, NCCN clinical practice guidelines in oncology. J Natl Compr Cancer Netw. 2018;16(7):874–901.
20. Xie H, Zhou X, Zhuo Z, et al. Effectiveness of MRI for the assessment of mesorectal fascia involvement in patients with rectal cancer: a systematic review and meta-analysis. Dig Surg. 2014;31(2):123–34.
21. Chaudhri S, Brown L, Hassan I, Horgan AF. Preoperative intensive, community-based vs. traditional stoma education: a randomized, controlled trial. Dis Colon Rectum. 2005;48(3):504–9.
22. Crooks S. Foresight that leads to improved outcome: stoma care nurses' role in siting stomas. Prof Nurse. 1994;10(2):89–92.

23. Nash GM, Weiser MR, Guillem JG, et al. Long-term survival after transanal excision of T1 rectal cancer. Dis Colon Rectum. 2009;52(4):577–82.
24. Berger NF, Sylla P. The role of Transanal endoscopic surgery for early rectal cancer. Clin Colon Rectal Surg. 2022;35(2):113–21.
25. Nascimbeni R, Burgart LJ, Nivatvongs S, Larson DR. Risk of lymph node metastasis in T1 carcinoma of the colon and rectum. Dis Colon Rectum. 2002;45(2):200–6.
26. Rogers AC, Winter DC, Heeney A, et al. Systematic review and meta-analysis of the impact of tumour budding in colorectal cancer. Br J Cancer. 2016;115(7):831–40.
27. You YN, Baxter NN, Stewart A, Nelson H. Is the increasing rate of local excision for stage I rectal cancer in the United States justified?: a nationwide cohort study from the National Cancer Database. Ann Surg. 2007;245(5):726–33.
28. Shaikh I, Askari A, Ouru S, et al. Oncological outcomes of local excision compared with radical surgery after neoadjuvant chemoradiotherapy for rectal cancer: a systematic review and meta-analysis. Int J Color Dis. 2015;30(1):19–29.
29. Heald RJ, Husband EM, Ryall RD. The mesorectum in rectal cancer surgery—the clue to pelvic recurrence? Br J Surg. 1982;69(10):613–6.
30. Lindsetmo RO, Joh YG, Delaney CP. Surgical treatment for rectal cancer: an international perspective on what the medical gastroenterologist needs to know. World J Gastroenterol. 2008;14(21):3281–9.
31. Baxter NN, Garcia-Aguilar J. Organ preservation for rectal cancer. J Clin Oncol. 2007;25(8):1014–20.
32. Yamamoto S, Watanabe M, Hasegawa H, et al. The risk of lymph node metastasis in T1 colorectal carcinoma. Hepato-Gastroenterology. 2004;51(58):998–1000.
33. Seitz U, Bohnacker S, Seewald S, et al. Is endoscopic polypectomy an adequate therapy for malignant colorectal adenomas? Presentation of 114 patients and review of the literature. Dis Colon Rectum. 2004;47(11):1789–96. discussion 1796–1787
34. Ueno H, Mochizuki H, Hashiguchi Y, et al. Risk factors for an adverse outcome in early invasive colorectal carcinoma. Gastroenterology. 2004;127(2):385–94.
35. Volk EE, Goldblum JR, Petras RE, Carey WD, Fazio VW. Management and outcome of patients with invasive carcinoma arising in colorectal polyps. Gastroenterology. 1995;109(6):1801–7.
36. Maeda K, Koide Y, Katsuno H. When is local excision appropriate for "early" rectal cancer? Surg Today. 2014;44(11):2000–14.
37. Bach SP, Hill J, Monson JR, et al. A predictive model for local recurrence after transanal endoscopic microsurgery for rectal cancer. Br J Surg. 2009;96(3):280–90.
38. Baron PL, Enker WE, Zakowski MF, Urmacher C. Immediate vs. salvage resection after local treatment for early rectal cancer. Dis Colon Rectum. 1995;38(2):177–81.
39. Friel CM, Cromwell JW, Marra C, et al. Salvage radical surgery after failed local excision for early rectal cancer. Dis Colon Rectum. 2002;45(7):875–9.
40. Garcia-Aguilar J, Renfro LA, Chow OS, et al. Organ preservation for clinical T2N0 distal rectal cancer using neoadjuvant chemoradiotherapy and local excision (ACOSOG Z6041): results of an open-label, single-arm, multi-institutional, phase 2 trial. Lancet Oncol. 2015;16(15):1537–46.
41. Rullier E, Vendrely V, Asselineau J, et al. Organ preservation with chemoradiotherapy plus local excision for rectal cancer: 5-year results of the GRECCAR 2 randomised trial. Lancet Gastroenterol Hepatol. 2020;5(5):465–74.
42. Lezoche E, Baldarelli M, Lezoche G, et al. Randomized clinical trial of endoluminal locoregional resection versus laparoscopic total mesorectal excision for T2 rectal cancer after neoadjuvant therapy. Br J Surg. 2012;99(9):1211–8.
43. Taira T, Nozawa H, Kawai K, et al. Oncological outcomes of pathological T1 lower rectal cancer patients with or without preoperative Chemoradiotherapy. In Vivo. 2020;34(6):3559–64.
44. Minsky BD. Conservative treatment of rectal cancer with local excision and postoperative radiation therapy. Eur J Cancer. 1995;31A(7–8):1343–6.
45. Taylor RH, Hay JH, Larsson SN. Transanal local excision of selected low rectal cancers. Am J Surg. 1998;175(5):360–3.

46. Lamont JP, McCarty TM, Digan RD, et al. Should locally excised T1 rectal cancer receive adjuvant chemoradiation? Am J Surg. 2000;180(6):402–5. discussion 405–406
47. Paty PB, Nash GM, Baron P, et al. Long-term results of local excision for rectal cancer. Ann Surg. 2002;236(4):522–9. discussion 529–530
48. Borstlap WAA, van Oostendorp SE, Klaver CEL, et al. Organ preservation in rectal cancer: a synopsis of current guidelines. Color Dis. 2017;
49. Borstlap WA, Tanis PJ, Koedam TW, et al. A multi-centred randomised trial of radical surgery versus adjuvant chemoradiotherapy after local excision for early rectal cancer. BMC Cancer. 2016;16:513.
50. Balyasnikova S, Read J, Tait D, et al. The results of local excision with or without postoperative adjuvant chemoradiotherapy for early rectal cancer among patients choosing to avoid radical surgery. Color Dis. 2017;19(2):139–47.
51. Al-Sawat A, Bae JH, Kim HH, et al. Short- and long-term outcomes of local excision with adjuvant radiotherapy in high-risk T1 rectal cancer patients. Ann Surg Treat Res. 2022;102(1):36–45.
52. Swanton C, Marcus S, Jayamohan J, et al. Can adjuvant pelvic radiation therapy after local excision or polypectomy for T1 and T2 rectal cancer offer an alternative option to radical surgery? Clin Transl Radiat Oncol. 2021;31:97–101.
53. Meyerhardt JA, Mangu PB, Flynn PJ, et al. Follow-up care, surveillance protocol, and secondary prevention measures for survivors of colorectal cancer: American Society of Clinical Oncology clinical practice guideline endorsement. J Clin Oncol. 2013;31(35):4465–70.
54. Morino M, Risio M, Bach S, et al. Early rectal cancer: the European Association for Endoscopic Surgery (EAES) clinical consensus conference. Surg Endosc. 2015;29(4):755–73.
55. Endreseth BH, Myrvold HE, Romundstad P, et al. Transanal excision vs. major surgery for T1 rectal cancer. Dis Colon Rectum. 2005;48(7):1380–8.
56. Garcia-Aguilar J, Mellgren A, Sirivongs P, et al. Local excision of rectal cancer without adjuvant therapy: a word of caution. Ann Surg. 2000;231(3):345–51.
57. Mellgren A, Sirivongs P, Rothenberger DA, Madoff RD, Garcia-Aguilar J. Is local excision adequate therapy for early rectal cancer? Dis Colon Rectum. 2000;43(8):1064–71. discussion 1071–1064
58. Chorost MI, Petrelli NJ, McKenna M, Kraybill WG, Rodriguez-Bigas MA. Local excision of rectal carcinoma. Am Surg. 2001;67(8):774–9.
59. van Oostendorp SE, Smits LJH, Vroom Y, et al. Local recurrence after local excision of early rectal cancer: a meta-analysis of completion TME, adjuvant (chemo)radiation, or no additional treatment. Br J Surg. 2020;107(13):1719–30.
60. Madbouly KM, Remzi FH, Erkek BA, et al. Recurrence after transanal excision of T1 rectal cancer: should we be concerned? Dis Colon Rectum. 2005;48(4):711–9. discussion 719–721
61. Tanaka S, Asayama N, Shigita K, et al. Towards safer and appropriate application of endoscopic submucosal dissection for T1 colorectal carcinoma as total excisional biopsy: future perspectives. Dig Endosc. 2015;27(2):216–22.
62. Kawachi H, Eishi Y, Ueno H, et al. A three-tier classification system based on the depth of submucosal invasion and budding/sprouting can improve the treatment strategy for T1 colorectal cancer: a retrospective multicenter study. Mod Pathol. 2015;28(6):872–9.
63. Kitajima K, Fujimori T, Fujii S, et al. Correlations between lymph node metastasis and depth of submucosal invasion in submucosal invasive colorectal carcinoma: a Japanese collaborative study. J Gastroenterol. 2004;39(6):534–43.
64. Asayama N, Oka S, Tanaka S, et al. Endoscopic submucosal dissection as total excisional biopsy for clinical T1 colorectal carcinoma. Digestion. 2015;91(1):64–9.
65. Saito Y, Sakamoto T, Nakajima T, Matsuda T. Colorectal ESD: current indications and latest technical advances. Gastrointest Endosc Clin N Am. 2014;24(2):245–55.
66. Kidane B, Chadi SA, Kanters S, Colquhoun PH, Ott MC. Local resection compared with radical resection in the treatment of T1N0M0 rectal adenocarcinoma: a systematic review and meta-analysis. Dis Colon Rectum. 2015;58(1):122–40.

67. Sajid MS, Farag S, Leung P, et al. Systematic review and meta-analysis of published trials comparing the effectiveness of transanal endoscopic microsurgery and radical resection in the management of early rectal cancer. Color Dis. 2014;16(1):2–14.
68. Lu JY, Lin GL, Qiu HZ, et al. Comparison of Transanal endoscopic microsurgery and Total Mesorectal excision in the treatment of T1 rectal cancer: a meta-analysis. PLoS One. 2015;10(10):e0141427.
69. Clancy C, Burke JP, Albert MR, O'Connell PR, Winter DC. Transanal endoscopic microsurgery versus standard transanal excision for the removal of rectal neoplasms: a systematic review and meta-analysis. Dis Colon Rectum. 2015;58(2):254–61.
70. Hyun JH, Alhanafy MK, Park HC, et al. Initial local excision for clinical T1 rectal cancer showed comparable overall survival despite high local recurrence rate: a propensity-matched analysis. Ann Coloproctol. 2022;38(2):166–75.
71. Bentrem DJ, Okabe S, Wong WD, et al. T1 adenocarcinoma of the rectum: transanal excision or radical surgery? Ann Surg. 2005;242(4):472–7. discussion 477–479
72. Huang A, Zhao H, Ling T, et al. Oncological superiority of extralevator abdominoperineal resection over conventional abdominoperineal resection: a meta-analysis. Int J Color Dis. 2014;29(3):321–7.
73. Negoi I, Hostiuc S, Paun S, Negoi RI, Beuran M. Extralevator vs conventional abdominoperineal resection for rectal cancer-a systematic review and meta-analysis. Am J Surg. 2016;212(3):511–26.

22 Can Total Mesorectal Excision Be Avoided in T2 Rectal Cancer?

Anthony Loria and Fergal J. Fleming

Introduction

In 2020, there were approximately 43,000 incident cases of rectal cancer in the United States and over 700,000 incident cases worldwide [1, 2]. Patients with clinical stage one rectal cancer (T1–2N0) represent approximately 25–30% of incident cases at the population level [3]. For patients with T2N0 disease, total mesorectal excision (TME) is the standard of care due to durable oncologic outcomes [4]. However TME can be associated with considerable morbidity. Balancing the risk of undertreatment with minimizing surgical morbidity has prompted a growing interest in using local excision among patients with T2N0 rectal cancer. Moreover, recent data on neoadjuvant chemoradiation followed by local excision is challenging the paradigm that TME is associated with superior oncologic outcomes in patients with T2N0 disease. This chapter aims to articulate the rationale for seeking alternatives to TME, weigh the contemporary evidence, and provide expert opinion on the rapidly advancing management of early (T1-T2, node-negative) rectal cancer.

Search Strategy

For this narrative review, a comprehensive literature search of PubMed identified studies comparing local excision with TME published between 2002 and 2023 (Table 22.1). Local excision in the context of early rectal (T1–2N0) cancer refers to transanal endoscopic microsurgery (TEMS) or transanal minimally invasive surgery

A. Loria · F. J. Fleming (✉)
Division of Colorectal Surgery, Department of Surgery, University of Rochester Medical Center, Rochester, NY, USA
e-mail: anthony_loria@urmc.rochester.edu; fergal_fleming@urmc.rochester.edu

K. Umanskiy, N. Hyman (eds.), *Difficult Decisions in Colorectal Surgery*, Difficult Decisions in Surgery: An Evidence-Based Approach,
https://doi.org/10.1007/978-3-031-42303-1_22

Table 22.1 PICO

P (patients)	I (intervention)	C (comparison)	O (outcomes)
T2N0 rectal cancer	TME	Local excision (TEMS, TAMIS)	Morbidity (short-term) Survival (overall, disease free) Patient reported

(TAMIS). The search included "rectal neoplasms," "natural orifice endoscopic surgery," "microsurgery," "minimally invasive surgical procedures," or "watchful waiting" [5]. Representative title or abstract limited terms included "early rectal cancer," "T1 rectal cancer," "T2 rectal cancer," "TEM," "local excision," "TAMIS," "EMR," among others. Non-English and non-comparative studies were excluded. The references were reviewed to identify additional studies not captured in the primary search.

Results

Difficulties in accurately staging early rectal cancer must be acknowledged. Tumor invasion (T) and nodal involvement (N) are assessed by either endorectal ultrasound (EUS) or magnetic resonance imaging (MRI) [4]. Unfortunately, for T2 lesions, MRI over stages 42% and EUS over stages 18% [6–8]. Similarly, accurately detecting nodal involvement is a diagnostic challenge. A meta-analysis found that the sensitivity and specificity for accurately detecting nodal involvement of EUS were 67% and 78%, and for MRI, they were 66% and 76% [6]. Consequently, European guidelines focus heavily on the area where MRI excels, tumor involvement of the circumferential resection margin [9].

TME Works: Why Replace it?

Benchmarking the short-term morbidity, functional, and oncologic outcomes associated with TME and local excision is essential. Expectedly, the short-term morbidity profile favors local excision. In a large retrospective study of 2124 patients with Stage I (T1–2N0) disease, 5.6% of patients who underwent local excision experienced a 30-day complication compared to 14.6% following TME ($p < 0.001$) [10]. Neoadjuvant therapy was less common in the era of those retrospective data, however, multi-institutional, randomized controlled trials suggest the postoperative morbidity following TME alone is higher than patients who receive neoadjuvant chemoradiation and local excision (50.6% vs. 20.7%, $p < 0.001$) [11]. Similarly, in a trial comparing neoadjuvant short-course radiation (SCRT) followed by local excision to TME alone, the rates of serious adverse events among the TME group were significantly higher than those who had SCRT followed by local excision (39% vs. 15%) [12]. Contemporary 30-day mortality rates following TME are low (approximately 1–1.5%), but it is notable that at 3-months post-TME, the mortality rate in four European nations ranged from 5.6–8.3% among patients 80 years or older with stage I rectal cancer [13, 14].

There is limited patient-reported outcome data focused exclusively on patients with T2N0 disease. Among patients with T1N0 disease, one study compared the quality of life of 17 patients who underwent local excision with 18 patients who underwent laparoscopic TME without an ostomy [15]. Questions regarding chemotherapy or stoma-related side effects were discarded, along with those related to sexual dysfunction, reportedly because few patients were sexually active. With these caveats, neither procedure showed a significant difference compared to preoperative status at 12 months in cancer-specific quality of life or colorectal-specific quality of life measured by the European Organization for Research and Treatment of Cancer (EORTC-QLQ-C30 and QLQ-CR38) [15]. Patients cite risk of needing an ostomy as a major concern during rectal cancer therapy. Even among patients with stage one disease, the contemporary rate of abdominoperineal resection is 21.5%, and an additional 12% undergo a Hartmann's procedure [3].

When neoadjuvant or adjuvant therapies are added, the patient-reported outcomes generally favor local excision. A study of patients with cT2–3 tumors (some with nodal involvement) who underwent neoadjuvant chemoradiation followed by local excision had significantly better global health status, emotional function, social function, body image, low anterior resection syndrome (LARS) scores, and fecal incontinence subscale scores compared to those who underwent TME [16]. Similarly, in a multicenter study of a heterogeneous group of patients (T2-T4, N1-N2, some with neoadjuvant therapy) who underwent local excision had significantly better mean constipation scores, less sensation of incomplete emptying, fewer second bowel movements within 15 minutes compared to those who had TME. Interestingly, patients who had local excision alone had the best patient-reported outcomes, followed by those who had a TME, then those who had a completion TME following local excision [17]. Elsewhere, a study comparing 35 patients (T1 n = 25; T2 n = 10) who underwent local excision with or without adjuvant chemotherapy compared to those who underwent TME (n = 32) found that 14.8% of patients who had local excision had LARS compared to 45.5% (p = 0.043) of those who underwent TME [18]. An analysis of the Transanal Endoscopic Microsurgery after Radiochemotherapy for Rectal Cancer (CARTs) study demonstrated that 48–68 months after local excision, 22% (7/32) of patients with cT1-3 N0 rectal cancer had no LARS, 28% (9/32) had minor LARS, and 50% (16/32) had major LARS [19]. Unfortunately, this study did not have LARS scores from before treatment to assess change associated with local excision.

Short-term morbidity and patient-reported outcomes notwithstanding, durable oncologic outcomes are why TME is the standard of care in patients with T2N0 disease [4]. In the Dutch TME trial, patients with Stage I disease (n = 243, cT1–2 N0) randomized to TME alone had a 10-year local recurrence rate of just 3% [20]. Similarly, in the OCUM study, out of 197 patients with cT2N0 disease who went straight to TME, the 5-year locoregional recurrence rate was 1.7% (95% CI, 0–3.7%) and the 5-year disease free survival 75.9% (95% CI, 69.8–82.0%) (personal communication with Professor T Junginger). Conversely, a pooled analysis including patients with a minimum of 3 years of follow-up who underwent local excision found a weighted average rate of local recurrence of 8.1% (n = 268/3050; 95%

confidence interval [CI], 6.6–9.9%) among those with pT1 disease and 28.9% for pT2 disease (n = 136/545; 95% CI, 22.3–36.4%) [5]. For patients who undergo a local excision with completion TME, the weighted local recurrence rate is 1.8% (n = 5/180; 95% CI, 1.2–6.5) for patients with pT1 disease and 4.1% (n = 5/123; 95% CI, 1.7–9.4%) for those with pT2 disease [5]. Finally, for those who underwent adjuvant chemoradiation after TME the weighted local recurrence was 4.8% for pT1 disease (n = 24/285; 95% CI 2.3–9.8%) and 14.7% for pT2 disease (11.2%–19.0%) [5]. In short, excellent surgical technique and high-quality TME are associated with exceptional oncological outcomes, and novel approaches in T2 disease seeking to increase the rates of organ preservation utilizing neoadjuvant therapy and local excision should be held to these standards.

Improving Oncologic Outcomes Associated with Local Excision

Recognizing that the oncologic benefits of TME come with higher rates of short-term morbidity, appreciable colostomy rates, and poorer patient-reported outcomes, investigators sought to improve the oncologic outcomes associated with local excision. Drawn by the successes of chemoradiation in locally advanced rectal cancer, favorable retrospective data, and the high rates of pathologic complete response following TME, the addition of neoadjuvant chemoradiation before local excision was the logical progression of subsequent trials. Here we will compare and contrast one post hoc analysis and randomized controlled trials comparing novel treatment modalities (neoadjuvant chemoradiation [or total neoadjuvant therapy] followed by local excision) to the current standard of care, TME. There are notable single-arm studies reporting oncologic and patient-reported outcomes following CRT followed by local excision or in case of poor response to TME, but these do not directly compare to TME [19, 21].

A post hoc analysis of patients with T2N0 disease from two separate trials was recently published [22]. This study is informative as it contrasts two management philosophies for early rectal cancer. This compared the survival and health-related quality of life between 79 patients with cT2N0 who underwent neoadjuvant chemoradiation (NCRT) followed by local excision (from ACOSOG Z6041) to 79 with pT2N0 who underwent upfront TME (from the Dutch TME trial) [22, 23]. The 5-year rate of local recurrence was 4.2% (CI, 1.4%–12.5%) in the NCRT-local excision group and 1.3% (CI, 0.2%–6.7%) in the TME group (hazard ratio, 5.42; 95% CI, 0.59–49.64, p = 0.14). Similarly, there was no difference between the groups in 5-year disease-free survival (88.2% vs. 88.3%), 5-year overall survival (90.3% vs. 88.4%), or 5-year relative survival (99.8% vs. 100%) [22]. One of the most notable differences between the two therapeutic approaches was the marked difference in sphincter preservation with a permanent ostomy rate of 51% in the subgroup from the Dutch TME trial compared to a 4% ostomy rate from ACOSOG Z6041 [21].

Table 22.2 summarizes the randomized controlled trials comparing neoadjuvant therapy followed by LE with the standard of care (TME) [11, 12, 24]. The randomized controlled trials differ in their inclusion criteria and neoadjuvant regimens but

Table 22.2 Randomized controlled trials comparing novel treatment modalities to standard of care

Study	GRECCAR2 [24]		TREC [12]		TAU-TEM [11]	
Quality	High		High		High	
Inclusion criteria	Responder to NCRT cT2–3 N0–1 ≤8 cm from anal verge, Lesion ≤4 cm diameter		cT1–2 N0 Lesion <3 cm diameter		cT2–3 N0 ≤10 cm of anal verge, lesion <4 cm diameter	
Intervention	TME Vs. Local excision		TME Vs. SCRT (25Gy) followed by local excision in 8–10 weeks		TME Vs. NCRT (DXT 50.4Gy with capecitabine) followed by local excision in 8 weeks	
Intention to treat or modified intention to treat	NCRT-TME (n = 71)	NCRT-LE (n = 74)	TME (n = 28)	SCRT-LE (n = 27)	TME (n = 81)	NCRT-LE (n = 81)
Grade ≥ 3 neoadjuvant toxicity[a]	10% (15/145)		—	15%	—	3.7%
30-day mortality[a]	0%	0%	0%	0%	1.2%	1.2%
30-day morbidity[a]	N = 61 10%	N = 53 6%[b]	39%	15%[b]	50.6%	20.7%[b]
Conversion to TME[a]	—	35%	—	30%	—	2.5%
Organ preservation[a]	12.7%	64%	3%	70%	0%	82.7%
Permanent ostomy[a]	7%	13%	14%	7%	19.8%	0%
pCR[a]	40% (57/141)		0%	26%	—	44.3%
Local recurrence	5 year 7%	5 year 7%	3 year 0%	3 year 11%[b]	N.A.	N.A.
Distant recurrence	19%	18%	7%	11%	N.A.	N.A.
Disease free survival	72%	70%	85%	76%	N.A.	N.A.
Overall survival	82%	84%	93%	88%	N.A.	N.A.
Cancer specific mortality	10%	7%	—	—	—	—

N.A. no oncologic data reported at the time of writing
[a]Short-term GRECCAR2 from PMID 28601342, and completion TME was performed in 27 of the 74 assigned to local excision
[b]Comparison between groups $p < 0.05$

are representative of novel treatment modalities for early rectal cancer. The first study with 5-year oncologic data was GRECCAR 2, which had oncological outcomes as secondary endpoints [24]. Here, adults with T2-T3 low rectal cancers were all treated with long-course neoadjuvant chemoradiation. Those who responded well to the neoadjuvant therapy (≤2 cm residual tumor at a 6–8 week post neoadjuvant MRI) were randomized to local excision or TME 8 weeks after chemotherapy. The 5-year local recurrence, metastasis, overall survival, and cancer-specific mortality were similar between the patients with NCRT+LE and the NCRT+TME groups (Table 22.2).

Neoadjuvant CRT is commonly used but is associated with substantial morbidity and even mortality, as seen in the CARTS study [19]. An alternative investigated in the TREC study is performing neoadjuvant short-course radiation (SCRT) followed by local excision [12]. The TREC study did include non-randomized patients whose treatment was determined by a multidisciplinary tumor board, but we will focus on the randomized patients. In the comparison of 28 patients randomized to TME compared to SCRT followed by TEM, there was no difference in 3-year overall (93% vs. 88%, $p = 0.35$) or 3-year disease-free survival (85% vs. 76%, $p = 0.12$), respectively. The most recent study (TAU-TEM) has published short-term outcomes, but no data are available to date on oncologic outcomes [11].

The high rates of pathologic complete response following neoadjuvant chemoradiation and the mixed data regarding patient-reported outcomes following NCRT + local excision have stimulated further investigation. Ongoing trials such as STAR-TREC (NCT02945566), GRECCAR12 (NCT02514278), OPERA (NCT02505750), and ReSARCh (NCT02710812) among others are assessing whether local excision can be avoided altogether with a watch and wait approach. Currently, there are minimal patient-reported outcomes data regarding the watch and wait strategy. The available studies assess patients with locally advanced rectal cancer and report comparisons between watch and wait to TME. One study compared 21 patients who underwent watch and wait to 21 who underwent sphincter preserving TME. Expectedly, 21 patients who had watch and wait matched to 21 who had TME had better bowel function on all of the subscales of the Memorial Sloan Kettering Cancer Center Bowel Function Instrument [25]. These results are corroborated elsewhere in a study of patients with locally advanced rectal cancer who received watch and wait compared to anterior resection [26]. A more appropriate comparison for patients who undergo watch and wait is to patients who receive local excision.

Recommendations Based on the Data

For a patient with cT2N0 rectal cancer who can tolerate surgery, or a patient where frequent surveillance for tumor recrudescence is impractical or impossible, a high quality TME is recommended to minimize their risk of recurrence and maximize their overall survival (Evidence: strong quality; Recommendation, strong). This is clearly the preferred approach in patients with T2N0 disease from the oncological standpoint.

In highly select patients with cT2N0 rectal cancer with prohibitively high-risk comorbidities or refuse TME, local excision can be considered (Evidence, moderate; Recommendation, weak). These high-risk patients should be carefully surveilled for potential completion TME salvage in the event of recrudescence. (Evidence, high quality; Recommendation, weak).

A Personal View of the Data

T2N0 Rectal Cancer: The Goldilocks Effect

Given the tremendous progress in reducing locoregional recurrence rates, we contend that the pressing issues in T2N0 rectal cancer management are now the risk of distant recurrence, minimizing acute and chronic treatment-related toxicities, and organ preservation. For patients with a T2N0 tumor, TME, often necessitating an abdominoperineal resection, may be 'too much' treatment. Conversely, local excision alone is clearly 'too little' treatment given the very high rates of locoregional recurrence. So, what is the 'just right' amount of therapy to reduce the locoregional risk of recurrence while minimizing toxicity and maximizing organ preservation?

Contemporary rectal cancer care is multidisciplinary and based on shared-decision making. Many patients, even those with a complete clinical response to neoadjuvant therapy, seek the most definitive treatment to "put the disease behind them." For them, a TME even with ypT0N0 is the appropriate treatment. However, it is possible to achieve durable oncologic outcomes and organ preservation using either NCRT-LE or TNT-WW [22, 27, 28]. Consider a 75-year-old male who lives independently with a 2 cm lesion 5 cm from the anal verge under local excision and pathology revealed a T2 tumor with clear margins positive for lymphovascular invasion tumor. The patient is interested in curative treatment but is concerned about complications leading to a loss of independence. In this case scenario without additional therapy, one in four patients (20–25%) will have a locoregional recurrence and 6–13% will have distant metastasis [5]. Adding adjuvant chemoradiation would offer approximately a 50% relative risk reduction in locoregional recurrence (10–12.5%) and distant recurrence (5–10%) [5]. A completion TME reduces the risk of locoregional recurrence to 4–5% and distant recurrence to 5–7% [5]. With proper counseling, we have employed each of these treatment approaches to good effect.

Another scenario is a 60-year-old female with a T2N0 tumor abutting the anal sphincter complex, who is keen to avoid a permanent colostomy, and has declined an upfront abdominoperineal resection. There is a reasonable body of data supporting the deployment of neoadjuvant therapy, possibly followed by local excision (NCRT-LE) ideally via a transanal endoscopic platform. This approach is associated with 60–80% organ preservation rates among patients who met post-treatment response criteria in clinical trials [11, 12, 24]. However, up to 10% of the patients in these studies required completion TME. The challenge of accurately identifying complete clinical responders to neoadjuvant therapy is a drawback of TNT-WW [29]. While NCRT-LE provides some reassurance that residual microscopic disease was removed, the relatively high rates of pathologic complete response in the trials (26–40%) and functional derangements (50% major LARS at 5 years in the CARTS study) highlight the urgent need to improve endoscopic, radiographic, and/or blood-based (ex. circulating cell-free DNA) methods of identifying complete clinical responders [19, 29]. There are very few patient-reported outcomes data comparing patients who had NCRT-LE and TNT-WW, and this area needs investigation. Presently, TNT-WW should be reserved for institutional review board approved protocols and is not the standard of care [30].

In conclusion, the management of early rectal cancer is rapidly advancing, and TME is an excellent option for most patients with T2N0 rectal cancer. Even patients with early disease who could be managed with TME alone should be presented in a tumor board setting adhering to evidence-based standards such as the National Accreditation Program for Rectal Cancer (NAPRC) standards [31]. However, clinicians should prepare for the growing trend toward organ preservation, particularly in light of the increasing adoption of TNT throughout the United States [32]. Surgeons should be at the forefront of investigations into pressing clinical questions regarding patient-reported outcomes, oncologic durability, and logistical or quality issues associated with the widespread implementation of organ preservation programs. Regardless, patients with T2N0 disease must be thoroughly counseled on the diagnostic uncertainty in early rectal cancer and all contemporary management options. If these patients remain highly committed to organ preservation, even potentially at the expense of oncologic outcomes, referral to experienced centers is recommended.

References

1. American Cancer Society. Colorectal Cancer Facts & Figures 2020–2022. Atlanta: American Cancer Society; 2020.
2. Sung H, Ferlay J, Siegel RL, Laversanne M, Soerjomataram I, Jemal A, Bray F. Global cancer statistics 2020: GLOBOCAN estimates of incidence and mortality worldwide for 36 cancers in 185 countries. CA Cancer J Clin. 2021;71(3):209–49. https://doi.org/10.3322/caac.21660. Epub 2021 Feb 4
3. Detering R, van Oostendorp SE, Meyer VM, van Dieren S, Bos ACRK, Dekker JWT, Reerink O, van Waesberghe JHTM, Marijnen CAM, Moons LMG, Beets-Tan RGH, Hompes R, van Westreenen HL, Tanis PJ, Tuynman JB, Dutch ColoRectal Audit Group*. MRIcT1-2 rectal cancer staging accuracy: a population-based study. Br J Surg. 2020;107(10):1372–82. https://doi.org/10.1002/bjs.11590. Epub 2020 Apr 16. PMID: 32297326; PMCID: PMC7496930
4. National Comprehensive Cancer Network. Rectal Cancer (Version 4.2022). https://www.nccn.org/guidelines/guidelines-detail?category=1&id=1461. Accessed Feb 27 2023.
5. van Oostendorp SE, Smits LJH, Vroom Y, Detering R, Heymans MW, Moons LMG, Tanis PJ, de Graaf EJR, Cunningham C, Denost Q, Kusters M, Tuynman JB. Local recurrence after local excision of early rectal cancer: a meta-analysis of completion TME, adjuvant (chemo)radiation, or no additional treatment. Br J Surg. 2020;107(13):1719–30. https://doi.org/10.1002/bjs.12040. Epub 2020 Sep 16. PMID: 32936943; PMCID: PMC7692925
6. Bipat S, Glas AS, Slors FJ, Zwinderman AH, Bossuyt PM, Stoker J. Rectal cancer: local staging and assessment of lymph node involvement with endoluminal US, CT, and MR imaging – a meta-analysis. Radiology. 2004;232(3):773–83. https://doi.org/10.1148/radiol.2323031368. Epub 2004 Jul 23

7. Sauer R, Liersch T, Merkel S, Fietkau R, Hohenberger W, Hess C, Becker H, Raab HR, Villanueva MT, Witzigmann H, Wittekind C, Beissbarth T, Rödel C. Preoperative versus postoperative chemoradiotherapy for locally advanced rectal cancer: results of the German CAO/ARO/AIO-94 randomized phase III trial after a median follow-up of 11 years. J Clin Oncol. 2012;30(16):1926–33. https://doi.org/10.1200/JCO.2011.40.1836. Epub 2012 Apr 23. PMID: 22529255
8. Mercury Study Group. Diagnostic accuracy of preoperative magnetic resonance imaging in predicting curative resection of rectal cancer: prospective observational study. BMJ. 2006;333(7572):779. https://doi.org/10.1136/bmj.38937.646400.55. Epub 2006 Sep 19. PMID: 16984925; PMCID: PMC1602032
9. Glynne-Jones R, Wyrwicz L, Tiret E, Brown G, Rödel C, Cervantes A, Arnold D, ESMO Guidelines Committee. Rectal cancer: ESMO Clinical Practice Guidelines for diagnosis, treatment and follow-up. Ann Oncol. 2018;29(Suppl 4):iv263. https://doi.org/10.1093/annonc/mdy161. Erratum for: Ann Oncol. 2017 Jul 1;28(suppl_4):iv22–iv40
10. You YN, Baxter NN, Stewart A, Nelson H. Is the increasing rate of local excision for stage I rectal cancer in the United States justified?: a nationwide cohort study from the National Cancer Database. Ann Surg. 2007;245(5):726–33. https://doi.org/10.1097/01.sla.0000252590.95116.4f. PMID: 17457165; PMCID: PMC1877081
11. Serra-Aracil X, Pericay C, Badia-Closa J, Golda T, Biondo S, Hernández P, Targarona E, Borda-Arrizabalaga N, Reina A, Delgado S, Vallribera F, Caro A, Gallego-Plazas J, Pascual M, Álvarez-Laso C, Guadalajara-Labajo HG, Mora-Lopez L. Short-term outcomes of chemoradiotherapy and local excision versus total mesorectal excision in T2-T3ab,N0,M0 rectal cancer: a multicentre randomised, controlled, phase III trial (the TAU-TEM study). Ann Oncol. 2023;34(1):78–90. https://doi.org/10.1016/j.annonc.2022.09.160. Epub 2022 Oct 8
12. Bach SP, Gilbert A, Brock K, Korsgen S, Geh I, Hill J, Gill T, Hainsworth P, Tutton MG, Khan J, Robinson J, Steward M, Cunningham C, Levy B, Beveridge A, Handley K, Kaur M, Marchevsky N, Magill L, Russell A, Quirke P, West NP, Sebag-Montefiore D, TREC collaborators. Radical surgery versus organ preservation via short-course radiotherapy followed by transanal endoscopic microsurgery for early-stage rectal cancer (TREC): a randomised, open-label feasibility study. Lancet Gastroenterol Hepatol. 2021;6(2):92–105. https://doi.org/10.1016/S2468-1253(20)30333-2. Epub 2020 Dec 11. PMID: 33308452; PMCID: PMC7802515
13. Ketelaers SHJ, Orsini RG, Burger JWA, Nieuwenhuijzen GAP, Rutten HJT. Significant improvement in postoperative and 1-year mortality after colorectal cancer surgery in recent years. Eur J Surg Oncol. 2019;45(11):2052–8. https://doi.org/10.1016/j.ejso.2019.06.017. Epub 2019 Jun 13
14. Claassen YHM, Bastiaannet E, van Eycken E, Van Damme N, Martling A, Johansson R, Iversen LH, Ingeholm P, Lemmens VEPP, Liefers GJ, Holman FA, Dekker JWT, Portielje JEA, Rutten HJ, van de Velde CJH. Time trends of short-term mortality for octogenarians undergoing a colorectal resection in North Europe. Eur J Surg Oncol. 2019;45(8):1396–402. https://doi.org/10.1016/j.ejso.2019.03.041. Epub 2019 Apr 9
15. Lezoche E, Paganini AM, Fabiani B, Balla A, Vestri A, Pescatori L, Scoglio D, D'Ambrosio G, Lezoche G. Quality-of-life impairment after endoluminal locoregional resection and laparoscopic total mesorectal excision. Surg Endosc. 2014;28(1):227–34. https://doi.org/10.1007/s00464-013-3166-2. Epub 2013 Sep 4
16. Brachet S, Meillat H, Chanez B, Ratone JP, Brunelle S, Tyran M, Poizat F, de Chaisemartin C, Lelong B. Case-matched comparison of functional and quality of life outcomes of local excision and total mesorectal excision following chemoradiotherapy for rectal cancer. Dis Colon Rectum. 2022;65(12):1464–74. https://doi.org/10.1097/DCR.0000000000002384. Epub 2022 Jul 27
17. Pucciarelli S, Giandomenico F, De Paoli A, Gavaruzzi T, Lotto L, Mantello G, Barba C, Zotti P, Flora S, Del Bianco P. Bowel function and quality of life after local excision or total mesorectal excision following chemoradiotherapy for rectal cancer. Br J Surg. 2017;104(1):138–47. https://doi.org/10.1002/bjs.10318. Epub 2016 Oct 5

18. Pacevicius J, Petrauskas V, Pilipavicius L, Dulskas A. Local excision ± Chemoradiotherapy vs. Total Mesorectal excision for early rectal cancer: case-matched analysis of long-term results. Front Surg. 2021;18(8):746784. https://doi.org/10.3389/fsurg.2021.746784. PMID: 34733880; PMCID: PMC8558343
19. Stijns RCH, de Graaf EJR, Punt CJA, Nagtegaal ID, Nuyttens JJME, van Meerten E, Tanis PJ, de Hingh IHJT, van der Schelling GP, Acherman Y, Leijtens JWA, Bremers AJA, Beets GL, Hoff C, Verhoef C, Marijnen CAM, de Wilt JHW, CARTS Study Group. Long-term oncological and functional outcomes of Chemoradiotherapy followed by organ-sparing Transanal endoscopic microsurgery for distal rectal cancer: the CARTS study. JAMA Surg. 2019;154(1):47–54. https://doi.org/10.1001/jamasurg.2018.3752. PMID: 30304338; PMCID: PMC6439861
20. van Gijn W, Marijnen CA, Nagtegaal ID, Kranenbarg EM, Putter H, Wiggers T, Rutten HJ, Påhlman L, Glimelius B, Van de Velde CJ. Dutch colorectal cancer group. Preoperative radiotherapy combined with total mesorectal excision for resectable rectal cancer: 12-year follow-up of the multicentre, randomised controlled TME trial. Lancet Oncol. 2011;12(6):575–82. https://doi.org/10.1016/S1470-2045(11)70097-3. Epub 2011 May 17
21. Garcia-Aguilar J, Renfro LA, Chow OS, Shi Q, Carrero XW, Lynn PB, Thomas CR Jr, Chan E, Cataldo PA, Marcet JE, Medich DS, Johnson CS, Oommen SC, Wolff BG, Pigazzi A, SM MN, Pons RK, Bleday R. Organ preservation for clinical T2N0 distal rectal cancer using neoadjuvant chemoradiotherapy and local excision (ACOSOG Z6041): results of an open-label, single-arm, multi-institutional, phase 2 trial. Lancet Oncol. 2015;16(15):1537–46. https://doi.org/10.1016/S1470-2045(15)00215-6. Epub 2015 Oct 22. PMID: 26474521; PMCID: PMC4984260
22. Lynn PB, Van der Valk MJM, Claassen YHM, Shi Q, Widmar M, Bastiaannet E, Van de Velde CJH, Garcia-Aguilar J. Chemoradiation and local excision versus total mesorectal excision for T2N0 rectal cancer: comparison of short- and long-term outcomes from 2 prospective studies. Ann Surg. 2023;277(1):e96–e102. https://doi.org/10.1097/SLA.0000000000005052. Epub 2021 Jul 2. PMID: 34225302; PMCID: PMC8658950
23. Kapiteijn E, Marijnen CA, Nagtegaal ID, Putter H, Steup WH, Wiggers T, Rutten HJ, Pahlman L, Glimelius B, van Krieken JH, Leer JW, van de Velde CJ, Dutch Colorectal Cancer Group. Preoperative radiotherapy combined with total mesorectal excision for resectable rectal cancer. N Engl J Med. 2001;345(9):638–46. https://doi.org/10.1056/NEJMoa010580.
24. Rullier E, Vendrely V, Asselineau J, Rouanet P, Tuech JJ, Valverde A, de Chaisemartin C, Rivoire M, Trilling B, Jafari M, Portier G, Meunier B, Sieleznieff I, Bertrand M, Marchal F, Dubois A, Pocard M, Rullier A, Smith D, Frulio N, Frison E, Denost Q. Organ preservation with chemoradiotherapy plus local excision for rectal cancer: 5-year results of the GRECCAR 2 randomised trial. Lancet Gastroenterol Hepatol. 2020;5(5):465–74. https://doi.org/10.1016/S2468-1253(19)30410-8. Epub 2020 Feb 7
25. Quezada-Diaz FF, Smith JJ, Jimenez-Rodriguez RM, Wasserman I, Pappou EP, Patil S, Wei IH, Nash GM, Guillem JG, Weiser MR, Paty PB, Garcia-Aguilar J. Patient-reported bowel function in patients with rectal cancer managed by a watch-and-wait strategy after neoadjuvant therapy: a case-control study. Dis Colon Rectum. 2020;63(7):897–902. https://doi.org/10.1097/DCR.0000000000001646. PMID: 32217857; PMCID: PMC7274891
26. Pascual-Russo A, Milito D, Facio L, Furia M, Forestier V, Iseas S, Méndez G, Coraglio M, Lumi CM, Masciangioli G, Mauriño E, Vázquez H. Better quality of life and reduced fecal incontinence in rectal cancer patients with the watch-and-wait follow-up strategy. Rev Gastroenterol Mex (Engl Ed). 2020 Aug 28:S0375-0906(20)30090-2. English, Spanish. https://doi.org/10.1016/j.rgmx.2020.06.0.
27. Garcia-Aguilar J, Patil S, Gollub MJ, Kim JK, Yuval JB, Thompson HM, Verheij FS, Omer DM, Lee M, Dunne RF, Marcet J, Cataldo P, Polite B, Herzig DO, Liska D, Oommen S, Friel CM, Ternent C, Coveler AL, Hunt S, Gregory A, Varma MG, Bello BL, Carmichael JC, Krauss J, Gleisner A, Paty PB, Weiser MR, Nash GM, Pappou E, Guillem JG, Temple L, Wei IH, Widmar M, Lin S, Segal NH, Cercek A, Yaeger R, Smith JJ, Goodman KA, Wu AJ, Saltz

LB. Organ preservation in patients with rectal adenocarcinoma treated with Total neoadjuvant therapy. J Clin Oncol. 2022;40(23):2546–56. https://doi.org/10.1200/JCO.22.00032. Epub 2022 Apr 28. PMID: 35483010; PMCID: PMC9362876

28. Fernandez LM, São Julião GP, Figueiredo NL, Beets GL, van der Valk MJM, Bahadoer RR, Hilling DE, Meershoek-Klein Kranenbarg E, Roodvoets AGH, Renehan AG, van de Velde CJH, Habr-Gama A, Perez RO, International Watch & Wait Database Consortium. Conditional recurrence-free survival of clinical complete responders managed by watch and wait after neoadjuvant chemoradiotherapy for rectal cancer in the International Watch & Wait Database: a retrospective, international, multicentre registry study. Lancet Oncol. 2021;22(1):43–50. https://doi.org/10.1016/S1470-2045(20)30557-X. Epub 2020 Dec 11
29. Nagtegaal ID, Glynne-Jones R. How to measure tumour response in rectal cancer? An explanation of discrepancies and suggestions for improvement. Cancer Treat Rev. 2020;84:101964. https://doi.org/10.1016/j.ctrv.2020.101964. Epub 2020 Jan 17
30. You YN, Hardiman KM, Bafford A, Poylin V, Francone TD, Davis K, Paquette IM, Steele SR, Feingold DL. On behalf of the clinical practice guidelines Committee of the American Society of colon and Rectal surgeons. The American Society of Colon and Rectal Surgeons clinical practice guidelines for the management of rectal cancer. Dis Colon Rectum. 2020;63(9):1191–222. https://doi.org/10.1097/DCR.0000000000001762.
31. Commission on Cancer National Accreditation Program for Rectal Cancer. Optimal Resources for Rectal Cancer Care: 2020 Standards. Accessed January 20, 2023.
32. Liu J, Ladbury C, Glaser S, Fakih M, Kaiser AM, Chen YJ, Williams TM, Amini A. Patterns of care for patients with locally advanced rectal cancer treated with total neoadjuvant therapy at predominately academic centers between 2016–2020: An NCDB Analysis. Clin Colorectal Cancer. 2023;5:S1533. https://doi.org/10.1016/j.clcc.2023.01.005. Epub ahead of print

Watch and Wait Versus Conventional Surgical Treatment in Rectal Cancer

23

Felipe F. Quezada-Diaz and J. Joshua Smith

Introduction

The standard of care for locally advanced rectal cancer (LARC) includes neoadjuvant long-course chemoradiotherapy (LCRT), total mesorectal excision (TME) and postoperative adjuvant chemotherapy [1]. However, over the past 2 decades, the treatment of locally advanced rectal cancer (LARC) has evolved in an attempt to balance between better survival outcomes and reducing long-term sequelae on the patient's quality of life (QoL) due to the toxicities associated with neoadjuvant treatment (NAT) [2].

Up to 20% of LARC patients treated with LCRT alone may develop a pathological complete response (i.e. absence of residual tumor cells at either the primary tumor site and the mesorectal nodes, pCR), but this can be as high as 40% in those treated with concomitant consolidative chemotherapy given after LCRT [3]. Patients with a pCR have improved survival rates, with lower than 5% of distant metastasis and 1% of locoregional failure [4].

Disclosure: Dr. Smith received travel funding from Intuitive Surgical Inc. (2015) and served as a clinical advisor for Guardant Health Inc. (2019) and Foundation Medicine Inc. (2022). He served as a consultant and speaker for Johnson & Johnson Inc. (2022) and GSK (2023).

F. F. Quezada-Diaz
Colorectal Unit, Department of Surgery, Complejo Asistencial Doctor Sótero del Río, Santiago, RM, Chile

J. J. Smith (✉)
Colorectal Service, Department of Surgery, Memorial Sloan Kettering Cancer Center, New York, NY, USA
e-mail: smithj5@mskcc.org

K. Umanskiy, N. Hyman (eds.), *Difficult Decisions in Colorectal Surgery*, Difficult Decisions in Surgery: An Evidence-Based Approach, https://doi.org/10.1007/978-3-031-42303-1_23

Given higher rates of tumor response with some NAT modalities, the need of TME in patients who achieve a pCR has been questioned, especially when surgery is associated with late bowel, sexual and genitourinary sequelae that significantly impairs the QoL of patients [5, 6].

A Watch-and-Wait strategy (WW) for rectal cancer has been advocated as a treatment alternative for selected LARC patients who achieved a clinical complete response (i.e., absence of detectable macroscopic tumor by clinical means, cCR). The implementation of a WW strategy depends on solving current challenges such as how to correctly identify the best candidates without compromising oncologic safety.

PICO table

Patients	Intervention	Comparator	Outcomes
Patients with locally advanced rectal cancer treated with Neoadjuvant Therapy	Clinical and Pathological Complete Response (cCR & pCR)	Total Mesorectal Excision	Organ preservation, overall/ disease specific survival, rate of local/systemic recurrence, quality of life

Search Strategy

A comprehensive literature search of Cochrane Database of Collected Research, EMBASE, MEDLINE, and PubMed was performed to identify all the English-language publications related to locally advanced rectal cancer treated with neoadjuvant therapy and watch and wait/organ preservation strategy from January 2004 until February 2023. The search term strategy included "rectal cancer", "neoadjuvant treatment", "organ preservation", "complete clinical response", "watch and wait" and "quality of life". We excluded studies that did not inform rates of watch and wait/organ preservation and included only rate of pathological complete response.

The references of the included studies were reviewed to identify additional studies that were incorporated as appropriate.

Results

Over the last 2 decades, several studies have reported a WW strategy for patients with LARC after NAT. Most of the data are retrospective case series with the methodological limitations associated with these types of studies [7–15]. A randomized controlled trial that compares a WW strategy versus TME after achieving a cCR after NAT is unlikely to be completed or accepted by patients, mainly due the higher rate of patients that refuse to undergo TME after achieving a cCR. According to patient-perspective focused studies, 83% of patients would consider a WW strategy if they achieved a cCR in spite of the potentially higher rate of local regrowth during the first 2 years of follow-up [16], with up to 30% of patients willing to sacrifice rates of long-term oncological cure in comparison with clinicians [17].

Several definitions of cCR and pCR exist and have been utilized in both case series and trials. While stricter criteria may increase the accuracy of individual patients selected for the WW strategy, more liberal criteria may risk worsening oncological outcomes. There is only one RCT that validated the use of a three-tier regression schema to assess response after NAT [18], including digital rectal exam, magnetic resonance imaging (MRI), and endoscopy. All 3 modalities combined report an accuracy of 98% to predict absence of tumor [19].

Enhancing response rates to NAT may be associated with higher number of patients undergoing WW. There is no consensus about which is the best way to enhance NAT response in LARC. Potential strategies that can be used include: (1) dose escalation of preoperative radiation therapy, (2) increasing the interval period after NAT and surgery and (3) administering consolidation chemotherapy after LCRT or SCRT rather than induction chemotherapy followed by LCRT.

Radiotherapy dose escalation strategies have utilized external beam radiotherapy, brachytherapy, contact radiotherapy and proton/iron beam radiotherapy. A report of nearly 3300 patients showed that the dose of NAT was a predictor of pCR [20]. Additionally, neoadjuvant brachytherapy or external radiation therapy boost did not add a significant benefit in survival or local recurrence when given after standard NA treatment and TME [21, 22]. The recent phase III OPERA trial that included early low rectal cancer (cT2, cT3a, cT3b with nodes smaller 8 mm), showed a 3-year organ preservation rate of 68% (CI 95% 54% to 85%) for tumors greater that 3 cm when treated with chemoradiotherapy and a prior boost of contact x-ray brachytherapy versus external beam boost [23]. A higher rate of 3-year organ preservation rate (97%) was observed in smaller tumors (<3 cm), but the benefit over local excision alone must be evaluated. In addition, this local therapy is associated with significant brachytherapy-induced rectal bleeding which requires local ablative intervention during the first 3 years post-treatment.

A longer delay interval between NAT and surgery is associated with higher rates of pCR/cCR. The Stockholm III trial showed that waiting 4 to 8 weeks after SCRT was associated with similar tumor regression rates compared to LCRT [24]. An analysis of a National Cancer Database including stage II and III rectal cancer patients undergoing LCRT suggested that any surgery interval longer than 8 weeks had higher odds of pCR (odd ratio 1.12, 95% CI 1.01 to 1.25) [25].

The concept of Total Neoadjuvant Therapy (TNT) implies the use of either SCRT or LCRT and moving the adjuvant dose of systemic chemotherapy into the realm of NA treatment. It seems that using a consolidation chemotherapy- based total neoadjuvant therapy (TNT) approach is associated with higher rates of response and organ preservation than using induction chemotherapy. The phase II German trial CAO/ARO/AIO-12 compared 4 cycles of FOLFOX before (induction) or after (consolidation) LCRT. They reported 17% (induction) and 25% (consolidation) pathological complete response rates, respectively [26]. Long term follow-up of this cohort showed similar results in favor of LCRT followed by consolidation chemotherapy as the preferred TNT sequence, especially if organ preservation is a priority [27]. Although no WW was offered, patients in the experimental arm of the RAPIDO Trial (SCRT followed by consolidation systemic chemotherapy) had higher rates of pCR (27.7% vs 13.8%, p-value<0,001) [28]. Updated 5-year data on the RAPIDO Trial showed that the experimental arm was associated with an increased risk of locoregional recurrence (10 vs 6%, p = 0.027) whereas the reduction in disease-related treatment failure and distant metastases remained similar [29]. The OPRA trial, in which patients were randomized to induction or consolidation TNT and then proceeded to surgery or WW depending on response, showed higher rates of organ preservation in the consolidation arm (58% vs 43%; P 0.01) [18]. These data suggest that higher rates of patients managed with WW may be achieved if consolidation chemotherapy is used over induction chemotherapy followed by LCRT. There is scarce evidence about the use of SCRT and consolidation chemotherapy as a WW strategy. In the STELLAR Trial which compared LARC patients treated with SCRT plus 4 cycles of CAPOX versus chemoradiation, 11.1% of patients in the TNT group had a cCR with almost all of them (9.4%) undergoing WW [30]. The early data of the phase II STAR-TREC Trial that compares TME vs SCRT-based organ preservation vs LCRT-based organ preservation strategies showed promising results with a 60% of organ preservation at 12 months [31]. A non-randomized single arm trial demonstrated that SCRT followed by 8 cycles of FOLFOX was associated with 68% a cCR at 1 year follow up [15]. Mismatch repair deficient tumors are have demonstrated better rates of response to NAT specifically to PD-1 blockade used in place of cytotoxic chemotherapy [32]. A summary of the most relevant WW studies incorporating a WW approach is presented in Table 23.1.

Neoadjuvant treatment, especially pelvic radiotherapy, may significantly affect the QoL in WW patients. In the Memorial Sloan Kettering published experience, WW patients report better bowel function when measured by the Memorial Sloan Kettering Cancer Center Bowel Function Instrument [33]. Hupkens et al., compared 47 WW patients with 41 patients after NAT and TME, showed that QoL was better in the WW group [34], but a third of the WW patients experienced major low anterior resection syndrome (LARS) as measured by the LARS Score.

Table 23.1 Summary of important WW studies for LARC patients treated with NAT

Study	n	NAT strategy	Study design	Regrowth, n(%)	Overall survival, (WW vs TME)	Quality of evidence
Habr-Gama et al., 2004 [7]	265	LCRT	Retrospective 71 (26.8%) cCR	2 (3%)	100% vs 88%	Low
Smith et al., 2012 [8]	79	LCRT	Retrospective 32 cCR vs 57 pCR	6 (18.8%)	97% vs 100%	Low
Habr-Gama et al., 2014 [9]	183	LCRT	Retrospective 90 (49%) cCR	28 (31%)	WW only OS: 91% DFS: 68%	Low
Appelt et al., 2015 [43]	51	LCRT (includes brachytherapy)	Prospective 40(78.4%) cCR	9 (22.5%)	WW Only OS: 100% DFS: 70%	Moderate
Lai et al., 2016 [11]	44 cCR	LCRT	Retrospective 18 WW vs 26 cCR TME	2(11%)	1005 vs 92.3%	Low
Martens et al., 2016 [10]	100	LRCT: 95% SCRT: 5%	Retrospective 82 (82%) 61 initial cCR 21 initial nCR	15(15%)	WW Only OS: 96.6% DFS: 80.6%	Low
Rebehan et al., OnCore, 2016 [44]	259	LCRT	Propensity Match 129 WW	44(34%)	96% vs 87%	Moderate
IWWD Consortium, 2018 [12]	1009	LCRT: 91%	Retrospective 808 cCR included	222 (25.2%)	WW only OS: 85% DFS: 94%	Low
Smith et al., 2019 [13]	249	LCRT: 31(27%) Induction: 47(42%) Consolidation: 33 (29%) Chemotherapy alone: 2(2%)	Retrospective 113 WW vs 136 pCR	22 (19.5%)	73% vs 94%	Low
Jimenez-Rodriguez et al., 2021 [14]	88	TNT Induction Chemotherapy (FOLFOX) + LCRT	Retrospective 32 cCR	2 (6%)	5-year overall survival HR 0.212 (95% CI 0.26-1.71, p=NS)	Low

(continued)

Table 23.1 (continued)

Study	n	NAT strategy	Study design	Regrowth, n(%)	Overall survival, (WW vs TME)	Quality of evidence
Kim et al., 2021 [15]	19	TNT SCRT + Consolidation chemotherapy	Retrospective 15 cCR 4 TME	5 (33.3%)	93% vs 67%	Very Low
Garcia-Aguilar et al., OPRA Trial, 2022 [18]	304	TNT Induction Chemotherapy + LCRT: 146 TNT LCRT + consolidation chemotherapy: 158	RCT 225 cCR Induction group: 105 Consolidation group: 120	75 Induction: 42/105 Consolidation: 33/120	DFS: 78% (Induction) vs 77% (Consolidation) Comparable OS	High
Bach et al., STAR-TREC Phase II, 2022 [31]	120	Organ Preservation: 80 (LCRT: 40/SCRT:40) TME: 40	RCT Organ Preservation: 48(60%)	NA	DFS 75.1% vs 91.2%	High
Cercek et al., 2022 [45]	12	Immunotherapy (Dorstalimab)	RCT 12 cCR (100%), only MMR deficient tumors	None (follow up 6 to 25 months)	100% (follow up 6 to 25 months)	High
Gerard et al., OPERA Trial, 2023 [23]	148	LCRT + External Beam Boost: 74 LCRT + Contact X-Ray Brachytherapy: 74	RCT External Beam Boost: 59% Contact X-Ray Brachytherapy: 81%	23% External Beam 15% Contact X-Ray Brachytherapy:	98% both groups	High

SCRT Short Course Radiotherapy, *LCRT* Long Course Radiotherapy, *OS* Overall Survival, *DFS* Disease Free survival, *IWWD* International Watch and Wait Database, *TNT* Total Neoadjuvant Therapy

Recommendation

WW should be part of the treatment discussion of LARC, considering increasing rates of cCR with new modalities of NAT, potential quality of life gains, avoidance of surgical morbidity, and patient preferences (evidence quality moderate, strong recommendation).

WW should be offered ideally in the context of a prospective trial, if possible, with a strict protocol and objective assessment standards (evidence quality moderate, strong recommendation). Currently,there are four ongoing trials incorporating WW for mismatch repair proficient tumors in the US, Europe, South America and Japan [35–37] (Table 23.2).

A standardized method for LARC response after NAT should be used, preferably the three-tiered regression schema from the OPRA trial which includes digital rectal exam, MRI and endoscopy (evidence quality moderate, weak recommendation).

For patients with LARC who want to maximize the rate of organ preservation, TNT-based on chemoradiation followed by consolidation chemotherapy should be recommended (evidence quality high, strong recommendation).

Patients with LARC and MMR-deficient tumors, immunotherapy should be considered as part of initial treatment with all patients with rectal cancer undergoing

Table 23.2 Ongoing rectal cancer Phase III RCT with cCR and WW approach as primary outcomes

Study	Estimated enrollment	Study design	Primary outcome	Secondary outcome
Yoshino et al., ENSEMBLE Trial [35]	608	TNT (SCRT + consolidation CAPOX vs SCRT + consolidation CAPOXIRI)	Organ Preservation adapted DFS at 3 years	ccR rate, recurrence(type), OS, distant metastases rate, QoL
Smith et al. (JANUS Trial [36]	312	TNT (LCRT + consolidation mFOLFOX6 vs LCRT + consolidation mFOLFIRINOX)	cCR rate at 5 years	DFS, Organ Preservation, OS, adverse events
Rödel et al., ACO/ARO/ AIO 18.1. Trial [37]	702	TNT (SCRT + Consolidation chemotherapy vs LCRT + Consolidation chemotherapy)	Organ preservation at 3 years	DFS, cCR, rate TME, local regrowth, rate salvage TME, local recurrence after TME, QoL
Habr-Gama A & Perez RO et al., CCHOWW Trial [45]	216 patients	TNT (LCRT + consolidation 4 cycles mFOLFOX6 or XELOX vs LCRT + consolidation 4 cycles capecitabine)	Decision to WW due to cCR/ near-complete response at 18 weeks from last date radiation	Surgery-free survival, TME-free survival, distant metastases free survival at 3 years, local regrowth-free survival and colostomy-free survival (all at 3 years)

SCRT Short Course Radiotherapy, *LCRT* Long Course Radiotherapy, *OS* Overall Survival, *DFS* Disease Free survival, *TNT* Total Neoadjuvant Therapy, *cCR* complete clinical response, *TME* Total Mesorrectal excision, *QoL* Quality of Life molecular determination of mismatch repair status prior to starting neoadjuvant therapy (evidence quality high, strong recommendation).

Personal View

Organ preservation is a valid treatment strategy for patients, who are willing to accept potentially worse oncological outcomes to achieve this goal. This approach is also in demand by patients and should be part of the modern colorectal surgeon's lexicon when treating and managing patients with rectal cancer.

Our strong preference is that a WW approach is completed in the context of a clinical trial if possible. Typical WW candidates usually are patients with mid-to-distal rectal adenocarcinomas considered for abdominoperineal resections preoperatively or very low stapled/handsewn colorectal/coloanal anastomoses which may significantly alter their QoL due to post-operative bowel dysfunction or permanent colostomy [38].

Currently, the most important challenge in WW is the correct selection of patients with cCR after NAT. In the perfect scenario, the correlation between patients with a pCR and cCR should be highly accurate before undergoing TME to safely offer WW. Real world data shows that up to 25–30% of patients with a cCR experienced a regrowth of the primary tumor [12], most of them during the first 2 years of follow up. Notably, up to 15% of patients with an cCR end up having a pCR [7, 19] in the pathology report.

One of the major uncertainties of WW is the long-term oncologic results [39]. Systematic reviews showed a local regrowth rate between 15.7% and 30% and that surgical salvage was not feasible in less that 5–8% of the patients [40, 41]. The International Watch and Wait Database (IWWD) [12] reported a 2-year cumulative incidence of local regrowth of 25.2%, with most of them diagnosed within the initial 2 years of surveillance. The available data from the OPRA trial shows that salvage surgery for those with local regrowth is feasible, that the oncologic outcomes are similar for those who underwent TME upfront versus at salvage for regrowth and that sphincter preservation rates were similar whether patients underwent TME upfront vs. at salvage (ref OPRA here) – the 5-year updates for this trial show stability on all outcomes reported at 3 years (data reported at ASCO 2023, Verheij F et al.).

An important concern in patients with apparent cCR, is a potential higher rate of distant metastasis after tumor regrowth. Data from a 10-year experience at Memorial hospital suggest a higher rate of distant metastases in patients with local regrowth when compared to those without local regrowth [13]. Data from the IWWD suggests the same pattern between local regrowth and distant metastases [12]. Jimenez-Rodriguez et al. reported a lower rate of local regrowth (6%) in patients treated with induction TNT by a single surgeon that actively performed WW [14]. Another publication from the IWWD showed that development of local regrowth at any time is a risk factor for distant metastases with this risk remaining higher for 5 years after development of local regrowth [42]. Still, whether removing the primary tumor after completion of NAT would have mitigated this risk is unknown, but this finding urges us to develop a WW strategy as part of a standardized clinical protocol. Data from prospective trials will better inform us on this subject and it is notable that the introduction of a WW strategy in OPRA was not associated with any oncologic detriment for the patients in either arm.

WW is a valid and feasible strategy for selected LARC patients, with the challenge still to identify sustained responders by clinical assessment. The OPRA trial was the first to integrate WW into a TNT strategy aimed at increasing response rates, but most of the current evidence for WW is retrospective, making prospectively collected data of great value. NOM or WW strategies should be part of the treatment discussion of LARC, considering patient interest, patient preference and acceptance of risk, along with the possible reduction in morbidity with avoidance of TME. Currently, the best way for patients to utilize WW strategies is in the context of a prospective trial, if possible, with a strict protocol and objective assessment standards.

References

1. National Comprehensive Cancer Network. NCCN guidelines: rectal cancer. [Internet]. [cited 2019 Jan 11]. Available from: www.nccn.org/professionals/physician_gls/pdf/rectal.pdf.
2. Smith JJ, Chow OS, Gollub MJ, Nash GM, Temple LK, Weiser MR, et al. Organ preservation in rectal adenocarcinoma: a phase II randomized controlled trial evaluating 3-year disease-free survival in patients with locally advanced rectal cancer treated with chemoradiation plus induction or consolidation chemotherapy, and total mesorectal excision or nonoperative management. BMC Cancer. 2015;15:767.
3. Garcia-Aguilar J, Chow OS, Smith DD, Marcet JE, Cataldo PA, Varma MG, et al. Effect of adding mFOLFOX6 after neoadjuvant chemoradiation in locally advanced rectal cancer: a multicentre, phase 2 trial. Lancet Oncol. 2015;16:957–66.
4. Maas M, Nelemans PJ, Valentini V, Das P, Rödel C, Kuo L-J, et al. Long-term outcome in patients with a pathological complete response after chemoradiation for rectal cancer: a pooled analysis of individual patient data. Lancet Oncol. 2010;11:835–44.
5. Ho VP, Lee Y, Stein SL, Temple LKF. Sexual function after treatment for rectal cancer: a review. Dis Colon Rectum. 2011;54:113–25.
6. Chen TY-T, Wiltink LM, Nout RA, Meershoek-Klein Kranenbarg E, Laurberg S, Marijnen CAM, et al. Bowel function 14 years after preoperative short-course radiotherapy and total mesorectal excision for rectal cancer: report of a multicenter randomized trial. Clin Colorectal Cancer. 2015;14:106–14.
7. Habr-Gama A, Perez RO, Nadalin W, Sabbaga J, Ribeiro U, Silva e Sousa AH, et al. Operative versus nonoperative treatment for stage 0 distal rectal cancer following chemoradiation therapy: long-term results. Ann Surg. 2004;240:711–7; discussion 717–718
8. Smith JD, Ruby JA, Goodman KA, Saltz LB, Guillem JG, Weiser MR, et al. Nonoperative management of rectal cancer with complete clinical response after neoadjuvant therapy. Ann Surg. 2012;256:965–72.
9. Habr-Gama A, Gama-Rodrigues J, São Julião GP, Proscurshim I, Sabbagh C, Lynn PB, et al. Local recurrence after complete clinical response and watch and wait in rectal cancer after neoadjuvant chemoradiation: impact of salvage therapy on local disease control. Int J Radiat Oncol Biol Phys. 2014;88:822–8.
10. Martens MH, Maas M, Heijnen LA, Lambregts DMJ, Leijtens JWA, Stassen LPS, et al. Long-term outcome of an organ preservation program after neoadjuvant treatment for rectal cancer. J Natl Cancer Inst. 2016;108:djw171.

11. Lai C-L, Lai M-J, Wu C-C, Jao S-W, Hsiao C-W. Rectal cancer with complete clinical response after neoadjuvant chemoradiotherapy, surgery, or "watch and wait". Int J Color Dis. 2016;31:413–9.
12. van der Valk MJM, Hilling DE, Bastiaannet E, Kranenbarg EM-K, Beets GL, Figueiredo NL, et al. Long-term outcomes of clinical complete responders after neoadjuvant treatment for rectal cancer in the International Watch & Wait Database (IWWD): an international multicentre registry study. Lancet. 2018;391:2537–45.
13. Smith JJ, Strombom P, Chow OS, Roxburgh CS, Lynn P, Eaton A, et al. Assessment of a Watch-and-Wait Strategy for Rectal Cancer in Patients With a Complete Response After Neoadjuvant Therapy. JAMA Oncol. 2019;5:e185896.
14. Jimenez-Rodriguez RM, Quezada-Diaz F, Hameed I, Kalabin A, Patil S, Smith JJ, et al. Organ preservation in patients with rectal cancer treated with total neoadjuvant therapy. Dis Colon Rectum. 2021;64:1463–70.
15. Kim H, Pedersen K, Olsen JR, Mutch MG, Chin R-I, Glasgow SC, et al. Nonoperative rectal cancer management with short-course radiation followed by chemotherapy: a nonrandomized control trial. Clin Colorectal Cancer. 2021;20:e185–93.
16. Gani C, Gani N, Zschaeck S, Eberle F, Schaeffeler N, Hehr T, et al. Organ preservation in rectal cancer: the patients' perspective. Front Oncol. 2019;9:318.
17. Kennedy ED, Borowiec AM, Schmocker S, Cho C, Brierley J, Li S, et al. Patient and physician preferences for nonoperative management for low rectal cancer: is it a reasonable treatment option? Dis Colon Rectum. 2018;61:1281–9.
18. Garcia-Aguilar J, Patil S, Gollub MJ, Kim JK, Yuval JB, Thompson HM, et al. Organ preservation in patients with rectal adenocarcinoma treated with total neoadjuvant therapy. J Clin Oncol. 2022;40:2546–56.
19. Maas M, Lambregts DMJ, Nelemans PJ, Heijnen LA, Martens MH, Leijtens JWA, et al. Assessment of clinical complete response after chemoradiation for rectal cancer with digital rectal examination, endoscopy, and MRI: selection for organ-saving treatment. Ann Surg Oncol. 2015;22:3873–80.
20. Hall MD, Schultheiss TE, Smith DD, Fakih MG, Wong JYC, Chen Y-J. Effect of increasing radiation dose on pathologic complete response in rectal cancer patients treated with neoadjuvant chemoradiation therapy. Acta Oncol. 2016;55:1392–9.
21. Appelt AL, Vogelius IR, Pløen J, Rafaelsen SR, Lindebjerg J, Havelund BM, et al. Long-term results of a randomized trial in locally advanced rectal cancer: no benefit from adding a brachytherapy boost. Int J Radiat Oncol Biol Phys. 2014;90:110–8.
22. Couwenberg AM, Burbach JPM, Berbee M, Lacle MM, Arensman R, Raicu MG, et al. Efficacy of dose-escalated chemoradiation on complete tumor response in patients with locally advanced rectal cancer (RECTAL-BOOST): a phase 2 randomized controlled trial. Int J Radiat Oncol Biol Phys. 2020;108:1008–18.
23. Gerard J-P, Barbet N, Schiappa R, Magné N, Martel I, Mineur L, et al. Neoadjuvant chemoradiotherapy with radiation dose escalation with contact x-ray brachytherapy boost or external beam radiotherapy boost for organ preservation in early cT2-cT3 rectal adenocarcinoma (OPERA): a phase 3, randomised controlled trial. Lancet Gastroenterol Hepatol. 2023; https://doi.org/10.1016/S2468-1253(22)00392-2.
24. Pettersson D, Lörinc E, Holm T, Iversen H, Cedermark B, Glimelius B, et al. Tumour regression in the randomized Stockholm III trial of radiotherapy regimens for rectal cancer. Br J Surg. 2015;102:972–8. discussion 978
25. Probst CP, Becerra AZ, Aquina CT, Tejani MA, Wexner SD, Garcia-Aguilar J, et al. Extended intervals after neoadjuvant therapy in locally advanced rectal cancer: the key to improved tumor response and potential organ preservation. J Am Coll Surg. 2015;221:430–40.
26. Fokas E, Allgäuer M, Polat B, Klautke G, Grabenbauer GG, Fietkau R, et al. Randomized phase II trial of chemoradiotherapy plus induction or consolidation chemotherapy as total neoadjuvant therapy for locally advanced rectal cancer: CAO/ARO/AIO-12. J Clin Oncol. 2019;37:3212–22.

27. Fokas E, Schlenska-Lange A, Polat B, Klautke G, Grabenbauer GG, Fietkau R, et al. Chemoradiotherapy plus induction or consolidation chemotherapy as total neoadjuvant therapy for patients with locally advanced rectal cancer: long-term results of the CAO/ARO/AIO-12 Randomized Clinical Trial. JAMA Oncol. 2021;8:e215445.
28. Bahadoer RR, Dijkstra EA, van Etten B, Marijnen CAM, Putter H, Kranenbarg EM-K, et al. Short-course radiotherapy followed by chemotherapy before total mesorectal excision (TME) versus preoperative chemoradiotherapy, TME, and optional adjuvant chemotherapy in locally advanced rectal cancer (RAPIDO): a randomised, open-label, phase 3 trial. Lancet Oncol. 2021;22:29–42.
29. Dijkstra EA, Nilsson PJ, Hospers GAP, Bahadoer RR, Meershoek-Klein Kranenbarg E, Roodvoets AGH, et al. Locoregional failure during and after short-course radiotherapy followed by chemotherapy and surgery compared to long-course chemoradiotherapy and surgery – a five-year follow-up of the RAPIDO trial. Ann Surg. 2023; https://doi.org/10.1097/SLA.0000000000005799.
30. Jin J, Tang Y, Hu C, Jiang L-M, Jiang J, Li N, et al. Multicenter, randomized, phase III trial of short-term radiotherapy plus chemotherapy versus long-term chemoradiotherapy in locally advanced rectal cancer (STELLAR). J Clin Oncol. 2022;40:1681–92.
31. Bach SP, de Wilt JHW, Peters F, Spindler K-LG, Appelt AL, Teo M, et al. STAR-TREC phase II: can we save the rectum by watchful waiting or transanal surgery following (chemo) radiotherapy versus total mesorectal excision for early rectal cancer? JCO Wolters Kluwer. 2022;40:3502.
32. de Rosa N, Rodriguez-Bigas MA, Chang GJ, Veerapong J, Borras E, Krishnan S, et al. DNA mismatch repair deficiency in rectal cancer: benchmarking its impact on prognosis, neoadjuvant response prediction, and clinical cancer genetics. J Clin Oncol. 2016;34:3039–46.
33. Quezada-Diaz FF, Smith JJ, Jimenez-Rodriguez RM, Wasserman I, Pappou EP, Patil S, et al. Patient-reported bowel function in patients with rectal cancer managed by a watch-and-wait strategy after neoadjuvant therapy: a case-control study. Dis Colon Rectum. 2020;63:897–902.
34. Hupkens BJP, Martens MH, Stoot JH, Berbee M, Melenhorst J, Beets-Tan RG, et al. Quality of life in rectal cancer patients after Chemoradiation: watch-and-wait policy versus standard resection – a matched-controlled study. Dis Colon Rectum. 2017;60:1032–40.
35. Yoshino T. A multicenter randomized phase iii study of short-term radiotherapy plus CAPOX and short-term radiotherapy plus CAPOXIRI as preoperative treatment for locally advanced rectal cancer [Internet]. clinicaltrials.gov; 2022 Dec. Report No.: NCT05646511. Available from: https://clinicaltrials.gov/ct2/show/NCT05646511
36. Alliance for Clinical Trials in Oncology. The Janus Rectal Cancer Trial: a randomized phase ii trial testing the efficacy of triplet versus doublet chemotherapy to achieve clinical complete response in patients with locally advanced rectal cancer [Internet]. clinicaltrials.gov; 2022 Nov. Report No.: NCT05610163. Available from: https://clinicaltrials.gov/ct2/show/NCT05610163
37. Rödel PD med C. Short-course radiotherapy versus chemoradiotherapy, followed by consolidation chemotherapy, and selective organ preservation for mri-defined intermediate and high-risk rectal cancer patients [Internet]. clinicaltrials.gov; 2022 Dec. Report No.: NCT04246684. Available from: https://clinicaltrials.gov/ct2/show/NCT04246684
38. Emmertsen KJ, Laurberg S. Rectal cancer function study group. Impact of bowel dysfunction on quality of life after sphincter-preserving resection for rectal cancer. Br J Surg. 2013;100:1377–87.
39. Park IJ, You YN, Agarwal A, Skibber JM, Rodriguez-Bigas MA, Eng C, et al. Neoadjuvant treatment response as an early response indicator for patients with rectal cancer. J Clin Oncol. 2012;30:1770–6.
40. Dossa F, Chesney TR, Acuna SA, Baxter NN. A watch-and-wait approach for locally advanced rectal cancer after a clinical complete response following neoadjuvant chemoradiation: a systematic review and meta-analysis. Lancet Gastroenterol Hepatol. 2017;2:501–13.
41. Martin ST, Heneghan HM, Winter DC. Systematic review and meta-analysis of outcomes following pathological complete response to neoadjuvant chemoradiotherapy for rectal cancer. Br J Surg. 2012;99:918–28.

42. Fernandez LM, São Julião GP, Renehan AG, Beets GL, Papoila AL, Vailati BB, et al. The risk of distant metastases in patients with clinical complete response managed by watch & wait after neoadjuvant therapy for rectal cancer: the influence of local regrowth in the international watch and wait database. Dis Colon Rectum. https://doi.org/10.1097/DCR.0000000000002494.
43. Appelt AL, Pløen J, Harling H, Jensen FS, Jensen LH, Jørgensen JCR, et al. High-dose chemoradiotherapy and watchful waiting for distal rectal cancer: a prospective observational study. Lancet Oncol. 2015;16:919–27.
44. Renehan AG, Malcomson L, Emsley R, Gollins S, Maw A, Myint AS, et al. Watch-and-wait approach versus surgical resection after chemoradiotherapy for patients with rectal cancer (the OnCoRe project): a propensity-score matched cohort analysis. Lancet Oncol. 2016;17:174–83.
45. Cercek A, Lumish M, Sinopoli J, Weiss J, Shia J, Lamendola-Essel M, et al. PD-1 blockade in mismatch repair-deficient, locally advanced rectal cancer. N Engl J Med. 2022;386:2363–76.

24 Which Patients Are the Right Candidates for Total Neoadjuvant Therapy (TNT)?

Maxwell D. Mirande and Scott R. Kelley

Introduction

Outcomes for locally advanced rectal cancer (LARC) have significantly improved over the past several decades with the introduction of total mesorectal excision (TME) and the addition of 5-fluorouracil (5-FU)-based neoadjuvant chemoradiotherapy (nCRT) [1–8] but have failed to improve overall survival (OS) due to distant metastases (DM) [4–9]. Distant recurrences occur in up to 30% and remain a significant cause of mortality for patients with LARC [9]. The addition of oxaliplatin to 5-FU-based chemotherapy (CT) has significantly improved disease-free survival (DFS) and OS in patients with stage II or III colon cancer [10]; however, an OS benefit has not been demonstrated for adjuvant chemotherapy (AC) use in LARC patients who have received nCRT [11, 12]. Delayed administration of AC and/or poor compliance affect up to 50% of patients, and are factors thought to contribute to this discrepancy. For these reasons, traditional trimodal therapy (nCRT, TME, AC) has been called into question and the concept of total neoadjuvant therapy (TNT) has emerged.

TNT is a novel approach which consists of the administration of multidrug systemic CT plus chemoradiotherapy (CRT) prior to surgery with the goal of reducing DM and maintaining local control in patients with LARC. TNT strategies comprise of either induction (prior to nCRT) or consolidation (after nCRT) CT. Proponents of TNT suggest the approach allows for earlier systemic treatment of occult

M. D. Mirande (✉)
Mayo Clinic, General Surgery, Rochester, MN, USA
e-mail: Mirande.Maxwell@mayo.edu

S. R. Kelley
Mayo Clinic, Colon and Rectal Surgery, Rochester, MN, USA
e-mail: kelley.scott@mayo.edu

K. Umanskiy, N. Hyman (eds.), *Difficult Decisions in Colorectal Surgery*, Difficult Decisions in Surgery: An Evidence-Based Approach,
https://doi.org/10.1007/978-3-031-42303-1_24

micrometastases leading to improved survival, better therapy compliance, better tumor response, and the potential for organ preservation. However, several questions remain regarding TNT including the optimal timing and protocol used, induction versus consolidation, variable tumor response, and possible overtreatment. Herein we review the literature and discuss which patients with LARC are the right candidates for TNT.

Search Strategy

Utilizing Embase and Medline databases, a search of the English literature was conducted using the terms rectal cancer, rectal neoplasms, total neoadjuvant therapy (TNT), chemoradiotherapy, induction chemotherapy, and consolidation chemotherapy. The search was limited to human studies over the last 10 years (2012–2022). Original studies evaluating outcomes of patients with LARC treated with TNT were included and manuscript reference lists were reviewed for additional articles (Tables 24.1). Studies from the same institution/author were excluded if previously reported. A total of nine studies were chosen for review.

Results

The Spanish GCR-3 multicenter phase II trial randomized 108 patients with cT3-T4, and/or N+ mid to distal rectal cancer into either a control (capecitabine plus oxaliplatin [CAPOX]-based long course CRT (LCCRT) followed by surgery and four cycles of CAPOX) or experimental arm (four cycles of induction CAPOX followed by the same LCCRT and surgery), with a primary endpoint of pathologic complete response (pCR) [13]. The experimental arm included more T4 and grade 3 tumors whereas the control arm had more tumors with a threatened circumferential resection margin (CRM). On an intention-to-treat analysis, induction CAPOX demonstrated a similar pCR, R0 resection, downstaging, and tumor regression rate. There was significantly higher compliance with induction CT as 94% received all four cycles ($p < 0.0001$) compared to 57% in the control arm. Additionally, there were no differences between the arms in grade 3 or 4 toxicities during CRT; however, there were significantly more grade 3 or 4 toxicities during AC when compared to induction CT (54% *v* 19%; $p = 0.0004$, respectively). With a median follow up of 69.5 months, no differences between the control and experimental arms were observed in 5-year cumulative LR (2% *v* 5%; $p = 0.61$), DM (21% *v* 23%; $p = 0.79$), DFS (64% *v* 62%; $p = 0.85$), or OS (78% *v* 75%; $p = 0.64$), respectively (Tables 24.2, 24.3, 24.4).

The Polish II study was one of the first multicenter phase III randomized trials to investigate short-course radiation (SCRT) plus consolidation CT [14]. A total of 515 patients with cT3-T4 rectal cancer were randomized to either the control arm (LCCRT with concomitant leucovorin, 5-FU, and oxaliplatin [FOLFOX]) or the experimental arm (SCRT plus three cycles of FOLFOX4), with a primary endpoint of R0 resection rate. The overall acute toxicity was lower in the experimental group than in the control (75% *v* 83%; $p = 0.006$), but similar grade 3 or 4 toxicities were observed between both groups (23% *v* 21%). No differences were seen in post-op complications (29% *v* 25%; $p = 0.18$) between the two groups. The R0 resection rate and pCR rates were also similar between both groups (77% *v* 71%; $p = 0.07$) and (16% *v* 12%; $p = 0.17$), respectively. At 3-years, the OS for the experimental arm was significantly higher at 73% versus 65% in the control arm (HR = 0.73, 95% CI 0.53–1.01; $p = 0.046$) but no differences were seen in 3-year LR, DM, or DFS. At 8-years, the difference in OS was no longer significant (HR = 0.90, 95% CI 0.70–1.15; $p = 0.38$) [15].

The phase II WAIT trial randomized 49 patients to either a control arm (LCCRT followed by surgery) or experimental arm (LCCRT plus three cycles of bolus 5-FU/leucovorin followed by surgery), with the primary endpoint of pCR [16]. Most patients were cT3 (86%) and 96% were considered node positive on MRI. A wait period of 10 weeks after completion of CRT was used. There were similar postoperative complications and length of stay between the two groups. The pCR was similar between both arms (16% *v* 25%; $p = 0.49$); however, this study was not powered to detect small differences.

The Korean Cancer Study Group (KCSG) CO 14–03 phase II randomized trial aimed to evaluate the efficacy of CAPOX consolidation CT [17]. A total of 108 patients with cT3-T4 rectal cancer were randomized into either the control arm (LCCRT followed by surgery) or the experimental arm (LCCRT followed by two cycles of CAPOX and surgery), with a primary endpoint of downstaging. The experimental arm had marginal improvements in pCR (13.6% *v* 5.8%; $p = 0.167$) and downstaging (36.4% *v* 21.2%; $p = 0.077$) compared to the control arm, but neither were significant. However, there was a high dropout rate of 13% with only 96 total patients undergoing surgery per protocol. Due to the dropout rate and safety concerns, a phase III trial using this strategy was discouraged.

The Chinese FOWARC study was a multicenter phase III randomized trial that compared LCCRT (control) versus five cycles of mFOLFOX6 with long-course radiation (exp. 1) versus five cycles of mFOLFOX6 alone (exp. 2) [18]. A total of 495 patients with stage II or III tumors within 12 cm of the anal verge were randomized with a primary endpoint of 3-year DFS. All groups underwent surgery 6–8 weeks following therapy and received postoperative AC. The pCR rate was 14.0%, 27.5%, and 6.6% for the control, exp. 1, and exp. 2 groups respectively (OR 0.428, 95% CI 0.237–0.776; $p = 0.005$). There was high treatment compliance (>90% of full-dose neoadjuvant CT) amongst the control (88.4%), exp. 1 (94.9%), and exp. 2 (94.5%) groups. At 3-years, there were no differences observed in DFS between the control (72.9%), exp. 1 (73.5%), and exp. 2 (73.5%) groups (log rank $p = 0.709$). The 3-year LR was rate was 8%, 7%, and 8.3% (log rank $p = 0.873$) and the 3-year OS was of 91.3%, 89.1%, and 90.7% (log rank $p = 0.971$), respectively. Although the exp. 2 group had inferior pCR, there was similar downstaging rates compared to the control group (35.5% *v* 37%) with less toxicity, complications, and no differences in DFS, LR, or OS. The role of neoadjuvant CT alone remains unclear but several ongoing studies, including the phase III randomized PROSPECT trial will provide additional insight [19].

The Swedish RAPIDO multicenter phase III trial randomized 912 patients with tumors less than 16 cm from the anal verge and MRI high-risk criteria (cT4a or cT4b, extramural vascular invasion, cN2, involved mesorectal fascia, or enlarged lateral lymph nodes considered to be metastatic) into either a control (LCCRT followed by surgery and optional adjuvant CAPOX or FOLFOX4) or experimental arm (SCRT followed by six cycles of CAPOX or nine cycles of FOLFOX4 followed by surgery), with a primary endpoint of 3-year disease-related treatment failure (DrTF) [20]. The experimental arm had a significantly higher pCR rate (28% *v* 14%; OR 2.37, 95% CI 1.67–3.37; $p < 0.0001$), fewer 3-year DrTF events (23.7% *v* 30.4%; HR = 0.75, 95% CI 0.60–0.95; $p = 0.019$), and a lower 3-year cumulative probability of DM (20.0% *v* 26.8%; HR = 0.69, 95% CI 0.54–0.90; $p = 0.0048$) compared to the control. The 3-year cumulative probability of locoregional failure (8.3% *v* 6.0%; $p = 0.12$) and OS (89.1% *v* 88.8%; $p = 0.59$) were similar between both arms, respectively. The authors concluded that SCRT followed by 18 weeks of consolidation CT before surgery can be considered as a new standard of treatment for patients with high-risk LARC and can potentially contribute to organ preservation.

The PRODIGE 23 trial is a multicenter phase III randomized trial that compared induction FOLFIRINOX (leucovorin, 5-FU, irinotecan, and oxaliplatin) to LCCRT [21]. A total of 461 patients with tumors within 15 cm of the anal verge and cT3 or cT4 were included. Patients were randomly assigned to either the experimental group (six cycles of FOLFIRINOX, followed by LCCRT, surgery, and adjuvant mFOLFOX6 or capecitabine) or the control group (LCCRT, surgery, and adjuvant mFOLFOX6 or capecitabine), with a primary endpoint of 3-year DFS. Like the RAPIDO trial, the experimental group had a significantly higher pCR rate (28% *v* 12%; $p < 0.001$). With a median follow-up of 46.5 months, the experimental group had improved 3-year DFS (76% *v* 69%; HR 0.69, 95% CI 0.49–0.97; $p = 0.034$) and 3-year metastasis-free survival (79% *v* 72%; HR 0.64, 95% CI 0.44–0.93; $p = 0.017$), with no differences in 3-year OS (91% *v* 88%, $p = 0.0773$). The authors concluded that induction FOLFIRINOX can be considered as one of the new standard-of-care treatment approaches for eligible patients with LARC.

The German CAO/ARO/AIO-12 trial is the first multicenter, phase II randomized trial to compare induction and consolidation CT [22]. Patients with cT3–4 and/or node positive tumors within 12 cm of the anal verge were included. A total of 306 were randomized into the induction CT group (three cycles of FOLFOX followed by LCCRT and surgery) or the consolidation CT group (LCCRT followed by three cycles of FOLFOX and surgery), with a primary endpoint of pCR. The trial demonstrated a higher pCR rate in the consolidation CT group (25% *v* 17%; OR 1.69, 95% CI 0.96–2.99; $p = 0.071$). It also showed that the treatment modality given first as part of TNT will likely always have higher compliance and lower toxicity. With a median follow-up of 43 months, the 3-year DFS was 73% in the induction group and 73% in the consolidation group ($p = 0.82$). The 3-year LR (6% *v* 5%; $p = 0.67$), 3-year DM (18% *v* 16%; $p = 0.52$), and 3-year OS (92% *v* 92%; $p = 0.81$) were all similar between both groups, respectively. The authors concluded that the consolidation TNT strategy was able to achieve higher pCR without compromising long-term oncologic outcomes, toxicity, or quality of life (QOL) and may be the best choice if organ preservation is a priority. The consolidation TNT regimen from this trial will be compared against the TNT regimen from the RAPIDO trial in the ACO/ARO/AIO-18.1 trial (NCT04246684), with 3-year DFS as the primary endpoint.

The OPRA trial is the first multicenter, phase II randomized trial evaluating TNT and a selective watch-and-wait (WW) strategy [23]. A total of 324 clinical stage II or III rectal cancer patients were randomized into the induction or consolidation CT groups, with a primary outcome of 3-year DFS. Patients were treated with either eight cycles of mFOLFOX6 or five cycles of CAPOX, and LCCRT. Tumor restaging was performed within 8 (+/−4) weeks after completion of TNT, and TME versus WW was offered based on tumor response. The trial demonstrated a 3-year DFS of 76% (95% CI, 69–84) for the induction and 76% (95% CI, 69–83) for the consolidation group. No differences were in seen in LR-free survival, DM-free survival, or OS between the two groups. Rectal preservation at 3 years was 41% (95% CI, 33–50) for the induction and 53% (95% CI, 45–62; $p = 0.1$) for the consolidation group. DFS was similar between patients who underwent initial TME and patients who underwent TME after tumor regrowth, thus demonstrating no apparent adverse impact on oncologic outcomes with WW.

Table 24.1 PICO table

Patients	Intervention	Comparator	Outcomes
Locally advanced rectal cancer (LARC)	Totally neoadjuvant therapy (TNT)	Trimodal therapy	Pathologic complete response (pCR) Recurrence Survival

Table 24.2 Trial characteristics

Author/Year/Study	Design	Treatment Arms	Median Follow-Up (month)	Primary End Point	Secondary End Points
Fernández-Martos/ 2015/ GCR-3	RCT phase II	**Con:** CRT (capecitabine/oxaliplatin) → surg → CAPOX × 4 **Exp:** CAPOX × 4 → CRT (capecitabine/ oxaliplatin) → surg	69.5	pCR	Toxicity, compliance, downstaging, R0 resection, 30-day complications, LR, DM, DFS, OS
Bujko/2016/ POLISH II	RCT phase III	**Con:** CRT (FOLFOX) → surg **Exp:** SCRT → FOLFOX4 × 3 → surg	35	R0 resection rate	Toxicity, 30-day and late complications, pCR, LR, DM, DFS, OS
Moore/2017/ WAIT	RCT phase II	**Con:** CRT (5-FU) → surg **Exp:** CRT (5-FU) → 5-FU/LV × 3 → surg	NR	pCR	LOS, 30-day complications
Kim/2018/ KCSG CO 14–03	RCT phase II	**Con:** CRT (capecitabine) → surg **Exp:** CRT (capecitabine) → CAPOX × 2 → surg	26	Downstaging rate to yp stage 0–1	pCR, LR, RFS, DFS, OS, safety profile, QOL
Deng/2019/ FOWARC	RCT phase III	**Con:** 5-FU × 5 + RT → surg → 5FU × 7 **Exp 1:** mFOLFOX6 × 5 + RT → surg → mFOLFOX6 × 7 **Exp 2:** mFOLFOX6 × 4–6 → surg → mFOLFOX6 × 6–8	45.2	3-yr DFS	Toxicity, response rate, pCR, R0 resection, sphincter-saving surgery, LR, OS, RFS, QOL
Bahadoer/2020/ RAPIDO	RCT phase III	**Con:** CRT (capecitabine) → surg → CAPOX × 8/ FOLFOX4 × 12 (optional) **Exp:** SCRT → CAPOX × 6/ FOLFOX4 × 9 → surg	55.2	3-yr DrTF	Compliance, toxicity, R0 resection, pCR, 30-day complications, LR, QOL, OS

Conroy/2021/ PRODIGE-23	RCT phase III	**Con:** CRT (capecitabine) → surg → mFOLFOX6 × 12/ capecitabine × 8 **Exp:** FOLFIRINOX × 6 → CRT (capecitabine) → surg → mFOLFOX6 × 6/capecitabine × 4	46.5	3-yr DFS	OS, MFS, CSS, LR, DM, pCR, R0 resection, complications, safety, QOL
Fokas/2022/ CAO/ARO/ AIO-12	RCT phase II	**Exp 1:** FOLFOX × 3 → CRT (5-FU) → surg **Exp 2:** CRT (5-FU) → FOLFOX × 3 → surg	43	pCR	DFS, LR, DM, OS, toxicity, QOL
Garcia-Aguilar/2022/ OPRA	RCT phase II	**Exp 1:** mFOLFOX6 × 8 or CAPOX × 5 → CRT (5-FU or capecitabine) → WW or surg **Exp 2:** CRT (5-FU or capecitabine) → mFOLFOX6 × 8 or CAPOX × 5 → WW or surg	36	3-yr DFS	TME-free survival, adverse events, LR, DM, OS, QOL

RCT Randomized control trial, *CRT* Chemoradiotherapy, *surg* Surgery, *CAPOX* Capecitabine and oxaliplatin, *pCR* Pathologic complete response, *LR* Local recurrence, *DM* Distant metastases, *DFS* Disease-free survival, *OS* Overall survival, *FOLFOX* Leucovorin calcium, 5-FU, and oxaliplatin, *SCRT* Short-course radiation, *QOL* Quality of life, *RFS* Relapse-free survival, *FOLFIRINOX* Leucovorin, 5-FU, irinotecan, and oxaliplatin, *MFS* Metastasis-free survival, *CSS* Cancer-specific survival, *WW* Watch-and-wait, *TME* Total mesorectal excision

Table 24.3 Patient characteristics

Study	Inclusion Criteria	N	Arms (N)	Gender (%) M:F	Median Age (range)
GCR-3	Distal/middle third, cT3-T4 and or N+	108	**Con:** (52) **Exp:** (56)	65:35 70:30	62 (42–75) 60 (38–76)
POLISH II	cT3-T4	515	**Con:** (254) **Exp:** (261)	67:33 70:30	60 60
WAIT	Non metastatic distal rectal LARC	49	**Con:** (24) **Exp:** (25)	75:25 72:28	61 60
KCSG CO 14–03	cT3-T4, N+	108	**Con:** (55) **Exp:** (53)	84:16 68:32	55 56
FOWARC	cT3-cT4, N+	495	**Con:** (158) **Exp 1:** (162) **Exp 2:** (163)	62:38 69:31 66:34	54 52 54
RAPIDO	High risk criteria on MRI (cT4a, CT4b, cN2)	912	**Con:** (450) **Exp:** (462)	69:31 65:35	62 (23–84) 62 (31–83)
PRODIGE-23	cT3-T4	461	**Con:** (230) **Exp:** (231)	68:32 65:35	62 (26–75) 61 (34–77)
CAO/ARO/AIO-12	cT3–4, N+	306	**Exp 1:** (156) **Exp 2:** (150)	68:32 67:33	60 62
OPRA	Stage II (cT3–4, N0) or Stage III (any T, N1–2)	324	**Exp 1:** (158) **Exp 2:** (166)	65:35 61:39	59 56

LARC Locally advanced rectal cancer, *MRI* Magnetic resonance imaging, *Con* Control, *Exp* Experimental

Table 24.4 Trial outcomes

Study	Arms (N)	Compliance with CT (%)	Grade 3–4 Toxicity (%)	Post-operative Complications No. (%)	pCR (%)	Local Recurrence (%)	Distant Recurrence (%)	DFS (%)	OS (%)
GCR-3	**Con:** (52)	57	54	21 (45)	13	2[a]	21[a]	64[a]	78[a]
	Exp: (56)	94	19	27 (51)	14	5[a]	23[a]	62[a]	75[a]
POLISH II	**Con:** (254)	–	21	49 (25)	12	–	25[b], 36[c]	52[b], 43[c]	65[b], 49[c]
	Exp: (261)		23	62 (29)	16	–	29[b], 34[c]	53[b], 41[c]	73[b], 49[c]
WAIT	**Con:** (24)	–	–	10 (42)	25	–	–	–	–
	Exp: (25)	–	–	13 (52)	16	–	–	–	–
KCSG CO 14–03	**Con:** (55)	–	4	2	6	–	–	–	–
	Exp: (53)	89	9	9	14	–	–	–	–
FOWARC	**Con:** (158)	88	–	–	14	8[b]	–	73[b]	91[b]
	Exp 1: (162)	95	–	–	28	7[b]	–	77[b]	89[b]
	Exp 2: (163)	94	–	–	7	8[b]	–	74[b]	91[b]
RAPIDO	**Con:** (450)	90	25	189 (47)	14	6[b]	27[b]	–	89[b]
	Exp: (462)	84	48	215 (50)	28	8[b]	20[b]	–	89[b]
PRODIGE–23	**Con:** (230)	79	74	–	12	4	25	69[b]	88[b]
	Exp: (231)	92	46	–	28	6	17	76[b]	91[b]
CAO/ARO/ AIO–12	**Exp 1:** (156)	93/92	37	42	17	6[b]	18[b]	73[b]	92[b]
	Exp 2: (150)	90/85	27	34	25	5[b]	16[b]	73[b]	92[b]
OPRA	**Exp 1:** (158)	83	71 (45)	–	12	7[b]/10[b*]	17[b]/17[b*]	76[b]	–
	Exp 2: (166)	81	63 (38)	–	16	11[b]/15[b*]	24[b]/21[b*]	76[b]	–

CT Chemotherapy, *pCR* Pathologic complete response, *DFS* Disease-free survival, *OS* Overall survival, *Con* Control, *Exp* Experimental

[a] Results at 5 years

[b] Results at 3 years

[c] Results at 8 years

[*] Patients who underwent total mesorectal excision after local regrowth

Recommendations Based on the Data

The administration of induction or consolidation CT as part of a TNT regimen should be considered for all patients with cT3–4 and/or N+ rectal cancer (high quality evidence, strong recommendation).

An oxaliplatin-based CT regimen (FOLFOX, CAPOX, FOLFIRINOX, etc.) rather than a fluoropyrimidine alone is recommended (high quality evidence, strong recommendation).

To achieve a higher pCR, consolidation rather than induction CT should be considered for treatment of cT3–4 and/or N+ rectal cancer (moderate evidence, moderate recommendation).

Currently there is insufficient evidence to recommend FOLFIRINOX or FOLFOXIRI over CAPOX or FOLFOX (high quality evidence, strong recommendation).

Currently, there is insufficient evidence to recommend the addition to bevacizumab to a TNT regimen (high quality evidence, strong recommendation).

A TNT approach increases tolerance and completion rates of CT (high quality evidence, strong recommendation).

Neoadjuvant radiotherapy (RT) (short or long course) should be offered as part of a TNT strategy for treatment of cT3–4 and/or N+ rectal cancer (high quality evidence, strong recommendation).

Short and long course RT protocols achieve similar rates of local control, sphincter preservation, DFS, and OS (high quality evidence, strong recommendation).

TNT is associated with higher rates of complete clinical response (cCR) and pCR (high quality evidence, strong recommendation).

Completion of TNT is associated with higher rates of DFS and lower rates of DM (high quality evidence, strong recommendation).

Treatment with TNT has not been shown to decrease rates of LR or increase rates of OS (high quality evidence, strong recommendation).

A Personal View of the Data

At Mayo Clinic, all rectal cancers are reviewed at a multidisciplinary rectal cancer conference (radiology, pathology, medical oncology, radiation oncology, colon and rectal surgery). We consider induction or consolidation oxaliplatin-based doublet CT (CAPOX or FOLFOX) combined with short or long course fluoropyrimidine-based (capecitabine or 5-FU) CRT for all patients with MRI cT3–4 and/or N+ rectal cancers. For lower-risk cancers (i.e., cT3N0 without high-risk features), we typically do not consider TNT since many of those patients will not need AC. For cT4, we consider triplet CT with FOLFIRINOX.

We typically start with 16 weeks of induction CT to treat micrometastatic disease and test tumor biology. Repeat imaging is performed around 8 weeks to determine response. If response is appropriate, induction CT is completed and followed by short or long course fluoropyrimidine-based CRT. For select patients without high-risk features (involved or threatened CRM, extramural venous invasion, N+ disease, extramesorectal adenopathy), SCRT followed by immediate surgery is typically pursued. For patients with high-risk features, fluoropyrimidine-based LCCRT is recommended. If the tumor is bulky or there is concern for organ preservation, we typically start with fluoropyrimidine-based LCCRT to shrink the size of the tumor and follow with consolidation CT.

No single protocol for TNT exists, which can make treatment selection challenging, and there is a risk of overtreatment. All patients should undergo immunohistochemical and microsatellite instability (MSI) testing since a substantial proportion who do not appropriately express mismatch repair proteins / are MSI-high will not respond to CT, and other treatment modalities should be considered. These patients should be reviewed at multidisciplinary tumor conferences and referred to centers capable of managing them.

Abstracted Recommendations

The administration of induction or consolidation CT as part of a TNT regimen should be considered for all patients with cT3–4 and/or N+ rectal cancer (high quality evidence, strong recommendation).

An oxaliplatin-based CT regimen (FOLFOX, CAPOX, FOLFIRINOX, etc.) rather than a fluoropyrimidine alone is recommended (high quality evidence, strong recommendation).

Neoadjuvant RT (short or long course) should be offered as part of a TNT strategy for treatment of cT3–4 and/or N+ rectal cancer (high quality evidence, strong recommendation).

Treatment with TNT has been shown to be associated with greater tolerance and completion of CT, more frequent cCR and pCR, less severe toxicity, higher rates of DM-free survival, longer DFS, and better QOL (high quality evidence, strong recommendation).

References

1. Heald RJ, Ryall RD. Recurrence and survival after total mesorectal excision for rectal cancer. Lancet. 1986;1(8496):1479–82.
2. Cedermark B, et al. Improved survival with preoperative radiotherapy in resectable rectal cancer. N Engl J Med. 1997;336(14):980–7.
3. Folkesson J, et al. Swedish rectal cancer trial: long lasting benefits from radiotherapy on survival and local recurrence rate. J Clin Oncol. 2005;23(24):5644–50.
4. Kapiteijn E, et al. Preoperative radiotherapy combined with total mesorectal excision for resectable rectal cancer. N Engl J Med. 2001;345(9):638–46.
5. van Gijn W, et al. Preoperative radiotherapy combined with total mesorectal excision for resectable rectal cancer: 12-year follow-up of the multicentre, randomised controlled TME trial. Lancet Oncol. 2011;12(6):575–82.
6. Bosset JF, et al. Chemotherapy with preoperative radiotherapy in rectal cancer. N Engl J Med. 2006;355(11):1114–23.

7. Gérard JP, et al. Preoperative radiotherapy with or without concurrent fluorouracil and leucovorin in T3-4 rectal cancers: results of FFCD 9203. J Clin Oncol. 2006;24(28):4620–5.
8. Sauer R, et al. Preoperative versus postoperative chemoradiotherapy for rectal cancer. N Engl J Med. 2004;351(17):1731–40.
9. Sauer R, et al. Preoperative versus postoperative chemoradiotherapy for locally advanced rectal cancer: results of the German CAO/ARO/AIO-94 randomized phase III trial after a median follow-up of 11 years. J Clin Oncol. 2012;30(16):1926–33.
10. André T, et al. Improved overall survival with oxaliplatin, fluorouracil, and leucovorin as adjuvant treatment in stage II or III colon cancer in the MOSAIC trial. J Clin Oncol. 2009;27(19):3109–16.
11. Breugom AJ, et al. Adjuvant chemotherapy after preoperative (chemo)radiotherapy and surgery for patients with rectal cancer: a systematic review and meta-analysis of individual patient data. Lancet Oncol. 2015;16(2):200–7.
12. Zhao L, et al. Oxaliplatin/fluorouracil-based adjuvant chemotherapy for locally advanced rectal cancer after neoadjuvant chemoradiotherapy and surgery: a systematic review and meta-analysis of randomized controlled trials. Color Dis. 2016;18(8):763–72.
13. Fernandez-Martos C, et al. Chemoradiation, surgery and adjuvant chemotherapy versus induction chemotherapy followed by chemoradiation and surgery: long-term results of the Spanish GCR-3 phase II randomized trial†. Ann Oncol. 2015;26(8):1722–8.
14. Bujko K, et al. Long-course oxaliplatin-based preoperative chemoradiation versus 5 × 5 Gy and consolidation chemotherapy for cT4 or fixed cT3 rectal cancer: results of a randomized phase III study. Ann Oncol. 2016;27(5):834–42.
15. Ciseł B, et al. Long-course preoperative chemoradiation versus 5 × 5 Gy and consolidation chemotherapy for clinical T4 and fixed clinical T3 rectal cancer: long-term results of the randomized polish II study. Ann Oncol. 2019;30(8):1298–303.
16. Moore J, et al. Prospective randomized trial of neoadjuvant chemotherapy during the 'wait period' following preoperative chemoradiotherapy for rectal cancer: results of the WAIT trial. Color Dis. 2017;19(11):973–9.
17. Kim SY, et al. A randomized phase 2 trial of consolidation chemotherapy after preoperative Chemoradiation therapy versus Chemoradiation therapy alone for locally advanced rectal cancer: KCSG CO 14-03. Int J Radiat Oncol Biol Phys. 2018;101(4):889–99.
18. Deng Y, et al. Neoadjuvant modified FOLFOX6 with or without radiation versus fluorouracil plus radiation for locally advanced rectal cancer: final results of the Chinese FOWARC trial. J Clin Oncol. 2019;37(34):3223–33.
19. Schrag D, et al. Challenges and solutions in the design and execution of the PROSPECT phase II/III neoadjuvant rectal cancer trial (NCCTG N1048/Alliance). Clin Trials. 2019;16(2):165–75.
20. Bahadoer RR, et al. Short-course radiotherapy followed by chemotherapy before total mesorectal excision (TME) versus preoperative chemoradiotherapy, TME, and optional adjuvant chemotherapy in locally advanced rectal cancer (RAPIDO): a randomised, open-label, phase 3 trial. Lancet Oncol. 2021;22(1):29–42.
21. Conroy T, et al. Neoadjuvant chemotherapy with FOLFIRINOX and preoperative chemoradiotherapy for patients with locally advanced rectal cancer (UNICANCER-PRODIGE 23): a multicentre, randomised, open-label, phase 3 trial. Lancet Oncol. 2021;22(5):702–15.
22. Fokas E, et al. Chemoradiotherapy plus induction or consolidation chemotherapy as Total neoadjuvant therapy for patients with locally advanced rectal cancer: long-term results of the CAO/ARO/AIO-12 randomized clinical trial. JAMA Oncol. 2022;8(1):e215445.
23. Garcia-Aguilar J, et al. Organ preservation in patients with rectal adenocarcinoma treated with Total neoadjuvant therapy. J Clin Oncol. 2022;40(23):2546–56.

Management of the Patient with Rectal Cancer Presenting with Synchronous Liver Metastases

25

Cimarron E. Sharon and Joshua I. S. Bleier

Introduction

With the incidence of colorectal (CRC) cancer rising [1, 2], notably among younger patients [3, 4], up to 25% are presenting with synchronous metastatic disease [5], most commonly in the liver [6]. Patients with synchronous metastatic disease and a rectal primary present a therapeutic dilemma, as no conventional approach exists, and treatment is often individualized.

Question: What is the best way to manage the patient with asymptomatic rectal cancer and synchronous liver metastases?

For patients with asymptomatic rectal cancer and synchronous liver metastases (SCRLM), treatment is typically multimodal, including a combination of chemotherapy, radiation, and surgical resection. With regards to the surgical strategy specifically, patients can undergo either a staged (i.e., proctectomy first or hepatectomy first) or combined approach, dependent on their tumor biology, response to chemotherapy/radiation, and the burden of metastatic disease. The goal of this chapter is to provide evidence-based recommendations to assist providers in caring for these complex patients.

C. E. Sharon
Department of Surgery, University of Pennsylvania, Perelman School of Medicine, Philadelphia, PA, USA
e-mail: Cimarron.sharon@pennmedicine.UPenn.edu

J. I. S. Bleier (✉)
Division of Colorectal Surgery, Department of Surgery, University of Pennsylvania, Perelman School of Medicine, Philadelphia, PA, USA
e-mail: Joshua.bleier@pennmedicine.upenn.edu

K. Umanskiy, N. Hyman (eds.), *Difficult Decisions in Colorectal Surgery*, Difficult Decisions in Surgery: An Evidence-Based Approach,
https://doi.org/10.1007/978-3-031-42303-1_25

Table 25.1 PICO table for rectal cancer and synchronous liver metastases

Patient Population	Intervention	Comparator	Outcomes
Patients with asymptomatic rectal cancer and synchronous liver metastases	Staged liver first resection	Combined rectal and liver resection	Morbidity Overall survival Disease-free survival

Search Strategy

A systematic review of the literature using PubMed was performed using search terms in various combinations of rectal cancer, liver metastases, hepatic metastases, synchronous resection, combined resection, staged resection, liver-first, imaging, diagnosis, chemotherapy, radiation, guidelines, and management. Articles were limited to peer reviewed reports in English published between 2010 and 2022, in order to provide an update to the chapter on this topic published in the 2017 edition of this textbook. Additional studies were identified from the references of the initial articles and were included as appropriate. Table 25.1 summarizes the population, intervention, comparator, and key outcomes (PICO) for the patient population.

Results

Initial Evaluation

Imaging

As discussed in previous chapters, imaging of the primary rectal tumor is best accomplished with pelvic magnetic resonance imaging (MRI) [7], which can assess tumor depth, presence of locoregional nodal disease, and the circumferential resection margin (CRM), all critical factors in preoperative planning [8, 9]. If MRI is contraindicated, then locoregional staging can be performed with an endorectal ultrasound (EUS) [7].

Assessment of distant metastatic disease should include a contrast-enhanced computed tomography (CT) scan of the chest, abdomen, and pelvis [7, 10]. In the assessment of liver metastases, specifically, a multiphasic CT scan (non-contrast followed by arterial, venous, and delayed phase intravenous contrast) is the diagnostic modality of choice [7, 11, 12]. For sub-centimeter liver lesions, and for evaluation after neoadjuvant chemotherapy, magnetic resonance imaging (MRI) is superior to CT [12, 13]. The role of positron emission tomography (PET)-CT in the evaluation of colorectal cancer metastases is to assess for extra-hepatic sites of disease, which if present, would preclude curative surgical resection [12, 14, 15].

Goals

Imaging evaluation of the rectal primary and the hepatic metastases assists in determining the resectability of the lesions. With regards to the hepatic lesions, knowledge of the number and size of the metastases, in addition to their lobar distribution and relationship to the vasculature, is imperative [7]. For hepatic metastases to be resectable, the liver remnant must encompass approximately 25% of the total liver volume, for patients without inherent liver disease [16]. Ascertaining resectability also drives the goals of treatment, whether curative or palliative in nature.

Multidisciplinary Team

Patient evaluation by a multidisciplinary team (MDT) assists in identifying treatment goals, in addition to course and strategy. Prior to initiation of therapy, whether in the form of systemic therapy or surgical resection, patients with SCRLM should be evaluated by an MDT [17]. This MDT typically consists of radiation and medical oncologists, pathologists, palliative care clinicians, and colorectal and hepatobiliary surgeons, who can jointly determine a patient's optimal first-line treatment [7, 12, 18, 19]. Patients with SCRLM who are evaluated by an MDT including a hepatobiliary surgeon have a higher resection rate and improved overall survival (OS) [18, 20].

Treatment

Neoadjuvant Treatment

While perioperative chemotherapy has notable advantages to resection alone [21], there is no consensus on timing, and the routine use of neoadjuvant chemotherapy (NCT) for patients with SCRLM is controversial. The advantage to NCT in these patients lies in the ability to downstage hepatic lesions to facilitate curative-intent surgical resection. However, the risks of NCT include chemotherapy-induced toxicities, most notably liver injury, which would complicate hepatic resection and increase the size of the required functional liver remnant (FLR) [22]. Further complications of NCT include disease progression during treatment which would prevent surgical resection, and disappearing liver lesions, wherein the macroscopic disease has regressed but the possibility of microscopic disease remains [22]. As such, the main advantage of NCT is for patients with unresectable hepatic disease to allow for tumor downstaging and conversion to resectability. For patients with unresectable or borderline resectable hepatic metastases, upfront resection of an asymptomatic rectal primary is not recommended due to the risk of perioperative morbidity which would delay necessary systemic therapy [7, 12, 23].

The NCT administered typically consists of a combination of systemic therapy and targeted biologic treatments, as recommended by the MDT. Current National Comprehensive Cancer Network (NCCN) guidelines [23] list FOLFIRI (5-fluorouracil, leucovorin, and irinotecan), FOLFOX (5-fluorouracil, leucovorin, and oxaliplatin), CAPEOX (capecitabine and oxaliplatin), or FOLFIRINOX (5-fluorouracil, leucovorin, irinotecan, and oxaliplatin) with or without bevacizumab (VEGF inhibitor) as treatment options for rectal cancer patients with initially unresectable liver metastases. Regardless of the type of NCT administered, patients should be re-evaluated every 2 months to assess tumor response/resectability and avoid any liver toxicity or disease progression which would render the metastases unresectable [24].

There is no clear consensus on the utility of pelvic radiation for patients with metastatic rectal cancer, despite its widespread use for locally advanced rectal cancer. Past studies have shown that for patients with metastatic rectal cancer the use of radiotherapy is associated with improved overall and disease-specific survival [25, 26]. According to NCCN guidelines, short course pelvic radiation should be considered in the setting of resectable liver metastases or after downstaging of initially unresectable lesions [23]. The main utility in radiotherapy lies in increased local control. However, most patients with SCRLM who develop recurrent disease do so distantly, indicating that radiation may be safely omitted in select patients [27]. For patients with lesions in the upper rectum or with a wide circumferential margin on imaging, either short course radiation can be utilized, or radiotherapy may be omitted [7, 28]. The choice to administer or omit radiotherapy is highly individualized and should be made in consultation with an MDT.

Surgery Summary

For the patient with asymptomatic rectal cancer and resectable synchronous liver metastases, three surgical options exist: the "classic" (rectal primary is resected first), the "reverse" (liver metastases are resected first), and the "synchronous" approach (rectal primary and liver metastases resected simultaneously) [7, 29, 30]. The goal of surgical resection is complete removal of disease while minimizing morbidity so as to not cause a delay in the initiation or resumption of systemic therapy [31]. As such, both patient comorbidities and the complication profile of the required procedure are taken into consideration when planning the optimal surgical approach. As with most treatment for patients with SCRLM, surgical planning is highly individualized and should include discussion with an MDT that includes a hepatobiliary surgeon. This chapter will address the three main surgical approaches and highlight patients who are the optimal candidates for each.

Notably, studies investigating the outcomes of the aforementioned surgical approaches include patients with synchronous liver metastases from both colon and rectal cancers, and the majority combine these patients when reporting outcomes. Additionally, the majority of reported data is retrospective in nature. Table 25.2 summarizes the results of notable publications, while also highlighting whether patients with rectal cancer were analyzed separately with regards to post-operative morbidity and long-term survival.

Rectum First

The "classic" approach where the rectal primary is resected first is rarely utilized for patients with asymptomatic rectal tumors, and its application has decreased overall in favor of the "reverse" or "synchronous" approach [30]. The rectum first strategy is more commonly used for patients with larger symptomatic primaries who also have a high burden of metastatic disease [7, 24]. When compared to the reverse

Table 25.2 Literature search results for studies comparing staged vs. combined liver resection for patients with rectal cancer and synchronous liver metastases

Study Author (year)	Patients (N)	Interventions (N)	Morbidity (%) p value	OS (p value)	DFS (p value)	Rectal cancer analyzed separately (Y/N)	Quality of Evidence
Chan (2022) [32]	CRC w/ SCRLM (125)	SR [16]LF [18] PF (75) No surgery [16]	SR vs. ST p = 0.66	PF [ref.] SR [HR 1.40, 95% CI 0.55–3.55, p = 0.78] LF [HR 0.87, 95% CI 0.32–2.34, p = 0.78]	35% overall cohort Between groups: p = 0.45	N	Low
Boudjema (2021) [33]	CRC w/ SCRLM (85)	SR [39] PF (46)	SR (18%) PF (22%) p = 0.70	2-year OS SR (87%) PF (70%) P = 0.05	2-year DFS SR (36%) PF (17%) P = 0.05	N	Moderate
Båverud Olsson (2021) [34]	CRC w/ SCRLM (238)	SR (60) LF (89) PF (51)	SR (53%) LF (33%) PF (8%) p = 0.033	5-year OS PF [ref.] LF [HR 1.06 (95% CI 0.63–1.78, p = 0.83] SR [HR 1.10, 95% CI 0.65–1.84, p = 0.72]	–	Y – Morbidity N – OS	Low

(continued)

Table 25.2 (continued)

Study Author (year)	Patients (N)	Interventions (N)	Morbidity (%) p value	OS (p value)	DFS (p value)	Rectal cancer analyzed separately (Y/N)	Quality of Evidence
Giuliante (2021) [35]	CRC w/ SCRLM (12,744)	SR (2393) PF (4415) LF (522)	SR (40%) PF (30%) LF (31%) p = 0.016[a]	5-year OS LF [ref] (51%) PF [HR 1.21, 95% CI 0.96–1.52, p = 0.10] (47%) SR [HR 1.30 (95% CI 1.02–1.66, p = 0.04] (45%)	5-year DFS SR (38%) PF (35%) LF (38%) p = 0.043	N	Low
Bogach (2020) [42]	CRC w/ SCRLM (1168)	SR (442) PF (619) LF (157)	SR (28%) ST (23%) p = 0.067	5-year OS SR (37.2%) ST (54.8%) p < 0.001	–	N	Low
Esposito [36] (2018)	CRC w/ SCRLM (653)	PF (587) LF (66)	–	5-year OS PF (75%) LF (62%) p = 0.77 After PSM p = 0.35	5-year DFS PF (24%) LF (33%) p = 0.01 After PSM P = 0.62	N	Low
Silberhumer [37] (2016)	CRC w/ SCRLM (429)	SR (320) ST (109)	–	5-year OS SR (38.5%) ST (38.9%) p = 0.52	5-year DFS SR (25.3%) ST (24.3%) p = 0.09	N	Low

CI confidence intervals, *CRC* colorectal cancer, *DFS* disease-free survival, *HF* hazard ratio, *LF* liver first, N no, OS overall survival, *PF* primary first, *PSM* propensity score matching, *SCRLM* synchronous colorectal liver metastases, *SR* synchronous resection, *ST* staged resection, *Y* yes method, resection of the primary tumor first is not associated with advantages in morbidity or overall survival (OS) [30, 32–37]. Additionally, a retrospective multicenter study by Esposito et al. [36] of 653 patients with SCRLM who underwent staged resection found no difference in recurrence-free survival between the patients who had the primary or the liver resected first following propensity score matching. Overall, patient selection for the rectum first strategy largely depends on the size and symptoms of the primary in addition to the burden of metastatic disease.

Liver First

When discussing the liver-first strategy, it should be put in the context that nearly all patients receive neoadjuvant chemotherapy. Resection of the liver first decreases the possibility that the metastases would progress to a degree that would preclude resectability, either due to the nature of the disease or from complications of the classic approach (e.g., anastomotic leaks) that would postpone the second procedure [38]. Additionally, it is hypothesized that further progression of metastatic disease originates from the liver [39], so it is advantageous to resect the metastases first to prevent further cancer spread. Thus, this strategy is best suited for patients with a higher metastatic burden or independently requiring a major hepatectomy [7] based on anatomic location of metastases. There is evidence that resection of the liver first is increasing in popularity [30, 40], which may be due to the increasing efficacy of systemic therapies, rendering more patients' metastases as resectable [14]. Conrad et al. [30] performed a single-center retrospective study of 268 patients with rectal cancer and SLM between 1999–2014, and they found that the proportion of patients undergoing the reverse approach increased from 6% from 1999–2003 and 38% from 2009–2014.

Synchronous Resection

Simultaneous resection of the rectal primary and hepatic metastases may be a safe option for patients who require low risk hepatectomies and proctectomies. Proper patient selection is critical, as patients who undergo synchronous resections have higher rates of post-operative morbidity compared to individual staged procedures [34, 35]. A study by Shubert et al. [41] utilized the American College of Surgeons National Surgical Quality Improvement Database (ACS NSQIP) to identify patients with SCRLM and classified their hepatectomies and colorectal resections as either low or high risk based on the rates of post-operative morbidity and mortality. Low risk procedures included partial and left hepatectomies and low anterior resections, while right hepatectomies, trisegmentectomies (extended right hepatectomies), and abdominal perineal resections were classified as high risk. They found that among patients who underwent a synchronous resection, the lowest risk of post-operative morbidity occurred in patients who received both a low risk hepatectomy and proctectomy. As such, optimal patient selection for a synchronous resection includes patients with a small burden of metastatic disease and a high rectal tumor.

Perioperative Outcomes

The CoSMIC trial [32] was the first prospective study to compare oncologic and perioperative outcomes for patients with SCRLM based on surgical sequence. The participants found that patients who underwent synchronous resections had higher rates of post-operative complications when compared to the classic and reverse resections individually. However, when the complications of each staged approach were summated, there was no difference in total complications between patients who underwent staged or synchronous resections ($p = 0.66$). There was also no difference in total critical care (5.6 days synchronous vs. 5.2 days staged, $p = 0.92$) or total inpatient stay (16.5 days synchronous vs. 16.8 days staged, $p = 0.91$). Notably, patients with staged vs. synchronous resections had no difference in anastomotic leak rate or stoma formation.

Recommendations

Imaging Evaluation

Initial imaging evaluation of the rectal primary should include a pelvic MRI, or an EUS if MRI is contra-indicated (quality of evidence: high, grade of recommendation: strong). A CT chest/abdomen/pelvis can evaluate for distant metastatic disease, with a multiphasic CT the modality of choice for optimal classification of hepatic metastases (quality of evidence: high, grade of recommendation: strong). PET-CT aids in identifying alternate sites of metastatic disease which would preclude resection of the hepatic metastases (quality of evidence: high, grade of recommendation: strong).

Neoadjuvant Treatment

For patients with borderline resectable or unresectable hepatic metastases, neoadjuvant chemotherapy (NCT) should be administered to downstage the hepatic lesions and increase the likelihood of subsequent resectability (quality of evidence: moderate, grade of recommendation: weak). Patients who receive NCT should be surveyed every 2 months to assess for disease response and avoid any disease progression or unnecessary liver toxicity (quality of evidence: high, grade of recommendation: strong). Perioperative chemotherapy is recommended for all patients with SCRLM, and those who do not receive neoadjuvant chemotherapy should be treated in the adjuvant setting (quality of evidence: high, grade of recommendation: strong). There is no consensus on the use of neoadjuvant pelvic radiotherapy, although short-course radiation may be considered for patients with resectable liver metastases (quality of evidence: moderate, grade of recommendation: weak).

Surgical Approach

The surgical approach is critically driven by patient characteristics. Primary assessment includes whether there are any symptomatic issues related to the primary tumor which may need to be addressed first. However, if the patient is largely asymptomatic, as in the focus of this chapter, we have more options in deciding how best to optimize treatment.

Essentially the need to separate the hepatectomy and proctectomy is largely driven by the complexity of the liver resection, with additional consideration given to the difficulty of the proctectomy and patient factors. Patients with a high burden of metastatic disease requiring a major hepatectomy should be offered a liver-first approach (quality of evidence: low, grade of recommendation: weak). Conversely, patients with larger or surgically complex rectal primaries are better candidates for a rectum-first approach (quality of evidence: low, grade of recommendation: weak). Patients who would require both a low risk hepatectomy and a straightforward proctectomy are more suitable for a synchronous resection (quality of evidence: low, grade of recommendation: weak).

A Personal View of the Data

As previously discussed, no prospective studies exist comparing the different surgical strategies for patients with SCRLM, making it challenging to interpret the data. Additionally, generalizability is difficult due to the heterogenous nature of this disease presentation. However, the management strategy at our institution draws from the literature and can be consolidated into a few key points:

1. As previously discussed, patients with SCRLM who are evaluated by an MDT including a hepatobiliary surgeon have a higher resection rate and improved overall survival (OS) [18, 20]. As such, in our institution all patients with SCRLM following diagnosis are evaluated by a MDT, including colorectal surgeons, hepatobiliary surgeons, medical and radiation oncologists, radiologists, palliative care physicians, and pathologists.
2. All patients are treated with neoadjuvant chemotherapy, with a regimen determined by the medical oncologists in the MDT. Generally, FOLFOX is administered as first line treatment. Our practice is to re-assess the liver response after 3–4 cycles to determine response and limit toxicity if the decision for surgery is made at that time.
3. Our approach to surgical strategy for patients with rectal cancer and synchronous liver metastases is represented in Fig. 25.1. Factors incorporated into our decision-making include primary tumor symptoms and risk of obstruction, assessment of resectability of liver metastases, and extent of liver resection required. Patients who undergo the rectum first strategy typically have a high-risk of impending obstruction from the primary in addition to a high burden of metastatic disease requiring a major hepatectomy. For patients without a risk of

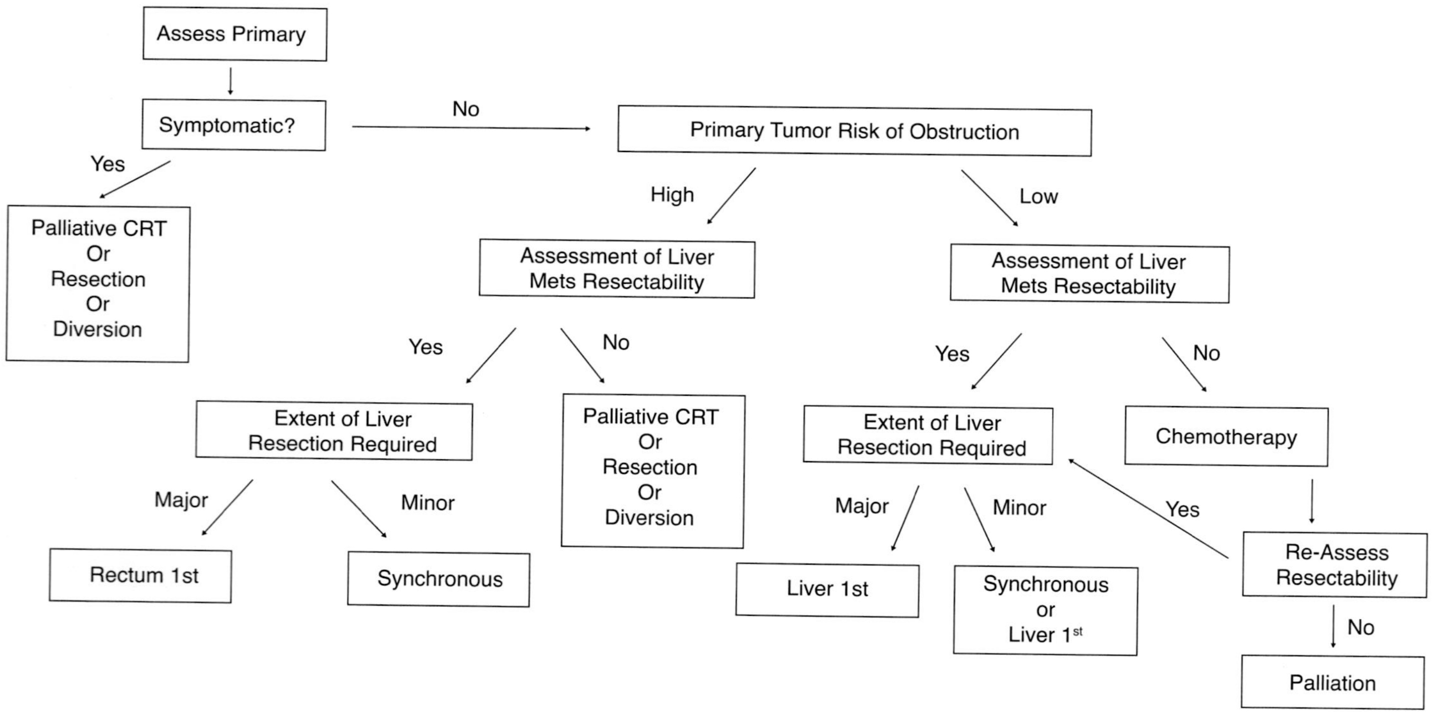

Fig 25.1 Flow chart depicting our approach to surgical and treatment decision-making for patients with rectal cancer and synchronous liver metastases. This flow chart is only intended to be a general recommendation. Every circumstance needs to be personalized on patient factors and the availability of personnel and specialists

obstruction and a high burden of metastatic disease, we typically proceed with a liver-first approach. Most patients who require a minor hepatectomy to clear metastatic disease are candidates for a synchronous approach.

Acknowledgements The authors wish to thank Dr. M. Kenneth Lee, MD for his assistance and input into the creation of our surgical strategy pathway.

References

1. Høydahl Ø, Edna TH, Xanthoulis A, Lydersen S, Endreseth BH. Long-term trends in colorectal cancer: incidence, localization, and presentation. BMC Cancer. 2020;20(1):1077. https://doi.org/10.1186/s12885-020-07582-x.
2. Sinicrope FA. Increasing incidence of early-onset colorectal cancer. N Engl J Med. 2022;386(16):1547–58. https://doi.org/10.1056/NEJMra2200869.
3. Loomans-Kropp HA, Umar A. Increasing incidence of colorectal cancer in young adults. J Cancer Epidemiol. 2019;2019:9841295. https://doi.org/10.1155/2019/9841295.
4. De Vera MA, Gill S, Ashamalla S, et al. Early-age-onset colorectal cancer in canada: evidence, issues and calls to action. Curr Oncol. 2022;29(5):3149–59. https://doi.org/10.3390/curroncol29050256.
5. Qiu M, Hu J, Yang D, Cosgrove DP, Xu R. Pattern of distant metastases in colorectal cancer: a SEER based study. Oncotarget. 2015;6(36):38658–66. https://doi.org/10.18632/oncotarget.6130.
6. Väyrynen V, Wirta EV, Seppälä T, et al. Incidence and management of patients with colorectal cancer and synchronous and metachronous colorectal metastases: a population-based study. BJS Open. 2020;4(4):685–92. https://doi.org/10.1002/bjs5.50299.
7. You YN, Hardiman KM, Bafford A, et al. The American society of colon and rectal surgeons clinical practice guidelines for the management of rectal cancer. Dis Colon Rectum. 2020;63(9):1191–222. https://doi.org/10.1097/DCR.0000000000001762.
8. Faletti R, Gatti M, Arezzo A, et al. Preoperative staging of rectal cancer using magnetic resonance imaging: comparison with pathological staging. Minerva Chir. 2018;73(1):13–9. https://doi.org/10.23736/S0026-4733.17.07392-8.
9. Xie H, Zhou X, Zhuo Z, Che S, Xie L, Fu W. Effectiveness of MRI for the assessment of mesorectal fascia involvement in patients with rectal cancer: a systematic review and meta-analysis. Dig Surg. 2014;31(2):123–34. https://doi.org/10.1159/000363075.
10. Choi DJ, Kwak JM, Kim J, Woo SU, Kim SH. Preoperative chest computerized tomography in patients with locally advanced mid or lower rectal cancer: its role in staging and impact on treatment strategy. J Surg Oncol. 2010;102(6):588–92. https://doi.org/10.1002/jso.21651.
11. Adam R, de Gramont A, Figueras J, et al. Managing synchronous liver metastases from colorectal cancer: a multidisciplinary international consensus. Cancer Treat Rev. 2015;41(9):729–41. https://doi.org/10.1016/j.ctrv.2015.06.006.
12. Vera R, González-Flores E, Rubio C, et al. Multidisciplinary management of liver metastases in patients with colorectal cancer: a consensus of SEOM, AEC, SEOR, SERVEI, and SEMNIM. Clin Transl Oncol. 2020;22(5):647–62. https://doi.org/10.1007/s12094-019-02182-z.
13. Scharitzer M, Ba-Ssalamah A, Ringl H, et al. Preoperative evaluation of colorectal liver metastases: comparison between gadoxetic acid-enhanced 3.0-T MRI and contrast-enhanced MDCT with histopathological correlation. Eur Radiol. Aug 2013;23(8):2187–96. https://doi.org/10.1007/s00330-013-2824-z.

14. Van Cutsem E, Cervantes A, Adam R, et al. ESMO consensus guidelines for the management of patients with metastatic colorectal cancer. Ann Oncol. 2016;27(8):1386–422. https://doi.org/10.1093/annonc/mdw235.
15. Maffione AM, Lopci E, Bluemel C, Giammarile F, Herrmann K, Rubello D. Diagnostic accuracy and impact on management of (18)F-FDG PET and PET/CT in colorectal liver metastasis: a meta-analysis and systematic review. Eur J Nucl Med Mol Imaging. 2015;42(1):152–63. https://doi.org/10.1007/s00259-014-2930-4.
16. Pawlik TM, Choti MA. Surgical therapy for colorectal metastases to the liver. J Gastrointest Surg. 2007;11(8):1057–77. https://doi.org/10.1007/s11605-006-0061-3.
17. Chiorean EG, Nandakumar G, Fadelu T, et al. Treatment of Patients With Late-Stage Colorectal Cancer: ASCO Resource-Stratified Guideline. JCO Glob Oncol. 2020;6:414–38. https://doi.org/10.1200/JGO.19.00367.
18. Engstrand J, Kartalis N, Strömberg C, et al. The impact of a hepatobiliary multidisciplinary team assessment in patients with colorectal cancer liver metastases: a population-based study. Oncologist. 2017;22(9):1067–74. https://doi.org/10.1634/theoncologist.2017-0028.
19. Lowes M, Kleiss M, Lueck R, et al. The utilization of multidisciplinary tumor boards (MDT) in clinical routine: results of a health care research study focusing on patients with metastasized colorectal cancer. Int J Color Dis. 2017;32(10):1463–9. https://doi.org/10.1007/s00384-017-2871-z.
20. Chen CH, Hsieh MC, Lao WT, Lin EK, Lu YJ, Wu SY. Multidisciplinary team intervention associated with improved survival for patients with colorectal adenocarcinoma with liver or lung metastasis. Am J Cancer Res. 2018;8(9):1887–98.
21. Schwarz RE, Berlin JD, Lenz HJ, Nordlinger B, Rubbia-Brandt L, Choti MA. Systemic cytotoxic and biological therapies of colorectal liver metastases: expert consensus statement. HPB (Oxford). 2013;15(2):106–15. https://doi.org/10.1111/j.1477-2574.2012.00558.x.
22. Guo M, Jin N, Pawlik T, Cloyd JM. Neoadjuvant chemotherapy for colorectal liver metastases: A contemporary review of the literature. World J Gastrointest Oncol. 2021;13(9):1043–61. https://doi.org/10.4251/wjgo.v13.i9.1043.
23. National Comprehensive Cancer Network Clinical Practice Guidelines - Rectal Cancer. National Comprehensive Cancer Network; 2022.
24. Adam R, De Gramont A, Figueras J, et al. The oncosurgery approach to managing liver metastases from colorectal cancer: a multidisciplinary international consensus. Oncologist. 2012;17(10):1225–39. https://doi.org/10.1634/theoncologist.2012-0121.
25. Takada T, Tsutsumi S, Takahashi R, et al. Control of primary lesions using resection or radiotherapy can improve the prognosis of metastatic colorectal cancer patients. J Surg Oncol. 2016;114(1):75–9. https://doi.org/10.1002/jso.24255.
26. Zhang CH, Pan YB, Zhang QW, et al. The influence of local therapy on the survival of patients with metastatic rectal cancer: a population-based, propensity-matched study. J Cancer Res Clin Oncol. 2017;143(9):1891–903. https://doi.org/10.1007/s00432-017-2442-2.
27. Butte JM, Gonen M, Ding P, et al. Patterns of failure in patients with early onset (synchronous) resectable liver metastases from rectal cancer. Cancer. 2012;118(21):5414–23. https://doi.org/10.1002/cncr.27567.
28. Martella A, Willett C, Palta M, Czito B. The selective use of radiation therapy in rectal cancer patients. Curr Oncol Rep. 2018;20(6):43. https://doi.org/10.1007/s11912-018-0689-7.
29. Baltatzis M, Chan AK, Jegatheeswaran S, Mason JM, Siriwardena AK. Colorectal cancer with synchronous hepatic metastases: systematic review of reports comparing synchronous surgery with sequential bowel-first or liver-first approaches. Eur J Surg Oncol. 2016;42(2):159–65. https://doi.org/10.1016/j.ejso.2015.11.002.
30. Conrad C, Vauthey JN, Masayuki O, et al. Individualized treatment sequencing selection contributes to optimized survival in patients with rectal cancer and synchronous liver metastases. Ann Surg Oncol. 2017;24(13):3857–64. https://doi.org/10.1245/s10434-017-6089-7.
31. Tzeng CW, Vauthey JN. Postoperative complications and oncologic outcomes after resection of colorectal liver metastases: the importance of staying on track. Ann Surg Oncol. 2013;20(8):2457–9. https://doi.org/10.1245/s10434-013-2974-x.

32. Chan AKC, Mason JM, Baltatzis M, Siriwardena AK, Collaborators C. Management of Colorectal Cancer with synchronous liver metastases: an inception cohort study (CoSMIC). Ann Surg Oncol. 2022;29(3):1939–51. https://doi.org/10.1245/s10434-021-11017-7.
33. Boudjema K, Locher C, Sabbagh C, et al. Simultaneous versus delayed resection for initially resectable synchronous colorectal cancer liver metastases: a prospective, open-label, randomized, controlled trial. Ann Surg. 2021;273(1):49–56. https://doi.org/10.1097/SLA.0000000000003848.
34. Båverud Olsson L, Buchli C, Villard C, Nilsson PJ. Differences in management and outcome for colon and rectal carcinoma with synchronous liver metastases: a population-based cohort study. Color Dis. 2021;23(4):860–7. https://doi.org/10.1111/codi.15468.
35. Giuliante F, Viganò L, De Rose AM, et al. Liver-first approach for synchronous colorectal metastases: analysis of 7360 patients from the LiverMetSurvey registry. Ann Surg Oncol. 2021;28(13):8198–208. https://doi.org/10.1245/s10434-021-10220-w.
36. Esposito F, Lim C, Sa Cunha A, et al. Primary tumor versus liver-first approach for synchronous colorectal liver metastases: an association Française de Chirurgie (AFC) multicenter-based study with propensity score analysis. World J Surg. 2018;42(12):4046–53. https://doi.org/10.1007/s00268-018-4711-x.
37. Silberhumer GR, Paty PB, Denton B, et al. Long-term oncologic outcomes for simultaneous resection of synchronous metastatic liver and primary colorectal cancer. Surgery. 2016;160(1):67–73. https://doi.org/10.1016/j.surg.2016.02.029.
38. Valdimarsson VT, Syk I, Lindell G, et al. Outcomes of liver-first strategy and classical strategy for synchronous colorectal liver metastases in Sweden. HPB (Oxford). 2018;20(5):441–7. https://doi.org/10.1016/j.hpb.2017.11.004.
39. Waisberg J, Ivankovics IG. Liver-first approach of colorectal cancer with synchronous hepatic metastases: A reverse strategy. World J Hepatol. 2015;7(11):1444–9. https://doi.org/10.4254/wjh.v7.i11.1444.
40. Brouquet A, Mortenson MM, Vauthey JN, et al. Surgical strategies for synchronous colorectal liver metastases in 156 consecutive patients: classic, combined or reverse strategy? J Am Coll Surg. 2010;210(6):934–41. https://doi.org/10.1016/j.jamcollsurg.2010.02.039.
41. Shubert CR, Habermann EB, Bergquist JR, et al. A NSQIP review of major morbidity and mortality of synchronous liver resection for colorectal metastasis stratified by extent of liver resection and type of colorectal resection. J Gastrointest Surg. 2015;19(11):1982–94. https://doi.org/10.1007/s11605-015-2895-z.
42. Bogach J, Wang J, Griffiths C, et al. Simultaneous versus staged resection for synchronous colorectal liver metastases: a population-based cohort study. Int J Surg. 2020;74:68–75. https://doi.org/10.1016/j.ijsu.2019.12.009.

Who Needs a Loop Ileostomy After Low Anterior Resection for Rectal Cancer?

26

L. Cunningham and E. Huang

Patient population	Intervention	Comparator	Outcomes studied
Patients after low anterior resection of the rectum for rectal cancer	Proximal diversion with ileostomy	No diversion	Leak rate, consequences

Introduction

The current surgical standard of care for rectal cancer is restorative anterior proctectomy. The most feared complication after low anterior resection (LAR) is anastomotic leak (AL), with its attendant consequences of pelvic sepsis and poor functional outcome. The overall published risk of anastomotic leak varies between 3 and 21% [1]. AL has a reported mortality of 2.1–22% and may require intervention with methods ranging from interventional radiologic drainage to reoperation [2]. Given the heterogeneity of what can be defined as anastomotic leak, a common definition and grading system was proposed by Rahbari et al., based on clinical symptoms and therapeutic interventions [3]. Later validation of this grading system found that some leaks, which were subclinical and discovered on routine workup for diverting ileostomy reversal, were not associated with significant impacts on postoperative course [4]. When assessing data on the impacts of AL, it is important to keep this in mind, as many studies do not document the distinction between AL that do and do not alter the clinical course.

In addition to immediate impact on a patient's clinical course, AL can have several significant consequences. Colonic conduit function after anastomotic leak is

L. Cunningham (✉) · E. Huang
Department of Surgery, The Ohio State University College of Medicine, Columbus, OH, USA
e-mail: lisa.cunningham@osumc.edu; emily.huang@osumc.edu

K. Umanskiy, N. Hyman (eds.), *Difficult Decisions in Colorectal Surgery*, Difficult Decisions in Surgery: An Evidence-Based Approach,
https://doi.org/10.1007/978-3-031-42303-1_26

significantly worse than in patients without leakage [2]. There is also concern regarding poorer oncologic outcomes after anastomotic leak, which may include increased rate of local recurrence and decreased disease-free and overall survival [5, 6]. This increase in cancer recurrence may be due to a delay or abandonment of the necessary adjuvant chemoradiotherapy [6]. Because of the serious morbidity associated with anastomotic leak, fecal diversion is typically considered worth the risk to minimize leak rates and the morbidity from such leaks. However, in recent years, data has emerged on the potential risks and drawbacks of diverting enterostomy, calling the dogma of mandatory fecal diversion after LAR into question. This chapter presents data that will be helpful in making this decision.

Methods

A detailed and updated search of the Embase-Medline and PubMed databases was conducted for medical literature. The following search terms were employed to identify relevant articles: ("rectal" OR "colon" OR "colorectal") AND ("resection" OR "low anterior resection" OR "proctectomy" OR "anastomosis" OR "coloproctostomy") AND ("ileostomy" OR "ostomy" OR "stoma" or "enterostomy" OR "colostomy" OR "diversion" OR "fecal diversion"). The title and abstract of English-language articles were screened for relevance. Relevant articles were reviewed in full.

Risks of Diverting Enterostomy

Despite the widespread use of fecal diversion, it is not without complications. These complications may include both short- and long-term problems and range from minor, requiring only local care, to major complications requiring reoperation and prolonged hospitalization [7, 8]. The most common complication after stoma construction is peristomal skin irritation [9]. While not necessarily defined by most members of the surgical community as a "major" complication, this can have implications for a patient's quality of life [10].

A retrospective review of ACS NSQIP data identified multiple complications that were increased in patients undergoing low anterior resection with fecal diversion [8]. Patients who underwent diversion were found to have a higher rate of progressive renal insufficiency (2.1% vs. 0.8%) without an increased risk of acute renal failure (1.3% vs. 0.7%). Using a risk adjusted model, this increased rate of renal insufficiency was 2.37 times more likely to occur in patients undergoing fecal diversion. Furthermore, patients with fecal diversion had a significantly higher rate of deep surgical site infections (7.5% vs 5.3%) and a higher rate of 30-day readmission (20.3% vs 11%). Although not specifically discussed in this study, the findings of renal insufficiency and readmission are not surprising following stoma creation, as one of the most commonly encountered problems with diverting ileostomy is high ostomy output with dehydration. This complication has a reported incidence of

1–16%, is most common 4–8 days postoperatively as bowel edema is resolving, and leads to electrolyte abnormalities, hypovolemia, and readmission [11]. Further out from the index operation, parastomal hernia occurs at a rate of 15–40% [12].

Diverting ileostomy has also been investigated as a risk factor associated with anastomotic stricturing, pelvic outlet problems, and LAR syndrome (LARS), which is a constellation of symptoms ranging from urgency and incontinence to emptying difficulties. This may be due to effects on the temporarily non-functioning rectum and pelvic floor during recovery and before ileostomy reversal. Two meta-analyses found both diverting ileostomy and AL to be risk factors for LARS (OR of 1.89 and 1.98 respectively, and OR 1.96 for diverting ileostomy) [13, 14]. Other risk factors included expected factors such as neoadjuvant radiation and low tumor [13]. Data from long term follow up of a single randomized trial of loop ileostomy vs. no diversion for LAR corroborate these findings. At 12 years, patients who had been randomly assigned to diverting loop ileostomy expressed increased incontinence for flatus and liquid stools, and worse overall low anterior resection syndrome score, but there were no differences in frequency, clustering, and urgency [15].

While ileostomy reversal is not a technically difficult procedure, it is not without risk. In a study from Pokorny et al. in 2006, 243 patients who underwent loop ileostomy closure were retrospectively reviewed for complications [7]. An overall complication rate of 19% was identified; 3% had anastomotic leak, 6% developed significant postoperative ileus, 1% had bleeding complications, and 9% had wound infections. In total, 4% of patients undergoing ileostomy closure required reoperation for their complication. Finally, although a diverting ileostomy is intended to be temporary, some patients do not undergo reversal due to factors that may include comorbidities or cancer progression. The literature suggests a non-reversal rate of up 3–32%, with one recent population-based study from Denmark indicating a rate of non-reversal of 25% at 3 years [16–18]. The risks of ileostomy creation clearly must be balanced against the risks it is intended to protect against.

Does Fecal Diversion Decrease Anastomotic Leak Rate?

The key question when considering fecal diversion following low anterior resection of the rectum is whether diversion changes the rate of anastomotic leak. Numerous retrospective studies over the years have reported mixed results, with the major limitation being that surgeons concerned about a LAR anastomosis will always favor the safety of temporary diversion.

There are several randomized trials of note that can inform decisions on fecal diversion. Graffner et al. were the first to design such a trial in 1983, when they randomized 50 patients to fecal diversion versus no diversion [19]. The rate of AL was low overall (4% vs. 12%), but stenosis was significantly more common in the diverted group (9/25 vs. 2/25), so the authors concluded that diversion should not routinely be used. The next study, performed in 1997 by Pakkastie et al., randomized 134 patients [20]. They reported a clinically detected AL rate of 16% vs. 32% in the diverted vs. non-diverted groups. Importantly, there was also a lower reoperation rate in the diverted group, as only one of three leaks required reoperation, compared to all six leaks in the non-diverted group.

Larger randomized studies subsequently addressed this issue. In 2007, Matthiessen et al. published data from a large multicenter trial in Sweden. 234 patients requiring LAR (tumor located at up to 15 cm from the anal verge) were randomized to diversion via ileostomy or transverse colostomy (n = 116) vs. no diversion (n = 118) [21]. AL was defined clinically, based on examination, endoscopic evaluation, or radiologic evaluation, but radiographically demonstrated leak (e.g., extravasation of contrast) without clinical symptoms was excluded. AL rate was significantly higher in patients in the non-diverted vs. the diverted group (28.2% vs. 10.3%; $p < 0.001$). Furthermore, there was a significantly higher rate of reoperation in the non-diverted group with overall 25.4% of patients requiring any reoperation versus 8.6% in the diverted group. Of note, a significant majority of patients in both arms of this study had undergone neoadjuvant radiotherapy (81.0% vs. 77.1%; $p < 0.001$). The authors concluded that defunctioning stoma absolutely does reduce symptomatic AL after LAR for cancer. Another study, published in 2008 by Chude et al., randomized 256 patients with tumors located at up to 5 cm from the anal verge, 120 to diversion and 136 to non-diversion [22]. Postoperatively, 12 of the 120 patients without diversion developed anastomotic leak (10%) vs. only 3 patients in the diverted group (2.2%). The study authors drew similar conclusions: that diversion was with minimal risk and significant benefit in prevention of AL. Another small, randomized study performed by Ulrich et al. was reported in 2009, from a single hospital in Germany [23]. This study design is of note as the authors initially intended to demonstrate similar risks in the case of diversion and non-diversion. 34 patients with low or mid rectal tumors undergoing LAR with a stapled colonic pouch were randomized intraoperatively to diversion or non-diversion, after a negative leak test by insufflation. Clinical signs were monitored postoperatively, and if CT demonstrated radiographic leak, the patient underwent laparotomy. Consistent with prior studies, there was a significantly higher rate of clinically detected anastomotic leaks in the non-diverted group (37.5%) compared to the diverted group (5.5%, $p = 0.02$). Due to the study design, all patients who developed a leak in the no stoma group required reoperation while none of the stoma patients with a leak returned to the OR. The outcome differences were in fact so dramatic that the study was terminated after 34 of the intended 40 patients were accrued.

A Cochran Database meta-analysis summarized these results in 2010 [24]. The meta-analysis found a dramatic reduction in AL using fecal diversion (RR 0.33; 95% CI [0.21, 0.53]). Furthermore, diverted patients had a decreased rate of urgent reoperation (RR 0.23; 95% CI [0.12, 0.42]). Despite these differences, there was no significant decrease in terms of overall mortality (RR 0.58; 95% CI [0.14, 2.33]). The reviewers concluded that fecal diversion is an effective method in reducing the rates of anastomotic leak in patients undergoing low anterior resection, and therefore diversion can be offered routinely. Limitations noted include the heterogeneity of definitions in the studies, and lack of reporting of long-term outcomes.

Since the Cochrane Review was completed, at least one further study has been performed in a prospective, randomized fashion [25]. Thoker et al. reported in 2014 on 78 patients undergoing LAR for rectal tumors 4–12 cm from the anal verge at a single hospital in India, who were randomized to ileostomy vs. no ileostomy. The authors focused on stoma-related outcomes, but unfortunately did not include information on use of neoadjuvant or adjuvant radiation therapy. Data revealed a lower leak rate in the diverted group (6% vs. 11%). Ileostomy predisposed patients to electrolyte imbalance in the postoperative period, as well as a significant overall stomal complication rate of 25.4%. The authors also found stoma closure to be associated with an overall complication rate of 67.7%.

More recent studies have examined the effects of wholesale policy changes on AL and diverting stoma formation. Blok et al. compared outcomes of patients undergoing LAR for low to mid rectal tumors at a single Dutch university hospital in an era of "highly selective diversion" vs. historical controls who underwent "routine diversion" [26]. The data are heterogeneous, as selection of diversion was left up to the surgeon, who selected for lower risk patients (e.g., higher tumors, no neoadjuvant long course radiation, healthy patient) to leave undiverted. The authors also incorporated a new practice pattern, transanal total mesorectal excision (TaTME), during the course of the data collection, which may confound results. They reported that stoma-related readmission and reoperation rate (including reversal) were significantly lower in their study group than in their control group (17% and 17%; vs. 84% and 86%; $p < 0.001$), and total hospital stay within 1 year was median 5 vs. 11 days, $p < 0.001$. AL rate was higher in the historical control group (20% vs. 8%), which also more frequently underwent long course chemoradiation (50% vs. 25%, $p = 0.016$). The findings do suggest that, when looking at the big picture of policy (mandatory vs. selective diversion), allowing surgeons to utilize diversion selectively might have significant benefits for patients.

Taken together, these data overall demonstrate that fecal diversion offers a clear benefit in LAR in lowering anastomotic leak rate and need for reoperation. While early retrospective studies arrived at varying conclusions, prospective randomized trials have all demonstrated a clear benefit to fecal diversion. Therefore, at this point, it is clear that at a population level, fecal diversion should be the default operation in combination with LAR. However, what these studies fail to address is which patients are at decreased risk of anastomotic leak and therefore could avoid defunctioning stoma placement.

Who Is at Highest Risk for Developing a Leak?

Patient factors associated with poor wound healing increase the risk of developing an anastomotic leak. Patients who are malnourished, on steroids, and obese, are at higher risk for developing an anastomotic leak [27]. Early retrospective analyses found specific rectal cancer factors associated with increased risk of AL: distance from anal verge was found to have the strongest association with leak rate (OR = 5.4–6 for anastomosis 5 cm from anal verge) [28, 29]. Further operative factors related to anastomotic leak included male gender (OR = 2.36), and intraoperative blood loss (OR = 1.05) [29]. Predictive risk score calculators may be useful in assessing patient and cancer-related factors. The REAL (REctal Anastomotic Leak) score was proposed by a collaborative study group based on meta-analysis of studies including 9735 patients, and utilizes 12 preoperative factors (interval from neoadjuvant therapy to surgery, short course radiotherapy, TNM staging, anastomotic distance from anal verge, patient age, gender, smoking status, BMI, diabetes, ASA grade, prior abdominal surgery, and hemoglobin) to calculate a patient's risk of AL [30].

Intraoperative assessment of the anastomosis may play an important role in reducing the leak rate and in deciding on the need for proximal diversion. Common methods of evaluating a colorectal anastomosis include air leak testing, saline leak, methylene blue leak tests and endoscopic assessment. Two randomized trials have evaluated the validity of performing an intraoperative leak test and have found that the risk of leak in those tested was significantly lower than the untested controls (5.8% versus 16%, $p < 0.05$) [31, 32]. Therefore, intraoperative leak testing should be performed and patients found to have concerning findings on exam should undergo repair, revision, and possibly fecal diversion.

A 2014 meta-analysis by Qin et al. included seven randomized controlled trials evaluating the role of preoperative radiotherapy as a risk factor for AL after LAR [33]. In the pooled studies, 1660 patients were included in the preoperative radiotherapy group and 1715 patients were included in the control group. In this analysis, rates of anastomotic leak were not increased in the preoperative radiotherapy group (OR = 1.02; CI 0.80, 1.30; $p = 0.88$). This analysis, however, is limited by the use of clinically detected anastomotic leaks in the individual trials making up the analysis, which may underreport anastomotic leaks that would be clinically significant if no defunctioning stoma were in place. Because it is not possible to directly measure the rate of clinically significant leaks in the presence of a defunctioning stoma, making strong recommendations in patients who received preoperative radiotherapy remains difficult. Short course chemoradiotherapy (delivery of neoadjuvant therapy over the course of 5 days vs. 25 fractions) has gained in popularity. The most direct comparison of relevant outcomes, a randomized controlled trial in which patients with T3 rectal adenocarcinoma within 12 cm of the anal verge were randomized to short course radiotherapy vs. long course chemoradiotherapy, demonstrated no significant difference in AL rate [34].

A new and growing body of evidence also points to the role gut microbiome in AL. A study by Shogan et al. in 2015 was one of the first to demonstrate the contribution of specific bacteria in development of AL [35]. This group noted that matrix metalloproteinase enzymes produced by Enterococcus faecalis were responsible for tissue degradation at the anastomosis in rats and found the same strains in anastomotic samples of patients undergoing colon resections. While research in this area is still ongoing, a substantial and growing body of literature suggests that environmental factors, including diet, antibiotics, bowel prep, and physiological stress from surgery, alter the microbiome to cause AL or worsened oncologic outcomes after colorectal surgery [36]. Upcoming microbiome sequencing technology may thus inform decisions about AL risk and diversion.

What Type of Diverting Ostomy Should We Use?

When considering fecal diversion, the two common options are loop ileostomy and loop colostomy. Four randomized trials have compared these two options to each other, with two studies favoring the use of loop colostomy [37, 38] and two favoring loop ileostomy [39, 40]. A 2007 Cochrane review found five randomized studies involving 334 patients: 168 undergoing loop Ileostomy and 166 undergoing loop colostomy [41]. There was a large and significant difference in stomal prolapse rates, with a rate of 2% in the ileostomy group vs. 19% in the colostomy group ($p < 0.01$); however, there were no other differences noted. Given the large difference in rates of prolapse, current recommendations are to create a loop ileostomy when possible.

Are There Benefits to Early Ileostomy Closure?

Most surgeons close a diverting ileostomy at 2–3 months after the initial LAR. Under traditional models of neoadjuvant chemoradiation and possible adjuvant chemotherapy, this occasionally caused considerable delay in closure, as patients might need to undergo uninterrupted adjuvant chemotherapy. Conversely, patients who developed stoma-related complications might be prevented from undergoing needed adjuvant therapy. There was thus significant interest in the possibility of early closure of diverting ileostomy, within 2 weeks of LAR. One multicenter randomized controlled trial from Denmark and Sweden addressed this question, finding that the mean number of complications up to 12 months of follow up after LAR was actually significantly lower in the early closure group vs. the control group undergoing ileostomy closure at 12 weeks (1.2 vs. 2.9, $p < 0.0001$) [42]. Cost analysis from this same trial demonstrated a mean cost savings of $3608 in favor of early closure [43]. Given the known functional impacts of delayed ileostomy closure including impaired bowel function, delaying ileostomy closure no longer than 6 months is recommended [44]. Total neoadjuvant therapy, in which both chemoradiotherapy and consolidation chemotherapy are delivered up-front before surgery, may help prevent prolonged interval to ileostomy closure after LAR.

Personal View of the Data

While proximal diversion is not without risks, the consequences of an anastomotic leak are significant enough that the benefits usually outweigh the risks. Therefore, proximal fecal diversion following anterior resection for rectal cancer should be considered standard practice in most patients. Some patients may be at low risk for developing an anastomotic leak, and consideration of patient factors such as age, sex, weight and smoking status, tumor factors, and intraoperative factors; as well as utilization of a risk calculator, may help determine those patients who are candidates for non-diversion. After creation, all colorectal anastomoses should be tested for the presence of an anastomotic leak. A positive test may necessitate a revision of the anastomosis and/or repair followed by proximal fecal diversion.

References

1. Karanjia ND, Corder AP, Bearn P, Heald RJ. Leakage from stapled low anastomosis after total mesorectal excision for carcinoma of the rectum. Br J Surg. 2005;81:1224–6.
2. Matthiessen P, Hallbook O, Andersson M, Rutegard J, Sjodahl R. Risk factors for anastomotic leakage after anterior resection of the rectum. Color Dis. 2004;6:462–9.
3. Rahbari NN, Weitz J, Hohenberger W, et al. Definition and grading of anastomotic leakage following anterior resection of the rectum: a proposal by the International Study Group of Rectal Cancer. Surgery. 2010;147:339–51.
4. Kulu Y, Ulrich A, Bruckner T, Contin P, Welsch T, Rahbari NN, Büchler MW, Weitz J. Validation of the international study Group of Rectal Cancer definition and severity grading of anastomotic leakage. Surgery. 2013;153:753–61.
5. Ha GW, Kim JH, Lee MR. Oncologic impact of anastomotic leakage following colorectal cancer surgery: a systematic review and meta-analysis. Ann Surg Oncol. 2017;24:3289–99.
6. Jung SH, Yu CS, Choi PW, Kim DD, Park IJ, Kim HC, Kim JC. Risk factors and oncologic impact of anastomotic leakage after rectal cancer surgery. Dis Colon Rectum. 2008;51:902–8.
7. Pokorny H, Herkner H, Jakesz R, Herbst F. Predictors for complications after loop stoma closure in patients with rectal cancer. World J Surg. 2006;30:1488–93.
8. Jafari MD, Halabi WJ, Jafari F, Nguyen VQ, Stamos MJ, Carmichael JC, Mills SD, Pigazzi A. Morbidity of diverting ileostomy for rectal cancer: analysis of the American College of Surgeons National Surgical Quality Improvement Program. Am Surg. 2013;79:1034–9.
9. Colwell JC, Goldberg M, Carmel J. The state of the standard diversion. J Wound Ostomy Continence Nurs. 2001;28:6–17.
10. Arumugam PJ, Bevan L, Macdonald L, Watkins AJ, Morgan AR, Beynon J, Carr ND. A prospective audit of stomas-analysis of risk factors and complications and their management. Color Dis. 2003;5:49–52.
11. Baker ML, Williams RN, Nightingale JMD. Causes and management of a high-output stoma. Color Dis. 2011;13:191–7.
12. Robertson I, Leung E, Hughes D, Spiers M, Donnelly L, Mackenzie I, Macdonald A. Prospective analysis of stoma-related complications. Color Dis. 2005;7:279–85.
13. Sun R, Dai Z, Zhang Y, Lu J, Zhang Y, Xiao Y. The incidence and risk factors of low anterior resection syndrome (LARS) after sphincter-preserving surgery of rectal cancer: a systematic review and meta-analysis. Support Care Cancer. 2021;29:7249–58.
14. Keane C, Sharma P, Yuan L, Bissett I, O'Grady G. Impact of temporary ileostomy on long-term quality of life and bowel function: a systematic review and meta-analysis. ANZ J Surg. 2020;90:687–92.
15. Gadan S, Floodeen H, Lindgren R, Matthiessen P. Does a Defunctioning stoma impair anorectal function after low anterior resection of the rectum for cancer? A 12-year follow-up of a randomized multicenter trial. Dis Colon Rectum. 2017;60:800–6.
16. Chow A, Tilney HS, Paraskeva P, Jeyarajah S, Zacharakis E, Purkayastha S. The morbidity surrounding reversal of defunctioning ileostomies: a systematic review of 48 studies including 6,107 cases. Int J Color Dis. 2009;24:711–23.
17. Alves A, Panis Y, Lelong B, Dousset B, Benoist S, Vicaut E. Randomized clinical trial of early versus delayed temporary stoma closure after proctectomy. Br J Surg. 2008;95:693–8.
18. Jørgensen JB, Erichsen R, Pedersen BG, Laurberg S, Iversen LH. Stoma reversal after intended restorative rectal cancer resection in Denmark: nationwide population-based study. BJS Open. 2020;4:1162–71.

19. Graffner H, Fredlund P, Olsson S-Å, Oscarson J, Petersson B-G. Protective colostomy in low anterior resection of the rectum using the EEA stapling instrument. Dis Colon Rectum. 1983;26:87–90.
20. Pakkastie TE, Ovaska JT, Pekkala ES, Luukkonen PE, Järvinen HJ. A randomised study of colostomies in low colorectal anastomoses. Eur J Surg. 1997;163:929–33.
21. Matthiessen P, Hallböök O, Rutegård J, Simert G, Sjödahl R. Defunctioning stoma reduces symptomatic anastomotic leakage after low anterior resection of the rectum for cancer. Ann Surg. 2007;246:207–14.
22. Chude GG, Rayate NV, Patris V, Koshariya M, Jagad R, Kawamoto J, Lygidakis NJ. Defunctioning loop ileostomy with low anterior resection for distal rectal cancer: should we make an ileostomy as a routine procedure? A prospective randomized study. Hepato-Gastroenterology. 2008;55:1562–7.
23. Ulrich AB, Seiler C, Rahbari N, Weitz J, Büchler MW. Diverting stoma after low anterior resection. Dis Colon Rectum. 2009;52:412–8.
24. Montedori A, Cirocchi R, Farinella E, Sciannameo F, Abraha I. Covering ileo- or colostomy in anterior resection for rectal carcinoma. Cochrane Database Syst Rev. 2010; https://doi.org/10.1002/14651858.CD006878.pub2.
25. Thoker M, Wani I, Parray FQ, Khan N, Mir SA, Thoker P. Role of diversion ileostomy in low rectal cancer: a randomized controlled trial. Int J Surg. 2014;12:945–51.
26. Blok RD, Stam R, Westerduin E, Borstlap WAA, Hompes R, Bemelman WA, Tanis PJ. Impact of an institutional change from routine to highly selective diversion of a low anastomosis after TME for rectal cancer. Eur J Surg Oncol. 2018;44:1220–5.
27. Hüser N, Michalski CW, Erkan M, Schuster T, Rosenberg R, Kleeff J, Friess H. Systematic review and meta-analysis of the role of Defunctioning stoma in low rectal cancer surgery. Ann Surg. 2008;248:52–60.
28. Bertelsen CA, Andreasen AH, Jørgensen T, Harling H. Anastomotic leakage after anterior resection for rectal cancer: risk factors. Color Dis. 2010;12:37–43.
29. Rullier E, Laurent C, Garrelon JL, Michel P, Saric J, Parneix M. Risk factors for anastomotic leakage after resection of rectal cancer. Br J Surg. 2003;85:355–8.
30. Arezzo A, Migliore M, Chiaro P, et al. The REAL (REctal anastomotic leak) score for prediction of anastomotic leak after rectal cancer surgery. Tech Coloproctol. 2019;23:649–63.
31. Beard JD, Nicholson ML, Sayers RD, Lloyd D, Everson NW. Intraoperative air testing of colorectal anastomoses: a prospective, randomized trial. Br J Surg. 2005;77:1095–7.
32. Ivanov D, Cvijanovic R, Gvozdenovic L. Intraoperative air testing of colorectal anastomoses. Srp Arh Celok Lek. 2011;139:333–8.
33. Qin C, Ren X, Xu K, Chen Z, He Y, Song X. Does preoperative radio(chemo)therapy increase anastomotic leakage in rectal cancer surgery? A meta-analysis of randomized controlled trials. Gastroenterol Res Pract. 2014;2014:1–7.
34. Ansari N, Solomon MJ, Fisher RJ, et al. Acute adverse events and postoperative complications in a randomized trial of preoperative short-course radiotherapy versus long-course Chemoradiotherapy for T3 adenocarcinoma of the rectum. Ann Surg. 2017;265:882–8.
35. Shogan BD, Belogortseva N, Luong PM, et al. Collagen degradation and MMP9 activation by enterococcus faecalis contribute to intestinal anastomotic leak. Sci Transl Med. 2015;7:286ra68.
36. Gaines S, Shao C, Hyman N, Alverdy JC. Gut microbiome influences on anastomotic leak and recurrence rates following colorectal cancer surgery. Br J Surg. 2018;105:e131–41.
37. Gooszen AW, Geelkerken RH, Hermans J, Lagaay MB, Gooszen HG. Temporary decompression after colorectal surgery: randomized comparison of loop ileostomy and loop colostomy. Br J Surg. 2003;85:76–9.
38. Law WL, Chu KW, Choi HK. Randomized clinical trial comparing loop ileostomy and loop transverse colostomy for faecal diversion following total mesorectal excision. Br J Surg. 2002;89:704–8.
39. Khoury GA, Lewis MC, Meleagros L, Lewis AA. Colostomy or ileostomy after colorectal anastomosis?: a randomised trial. Ann R Coll Surg Engl. 1987;69:5–7.

40. Williams NS, Nasmyth DG, Jones D, Smith AH. De-functioning stomas: a prospective controlled trial comparing loop ileostomy with loop transverse colostomy. Br J Surg. 2005;73:566–70.
41. Güenaga KF, Lustosa SA, Saad SS, Saconato H, Matos D. Ileostomy or colostomy for temporary decompression of colorectal anastomosis. Cochrane Database Syst Rev. 2007;2010:CD004647. https://doi.org/10.1002/14651858.CD004647.pub2.
42. Danielsen AK, Park J, Jansen JE, Bock D, Skullman S, Wedin A, Marinez AC, Haglind E, Angenete E, Rosenberg J. Early closure of a temporary ileostomy in patients with rectal cancer: a multicenter randomized controlled trial. Ann Surg. 2017;265:284–90.
43. Park J, Angenete E, Bock D, et al. Cost analysis in a randomized trial of early closure of a temporary ileostomy after rectal resection for cancer (EASY trial). Surg Endosc. 2020;34:69–76.
44. Vogel I, Reeves N, Tanis PJ, Bemelman WA, Torkington J, Hompes R, Cornish JA. Impact of a defunctioning ileostomy and time to stoma closure on bowel function after low anterior resection for rectal cancer: a systematic review and meta-analysis. Tech Coloproctol. 2021;25:751–60.

Reoperative Surgery for Locally Recurrent Rectal Cancer

27

Nicholas P. McKenna and Robert R. Cima

Introduction

Locoregional rectal cancer recurrence rates have decreased from as high as 30% to less than 10% since the widespread adoption of total mesorectal excision along with administration of neoadjuvant or adjuvant chemoradiotherapy [1–4]. Locoregional recurrences treated with chemoradiation alone have poor outcomes, with a median survival of only 12 to 24 months [5–7]. However, the combination of preoperative chemoradiation or re-irradiation, an R0 resection, and intraoperative radiation therapy (IORT) when indicated can significantly improve outcomes. Patients with locoregional recurrences undergoing this multimodal treatment approach have 5-year survival between 37% and 57% [7, 8].

Reoperative surgery for locally recurrent rectal cancer is associated with major morbidity rates ranging from 15% to 68% and mortality rates of up to 10% [9]. Therefore, patient selection is critical to ensure that only patients with a reasonable chance for an R0 resection undergo such an extensive operation. Additional important considerations are ensuring the patient is optimized from a nutritional standpoint, is not smoking, the resection of local recurrence is technically feasible, and that any metastatic disease is controlled or controllable. The latter two factors influence whether the **operation** is curative or palliative. Optimally, the patient's case is reviewed by a multidisciplinary team to ensure that appropriate preoperative therapy is provided. Given the complexity of these cases, care should provided at a tertiary referral center with the resources and experience to perform an R0 multivisceral resection as well as manage potentially significant postoperative complications [10].

N. P. McKenna · R. R. Cima (✉)
Mayo Clinic, Division of Colon and Rectal Surgery, Rochester, MN, USA
e-mail: McKenna.Nicholas@mayo.edu; cima.robert@mayo.edu

K. Umanskiy, N. Hyman (eds.), *Difficult Decisions in Colorectal Surgery*, Difficult Decisions in Surgery: An Evidence-Based Approach,
https://doi.org/10.1007/978-3-031-42303-1_27

Table 27.1 PICO question search strategy for the chapter

Patients	Intervention	Comparator	Outcomes
Patients with recurrent rectal cancer	Surgery	Palliative treatment Non-treatment	Survival Cure Morbidity Quality of life

Search Strategy

PubMed was utilized to conduct a review of the English literature on recurrent rectal cancer. Search terms used included "recurrent rectal cancer," "locally recurrent rectal cancer," and "intraoperative radiation therapy." Original studies were used where possible and supplemented by meta-analyses. Reference lists in systematic reviews were used to identify additional manuscripts. Manuscripts published between 1986 and 2022 were assessed with a focus on the last 10 years (Table 27.1).

Results

Diagnosis

Data on diagnosis of locoregional recurrence of rectal cancer is heterogeneous, with some studies describing over 65% of patients diagnosed due to symptoms [7, 11], while others describe the majority of recurrences diagnosed based on routine surveillance imaging and carcinoembryonic antigen (CEA) levels [12]. All patients with a confirmed recurrence require a full staging workup, including cross-sectional imaging, a colonoscopy, and a CEA level. Cross-sectional imaging should include CT scan of the chest, abdomen, and pelvis, as well as a pelvic MRI. Chest and abdominal imaging are useful for the detection of distant recurrence, while CT and MRI of the pelvis define the anatomic relationships of the locoregional recurrence. MRI is particularly useful since it allows better soft-tissue resolution and can distinguish recurrent rectal cancer from presacral scar [13]. Tissue diagnosis via colonoscopy if a luminal recurrence or via CT-guided biopsy is important before committing to an operation. If biopsies are non-diagnostic, PET CT is also often helpful to distinguish fibrosis from recurrence. It may also detect distant metastatic disease missed by CT scan.

Classification Systems and Outcomes

Once a recurrence is diagnosed, there are numerous classification systems to describe the recurrence pattern without clear superiority of one system [14]. The Memorial Sloan Kettering system is based on anatomical compartments (axial, anterior, posterior, or pelvic sidewall). Axial recurrences can be anastomotic (patients status post low anterior resection), perineal (patients status post abdominoperineal resection), or local recurrence after transanal or transsphincteric excision. Anterior recurrences involve the urogenital structures while posterior recurrences involve the sacrum and/or coccyx. Lateral recurrences involve the pelvic sidewall bones, musculature, or sidewall structures [15]. In studies that have used the Memorial Sloan Kettering system to evaluate surgical outcomes, R0 resections were more common for axial recurrences compared all other compartments [15–17]. Iliac vessel involvement was also specifically associated with decreased R0 resections rates [15]. Yamada et al. proposed a system based on the pattern of pelvic invasion – localized type, sacral invasive type, and lateral invasive type [18]. Like the Memorial Sloan Kettering system axial compartment recurrence type, survival was best with the local invasive type [18–20]. The Mayo Clinic system uses sites of fixation [from 0 sites of fixation (F0) to 3–4 sites of fixation (F3)] and symptoms [no symptoms or pain (S0) to symptomatic and painful (S2)] to classify recurrence [21]. Survival has been shown to decrease with both increasing sites of fixation and increasing symptoms and pain [8, 21–23]. Additional classification systems exist and are largely based on the pattern of pelvic invasion [23, 24]. The common theme amongst all recurrence classification systems is that axial or local recurrences and therefore less points of fixation are associated with either improved rates of R0 resection, survival, or both. No comparisons between the classification systems exist to determine whether one is more prognostic than others.

Treatment and Oncologic Outcomes

Since an R0 resection is the most consistent favorable factor for survival, it is critically important to maximize the chances of this. Multimodal therapy with a combination of chemotherapy, chemoradiotherapy, and surgery have shown the best outcomes compared to surgery alone or radiotherapy alone [25–27]. Specific treatment received and the sequence of treatment depends on several factors related to the extent of the local recurrence and prior treatment received.

The patients who are radiation naïve, should receive a full course of chemoradiation following the same protocols used for locally advanced rectal cancer with 50 to 50.4 Gy in 25–28 fractions with radiosensitizing chemotherapy [28]. Patients who previously received radiation can typically receive up to 30.4–39 Gy in additional radiation with acceptable toxicity [29–31]. Re-irradiation may be better tolerated moving forward with increased use of intensity-modulated radiation therapy [32], which allows precise dose delivery [33]. Hyperfractionated radiotherapy may also reduce the late toxicity of reirradiation [34].

Receipt of radiation or re-irradiation is essential as pooled data from the Mayo Clinic, Rochester and the Catharina Hospital, Eindhoven showed lower rates of R0 resections in patients who never received either radiation or re-irradiation (25.9%) versus those who received full course (50.2%) or re-irradiation (43.0%) in the largest series to date (n = 565) [25]. Additionally, neoadjuvant chemoradiation and re-irradiation are associated with improved 3-year overall survival (full course 49.3%, re-irradiation 47.6%, no radiation 25.0%) and 3-year local control (full course

69.0%, re-irradiation 48.9%, no radiation 37.6%) compared to patients who were not re-irradiated [35]. Lastly, in a recent systematic review of studies from 1999 to 2021, the highest proportion of R0 resections were observed in patients treated with neoadjuvant chemoradiotherapy compared to neoadjuvant radiotherapy or adjuvant chemoradiotherapy [36].

Recently, Catharina Hospital, Eindhoven published their results of adding induction chemotherapy to the treatment regimen for recurrent rectal cancer with the goal of improved downsizing the local recurrence and increasing pathologic complete response rates. The regimen consists of either 3 cycles of CAPOX (capecitabine and oxaliplatin) or 4 cycles of FOLFOX (leucovorin, 5-fluorouraicl, oxaliplatin) followed by radiation or re-irradiation as described above. If on restaging imaging a patient had a good response to chemotherapy, consolidation chemotherapy is considered during the interval between radiation and surgery.

With this regimen, they achieved a 17% completely pathologic response [37, 38]. This is better than reported complete pathologic response rates of 8%–12% with radiotherapy alone [39–41]. Mayo Clinic employs a similar protocol with 4 cycles of FOLFOX followed by re-staging imaging with PET-CT and musculoskeletal protocol MRI followed by radiation or re-irradiation [42].

With respect to long-term outcomes, patients in the Catharine Hospital experience with a complete pathologic response had a 3-year overall survival of 92%. Since all patients with a complete response have an R0 resection, by definition, the authors also studied patients with a good response to neoadjuvant therapy and R0 resection. These patients did better than patients with a poor response and R0 resection in both overall survival and local disease-free interval. Interestingly, patients with a poor response but an R0 resection had outcomes similar to patients without an R0 resection for both local-recurrence free survival and metastasis-free survival. Toxicity from chemotherapy was acceptable with 10% of patients experiencing grade 3–4 toxicity and no grade 5 events.

No other institutions have reported outcomes of induction chemotherapy for locally recurrent chemotherapy yet, but the results from Catharina Hospital are promising. They also are in line with the increasing utilization of total neoadjuvant therapy for primary locally advanced rectal cancer [43], which is addressed in a separate chapter. Randomized controlled trials comparing neoadjuvant chemotherapy followed by pelvic re-irradiation versus neoadjuvant chemotherapy alone (GRECCAR 15) and neoadjuvant chemotherapy followed by pelvic re-irradiation versus neoadjuvant chemoradiotherapy (PelvEx II) are currently recruiting patients with recurrent rectal cancer [44, 45]. Therefore, higher-level evidence on preoperative therapy for recurrent rectal cancer may be available in the future.

Intraoperative radiation therapy can be added after surgical resection to overcome the dose tolerance of normal tissue to external beam radiation and re-irradiation. Outcomes with the use of IORT are generally favorable in terms of local control and survival without a concomitant increase in morbidity [25, 46–50]. At the Mayo Clinic and Catharina Hospital, IORT is delivered via a dedicated linear accelerator in the operating room [25, 51]. The IORT dose is determined intraoperatively based on frozen section pathologic margins and the radiation dose the patient received preoperatively. For patients who received 45–54 Gy preoperatively, IORT consisted of 10–12.5 Gy for R0 but close margins, 12.5–15 Gy for R1 resections, and 15–20 Gy for R2 resections. In patients who were re-irradiated with 30 Gy, IORT dose was 15–20 Gy typically [42, 51]. This dosing pattern is in line with the European Society Radiation Oncology – The Advisory Committee for Radiation Oncology Practice IORT recommendations [52].

Data on the benefit of IORT are all limited by the lack of any randomized trials comparing the receipt versus omission. The time between completion of neoadjuvant radiation and surgery with IORT has also been debated to maximize the chance of an R0 resection but minimize the chances of a local re-recurrence. In pooled data from Catharine Hospital and the Mayo Clinic of 565 patients, they identified 5–7 weeks after completion of radiation as the optimal window. This window is based on prior analysis showing significant downstaging of rectal cancers at 4–6 weeks after completion of chemoradiation [53–56] and an increase in local recurrence when surgery and IORT delivery was delayed past 7 weeks [25].

Nutritional Status and Postoperative Morbidity

If a patient is to be considered a candidate for reoperative surgery, they must also be physiologically fit enough to undergo reoperative surgery that often requires multivisceral resection. The prevalence of malnutrition amongst cancer patients has become more evident in recent years [57], with malnutrition diagnosed in 15% to33% of patients with either locally advanced or recurrent rectal cancer set to undergo pelvic exenteration [58–60]. Major complications occur after up to 36% of exenterative surgery cases for recurrent rectal cancer and malnutrition is a leading risk factor [59]. There is limited data on specific complications after reoperation for recurrent rectal cancer but one study from 2003 found that the most common complications were pelvic abscesses, bowel obstructions, and perineal wound healing issues [8]. Perineal wound healing becomes a major source of morbidity due to the size of the perineal defect and the amount of radiation received preoperatively. Use of a tissue flap to fill the dead space in the pelvis and potentially reduce perineal wound issues is critical [61, 62]. Multiple flap options exist with omental flaps and vertical rectus abdominis myocutaneous flaps utilized most often [63, 64].

To further mitigate risk, prehabilitation before surgery is an option. Prehabilitation has been shown to reduce the risk of morbidity and length of stay after colorectal cancer operations but has not been studied in patients with recurrent rectal cancer [65, 66]. Given the high rates of major morbidity after pelvic exenteration, this area deserves further study. The neoadjuvant chemotherapy and radiation regimens for recurrent rectal cancer allow a natural window for prehabilitation to occur.

Patients Ineligible for Curative Surgery

In patients who are not candidates for a curative operation, attempts at operations that will result in an R2 resection should be avoided. Various options for palliation exist depending on the primary symptoms the patient is experiencing. Radiation and

Table 27.2 Summary of Outcomes after Neoadjuvant Treatment and Surgery for Recurrent Rectal Cancer

Study	Patients, n	Intervention and outcome	Results	Quality of Evidence
Holman et al. [25]	565	No preoperative treatment versus re-irradiation versus full-course radiotherapy and R0 resection rate	R0 resection rate 26% versus 43% versus 50%, $p < 0.0001$	Moderate
Harris et al. [27]	533	Surgical margin impact on 5-year survival	5-year survival 44% for R0 versus 26% and 10% for R1 and R2	Moderate
Dresen et al. [35]	147	Preoperative radiation and survival	3-year overall survival (full course 49.3%, re-irradiation 47.6%, no radiation 25.0%) and 3-year local control (full course 69.0%, re-irradiation 48.9%, no radiation 37.6%)	Moderate
Voogt et al. [38]	132	Pathologic response rate after induction chemotherapy and chemo(re)irradiation	17% complete pathologic response	Moderate
Voogt et al. [38]	132	3-year survival in complete versus non-complete responders	92% vs 57% in complete versus non-complete responders, $p = 0.045$	Moderate
Ansell et al. [42]	267	Survival for re-resection of positive intraoperative margins	Overall survival 4.4 years for R0 versus 2.7 years for R1 to R0 and 2.9 years for R1 to R1	Moderate

re-irradiation have been shown to have favorable outcomes with respect to pain and pelvic symptoms while avoiding the morbidity of surgery [67]. For patients presenting with malignant bowel obstruction and unresectable disease, both self-expanding metal stents and colonic diversion are options for palliation and choice depends on the specific clinical circumstances [68]. Again, as an R0 resection is the most consistent favorable prognostic factor, extensive operations should not be undertaken if this is not the likely outcome (Table 27.2).

Recommendations Based on the Data

Recommendations on the workup and medical and surgical management of recurrent rectal cancer are limited by the existing data, which are primarily retrospective, single institution studies. Fortunately, in the future with two randomized control trials actively recruiting, higher level evidence may be available on how to optimally treat patients preoperatively.

Work up of patients with suspected rectal cancer recurrence should include pelvic MRI to assess anatomical relationships of the recurrence. Patients also need a

CT of the chest and abdomen to assess for distant metastases. For equivocal findings on imaging, PET-CT and/or percutaneous biopsy can be performed. (Evidence: moderate; Recommendation: strong).

Based on the MRI finding and the patient symptoms, recurrence can be anatomically defined based on the classification system of the surgeon's choice. This will help determine the probability of an R0 resection and whether surgery is a potential eventual treatment option. (Evidence: moderate; Recommendation: strong).

Neoadjuvant chemotherapy should likely be administered to all patients based on increased rates of R0 resections and complete pathologic response. Patients who are radiologically naïve should receive 50.4 Gy of chemoradiotherapy. Patients who received neoadjuvant chemoradiation before their initial surgery should be re-irradiated with up to 30 Gy. (Evidence: weak; Recommendation: strong).

After completion of neoadjuvant therapy, re-staging should occur with surgery planned for 5–7 weeks after completion of therapy if an R0 resection is felt to be possible. IORT can be planned if a threatened margin is likely. (Evidence: weak; Recommendation: strong).

R0 resections provide the best chance at long-term survival. IORT can supplement an R1 resection but does not provide equivalent survival to an R0 resection. R2 resections result in significant morbidity with no survival benefit and should not be pursued. (Evidence: moderate; Recommendation: strong).

Malnutrition is prevalent amongst patients with recurrent rectal cancer and is a major risk factor for postoperative morbidity. Prehabilitation may be able to reduce some of the associated morbidity, while myocutaneous flaps to exclude the pelvis help with perineal wound healing issues. (Evidence: moderate; Recommendation: weak).

In patients with a recurrence that is unresectable or who are not candidates for curative surgery for physiologic reasons, palliation may be offered with a variety of modalities available depending on specific symptoms. (Evidence: moderate; Recommendation: strong).

A Personal View of the Data

Patients referred to Mayo Clinic, Rochester for locally recurrent rectal cancer are initially evaluated with a musculoskeletal protocol MRI of the pelvis as well as a CT scan of the chest, abdomen, and pelvis. For equivocal cases on MRI, a PET-CT is obtained. The pelvic MRI will allow the recurrence to be classified by the surgeon's system of choice. At Mayo Clinic, the Mayo Clinic system is used. This will guide the decision of whether a recurrence is potentially anatomically resectable to an R0 margin with acceptable postoperative outcomes. The chest, abdomen, and pelvis CT will identify any distant metastatic disease that may influence the decision to operate or not. The operation will likely require a multi-disciplinary team, so urology, gynecology, vascular surgery, radiation oncology, and plastic surgery should be coordinated as needed preoperatively depending on the tumor's anatomic relationships.

Like Catharina Hospital, we have begun administering 4 cycles of FOLFOX to patients before restaging with pelvic MRI. External beam chemoradiotherapy is then used with the dose delivered based on prior receipt of radiation or not. For radiotherapy naive patients, long-course chemoradiotherapy with 50.4 Gy is given. For patients who previously received chemoradiotherapy for their primary cancer, a reduced dose of 30 Gy is given along with radiosensitizing chemotherapy. After an additional 5–7 weeks, patients are again restaged, and if they are still appropriate for surgery, resection is undertaken. The decision to use IORT or not is based on final margin status on intraoperative frozen pathology.

References

1. Swedish Rectal Cancer T, Cedermark B, Dahlberg M, Glimelius B, Pahlman L, Rutqvist LE, et al. Improved survival with preoperative radiotherapy in resectable rectal cancer. N Engl J Med. 1997;336(14):980–7.
2. Kapiteijn E, Marijnen CA, Colenbrander AC, Klein Kranenbarg E, Steup WH, van Krieken JH, et al. Local recurrence in patients with rectal cancer diagnosed between 1988 and 1992: a population-based study in the West Netherlands. Eur J Surg Oncol. 1998;24(6):528–35.
3. Sebag-Montefiore D, Stephens RJ, Steele R, Monson J, Grieve R, Khanna S, et al. Preoperative radiotherapy versus selective postoperative chemoradiotherapy in patients with rectal cancer (MRC CR07 and NCIC-CTG C016): a multicentre, randomised trial. Lancet. 2009;373(9666):811–20.
4. MacFarlane JK, Ryall RD, Heald RJ. Mesorectal excision for rectal cancer. Lancet. 1993;341(8843):457–60.
5. Rhomberg W, Eiter H, Hergan K, Schneider B. Inoperable recurrent rectal cancer: results of a prospective trial with radiation therapy and razoxane. Int J Radiat Oncol Biol Phys. 1994;30(2):419–25.
6. Ito Y, Ohtsu A, Ishikura S, Boku N, Nihei K, Ogino T, et al. Efficacy of chemoradiotherapy on pain relief in patients with intrapelvic recurrence of rectal cancer. Jpn J Clin Oncol. 2003;33(4):180–5.
7. Palmer G, Martling A, Cedermark B, Holm T. A population-based study on the management and outcome in patients with locally recurrent rectal cancer. Ann Surg Oncol. 2007;14(2):447–54.
8. Hahnloser D, Nelson H, Gunderson LL, Hassan I, Haddock MG, O'Connell MJ, et al. Curative potential of multimodality therapy for locally recurrent rectal cancer. Ann Surg. 2003;237(4):502–8.
9. Nielsen MB, Laurberg S, Holm T. Current management of locally recurrent rectal cancer. Color Dis. 2011;13(7):732–42.
10. Harji DP, Griffiths B, McArthur DR, Sagar PM. Current UK management of locally recurrent rectal cancer. Color Dis. 2012;14(12):1479–82.
11. Waldenstedt S, Haglind E, Angenete E. Symptoms and diagnosis of local recurrence after rectal cancer treatment. Acta Oncol. 2022;69:1043–9.
12. Wieldraaijer T, Bruin P, Duineveld LAM, Tanis PJ, Smits AB, van Weert H, et al. Clinical pattern of recurrent disease during the follow-up of Rectal carcinoma. Dig Surg. 2018;35(1):35–41.
13. Schaefer O, Langer M. Detection of recurrent rectal cancer with CT. MRI and PET/CT Eur Radiol. 2007;17(8):2044–54.
14. Rokan Z, Simillis C, Kontovounisios C, Moran BJ, Tekkis P, Brown G. Systematic review of classification systems for locally recurrent rectal cancer. BJS Open. 2021;5(3)
15. Moore HG, Shoup M, Riedel E, Minsky BD, Alektiar KM, Ercolani M, et al. Colorectal cancer pelvic recurrences: determinants of resectability. Dis Colon Rectum. 2004;47(10):1599–606.

16. Iversen H, Martling A, Johansson H, Nilsson PJ, Holm T. Pelvic local recurrence from colorectal cancer: surgical challenge with changing preconditions. Color Dis. 2018;20(5):399–406.
17. Zhao J, Du CZ, Sun YS, Gu J. Patterns and prognosis of locally recurrent rectal cancer following multidisciplinary treatment. World J Gastroenterol. 2012;18(47):7015–20.
18. Yamada K, Ishizawa T, Niwa K, Chuman Y, Akiba S, Aikou T. Patterns of pelvic invasion are prognostic in the treatment of locally recurrent rectal cancer. Br J Surg. 2001;88(7):988–93.
19. Kanemitsu Y, Hirai T, Komori K, Kato T. Prediction of residual disease or distant metastasis after resection of locally recurrent rectal cancer. Dis Colon Rectum. 2010;53(5):779–89.
20. Bird TG, Ngan SY, Chu J, Kroon R, Lynch AC, Heriot AG. Outcomes and prognostic factors of multimodality treatment for locally recurrent rectal cancer with curative intent. Int J Color Dis. 2018;33(4):393–401.
21. Suzuki K, Dozois RR, Devine RM, Nelson H, Weaver AL, Gunderson LL, et al. Curative reoperations for locally recurrent rectal cancer. Dis Colon Rectum. 1996;39(7):730–6.
22. Valentini V, Morganti AG, De Franco A, Coco C, Ratto C, Battista Doglietto G, et al. Chemoradiation with or without intraoperative radiation therapy in patients with locally recurrent rectal carcinoma: prognostic factors and long term outcome. Cancer. 1999;86(12):2612–24.
23. Boyle KM, Sagar PM, Chalmers AG, Sebag-Montefiore D, Cairns A, Eardley I. Surgery for locally recurrent rectal cancer. Dis Colon Rectum. 2005;48(5):929–37.
24. Georgiou PA, Tekkis PP, Constantinides VA, Patel U, Goldin RD, Darzi AW, et al. Diagnostic accuracy and value of magnetic resonance imaging (MRI) in planning exenterative pelvic surgery for advanced colorectal cancer. Eur J Cancer. 2013;49(1):72–81.
25. Holman FA, Bosman SJ, Haddock MG, Gunderson LL, Kusters M, Nieuwenhuijzen GA, et al. Results of a pooled analysis of IOERT containing multimodality treatment for locally recurrent rectal cancer: results of 565 patients of two major treatment centres. Eur J Surg Oncol. 2017;43(1):107–17.
26. You YN, Skibber JM, Hu CY, Crane CH, Das P, Kopetz ES, et al. Impact of multimodal therapy in locally recurrent rectal cancer. Br J Surg. 2016;103(6):753–62.
27. Harris CA, Solomon MJ, Heriot AG, Sagar PM, Tekkis PP, Dixon L, et al. The outcomes and patterns of treatment failure after surgery for locally recurrent rectal cancer. Ann Surg. 2016;264(2):323–9.
28. Wo JY, Anker CJ, Ashman JB, Bhadkamkar NA, Bradfield L, Chang DT, et al. Radiation therapy for rectal cancer: executive summary of an ASTRO clinical practice guideline. Pract Radiat Oncol. 2021;11(1):13–25.
29. Youssef FF, Parikh PJ, DeWees TA, Mutch MG, Tan BR Jr, Grigsby PW, et al. Efficacy and toxicity of rectal cancer reirradiation using IMRT for patients who have received prior pelvic radiation therapy. Adv Radiat Oncol. 2016;1(2):94–100.
30. Ng MK, Leong T, Heriot AG, Ngan SY. Once-daily reirradiation for rectal cancer in patients who have received previous pelvic radiotherapy. J Med Imaging Radiat Oncol. 2013;57(4):512–8.
31. Das P, Delclos ME, Skibber JM, Rodriguez-Bigas MA, Feig BW, Chang GJ, et al. Hyperfractionated accelerated radiotherapy for rectal cancer in patients with prior pelvic irradiation. Int J Radiat Oncol Biol Phys. 2010;77(1):60–5.
32. Wegner RE, Abel S, White RJ, Horne ZD, Hasan S, Kirichenko AV. Trends in intensity-modulated radiation therapy use for rectal cancer in the neoadjuvant setting: a National Cancer Database analysis. Radiat Oncol J. 2018;36(4):276–84.
33. Jabbour SK, Patel S, Herman JM, Wild A, Nagda SN, Altoos T, et al. Intensity-modulated radiation therapy for rectal carcinoma can reduce treatment breaks and emergency department visits. Int J Surg Oncol. 2012;2012:891067.
34. Tao R, Tsai CJ, Jensen G, Eng C, Kopetz S, Overman MJ, et al. Hyperfractionated accelerated reirradiation for rectal cancer: an analysis of outcomes and toxicity. Radiother Oncol. 2017;122(1):146–51.
35. Dresen RC, Gosens MJ, Martijn H, Nieuwenhuijzen GA, Creemers GJ, Daniels-Gooszen AW, et al. Radical resection after IORT-containing multimodality treatment is the most important determinant for outcome in patients treated for locally recurrent rectal cancer. Ann Surg Oncol. 2008;15(7):1937–47.

36. Fadel MG, Ahmed M, Malietzis G, Pellino G, Rasheed S, Brown G, et al. Oncological outcomes of multimodality treatment for patients undergoing surgery for locally recurrent rectal cancer: a systematic review. Cancer Treat Rev. 2022;109:102419.
37. Voogt ELK, van Zoggel D, Kusters M, Nieuwenhuijzen GAP, Bloemen JG, Peulen HMU, et al. Improved outcomes for responders after treatment with induction chemotherapy and chemo(re) irradiation for locally recurrent Rectal Cancer. Ann Surg Oncol. 2020;27(9):3503–13.
38. van Zoggel D, Bosman SJ, Kusters M, Nieuwenhuijzen GAP, Cnossen JS, Creemers GJ, et al. Preliminary results of a cohort study of induction chemotherapy-based treatment for locally recurrent rectal cancer. Br J Surg. 2018;105(4):447–52.
39. Wiig JN, Larsen SG, Dueland S, Giercksky KE. Clinical outcome in patients with complete pathologic response (pT0) to preoperative irradiation/chemo-irradiation operated for locally advanced or locally recurrent rectal cancer. J Surg Oncol. 2005;92(1):70–5.
40. Sorrentino L, Belli F, Valvo F, Villa S, Guaglio M, Scaramuzza D, et al. Neoadjuvant (re) chemoradiation for locally recurrent rectal cancer: impact of anatomical site of pelvic recurrence on long-term results. Surg Oncol. 2020;35:89–96.
41. Yu SK, Bhangu A, Tait DM, Tekkis P, Wotherspoon A, Brown G. Chemoradiotherapy response in recurrent rectal cancer. Cancer Med. 2014;3(1):111–7.
42. Ansell J, Perry WRG, Mathis KL, Grass F, Yonkus JA, Hallemeier CL, et al. Re-resection of microscopically positive margins found on intraoperative frozen section analysis does not result in a survival benefit in patients undergoing surgery and intraoperative radiation therapy for locally recurrent Rectal Cancer. Dis Colon Rectum. 2022;65(9):1094–102.
43. Babar L, Bakalov V, Abel S, Ashraf O, Finley GG, Raj MS, et al. Retrospective review of total neoadjuvant therapy. World J Gastrointest Oncol. 2019;11(10):857–65.
44. Denost Q, Frison E, Salut C, Sitta R, Rullier A, Harji D, et al. A phase III randomized trial evaluating chemotherapy followed by pelvic reirradiation versus chemotherapy alone as preoperative treatment for locally recurrent rectal cancer – GRECCAR 15 trial protocol. Color Dis. 2021;23(7):1909–18.
45. PelvEx C. Induction chemotherapy followed by chemoradiotherapy versus chemoradiotherapy alone as neoadjuvant treatment for locally recurrent rectal cancer: study protocol of a multicentre, open-label, parallel-arms, randomized controlled study (PelvEx II). BJS Open. 2021;5(3)
46. Kishan AU, Voog JC, Wiseman J, Cook RR, Ancukiewicz M, Lee P, et al. Standard fractionation external beam radiotherapy with and without intraoperative radiotherapy for locally recurrent rectal cancer: the role of local therapy in patients with a high competing risk of death from distant disease. Br J Radiol. 2017;90(1076):20170134.
47. Hyngstrom JR, Tzeng CW, Beddar S, Das P, Krishnan S, Delclos ME, et al. Intraoperative radiation therapy for locally advanced primary and recurrent colorectal cancer: ten-year institutional experience. J Surg Oncol. 2014;109(7):652–8.
48. Alektiar KM, Zelefsky MJ, Paty PB, Guillem J, Saltz LB, Cohen AM, et al. High-dose-rate intraoperative brachytherapy for recurrent colorectal cancer. Int J Radiat Oncol Biol Phys. 2000;48(1):219–26.
49. Lindel K, Willett CG, Shellito PC, Ott MJ, Clark J, Grossbard M, et al. Intraoperative radiation therapy for locally advanced recurrent rectal or rectosigmoid cancer. Radiother Oncol. 2001;58(1):83–7.
50. Mirnezami R, Chang GJ, Das P, Chandrakumaran K, Tekkis P, Darzi A, et al. Intraoperative radiotherapy in colorectal cancer: systematic review and meta-analysis of techniques, long-term outcomes, and complications. Surg Oncol. 2013;22(1):22–35.
51. Haddock MG, Miller RC, Nelson H, Pemberton JH, Dozois EJ, Alberts SR, et al. Combined modality therapy including intraoperative electron irradiation for locally recurrent colorectal cancer. Int J Radiat Oncol Biol Phys. 2011;79(1):143–50.
52. Calvo FA, Sole CV, Rutten HJ, Dries WJ, Lozano MA, Cambeiro M, et al. ESTRO/ACROP IORT recommendations for intraoperative radiation therapy in locally recurrent rectal cancer. Clin Transl Radiat Oncol. 2020;24:41–8.
53. Horn A, Morild I, Dahl O. Tumour shrinkage and down staging after preoperative radiation of rectal adenocarcinomas. Radiother Oncol. 1990;18(1):19–28.

54. Berger C, de Muret A, Garaud P, Chapet S, Bourlier P, Reynaud-Bougnoux A, et al. Preoperative radiotherapy (RT) for rectal cancer: predictive factors of tumor downstaging and residual tumor cell density (RTCD): prognostic implications. Int J Radiat Oncol Biol Phys. 1997;37(3):619–27.
55. Randomised trial of surgery alone versus surgery followed by radiotherapy for mobile cancer of the rectum. Medical Research Council Rectal Cancer working party. Lancet. 1996;348(9042):1610–4.
56. Lim SB, Choi HS, Jeong SY, Kim DY, Jung KH, Hong YS, et al. Optimal surgery time after preoperative chemoradiotherapy for locally advanced rectal cancers. Ann Surg. 2008;248(2):243–51.
57. McKenna NP, Bews KA, Al-Refaie WB, Colibaseanu DT, Pemberton JH, Cima RR, et al. Assessing malnutrition before major oncologic surgery: one size does not fit all. J Am Coll Surg. 2020;230(4):451–60.
58. Beaton J, Carey S, Solomon MJ, Tan KK, Young J. Preoperative body mass index, 30-day postoperative morbidity, length of stay and quality of life in patients undergoing pelvic exenteration surgery for recurrent and locally-advanced rectal cancer. Ann Coloproctol. 2014;30(2):83–7.
59. van Rees JM, Visser E, van Vugt JLA, Rothbarth J, Verhoef C, van Verschuer VMT. Impact of nutritional status and body composition on postoperative outcomes after pelvic exenteration for locally advanced and locally recurrent rectal cancer. BJS Open. 2021;5(5)
60. Hogan S, Steffens D, Vuong K, Rangan A, Solomon M, Carey S. Preoperative nutritional status impacts clinical outcome and hospital length of stay in pelvic exenteration patients – a retrospective study. Nutr Health. 2022;28(1):41–8.
61. Spasojevic M, Mariathasan AB, Goscinski M, Thorgersen EB, Solbakken AM, Gullestad HP, et al. Vertical rectus abdominis musculocutaneous flap repair improves perineal wound healing after abdominoperineal resection for irradiated locally advanced rectal cancer. Ann Surg Oncol. 2018;25(5):1357–65.
62. Houdek MT, Bakri K, Tibbo ME, Wagner ER, Rose PS, Sim FH, et al. Outcome and complications following vertical rectus abdominis myocutaneous flap surgery to reconstruct sacrectomy defects. Plast Reconstr Surg. 2018;142(5):1327–35.
63. Killeen S, Devaney A, Mannion M, Martin ST, Winter DC. Omental pedicle flaps following proctectomy: a systematic review. Color Dis. 2013;15(11):e634–45.
64. Witte DYS, van Ramshorst GH, Lapid O, Bouman MB, Tuynman JB. Flap reconstruction of perineal defects after pelvic exenteration: a systematic description of four choices of surgical reconstruction methods. Plast Reconstr Surg. 2021;147(6):1420–35.
65. Lambert JE, Hayes LD, Keegan TJ, Subar DA, Gaffney CJ. The impact of Prehabilitation on patient outcomes in hepatobiliary, colorectal, and upper gastrointestinal Cancer surgery: a PRISMA-accordant meta-analysis. Ann Surg. 2021;274(1):70–7.
66. Bojesen RD, Grube C, Buzquurz F, Miedzianogora REG, Eriksen JR, Gogenur I. Effect of modifying high-risk factors and prehabilitation on the outcomes of colorectal cancer surgery: controlled before and after study. BJS Open. 2022;6(3)
67. Cameron MG, Kersten C, Vistad I, Fossa S, Guren MG. Palliative pelvic radiotherapy of symptomatic incurable rectal cancer – a systematic review. Acta Oncol. 2014;53(2):164–73.
68. Ronnekleiv-Kelly SM, Kennedy GD. Management of stage IV rectal cancer: palliative options. World J Gastroenterol. 2011;17(7):835–47.

Part IV

Anal Dysplasia/Cancer

28 Intensive vs Conservative Management of Patients with Low Grade Squamous Intraepithelial Lesions

Ray Ramirez, Nell Maloney Patel, and Joseph Terlizzi

Introduction

Anal cancer is preceded by anal intraepithelial neoplasia (AIN) in the same way that cervical intraepithelial neoplasia precedes cervical cancer. A classification system, similar to that of cervical pathology, has been developed using the Bethesda system terminology AIN I, II, and III, where AIN 1 is "low-grade squamous intraepithelial lesion (LSIL)" and AIN II and III is "high grade squamous intraepithelial lesions (HSIL)" [1]. While HSIL, the direct anal squamous cell carcinoma precursor is considered premalignant, LSIL is not. However, LSIL is a marker for concurrent HSIL and the development of HSIL in the future. It has been hypothesized that LSIL is associated with low-risk HPV genotypes and HSIL is associated with high-risk HPV genotypes [1, 2]. While the risk of anal cancer is low overall, it is significantly increased in certain populations. These populations include people with high-risk sexual behaviors (men who have sex with men (MSM), receptive anal intercourse, or a history of multiple sexual partners), persons living with HIV (PLHIV), other immunocompromised individuals such as solid organ transplant recipients (SOTRs) or those with autoimmune diseases, and women diagnosed with HPV-related gynecological (pre)cancers [3]. AIN is a disease with an overall

R. Ramirez (✉)
Rutgers Robert Wood Johnson Medical School, Surgery, New Brunswick, NJ, USA
e-mail: rr1156@rwjms.rutgers.edu

N. M. Patel
Rutgers Robert Wood Johnson Medical School, Colon and Rectal Surgery, Westfield, NJ, USA
e-mail: malonene@rutgers.edu

J. Terlizzi
Mount Sinai School of Medicine, Surgery, New York, NY, USA

K. Umanskiy, N. Hyman (eds.), *Difficult Decisions in Colorectal Surgery*, Difficult Decisions in Surgery: An Evidence-Based Approach,
https://doi.org/10.1007/978-3-031-42303-1_28

Table 28.1 Incidence of anal cancer in high risk populations [3]

Population	Incidence rates of anal cancer
MSM with HIV	85/100,000 py (95% CI = 82–89)
Non-MSM with HIV	32/100,000 py (95% CI = 30–35)
Females with HIV	22/100,000 py (95% CI = 19–24)
HIV-negative MSM	19/100,000 py (95% CI = 10–36)
Women with Cervical Cancer	9/100,000 py (95% CI = 8–12)
Women with Precancerous Cervical Lesions	6/100,000 py (95% CI = 5–7)
Women with Vulvar Cancer	48/100,000 py (95% CI = 38/61)
Women with Vaginal Cancer	10/100,000 py (95% CI = 3–30)
Solid Organ Transplant Recipients	13/100,000 py (95% CI = 12–15)
Autoimmune Disorders	10/100,000 py (95% CI = 5–19)
Ulcerative Colitis	6/100,000 py (95% CI = 3–11)
Crohn's Disease	3/100,000 py (95% CI = 2–4)

Table 28.2 PICO question

Patients	Intervention	Comparator	Outcome
Patients with low grade squamous anal intraepithelial neoplasia	Topical therapy and/or local ablative therapy	Surveillance	Progression to high-grade AIN

predicted incidence of approximately 1–2 cases per 100,000 person-years (py) [3], it is often difficult to study and assess (Table 28.1).

Because AIN remains relatively rare and requires a level of expertise to diagnose and treat, it is currently recommended that patients with AIN be referred to expert centers for high resolution anoscopy and any associated treatments [1] (Table 28.2).

Search Strategy

A comprehensive literature search of Cochrane Database of Collected Research, EMBASE, and PubMed was performed to identify all of the English-language publications related to management of patients with low grade squamous intraepithelial lesions and recurrence from 2000 to 2022. Because of the low volume of studies looking specifically at LSIL, anal cancer and HSIL were included. Key search terms included the following: "AIN low-grade, "anal LSIL", "anal HSIL," and "anal cancer." Studies were excluded if they had no mention of LSIL or treatment of LSIL/HSIL. Only the most recent study was included if similar studies from the same institution were encountered. The references of the included studies were reviewed to identify additional studies that were incorporated as appropriate.

Results

Over the past two decades, there have been very few studies reported on LSIL and its progression to HSIL. However, within these studies, there is no mention of treatment to prevent further progression of disease from LSIL to HSIL. There have been three studies which specifically looked at LSIL progression to HSIL in MSM LWHIV. All three studies employed anal cytology and HPV testing. Results of the anal cytology were classified as normal, atypical squamous cells of undetermined significance (ASCUS), LSIL, HSIL, or squamous-cell carcinoma, in accordance with the Bethesda classification. High resolution anoscopy (HRA) with biopsy was performed after the anal pap smear. In HIV-infected MSM, Burgos *et al* reported a progression rate of LSIL to HSIL to be 10.5 cases/100 person-years [4]. A similar rate was found in de Pokomandy with 10.7 cases/100 person-years and Tong reported rate of 13.1 cases/100 person-years [5, 6]. Together these three studies suggest that while LSIL has the potential to progress to HSIL, the overall rate of progression is relatively low.

The endpoint for all three studies was HSIL diagnosed histologically via a biopsy. This was compared to all participants initial pap smear/biopsy to show progression of disease [4–6].

Study	Patients (N)	Progression to HSIL	Cumulative Incidence of HSIL	Median Follow-Up	Quality of Evidence
Burgos [4]	556 HIV-infected MSM	10.5 cases/100 person-years	16.2% at 24 months and 24.5% at 36 months	26.4 months	High
de Pokomandy [5]	157 HIV-infected MSM	10.7 cases/100 person-years	23.1% at 24 months and 36.6% at 36 months	38 months	Moderate
Tong [6]	152 HIV-infected MSM	13.1 cases/100 person-years	16.2% at 24 months and 24.5% at 36 months	13.2 months	Moderate

Looking at the risk of LSIL progression to HSIL, practitioners can better identify the need to treat LSIL or simply to surveil it. The Anal Cancer HSIL Outcomes Research (ANCHOR) trial is the only randomized controlled trial studying the treatment of HSIL and has demonstrated that treating HSIL significantly reduced the incidence of anal squamous cell carcinoma in PLWHIV compared with active monitoring via regular exams (including anal cytology combined with HRA and biopsy of any concerning lesions) [7, 8].

Recommendations

Certain individuals are at significantly increased risk of anal cancer and should undergo anal dysplasia screening. ANCHOR has shown that treating HSIL prevents SCC. All HSIL should be treated (Evidence high; recommendations high). However, LSIL, while a risk factor for HSIL, is caused by low-risk HPV infection and is not a direct SCC precursor. Patients with LSIL should undergo close surveillance, but we do not recommend routinely treating LSIL (Evidence: low; Recommendation: moderate).

Patients with LSIL should undergo close surveillance with digital anorectal examination, anal cytology, high-risk HPV testing and HRA at regular intervals (Evidence: low; Recommendation: moderate).

All patients with HSIL should be treated with topical therapy and/or local ablative therapy (Evidence high; recommendations high).

Personal View

LSIL is not the direct SCC precursor and does not require treatment. If patients have symptomatic LSIL (itching, palpable lesions, etc.) treatment is justified. Patients with LSIL must be screened for HSIL with digital anorectal examination, anal cytology, high-risk HPV testing and HRA at regular intervals. For higher risk patients (increasing age, people with high-risk sexual behaviors (MSM, receptive anal intercourse, or a history of multiple sex partners), persons living with HIV (PLHIV), other immunocompromised individuals such as solid organ transplant recipients (SOTRs) or autoimmune diseases, and women diagnosed with HPV-related gynecological (pre)cancers)) with LSIL, screening intervals may be shortened. All HSIL should be treated.

References

1. Roberts JR, Siekas LL, Kaz AM. Anal intraepithelial neoplasia: a review of diagnosis and management. World J Gastrointest Oncol. 2017;9(2):50. https://doi.org/10.4251/wjgo.v9.i2.50.
2. Stanley MA, Winder DM, Sterling JC, Goon PKC. HPV infection, anal intra-epithelial neoplasia (AIN) and anal cancer: current issues. BMC Cancer. 2012;12(1) https://doi.org/10.1186/1471-2407-12-398.
3. Clifford GM, Georges D, Shiels MS, et al. A meta-analysis of anal cancer incidence by risk group: toward a unified anal cancer risk scale. Int J Cancer. 2021;148:38–47. https://doi.org/10.1002/ijc.33185.

4. Burgos J, Curran A, Tallada N, Guelar A, Navarro J, Landolfi S, Villar J, Crespo M, Ribera E, Falcó V. Risk of progression to high-grade anal intraepithelial neoplasia in HIV-infected MSM. AIDS. 2015;29(6):695–702.
5. de Pokomandy A, Rouleau D, Ghattas G, Trottier H, Vézina S, Coté P, et al. HAART and progression to high-grade anal intraepithelial neoplasia in men who have sex with men and are infected with HIV. Clin Infect Dis. 2011;52:1174–81.
6. Tong WW, Jin F, McHugh LC, Maher T, Sinclair B, Grulich AE, et al. Progression to and spontaneous regression of high-grade anal squamous intraepithelial lesions in HIV-infected and un-infected men. AIDS. 2013;27:2233–43.
7. Palefsky JM, Lee JY, Jay N, Goldstone SE, Darragh TM, et al. ANCHOR investigators group. Treatment of anal highgrade squamous intraepithelial lesions to prevent anal cancer N. Engl. J. Med. 2022;386(24):2273–82. https://doi.org/10.1056/NEJMoa2201048. https://anchorstudy.org/.
8. Jones MP, Carroll S, Martin J, Hillman R, Grulich A, O'Connell D, Young C, Poynten IM. Management of early anal cancer: need for guidelines and standardisation. Int J Color Dis. 2017;32(12):1719–24. https://doi.org/10.1007/s00384-017-2913-6.

29 How Aggressive Should We Be in Management of Patients with High Grade Squamous Intraepithelial Lesion?

Kinga S. Olortegui

Introduction

Anal squamous intraepithelial neoplasia is a rare lesion, but increasingly encountered by the colorectal surgeon [1]. Expert consensus supports expectant management for patients with low grade squamous intraepithelial lesions. High grade squamous intraepithelial lesions (HSIL or HGSIL, or anal intraepithelial neoplasia grade II or III) present a significant clinical challenge. HSIL may be found during recommended screening in a high-risk population [2, 3]. Frequently, lesions are identified incidentally during excision of condyloma or upon pathology review after hemorrhoidectomy. [4] Occasionally, HSIL may be visually identified at colonoscopy, particularly during retroflexion [5]. Once found, there is little guidance on how aggressively these lesions should be treated, and this has been a major area of debate among colorectal surgeons [6]. Historically, the rate of progression from HSIL to anal squamous cell cancer (SCC) was thought to be quite low, but a review of 2074 patients with AIN III in the Surveillance, Epidemiology, and End Research (SEER) database between 1973 and 2014 found the rate to be 1.9% per year, for an overall rate of 9.5% at 5 years [7]. Of patients who developed anal cancer in this study, nearly one third had stage T2 or higher tumors at time of diagnosis. A limitation of the study was that HIV status was unknown, and this subgroup is known to be at higher risk of anal SCC [8–10]. In fact, HSIL or anal SCC has been shown to correlate with the CD4/CD8 cell ratio, suggesting that treatment and control of HIV is an important contributor to decreasing risk of cancer in this population [11]. While this study showed an alarmingly high rate of anal SCC, another recent study

K. S. Olortegui (✉)
Section of Colon & Rectal Surgery, Department of Surgery, UChicago Medicine, Chicago, IL, USA
e-mail: kskowron@bsd.uchicago.edu

K. Umanskiy, N. Hyman (eds.), *Difficult Decisions in Colorectal Surgery*, Difficult Decisions in Surgery: An Evidence-Based Approach,
https://doi.org/10.1007/978-3-031-42303-1_29

specifically of HIV-positive patients, also using the SEER database but using a more narrow and recent timeframe (2000–2011), showed an incidence of anal SCC of 1.2% at 1 year and 5.7% at 5 years [12].

Of course, no one wants to miss an opportunity to prevent progression to an anal cancer. Yet, aggressive treatments can be highly morbid. Aggressive surveillance programs come at a personal cost to the patient, time off work for procedures and emotional distress at the prospect of developing cancer [13]. This leads us to the question, are aggressive treatments strategies for HSIL justified?

PICO table

Patients	Intervention	Comparator	Outcome
Patients with high grade anal intraepithelial neoplasia	Ablation	Expectant management	Recurrence of dysplasia or progression to anal cancer

Search Strategy

A literature search was conducted using PubMed and Google Scholar to identify all English language publications regarding anal intraepithelial neoplasia treatment from 2017–2022. A strict time interval was chosen, as older studies were extensively reviewed in a prior edition of this book on a similar topic [14]. The search was conducted using following terms: "anal intraepithelial neoplasia," "anal high grade squamous intraepithelial lesion," "anal Bowen's disease" and "perianal Bowen's disease," "anal HSIL," and "AIN." Studies were excluded if they did not describe treatment patterns and algorithms. References of studies identified were reviewed to identify any historic studies of interest.

Results

As mentioned in the introduction, high risk populations should be aggressively screened for anal cancer and anal dysplasia. The options for treatment for anal dysplasia once it is diagnosed vary considerably, and will be reviewed here, beginning with the least invasive, through the most invasive.

The 2018 Clinical Practice Guidelines of the American Society of Colon and Rectal Surgeons (ASCRS) recommend that patients who are diagnosed with anal dysplasia (HSIL or AIN III) be followed clinically at regular intervals, with history and physical exam [6]. These recommendations are based upon the fact that the rate of progression from HSIL to anal SCC is poorly understood. In fact, in a study of 574 patients with HIV who underwent anal cancer screening, authors describe an incidence of 12.5% of HSIL [15]. In this study, only 6 cancers were detected, of which 2 had a prior history of HSIL. Importantly, 24% of patients with HSIL demonstrated spontaneous regression (to normal exam or LSIL). Many observational studies support the use of expectant management after diagnosis of HSIL. The exact interval for surveillance visits is not specified, as various studies have reported different follow up strategies. In a report of the University of California, San Francisco Anal Neoplasia Study and Anal Neoplasia Clinic, approximately 2,000 men with HIV were followed over time [16]. Initial lesions were treated with 85% trichloroacetic acid if they were small, and excision / ablation if they were larger. Those who declined therapy, had extensive lesions, or developed recurrent HSIL were followed with digital exam and high resolution anoscopy every 3–4 months. The vast majority of patients who developed anal SCC had tumors detectable on digital exam alone. In another report of 341 patients with HSIL and HIV followed by a single surgeon for over 20 years, anal cancer was detected at a rate of 1.3% per patient-year [17]. The follow up strategy included a history and exam (visual and digital) every 6 months. In a large retrospective review of nearly 6 million patients treated in the Kaiser Permanente Southern California healthcare system, patients were followed with exam and referred for excision or fulguration of grossly abnormal or symptomatic lesions only. [18]. 90.7% of anal cancers were diagnosed in patients without HIV or prior high-risk lesions. The cumulative incidence of anal cancer among patients with prior anal dysplasia was 0.69% (6 out of 872 patients). Therefore, a minimum follow up strategy of anal exam (including digital exam) with office anoscopy (high resolution or basic) at an interval of 3–6 months is reasonable and supported by data.

Numerous studies have described the use of topical therapies for chemical ablation of HSIL. Topical therapies are an attractive option, as they reduce the need for invasive procedures, and can typically be applied in the privacy of one's home. They certainly are not without side effects, and can cause pain and bleeding which may limit compliance with this treatment option. The agents described include 5% imiquimod, 1% cidofovir, 5-fluorouracil (5-FU), and 80% trichloracetic acid (TCA), based upon small, but randomized clinical trials or case series in the late 2000s and early 2010s. A recent systematic review evaluated these studies together [19]. Unfortunately, the vast majority of such studies suffered from a significant degree of bias. Compliance rates were quite good, at least 79%, though many studies reported 100% compliance. The ranges for the rate of complete response were 14–74% for imiquimod, 15–59% for cidofovir, 9–86% for 5-FU, and 28–72% for TCA. Rates of recurrence ranged from 16–71% for imiquimod, unknown-12% for cidofovir, 0–58% for 5-FU, and 15–28% for TCA. Obviously, such wide ranges should raise suspicion about the true result. Furthermore, many of these therapies are not FDA-approved for treatment of anal HSIL, and depending on the patient's insurance status, may be prohibitively expensive. Therefore, topical ablation can be used safely and is generally well-tolerated, but the effectiveness is really unknown.

The next category of treatment options for HSIL is that of physical ablation. Methods typically used for this include electrocautery, infrared coagulation and laser. As with chemical ablation, reports of physical ablation began to appear in large numbers in the late 2000s and frequently in the 2010s. These were largely retrospective reviews of single institution experiences. This is also true of the majority of the more recent literature on this topic. Electrocautery is by far the most common technique used, and newer literature explores other options. For example, a retrospective review of 81 patients treated with infrared coagulation via high resolution anoscopy demonstrated a recurrence rate of 25% at a median of 6 months of follow up. [20] Two recent reports have described the use of radiofrequency ablation (RFA) as another option for treatment of HSIL. A small single-institution study of 21 patients treated with RFA showed a relatively high rate of recurrence of 29% at 1 year [21]. A retrospective review of 12 patients demonstrated a 58% response rate; the remaining patients were retreated with electrocautery and achieved disease eradication at 1 year from treatment [22]. Case reports have also described the use nitrous oxide cryoablation as another method for ablation [23]. Such novel therapies thus far lack high quality evidence to support their use, and therefore electrocautery remains the favored method for mechanical destruction of HSIL. Finally, the results of the much-awaited Anal Cancer-HSIL Outcomes Research (ANCHOR) trial have been published this year [24]. This was a large, phase 3 randomized, controlled trial comparing ablation of HSIL with active monitoring. Patients with HIV were invited to participate in a screening protocol, in which they underwent a physical exam, anal swab for cytology, and high resolution anoscopy (HRA). Any suspicious lesions at HRA were biopsied. If HSIL was confirmed, patients were invited to participate in the study. 10,723 patients were screened, of which 4,459 patients were randomized at 25 U.S. sites between September 2014 and August 2021, 2,237 in the treatment group and 2,222 in the monitoring group. Patients in the treatment arm underwent immediate treatment with a goal of eradication of HSIL. The treatments included were ablation using with infrared coagulation, electrocautery and laser, excision or ablation under anesthesia, or topical treatments. Patients in the active monitoring arm underwent HRA every 6 months; any visible lesions were biopsied annually to confirm HSIL and exclude anal cancer. Patients in either arm with concerning lesions were followed more closely (every 3 months), and any lesions suspicious for cancer were biopsied. Patients found to have cancer were removed from the trial and referred for treatment. 4,446 patients were ultimately analyzed, 2227 in the treatment group and 2219 in the monitoring group, with a median 25.3 and 27.2 months of follow up, respectively. The vast majority of patients in the treatment arm underwent office-based electrocautery ablation (83.6%). 86.3% of patients received only one type of ablative treatment, and 10.5% received two methods. There were 9 patients with SCC in the treatment group, and 21 in the monitoring group. This translated to a cumulative incidence of anal cancer at 48 months of 0.9% in the treatment group and 1.8% in the monitoring group, or a difference in incidence between groups of about 0.2% per year. While this study showed a statistically-significant reduction in progression from HSIL to anal cancer with aggressive treatment of HSIL over monitoring, the incidence of anal cancer in both groups was quite low. The number needed to treat to prevent one patient developing anal cancer is 111 ablations. With considerable cost, commitment from patients and pain, it remains a question whether this approach is justified.

One point of variability between the various techniques used for screening and treatment is the use of HRA, as seen in the ANCHOR study above. HRA is performed in the office or operating room using a magnification anoscope and a topical agent, usually acetic acid or Lugol's solution, to aid in the visualization of

HSIL. Numerous studies have discussed using HRA as a screening tool to identify HSIL, and have shown it to be superior to cytology for detection of HSIL. However, once HSIL is diagnosed, it is not clear that HRA is superior to standard anoscopy for treatment of HSIL lesions, as no high quality comparative studies in this context exist; several recent studies confirm a low rate of progression to cancer in cohorts followed with standard anoscopy [25–28]. The ASCRS clinical practice guidelines leave this as an optional method of surveillance. [6] What is clear, is that patients should be followed with some type of anoscopy, and any visible or palpable lesions should be treated.

For completeness of discussion, we will review the historical option of wide excision of HSIL. This was a common practice described in the 1990s. In survey of 642 ASCRS members in 2000, 96% used wide local excision for small lesions of HSIL and 87% used it for large lesions [29]. Full thickness excision of lesion and surrounding skin was carried out, often requiring skin flap coverage. Scholefield, et al. described 27 patients with AIN III treated with excision; they report a recurrence rate of 30% and progression to cancer in 9% [30]. Brown, et al. described surgical excision in 34 patients, with a recurrence rate of 18% with a median 41 months of follow up. [31] Importantly, only 14% of patients in this study achieved negative margins (free of high grade AIN). This study reported no progression to cancer, but a nearly 10% risk of anal stenosis or fecal incontinence. Due to the high risk of morbidity for little to no benefit over less invasive options, wide surgical excision is no longer recommended.

Another exciting option which came and went was the HPV vaccine used as an adjuvant treatment for HSIL. Vaccination against the human papillomavirus (HPV) has dramatically decreased the rate of HPV-associated squamous cell cancers, such as cervical, head and neck, and anal cancer. Vaccination of patients not infected with the HPV virus has shown to decrease the rate of HSIL as well in an industry-sponsored trial [32]. However, two double-blinded, randomized, controlled trials of patients with HIV have now shown that patients treated for HSIL prior to vaccination were not less likely to have HSIL recurrence (63% recurrence in the vaccinated group versus 57% in the placebo group in one study, and 68.8% versus 61.3% in the other) [33, 34]. Therefore, vaccination as an adjuvant treatment for HSIL is not recommended.

Recommendations

Based upon the above discussion, treatment or follow up for HSIL is important in the prevention of progression to anal SCC, based upon moderate-quality evidence. The challenge with this disease for the clinician is the lack of standardized follow up intervals for HSIL, or for surveillance after ablation of HSIL, as those which exist for cancer, guided by the National Comprehensive Cancer Network. There is also a paucity of data for treatment of HSIL in patients without HIV, compared with the HIV-positive population.

Personal View

In my practice, I do not typically perform primary screening for anal dysplasia, but work closely with specialists who do. Patients are referred to our clinic from a screening program with a lesion noted on digital exam or anoscopy, or a positive anal Pap smear. Other patients present with bothersome anal lesions. Rarely, distal rectal or anal lesions are biopsied at colonoscopy, resulting in a diagnosis of HSIL. In all of these cases, I recommend a careful anal exam under anesthesia in the operating room. I use high magnification loupes, and stain the anal canal with acetic acid to assist with identification of HSIL. Lesions are biopsied to confirm the diagnosis, and ablated with electrocautery. Patients are then entered into a follow up program, which I will detail below. Occasionally, patients are found to have HSIL incidentally on pathologic evaluation after hemorrhoidectomy or excision of condylomas. These patients are similarly entered into the below follow up program.

The intensity of follow up after the initial encounter for HSIL depends upon each patient's risk factors and personal risk tolerance. Patients without obvious immunosuppression are tested for HIV, as this clearly affects their risk of future anal cancer; any patient diagnosed with HIV is referred for treatment. Patients who are smoking are referred for smoking cessation [9, 35]. Patients who are immunosuppressed due to transplantation have been shown to be at higher risk for HSIL [36]. When they are diagnosed with HSIL, I discuss the diagnosis with their transplant medicine team, and discuss whether there is room to reduce the degree of immunosuppression without compromise to the transplant.

For patients who are not immunosuppressed, I typically recommend office anoscopy and digital exam at 6 months, and a surveillance biopsy / ablation at 12 months. If there is no recurrent or residual HSIL, then I recommend annual office exam and anoscopy. If there is recurrent HSIL, then we repeat the follow up and surveillance pattern.

For patients who are immunosuppressed (HIV positive, transplant, inflammatory bowel disease on immunosuppression, etc.), I recommend an office exam in 3 months, and surveillance biopsy / ablation at 6 months. If there is no HSIL at that point, I recommend office exam and anoscopy every 6 months. If there is recurrent HSIL, we repeat the follow up and surveillance pattern, but in that case, I prescribe a course of imiquimod prior to the next visit. I find that this is generally well-tolerated, and based upon the above data, it may be helpful, particularly in a high-risk population. I have a frank conversation with patients about the limited utility of this method of ablation compared with electrocautery, and discuss with them that if the cost is prohibitive or if they experience any side effects, we would not use this modality.

If at any point there is a visible or palpable lesion at the office visit, I recommend repeat biopsy and ablation. If HSIL is confirmed, the follow up plan restarts. Of course, any patient found to have anal cancer is referred for appropriate treatment.

Particularly for patients without immunosuppression, we discuss the overall low risk of SCC, paucity of data and variability in treatment and surveillance options. If patients are less risk averse, and more concerned with missing work for procedures or having pain from biopsies, we may forgo the surveillance biopsy visit and follow with office exam and standard anoscopy instead. What is clear from the data is that some type of treatment and follow up is necessary, and I do my best to tailor this for each individual patient.

References

1. Shiels MS, Kreimer AR, Coghill AE, et al. Anal cancer incidence in the United States, 1977–2011: distinct patterns by histology and behavior. Cancer Epidemiol Biomark Prev. 2015;24:1548–56.
2. Milanés Guisado Y, Sotomayor C, Fontillón M, et al. Incidence rate and risk factors for anal squamous cell carcinoma in a cohort of people living with HIV from 2004 to 2017: implementation of a screening program. Dis Colon Rectum. 2022;65:28–39.
3. Revollo B, Videla S, Llibre JM, et al. Routine screening of anal cytology in persons with human immunodeficiency virus and the impact on invasive anal cancer: a prospective cohort study. Clin Infect Dis. 2020;71:390–9.
4. Peixoto A, Silva M, Castro R, et al. Anal condylomas: predictors of recurrence and progression to high-grade dysplasia/carcinoma in situ. J Gastrointest Oncol. 2017;8:1114–5.
5. Voss JK, Kurdi AT, Neto MB, et al. Detection of anal intraepithelial neoplasia and anal squamous cell carcinoma on colonoscopy. ACG Case Rep J. 2022;9:e00792.
6. Stewart DB, Gaertner WB, Glasgow SC, et al. The American Society of Colon and Rectal Surgeons clinical practice guidelines for anal squamous cell cancers (revised 2018). Dis Colon Rectum. 2018;61:755–74.
7. Lee GC, Kunitake H, Milch H, et al. What is the risk of anal carcinoma in patients with anal intraepithelial neoplasia III? Dis Colon Rectum. 2018;61:1350–6.
8. Frisch M, Biggar RJ, Goedert JJ. Human papillomavirus-associated cancers in patients with human immunodeficiency virus infection and acquired immunodeficiency syndrome. J Natl Cancer Inst. 2000;92:1500–10.
9. Gaisa M, Ita-Nagy F, Sigel K, et al. High rates of anal high-grade squamous intraepithelial lesions in HIV-infected women who do not meet screening guidelines. Clin Infect Dis. 2017;64:289–94.
10. Faber MT, Frederiksen K, Palefsky JM, Kjaer SK. Risk of anal cancer following benign anal disease and anal cancer precursor lesions: a Danish Nationwide cohort study. Cancer Epidemiol Biomark Prev. 2020;29:185–92.
11. Sanger CB, Xu Y, Carchman E, et al. Prevalence of high-grade anal dysplasia and anal cancer in veterans living with HIV and CD4/CD8 ratio as a marker for increased risk: a regional retrospective cohort study. Dis Colon Rectum. 2021;64:805–11.
12. Arens Y, Gaisa M, Goldstone SE, et al. Risk of invasive anal cancer in HIV-infected patients with high-grade anal dysplasia: a population-based cohort study. Dis Colon Rectum. 2019;62:934–40.
13. Chesson HW, Laprise J-F, Brisson M, et al. The estimated lifetime medical cost of diseases attributable to human papillomavirus infections acquired in 2018. Sexual Trans Dis. 2021;48:278–84.
14. Lightner AL, Welton ML. Anal dysplasia/cancer: Management of Patients with AIN 3. In: Hyman N, Umanskiy K, editors. Difficult decisions in colorectal surgery. Difficult decisions in surgery: an evidence-based approach. Cham: Springer International Publishing; 2017. p. 255–65.
15. Tong WWY, Jin F, McHugh LC, et al. Progression to and spontaneous regression of high-grade anal squamous intraepithelial lesions in HIV-infected and uninfected men. AIDS. 2013;27:2233–43.

16. Berry JM, Jay N, Cranston RD, et al. Progression of anal high-grade squamous intraepithelial lesions to invasive anal cancer among HIV-infected men who have sex with men. Int J Cancer. 2014;134:1147–55.
17. Cajas-Monson LC, Ramamoorthy SL, Cosman BC. Expectant Management of High-Grade Anal Dysplasia in people with HIV: long-term data. Dis Colon Rectum. 2018;61:1357–63.
18. Tomassi MJ, Abbas MA, Klaristenfeld DD. Expectant management surveillance for patients at risk for invasive squamous cell carcinoma of the anus: a large US healthcare system experience. Int J Color Dis. 2019;34:47–54.
19. Brogden DRL, Walsh U, Pellino G, et al. Evaluating the efficacy of treatment options for anal intraepithelial neoplasia: a systematic review. Int J Color Dis. 2021;36:213–26.
20. Corral J, Parés D, García-Cuyás F, et al. Incidence of recurrent high-grade anal dysplasia in HIV-1-infected men and women following infrared coagulation ablation: a retrospective cohort study. Pathogens. 2021;10:208.
21. Goldstone RN, Hasan SR, Drury S, et al. A trial of radiofrequency ablation for anal intraepithelial neoplasia. Int J Color Dis. 2017;32:357–65.
22. Vergara-Fernandez O, Solórzano-Vicuña D, Coss-Adame E, Trejo-Avila M. Outcomes of radiofrequency ablation for anal high-grade squamous intraepithelial lesions. Tech Coloproctol. 2021;25:701–7.
23. Kerdsirichairat T, Voltaggio L, Rifkin S, Canto MI. Multifocal nitrous oxide Cryoballoon ablation for high-grade anal intraepithelial neoplasia. Am J Gastroenterol. 2019;114:1194–4.
24. Palefsky JM, Lee JY, Jay N, et al. Treatment of anal high-grade squamous intraepithelial lesions to prevent anal cancer. N Engl J Med. 2022;386:2273–82.
25. Gudur A, Shanmuganandamurthy D, Szep Z, Poggio JL. An update on the current role of high resolution Anoscopy in patients with anal dysplasia. Anticancer Res. 2019;39:17–23.
26. McCutcheon T, Hawkins AT, Muldoon RL, et al. Progression of anal intraepithelial neoplasia in HIV-positive individuals: predisposing factors. Tech Coloproctol. 2019;23:325–32.
27. Gardner IH, Watson KM, Nguyen D, et al. Progression of anal intraepithelial neoplasia to cancer is low with Anoscopy surveillance and treatment. J Gastrointest Surg. 2022;26:929–31.
28. Fazendin EA, Crean AJ, Fazendin JM, et al. Condyloma Acuminatum, anal intraepithelial neoplasia, and anal cancer in the setting of HIV: do we really understand the risk? Dis Colon Rectum. 2017;60:1078–82.
29. Cleary RK, Schaldenbrand JD, Fowler JJ, et al. Treatment options for perianal Bowen's disease: survery of American Society of Colon and Rectal Surgeons members. Am Surg. 2000;66:686–8.
30. Scholefield JH, Ogunbiyi OA, Smith JHF, et al. Treatment of anal intraepithelial neoplasia. Br J Surg. 2005;81:1238–40.
31. Brown SR, Skinner P, Tidy J, et al. Outcome after surgical resection for high-grade anal intraepithelial neoplasia (Bowen's disease). Br J Surg. 1996;86:1063–6.
32. Palefsky JM, Giuliano AR, Goldstone S, et al. HPV vaccine against anal HPV infection and anal intraepithelial neoplasia. N Engl J Med. 2011;365:1576–85.
33. Wilkin TJ, Chen H, Cespedes MS, et al. A randomized, placebo-controlled trial of the Quadrivalent human papillomavirus vaccine in human immunodeficiency virus-infected adults aged 27 years or older: AIDS Clinical Trials Group protocol A5298. Clin Infect Dis. 2018;67:1339–46.
34. Gosens KCM, van der Zee RP, van Heukelom MLS, et al. HPV vaccination to prevent recurrence of anal intraepithelial neoplasia in HIV+ MSM. AIDS. 2021;35:1753–64.
35. Gaisa MM, Liu Y, Deshmukh AA, et al. Electrocautery ablation of anal high-grade squamous intraepithelial lesions: effectiveness and key factors associated with outcomes. Cancer. 2020;126:1470–9.
36. Albuquerque A, Stirrup O, Nathan M, Clifford GM. Burden of anal squamous cell carcinoma, squamous intraepithelial lesions and HPV16 infection in solid organ transplant recipients: a systematic review and meta-analysis. Am J Transplant. 2020;20:3520–8.

30 Observation Versus Chemoradiotherapy for Management of Superficial Anal Cancer

Martin Uwah, Cory Nonnemacher, Erin King-Mullins, and Valentine N. Nfonsam

Background

The evolution in management of anal squamous cell carcinoma (ASCC) away from abdominoperineal resection in the mid-1900s was prompted by an unacceptable 5-year mortality rate, as well as the morbidity secondary to the operation [1]. This changed in 1974 when Nigro *et al* published their preliminary report on the use of combined chemotherapy and radiation for management of anal cancer which showed promising results [2]. Nigro updated his recommendations in 1984 after having managed 104 patients with radio sensitizing chemotherapy and radiation, which suggested this treatment to be at least as effective as radical surgery [3]. These recommendations from Nigro and his colleagues paved the way for chemotherapy and radiation to be the treatment of choice for ASCC, and a randomized trial in 1996 by the United Kingdom Coordinating Committee of Cancer Research (UKCCCR) confirmed these results. Their conclusion lead to a new standard of care, The Nigro Protocol, comprised of radiotherapy in combination with 5-Fluorouracil and Mitomycin [4]. Further studies have gone on to investigate

M. Uwah
University of Chicago, Department of Colon and Rectal Surgery, Chicago, IL, USA

C. Nonnemacher
Atrium Health Navicent, Department of General Surgery, Macon, GA, USA

E. King-Mullins
Colorectal Wellness Center, Fayetteville, GA, USA

V. N. Nfonsam (✉)
LSU Health Department of Surgery, Louisiana State University, New Orleans, LA, USA
e-mail: vnfons@lsuhsc.edu

K. Umanskiy, N. Hyman (eds.), *Difficult Decisions in Colorectal Surgery*, Difficult Decisions in Surgery: An Evidence-Based Approach,
https://doi.org/10.1007/978-3-031-42303-1_30

alternative regimens with other agents or with induction chemotherapy prior to radiation without improvement in disease free survival [5].

Defining the Problem

While combined chemotherapy and radiation remains the gold standard for invasive anal ca, there are variations in practice patterns which are worth exploring. Surgery as the upfront treatment of low-grade tumors with certain characteristics has entered the algorithm of management and has become progressively more prevalent.

Superficially invasive squamous cell carcinoma is a minimally invasive tumor defined as having an invasive depth of <3 mm from the basement membrane, a horizontal spread of <7 mm and on pathology has histologically negative margins [6]. The guidelines on managing patients with primary findings of superficially invasive squamous cell carcinoma (SISCCA) of the anus or perianal area are not very robust. One of the most challenging scenarios, that is unfortunately very common, is incidental findings of superficially invasive squamous cell carcinoma in patients who underwent a hemorrhoidectomy or anorectal procedure. In most cases most of the tumor has been excised with very minimal residual tumor or there is a positive resection margin. The challenge, with no significant clear guidelines, is how to manage these patients. Some have argued that re-resection is adequate, and others have advocated for a more aggressive treatment approach of chemoradiation.

PICO table

Patients	Intervention	Comparator	Outcome
Patients with superficially invasive squamous cell carcinoma of the anus	Surgical excision	Chemoradiotherapy with or without surgical excision	Overall survival, disease-free survival, loco-regional recurrence

Treatment Decisions

When deciding the most appropriate management of SISCCA, we can infer from our knowledge of how we manage other low-grade tumors and use that as a treatment roadmap. Surgical resection of T1N0M0 tumors has been accepted as treatment without neoadjuvant or adjuvant chemoradiation. A retrospective cohort study using National Cancer Database and a joint program between the American College of Surgeons commission on cancer and the American Cancer Society evaluated T1N0M0 patients undergoing surgery versus chemoradiation [7]. The authors noted on their assessment after significant literature review that most landmark trials supporting chemoradiation dealt with tumors that were T2 and above, with many trials excluding T1 tumors. Nigro's reports and the previously mentioned UKCCCR trials did not include T1 tumors and yet are often cited as justification for treatment with chemoradiation for all ASCC. Multiple conclusions were drawn from this joint study.

1. Those who underwent excision had smaller tumor sizes with 41.6% of tumors <1 cm while 21.5% of those undergoing chemoradiation had sub centimeter tumors.
2. Tumors undergoing excision were more often well-differentiated, with 36.2% being well differentiated compared to 11.8%
3. Trends from 2004 to 2012 showed a higher tendency to perform local excision.
4. 5-year survival was the same in both cohorts (85.3% versus 86.8%)

In this study, the authors did not draw the specific conclusion that surgery should be the standard treatment for T1 tumors but do outline that surgical intervention on these tumors is noninferior and is becoming a more popular treatment option. Data from this study was cited in the National Comprehensive Cancer Network (NCCN) guidelines. Current NCCN recommendations support excision of well and moderately differentiated T1N0, stage I, perianal (anal margin) tumors with a 1 cm margin if the sphincter can be preserved [8]. These recommendations are specific to tumors of the perianal skin and exclude those of the anal canal.

Translating this data to the management of SISSCA, it is important to understand how SISSCA can differ from what is currently understood to be acceptable. The aforementioned research and NCCN guidelines do not give specific recommendations on the incidentally excised SISSCA which is the target in question for this chapter. SISSCA lesions do classify as T1 lesions given their size, but incidentally resected lesions may not result in achieving the recommended oncologic margins. The other critical difference is in the anatomic location of these lesions. The literature surrounding the resection of T1N0 lesions centers around the lesions being of the anal margin and excluding the anal canal. Depending on the location of incidental cancer within the specimen, a hemorrhoid for example, the tumor may instead involve the anal canal which has no good data. Lack of orientation of the specimen in non-hemorrhoidectomy specimens can lead to a diagnostic dilemma regarding margins. Extrapolating from the accepted T1N0 data to the management of SISSCA may requires accepting that tumors arising from the anal canal may be treated as anal margin tumors but this is not completely clear in the literature.

As previously mentioned, the combination 5-FU chemotherapy, mitomycin C and radiotherapy (CRT) is well established as the primary treatment regimen for anal squamous cell carcinoma with complete tumor regression in 80–90% of patients. We have also established that there are, however, subsets of these patients in whom the standard application of CRT can be challenged--early-stage anal cancer. This understudied population includes those with SISCCA as well as T1N0 perianal tumors (PAT) which replaces the previously used term anal margin, pigmented skin immediately surrounding the anal orifice, extending to a radius of 5 cm. The distinction between these tumors and anal canal tumors (ACT), tumors arising proximal to the anal margin and located within the canal, may prove critical in assessing prognosis and management.

Previous studies including NIGRO's and the UKCCCR had advocated for chemoradiation treatment for all stages of PAT and ACT even without strong evidence of their utility. However, this blanket treatment of these cancers has been challenged by recent studies advocating for surgical resection in early cancers [7, 9]. The rationale for the consideration of local excision in early-stage anal cancer is informed by several factors. While CRT offers both good local tumor control and sphincter preservation, it is also associated with multiple severe early and late adverse effects such as toxic gastrointestinal tract and hematologic effects, infections, proctitis, impotence, dyspareunia, skin dermatitis, anal and vaginal stenosis, incontinence, fecal urgency. Additionally, most of the data regarding CRT is from data of intermediate to more locally advanced diseases. The question remains if definitive CRT is necessary for all patients with early-stage disease. Several studies have looked at the safety, survival, and oncologic outcomes of CRT in early-stage disease. Chai et al. performed a retrospective cohort study that analyzed 2243 patients in the National Cancer Database (2004–2012) between the ages of 18 and 80 years who were diagnosed with T1N0M0 Squamous Cell Cancer of the Anal Canal (SCCAC) [7]. They noted a statistically significant increase in the use of local excision during the study period (17.3% in 2004 to 30.8% in 2012; $P < .001$). This increased use was observed among patients with primary tumors less than or equal to 2 cm ($P < .001$). No statistically significant difference in 5-year overall survival for the two different management strategies (85.3% for local excision; 86.8% for CRT; $P = .93$). These findings remained robust when stratifying patients by tumor size and when patients who underwent abdominoperineal resection after CRT were excluded. The study concluded that with no clear difference in overall survival, local excision should be considered as a viable approach in the appropriate patient population.

Maccabe *et. al* assessed both survival outcomes and determine factors associated with R1 excision examining 367 consecutive patients identified with anal cancer between 2007 to 2019 [10]. Thirty-nine of these patients (10.6%) with complete follow-up data underwent local resection. These patients were further subdivided into two groups: 24 patients with perianal tumors (PAT) and 15 patients with anal canal tumors (ACT). R1 resections were observed in 27 patients (69.2%) with more frequency in ACTs than PATs (93.3% vs. 54.2%, $P = 0.006$). This study concluded similarly that local excision (LE) alone is a viable treatment strategy for early SCCAC with the caveat that it is considered in perianal tumors and not of the anal canal. Long-term outcomes were observed to be acceptable even in the setting of an R1 resection with the use of adjuvant chemoradiotherapy.

An integrated protocol clinical trial with 3 separate arms has been designed as a non-randomized phase II multi-center trial of patients with T1N0 anal margin cancers [11]. It aims to recruit subjects having undergone LE with a goal of demonstrating a 3-year locoregional failure rate of <10% following frequent clinical assessments and pelvic magnetic resonance imaging. The strategy of low dose CRT for margins less than or equal to 1 millimeter will discourage *ad hoc* use of post-excision CRT and repeat excisions. The study hopes to address the concerns regarding the significant morbidity of conventional CRT by employing lower doses of radiotherapy, based on the findings of several published studies [12]. Interestingly, the inclusion criteria was widened to include the piecemeal excisions that often occur in clinical practice. For example, patients who incidentally present with malignancy following hemorrhoidectomy will be included. Additionally, patients with superficially invasive squamous cell carcinoma of the anus (SISCCA) as defined by the Lower Anogenital Squamous Terminology (LAST) consensus also be included [6]. Given the current heterogeneity in management of this understudied group, continued prospective studies will be crucial in establishing a more defined treatment algorithm.

Conclusion and Personal View of the Literature

The determination of treatment options for patients with SISCCA or early anal and perianal CA is truly a difficult decision. This difficulty is accentuated when these pathologic findings are incidental after a hemorrhoidectomy or anorectal surgery. The debate for local excision versus CRT persists but a preponderance of available retrospective cohort studies points to the consideration for local excision alone as a better alternative to chemoradiation for patients with early-stage anal cancer. The authors, therefore, propose the following recommendations:

- T1N0 perianal tumors can be locally excised while ensuring adequate margins of 1 cm if possible [6].
- T1N0 anal canal tumors should be treated with primary CRT and local excision should not be considered given the high likelihood of inadequate margins. Interestingly, the rate of local recurrence in ACTs, even with R1/Rx resection has been shown to be 9%, suggesting that the effectiveness of adjuvant therapy was not significantly undermined. Maccabe *et al* showed that those ACTs that got re-resected, even to an R0, recurred locally suggesting that resection may not be a viable option for any squamous cell tumors located in the anal canal [10].
- In the setting of an R1 resection of either variety of tumor, an acceptably low rate of local regional recurrence can still be achieved by employing adjuvant CRT.
- Any consideration of wide local excision alone should include multidisciplinary evaluation and discussion along with appropriate surveillance.

Hopefully, current ongoing clinical trials will provide answers and make treatment decisions for early anal and perianal cancers less difficult.

References

1. Pessia B, Romano L, Giuliani A, Lazzarin G, Carlei F, Schietroma M. Squamous cell anal cancer: Management and therapeutic options. Ann Med Surg (Lond). 2020;55:36–46.
2. Nigro ND. An evaluation of combined therapy for squamous cell cancer of the anal canal. Dis Colon Rectum. 1984;27(12):763–6.
3. Nigro ND, Vaitkevicius VK, Considine B Jr. Combined therapy for cancer of the anal canal: a preliminary report. Dis Colon Rectum. 1974;17(3):354–6.
4. Epidermoid anal cancer: results from the UKCCCR randomised trial of radiotherapy alone versus radiotherapy, 5-fluorouracil, and mitomycin. UKCCCR Anal Cancer Trial Working Party. UK Co-ordinating Committee on Cancer Research. Lancet. 1996;348(9034):1049–54.

5. Ajani JA, Winter KA, Gunderson LL, Pedersen J, Benson AB 3rd, Thomas CR Jr, Mayer RJ, Haddock MG, Rich TA, Willett C. Fluorouracil, mitomycin, and radiotherapy vs fluorouracil, cisplatin, and radiotherapy for carcinoma of the anal canal: a randomized controlled trial. JAMA. 2008;299(16):1914–21.
6. Darragh TM, Colgan TJ, Cox JT, et al. The lower anogenital squamous terminology standardization project for HPV-associated lesions: background and consensus recommendations from the College of American Pathologists and the American Society for Colposcopy and Cervical Pathology. J Low Genit Tract Dis. 2012;16:205–42.
7. Chai CY, Tran Cao HS, Awad S, Massarweh NN. Management of Stage I Squamous Cell Carcinoma of the Anal Canal. JAMA Surg. 2018;153(3):209–15.
8. NCCN Clinical Practice Guidelines in Oncology (NCCN Guidelines®) for Anal Cancer V.2.2023. © National Comprehensive Cancer Network, Inc. 2023. All rights reserved.
9. Chakrabarti S, Jin Z, Huffman BM, Yadav S, Graham RP, Lam-Himlin DM, Lightner AL, Hallemeier CL, Mahipal A. Local excision for patients with stage I anal canal squamous cell carcinoma can be curative. J Gastrointest Oncol. 2019;10(2):171–8.
10. Maccabe TA, Parwaiz I, Longman RJ, Thomas MG, Messenger DE. Outcomes following local excision of early anal squamous cell carcinomas of the anal canal and perianal margin. Colorectal Dis. 2021;23:689–97.
11. PLATO_trial. PersonaLising Anal cancer radioTherapy dOse– Incorporating ACT3, ACT4 and ACT5.
12. Hatfield P, Cooper R, Sebag-Montefiore D. Involved-field, low-dose chemoradiotherapy for early-stage anal carcinoma. Int J Radiat Oncol Biol Phys. 2008;70:419–24.

31 Is High Resolution Anoscopy Superior to Direct Evaluation of Anal Dysplasia?

Maria Abou Khalil and Sender Liberman

Introduction

While overall rare, anal squamous cell carcinoma is a potentially debilitating condition commonly encountered in a colorectal surgery practice. The incidence of this malignancy has been increasing, with age-adjusted rates for new anal cancer diagnosis rising on average 2.2% each year in the past decade [1]. It shares many epidemiologic, virologic and pathologic similarities with its gynecological counterpart: cervical squamous cell cancer. This is particularly true of the pathophysiology, thought to be related in the overwhelming majority of cases to infection with human papillomavirus (HPV) and the natural history of the disease evolving from precursor lesions [2, 3]. However, while guidelines and screening programs for cervical squamous cell cancer prevention and high-grade lesions exist and are well established, this public health parallel has not transpired for the management of precursor lesions in the anorectal area. This is likely multifactorial, owing amongst other reasons to the lower progression from anal dysplastic lesions to squamous cell carcinoma in the anus compared with the cervix, the lack of good quality public health data demonstrating the benefit of screening program, and the inability to define what type of screening tools to use for diagnosis and management of pre-malignant anal lesions [4].

High resolution anoscopy is a procedure very similar to colposcopy employed in screening, diagnosis and treatment of precursor and malignant lesions. The primary

M. Abou Khalil
McGill University Health Center, Montreal, QC, Canada
e-mail: maria.aboukhalil@mcgill.ca

S. Liberman (✉)
McGill University Health Centre, Colon & Rectal Surgery, Montreal, QC, Canada
e-mail: sender.liberman@mcgill.ca

K. Umanskiy, N. Hyman (eds.), *Difficult Decisions in Colorectal Surgery*, Difficult Decisions in Surgery: An Evidence-Based Approach,
https://doi.org/10.1007/978-3-031-42303-1_31

aim of this chapter is to review the role of high resolution anoscopy as compared to standard care with physical examination and direct anoscopy in patients with dysplastic anal lesions with regards to recurrence of these lesions or progression to cancer.

PICO Table

Patients	Intervention	Comparator	Outcome
Patients with dysplastic anal lesions	High resolution anoscopy	Conventional direct anoscopy	Recurrence of dysplasia, progression to cancer

Methodology

An electronic PubMed database using the search terms "anal cancer", "anal squamous carcinoma", "high resolution anoscopy", "anal dysplasia" was performed limiting the search to the years 2010–2022. Papers assessing the role of high resolution anoscopy in the identification and treatment of precursor lesions were reviewed.

Anal Dysplasia and High-Risk Groups

The Lower Anogenital Squamous Terminology (LAST) standardization consensus project was a multi-societal effort to unify the terminology for HPV-associated squamous lesions of the lower anogenital tract [5]. The goal was to improve communications across pathologists and clinicians across various specialties caring for patients with lesions. With regards to dysplastic lesions, they were separated into low or high-grade squamous intraepithelial lesions, respectively LSIL or HSIL. Anal intraepithelial neoplasia (AIN) was the terminology used previously for dysplastic lesions of the anal canal. In the newest terminology, LSIL corresponds to AIN I or anal condylomas, and HSIL corresponds to the higher dysplastic lesions AIN-2 and 3. Cytologic classification of lesions in the anal canal include atypical squamous cells of undetermined significance (ASCUS), atypical squamous cells, cannot rule out HSIL, LSIL, and HSIL.

Whether or not all anal dysplastic lesions develop into malignant ones and the rate at which they do is a matter of debate. Establishing this is important to identify screening and treatment guidelines. This contrasts with the dysplastic lesion for cervical cancer which have known rates of progression to cervical cancer from precursor lesions. In the anal region, LSIL is thought to be a marker of the risk for future HSIL diagnosis rather than a direct precursor for anal malignancy. The risk of progression to HSIL has been associated with some patient and viral factors. For example, infection with certain high-risk HPV-subtypes (particularly types 16 and 18) has been associated with increased risk of HSIL [6]. It has also been reported close to 50% of LSIL will spontaneously regress, a finding that is well described for cervical lesions [7].

Contrary to LSIL, HSIL is considered a true precursor to anal SCC. Berry et al. showed the malignant potential of HSIL and demonstrated evidence for progression to anal SCC in men who have sex with men (MSM) [8]. While regression of HSIL does occur, it seems to be less likely than LSIL, again especially when linked to certain HPV genotypes like HPV-16 [9].

In one of the largest cohort studies available, Arens et al. evaluated the risk of progression from anal dysplasia to invasive anal cancer using the SEER database over an 11-year period [10]. They reported an incidence of anal cancer of 1.2% and 5.7% at 1 and 5-years following AIN 3 diagnosis, respectively. In their analysis, this risk did not differ by treatment status for AIN (surgical or non-surgical) or surveillance denoting anal cytology done 30 days later. This study was limited by the significant heterogeneity in the terminology (the use of AIN 3 in the SEER database preceded the LAST project), population, and follow-up times. Rates of progression reported in the literature have varied from 0–1.2% at 1 year and 1.7–13% at 5-years following the diagnosis of precursor lesions [9, 11–13].

As alluded to earlier, there are important risk factors for both the development of anal dysplasia and progression to anal cancer. The imbalance with which certain at-risk groups are affected results in difficulty to study these issues on a large scale and create screening and management guidelines. The development of anal dysplasia being so closely related to infection with HPV infection, it goes without saying that they share many risk factors. In addition, factors that cause HPV virus persistence and non-clearance also increase the risk of anal dysplasia, and are likely closely linked to the development of anal cancer. Common risk factors for HPV infection and persistence include immunosuppression, infection with multiple HPV subtypes (particularly oncogenic subtypes 16/18), increasing age, number of sexual partners and younger age at sexual activity [14–16]. An important at risk-group for anal dysplasia are patients who have had history previous HPV-associated lesions especially gynecological or perineal disease [17–19].

Rates of anal dysplasia are particularly high in Human Immunodeficiency Virus (HIV) positive patients [20]. While this increased risk in HIV positive individuals is true regardless of sexual behaviors, men who have sex with men (MSM) are a particularly high-risk group [21, 22]. The incidence of anal cancer in the HIV positive population is estimated to be 28 times that of the general population, with an incidence of 35 per 100,000 cases [23–26]. This risk increases up to 40-fold for MSM compared to the general population [27]. Owing to advances in HIV care, it has become a chronic disease with concerns shifting from acute opportunistic illnesses to chronic illnesses, in particular HPV-related anal dysplasia/cancer.

Given the above, the overwhelming majority of studies evaluating the natural history of anal dysplasia especially concerning the benefit of interventions in preventing or halting progression to neoplasia have targeted these groups of high-risk individuals. The rest of this chapter will focus on these patient populations, limiting conclusions that can be generalized to the low-risk population.

High Resolution Anoscopy

High resolution anoscopy (HRA) is a specialized technique that uses magnification, lighting, and staining to thoroughly evaluate the anal canal mucosa and identify suspect lesions. Necessary equipment include a colposcope or an anoscope with lighting and magnification, an electrosurgical unit, biopsy capability, and staining usually with acetic acid and/or Lugol's solution. It is in essence the equivalent of a colposcopic examination, in the anal canal.

It can be performed in the office setting or in the operating room. Office evaluations and treatments under local anesthesia are feasible in the majority of cases, obviating the need for general anesthesia and use of operating room resources. A recent review of close to four hundred patient experience surveys from a HRA referral center the United Kingdom described good, patient satisfaction and low problematic pain scores with the office-based procedures [28].

The uptake of high resolution anoscopy has been much slower than that of colposcopy. HRA is a specialized skill with a learning curve especially relating to lesion identification [29]. Hillman et al. proposed a minimum of 50 HRA per year with identification of at least 20 cases of HSIL as a quality assurance metric, and identified that this skill improves over time [4, 29]. Siegenbeek van Heukelom et al. analyzed rates of HSIL detection of 7 anoscopists performing HRA in HIV positive MSM and found that over time, there was an increased HSIL detection rate and concluded that HSIL detection rate and mean HSIL rate per biopsy can also be used as a quality assurance metric for HRA [30]. Several attempts have been made to unify nomenclature and identify certain features that increase the positive predictive value of picking up HSILs, and identifying areas that need to be biopsied. These descriptors include amongst others lesion contour, mosaic pattern, vascular punctation/irregular vascularization patterns and Lugol negative staining [31, 32]. There is also data to support the growing role of artificial intelligence for lesion identification in HRA, with the potential for an improved learning curve for lesion identification and better accuracy [33]. While scarce, studies evaluating the impact of introduction of HRA programs are important. A recent such publication by Squeo et al. concluded that the establishment of a HRA program was associated with increased identification and treatment of high-grade anal lesions among women living with HIV [34]. The identification of HSIL was specifically higher when HRA was performed as compared to when anoscopy was performed without the use of a colposcope or dyes. While the non-randomized historical design and small sample size limit the definitive comparison between routine anoscopy/EUA and HRA, this is similar to other studies evaluating this topic [35–37].

Treatment Options

After identification of anal dysplastic lesions, a decision should be made with regards to both treatment and follow-up. There is a wide spectrum of options available, from observation alone to more aggressive and less performed wide local excisions.

The finding of LSIL lesions generally does not warrant treatment as close to half of the lesions may regress spontaneously. However, taking into account the patient's risk factor profile is important and will impact the decision to treat and how closely to survey these patients. Upon the finding of HSIL, treatment options include ablative and local therapies. Ablative therapies include electrocautery/hyfrecation, laser ablation, or infrared coagulation. While all these options are generally similar with regards to efficacy, there appears to be a superiority of electrocautery when compared to topical treatments with 5-fluorouracil and imiquimod with improved response and fewer side effects. A randomized controlled trial by Richel et al. randomized HIV+ MSM with dysplasia diagnosed on HRA to provider administered electrosurgical ablation using HRA versus patient applied topical fluorouracil or imiquimod [38]. In 388 patients randomized, electrocautery was better at the treatment of anal intraepithelial neoplasia compared to topical fluorouracil or imiquimod, but recurrence rates were substantial with more than 50% of patients having a recurrence.

The ANCHOR Trial

Whether or not treatment of HSIL decreases the risk of progression to anal SCC and the risk of recurrent HSIL is a matter of debate. This was the main question raised by the ANCHOR trial.

This eagerly awaited and recently published study is a phase III randomized controlled trial which included patients enrolled across twenty-five sites in the United States [39]. The main objective of the study was to establish the efficacy of ablation of HSIL lesions in preventing progression to anal cancer, evaluated as a time-to-event analysis for progression to anal cancer. Patients living with HIV and aged 35 and older were invited for anal HSIL screening with anal cytology and underwent physical examination and HRA. All physicians participating in the trial were well versed with HSIL management and HRA. Patients with a history of anal cancer or who were found to have anal cancer at presentation were excluded. Patients with biopsy proven HSIL were randomly assigned to immediate treatment or active monitoring. For patients in the treatment group, management was selected by the treating physician from a list of protocol approved therapies and included both ablative (infrared coagulation, electrocautery and laser) and topical (imiquimod and fluorouracil) treatment options. Patients returned for repeat HRA and at least every 6 months after randomization after all HSIL was eradicated. The identification of recurrent HSIL at follow-up mandated treatment until resolution. The active monitoring arm had repeat HRA every 6 months after randomization and visible lesions were biopsied annually to confirm HSIL persistence and assess anal cancer progression.

Of close to 9500 patients screened for HSIL, 4459 patients met the inclusion criteria and underwent randomization. The majority of patients in the treatment group had office-based electrocautery ablation (1862(83.6%)). Overall median follow-up was 27.2 months for the active monitoring group and 25.3 months. During the follow-up period, 9 patients developed invasive anal cancer compared to 21 patients in the active monitoring group, with rates of progression of 173/100,000 person-years (95%CI 90–332) compared to 402/100,000 person-years (95%CI 262–616), respectively. The treatment arm witnessed an impressive 57% (95%CI 6–80) reduction in the risk of anal cancer (*p* 0.029). Interestingly, the results identified that progression to anal cancer was associated with lesion size but not related to CD4 count.

Some noteworthy findings of the study include the high rate of detection of anal cancer in the active monitoring group with 402 cases/100,000 person-years, which is much higher than the estimates found in previously published registries [40]. As the authors discuss, this could be explained by patients history of smoking and reported male-to-male sexual contact, as well as the screening/preventative nature of this study. One of the limitations mentioned in the discussion raises the important point of replicability: the authors question the replicability of the results in settings where HRA and treatments are performed by less qualified physicians or physicians with different clinical support systems in place.

The high rate of progression from HSIL to anal cancer in this population highlights the need to set-up screening, treatment, and follow-up algorithms for these high-risk patients as a public health preventative intervention. There still is a gap in the knowledge on how to appropriately screen patients-and which patients- for precursor lesions. Anal cytology and anal HPV testing and genotyping may have a role but have limitations [41].

Conclusions

The role high resolution anoscopy plays in the management of anal dysplastic lesions was reviewed in this chapter. This is an especially important topic to review at this time given the significant findings of the recently published ANCHOR trial, which showed an impressive reduction in progression to anal cancer in patients with HIV positive HSIL using HRA-guided investigations and treatments as compared to active monitoring alone. While there is still no gold standard for screening or treatments of patients with anal dysplastic lesions, HRA is emerging as a central component in the management of patients with anal dysplastic lesions, particularly patient who belong to high-risk groups like HIV positive patients, MSM, or patients with gynecological HPV-associated lesions. While HRA is more costly and technically challenging than routine anoscopic examinations and digital rectal examinations, this has also been found to be cost-effective in certain situations. A cost effectiveness analysis using a decision-analytic model of the natural history of anal carcinoma and HSIL management strategies concluded that for HIV-positive MSM aged 38 or above, using treatment with adjuvant quadrivalent HPV vaccination is likely to be cost-effective, while a conservative approach with no treatment is likely to be cost-effective in younger patients [42]. In this paper, the authors compared a do nothing strategy, where given not all patients with HSIL develop anal cancer, diagnosis of anal cancer would be based on symptoms alone; active monitoring where patients would be examined using digital rectal examinations and HRA-guided biopsy for early anal cancer; treatment for HSIL where patients would be treated and followed using digital rectal examination and HRA annually; and treatment plus adjuvant quadrivalent HPV vaccination where patients would receive the vaccine on top of treatment of HSIL lesions and monitoring. HPV vaccination and catch-up vaccination in high-risk groups has been shown to reduce HPV-seropositivity [14, 42–44]. As data emerges linking increased vaccination with decreased incidence rates of anal dysplastic lesions, future research will elucidate and identify high-risk patients who will benefit from heightened screening and close follow-up with HRA [45].

We believe the first step in the management of patients at risk for anal dysplasia/SCC should be patient risk stratification. Patients at high risk for finding HSIL should be offered screening with anal pap smear or HRA. While HRA may not be available at all institutions given the associated limitations with access to a platform or lack of training, referral to gynecologic clinic with colposcopic abilities is an option, or referral to other centers with HRA capabilities is warranted.

With the growing use of HRA, we believe it should be in the armamentarium of a colorectal surgical practice in areas with high-risk populations.

References

1. Cancer SSFS-A. [Available from: https://seer.cancer.gov/statfacts/html/anus.html
2. De Vuyst H, Clifford GM, Nascimento MC, Madeleine MM, Franceschi S. Prevalence and type distribution of human papillomavirus in carcinoma and intraepithelial neoplasia of the vulva, vagina and anus: a meta-analysis. Int J Cancer. 2009;124(7):1626–36.
3. Videla S, Darwich L, Canadas MP, Coll J, Pinol M, Garcia-Cuyas F, et al. Natural history of human papillomavirus infections involving anal, penile, and oral sites among HIV-positive men. Sex Transm Dis. 2013;40(1):3–10.
4. Hillman RJ, Cuming T, Darragh T, Nathan M, Berry-Lawthorn M, Goldstone S, et al. 2016 IANS international guidelines for practice standards in the detection of anal cancer precursors. J Low Genit Tract Dis. 2016;20(4):283–91.
5. Darragh TM, Colgan TJ, Cox JT, Heller DS, Henry MR, Luff RD, et al. The lower anogenital squamous terminology standardization project for HPV-associated lesions: background and consensus recommendations from the College of American Pathologists and the American Society for Colposcopy and Cervical Pathology. Arch Pathol Lab Med. 2012;136(10):1266–97.
6. Liu Y, Sigel K, Gaisa MM. Human papillomavirus genotypes predict progression of anal low-grade squamous intraepithelial lesions. J Infect Dis. 2018;218(11):1746–52.
7. Jongen VW, Richel O, Marra E, Siegenbeek van Heukelom ML, van Eeden A, de Vries HJC, et al. Anal squamous intraepithelial lesions (SILs) in human immunodeficiency virus-positive men who have sex with men: incidence and risk factors of SIL and of progression and clearance of low-grade SILs. J Infect Dis. 2020;222(1):62–73.
8. Berry JM, Jay N, Cranston RD, Darragh TM, Holly EA, Welton ML, et al. Progression of anal high-grade squamous intraepithelial lesions to invasive anal cancer among HIV-infected men who have sex with men. Int J Cancer. 2014;134(5):1147–55.
9. Tong WW, Jin F, McHugh LC, Maher T, Sinclair B, Grulich AE, et al. Progression to and spontaneous regression of high-grade anal squamous intraepithelial lesions in HIV-infected and uninfected men. AIDS. 2013;27(14):2233–43.
10. Arens Y, Gaisa M, Goldstone SE, Liu Y, Wisnivesky J, Sigel CS, et al. Risk of invasive anal cancer in HIV-infected patients with high-grade anal dysplasia: a population-based cohort study. Dis Colon Rectum. 2019;62(8):934–40.
11. Scholefield JH, Castle MT, Watson NF. Malignant transformation of high-grade anal intraepithelial neoplasia. Br J Surg. 2005;92(9):1133–6.

12. Goldstone SE, Johnstone AA, Moshier EL. Long-term outcome of ablation of anal high-grade squamous intraepithelial lesions: recurrence and incidence of cancer. Dis Colon Rectum. 2014;57(3):316–23.
13. Cachay E, Agmas W, Mathews C. Five-year cumulative incidence of invasive anal cancer among HIV-infected patients according to baseline anal cytology results: an inception cohort analysis. HIV Med. 2015;16(3):191–5.
14. Tota JE, Giuliano AR, Goldstone SE, Dubin B, Saah A, Luxembourg A, et al. Anogenital human papillomavirus (HPV) infection, Seroprevalence, and risk factors for HPV Seropositivity among sexually active men enrolled in a global HPV vaccine trial. Clin Infect Dis. 2022;74(7):1247–56.
15. Daling JR, Madeleine MM, Johnson LG, Schwartz SM, Shera KA, Wurscher MA, et al. Human papillomavirus, smoking, and sexual practices in the etiology of anal cancer. Cancer. 2004;101(2):270–80.
16. Albuquerque A, Cappello C, Cuming T, De Masi A, Bowring J, Rosenthal AN, et al. Anal high-grade squamous intraepithelial lesions in pharmacologically immunocompromised patients followed in a referral center. Dis Colon Rectum. 2018;61(11):1267–72.
17. Lin C, Slama J, Gonzalez P, Goodman MT, Xia N, Kreimer AR, et al. Cervical determinants of anal HPV infection and high-grade anal lesions in women: a collaborative pooled analysis. Lancet Infect Dis. 2019;19(8):880–91.
18. Gilbert DCWK, Langley RE, Vale CL. Increased risk of second cancers at sites associated with HPV after a prior HPV-associated malignancy, a systematic review and meta-analysis. Br J Cancer. 2019 Jan;120(2):256–68.
19. Albuquerque A, Stockdale CK, Heller D, Bornstein J, Roberts JM, Preti M, et al. Vulvar high-grade squamous intraepithelial lesions and Cancer as a risk factor for anal cancer: a review. J Low Genit Tract Dis. 2022;26(1):32–7.
20. Kelly H, Chikandiwa A, Alemany Vilches L, Palefsky JM, de Sanjose S, Mayaud P. Association of antiretroviral therapy with anal high-risk human papillomavirus, anal intraepithelial neoplasia, and anal cancer in people living with HIV: a systematic review and meta-analysis. Lancet HIV. 2020;7(4):e262–e78.
21. Machalek DA, Grulich AE, Jin F, Templeton DJ, Poynten IM. The epidemiology and natural history of anal human papillomavirus infection in men who have sex with men. Sex Health. 2012;9(6):527–37.
22. Machalek DA, Poynten M, Jin F, Fairley CK, Farnsworth A, Garland SM, et al. Anal human papillomavirus infection and associated neoplastic lesions in men who have sex with men: a systematic review and meta-analysis. Lancet Oncol. 2012;13(5):487–500.
23. Johnson LG, Madeleine MM, Newcomer LM, Schwartz SM, Daling JR. Anal cancer incidence and survival: the surveillance, epidemiology, and end results experience, 1973–2000. Cancer. 2004;101(2):281–8.
24. Shiels MS, Goedert JJ, Engels EA. Recent trends and future directions in human immunodeficiency virus-associated cancer. Cancer. 2010;116(23):5344–7.
25. Diamond C, Taylor TH, Aboumrad T, Bringman D, Anton-Culver H. Increased incidence of squamous cell anal cancer among men with AIDS in the era of highly active antiretroviral therapy. Sex Transm Dis. 2005;32(5):314–20.
26. Colon-Lopez V, Shiels MS, Machin M, Ortiz AP, Strickler H, Castle PE, et al. Anal cancer risk among people with HIV infection in the United States. J Clin Oncol. 2018;36(1):68–75.
27. Silverberg MJ, Lau B, Justice AC, Engels E, Gill MJ, Goedert JJ, et al. Risk of anal cancer in HIV-infected and HIV-uninfected individuals in North America. Clin Infect Dis. 2012;54(7):1026–34.
28. De-Masi A, Davis E, Cuming T, Chindawi N, Pesola F, Cappello C, et al. The acceptability of high resolution anoscopy examination in patients attending a tertiary referral centre. BMC Cancer. 2018;18(1):554.
29. Hillman RJ, Gunathilake MP, Jin F, Tong W, Field A, Carr A. Ability to detect high-grade squamous anal intraepithelial lesions at high resolution anoscopy improves over time. Sex Health. 2016;13(2):177–81.

30. Siegenbeek van Heukelom ML, Marra E, Cairo I, Van Eeden A, Schim van der Loeff MF, De Vries HJC, et al. Detection rate of high-grade squamous intraepithelial lesions as a quality assurance metric for high-resolution anoscopy in HIV-positive men. Dis Colon Rectum. 2018;61(7):780–6.
31. Camus M, Lesage AC, Flejou JF, Hoyeau N, Atienza P, Etienney I. Which lesions should be biopsied during high-resolution anoscopy? Prospective descriptive study of simple morphological criteria. J Low Genit Tract Dis. 2015;19(2):156–60.
32. Jay N, Berry JM, Miaskowski C, Cohen M, Holly E, Darragh TM, et al. Colposcopic characteristics and Lugol's staining differentiate anal high-grade and low-grade squamous intraepithelial lesions during high resolution Anoscopy. Papillomavirus Res. 2015;1:101–8.
33. Saraiva MM, Spindler L, Fathallah N, Beaussier H, Mamma C, Quesnee M, et al. Artificial intelligence and high-resolution anoscopy: automatic identification of anal squamous cell carcinoma precursors using a convolutional neural network. Tech Coloproctol. 2022;26(11):893–900.
34. Squeo GC, Geba MC, Kane WJ, Thomas TA, Newberry Y, Wang XQ, et al. Impact of a high-resolution anoscopy clinic on management of anal dysplasia in women living with HIV. Am Surg. 2022:31348221129508.
35. Pineda CE, Berry JM, Jay N, Palefsky JM, Welton ML. High-resolution anoscopy targeted surgical destruction of anal high-grade squamous intraepithelial lesions: a ten-year experience. Dis Colon Rectum. 2008;51(6):829–35; discussion 35–7.
36. Pernot S, Boucheron P, Pere H, Lucas ML, Veyer D, Fathallah N, et al. Comparison of anal cancer screening strategies including standard anoscopy, anal cytology, and HPV genotyping in HIV-positive men who have sex with men. Br J Cancer. 2018;119(3):381–6.
37. Wells JS, Holstad MM, Thomas T, Bruner DW. An integrative review of guidelines for anal cancer screening in HIV-infected persons. AIDS Patient Care STDs. 2014;28(7):350–7.
38. Richel O, de Vries HJ, van Noesel CJ, Dijkgraaf MG, Prins JM. Comparison of imiquimod, topical fluorouracil, and electrocautery for the treatment of anal intraepithelial neoplasia in HIV-positive men who have sex with men: an open-label, randomised controlled trial. Lancet Oncol. 2013;14(4):346–53.
39. Palefsky JM, Lee JY, Jay N, Goldstone SE, Darragh TM, Dunlevy HA, et al. Treatment of anal high-grade squamous intraepithelial lesions to prevent anal Cancer. N Engl J Med. 2022;386(24):2273–82.
40. Holly EA, Whittemore AS, Aston DA, Ahn DK, Nickoloff BJ, Kristiansen JJ. Anal cancer incidence: genital warts, anal fissure or fistula, hemorrhoids, and smoking. J Natl Cancer Inst. 1989;81(22):1726–31.
41. Clarke MA, Wentzensen N. Strategies for screening and early detection of anal cancers: a narrative and systematic review and meta-analysis of cytology, HPV testing, and other biomarkers. Cancer Cytopathol. 2018;126(7):447–60.
42. Deshmukh AA, Chiao EY, Cantor SB, Stier EA, Goldstone SE, Nyitray AG, et al. Management of precancerous anal intraepithelial lesions in human immunodeficiency virus-positive men who have sex with men: clinical effectiveness and cost-effectiveness. Cancer. 2017;123(23):4709–19.
43. Goldstone SE, Giuliano AR, Palefsky JM, Lazcano-Ponce E, Penny ME, Cabello RE, et al. Efficacy, immunogenicity, and safety of a quadrivalent HPV vaccine in men: results of an open-label, long-term extension of a randomised, placebo-controlled, phase 3 trial. Lancet Infect Dis. 2022;22(3):413–25.
44. Poynten IM, Tabrizi SN, Jin F, Templeton DJ, Machalek DA, Cornall A, et al. Vaccine-preventable anal human papillomavirus in Australian gay and bisexual men. Papillomavirus Res. 2017;3:80–4.
45. Berenson AB, Guo F, Chang M. Association of human papillomavirus vaccination with the incidence of squamous cell carcinomas of the anus in the US. JAMA Oncol. 2022;8(4):1–3.

Part V

Benign Colon Disease

Surgical Management Options in Severe *C Difficile* Colitis

32

Allison M. Ammann and Ian M. Paquette

Introduction

Clostridioides difficile (*C. difficile*), previously known as *Clostridium difficile,* is a spore-forming, anaerobic gram-positive toxin-producing bacillus that is found to be part of normal large intestinal flora, but can become pathogenic when the microbiome is altered [1]. It is the most implicated cause of antibiotic-associated diarrhea with approximately half a million infections in the United States each year according to the Centers for Disease Control [2]. Alterations in the normal microbial flora of the large intestine, most often due to antibiotic use or immunosuppression, results in increased susceptibility to *C. difficile* infection [3]. Clinical manifestations of *C. difficile* infection (CDI) can range from asymptomatic carriers to mild CDI with watery diarrhea and crampy abdominal pain to severe, fulminant colitis with multi-organ failure. Severity of infection also depends on the virulence of the strain implicated, with more virulent strains resulting in more severe infections [4]. Recent collaborative efforts and practice measures including antibiotic stewardship programs have been implemented to reduce the rate of CDI, but it remains a significant source of morbidity and mortality for hospitalized patients due to recurrent and resistant infections [3].

A. M. Ammann
University of Cincinnati College of Medicine, Surgery, Cincinnati, OH, USA
e-mail: ammannao@ucmail.uc.edu

I. M. Paquette (✉)
Chief of the Division of Colon and Rectal Surgery, University of Cincinnati College of Medicine, Cincinnati, OH, USA
e-mail: ian.paquette@uc.edu

K. Umanskiy, N. Hyman (eds.), *Difficult Decisions in Colorectal Surgery*, Difficult Decisions in Surgery: An Evidence-Based Approach,
https://doi.org/10.1007/978-3-031-42303-1_32

Management of CDI relies on cessation of the offending antibiotics, and treatment with oral vancomycin or fidaxomicin as first line treatment. The workup includes laboratory evaluation focusing on presence of leukocytosis (>15 × $10^3/mm^3$) or other organ failure, physical examination, and imaging to evaluate colonic dilation or inflammation. Most patients, approximately 95–99%, with CDI will not require surgical intervention. Surgical intervention is reserved for patients with colonic perforation or severe colitis that does not improve with medical therapy and the decision to operate on severe CDI is provider-specific and often guided by experience [3, 5]. The historically recommended and most commonly performed procedure for severe-complicated *C. difficile* colitis is timely total abdominal colectomy (TAC) with end ileostomy as this procedure provides optimum source control [3, 6, 7]. Unfortunately, mortality rates following this procedure remain high and range from 34% to 57% with predictors of mortality including patient factors such as age, immunosuppression, and preoperative clinical signs of end organ damage [3, 8]. Additionally, patients undergoing laparotomy and TAC often require permanent end ileotomy, which can be associated with significant morbidity [9]. Thus it is important to proceed to surgical intervention at the correct time, as surgery too early can lead to unnecessary morbidity, where surgery performed too late increases the likelihood of mortality.

The previous edition of this text focused on the indications for surgical management of CDI and focused primarily on TAC with end ileostomy, which has been repeatedly shown to be superior to segmental colectomy. An alternative approach to the treatment of severe CDI is a loop ileostomy (LI) with antegrade colonic lavage using high-volume polyethylene glycol or electrolyte solution followed by postoperative antegrade vancomycin enemas. This was originally described by Neal et al. in 2011. The authors demonstrated that LI was a safe alternative operative approach in the surgical treatment of severe, fulminant CDI with evidence of decreased mortality in those receiving LI and colonic lavage compared to TAC [9, 10]. However, strong evidence supporting the safety and efficacy of LI is lacking and controversy still exists regarding the benefit in mortality of this approach compared to TAC with end ileostomy. The patient population of interest is indicated in Table 32.1.

Table 32.1 PICO table

P (Patient Population)	I (Intervention)	C (Comparator)	O (Outcomes)
Patients with severe *Costridioides difficile* colitis	Surgery	No surgery	Morbidity, mortality, quality of life

Search Strategy

A comprehensive search of PubMed and MEDLINE was performed to identify all English-language publications related to the operative management and outcomes related to C. difficile colitis from January 1st, 2015–August 1st, 2022. Published information was graded according to the GRADE guidelines. Key search terms included the following: "*Clostridioides difficile*", "*Costrisium difficile*", "surgery", and "outcomes". Evidence was generally moderate to low due to the retrospective nature of the published results available. Case reports, and reviews not containing original data were also excluded.

Results

Overall evidence is on this subject was low due to the retrospective nature of these studies with no identified randomized controlled trials (RCT) (Table 32.2). We updated the available clinical evidence presented since the previous version of this chapter was published. No high-level evidence regarding surgical technique is available. In fact, recent RCT aimed at examining outcomes between TAC and LI terminated early due to paucity of eligible patients or slow accrual [11]. The overall mortality rate for patients with severe CDI managed surgically was found in the studies we examined to be between 30% and 32%. Mortality for patients undergoing TAC ranged from 23% to 40% while the mortality for patients undergoing LI was between 17% and 36%.

Ferrada et al. retrospectively compared the outcomes of patients with CDI in this multi-center study following surgery (TAC vs LI) and found that adjusted mortality, controlled for pre-procedure confounders, was lower in the LI group (17.2% vs 39.7%, $p = 0.002$) [10]. This was the only study examined in this text to show a mortality benefit for LI and antegrade colonic lavage. Hall et al. queried the ACS-NSQIP database for patients undergoing LI or TAC. In this study, which is the largest to date comparing outcomes between LI and TAC in patients undergoing surgery for CDI, the authors found no mortality difference between the two approaches. However, patients who underwent LI had lower median operative times (1.6 h vs. 2.2 h, $p < 0.0001$), experienced fewer post-operative complications (72% vs 87%, $p = 0.021$) and had less frequent blood transfusions (19% vs 54%, $p < 0.0001$). Interestingly, the reoperation rates were similar for patients undergoing LI compared to TAC (9% vs. 11%, $P > 0.05$) [12]. Fashandi et al. retrospectively reviewed patients at a single institution who underwent either TAC or LI and colonic lavage for CDI and found no difference in mortality (30% vs. 23%, $p = 1.0$) [13]. Although this study was limited by a small sample size and single institution analysis, a majority (83%) of patients who underwent LI had return of intestinal continuity and all had colonic preservation. Juo et al. examined the Healthcare Cost and Utilization Project Nationwide Inpatient Sample (NIS) for patients undergoing either TAC or LI in the US to evaluate trends in the surgical treatment of fulminant *C. difficile* colitis. They found that the proportion treated with LI doubled over the study period

Table 32.2 Summary of studies

Year	Study	Design	Study Type	Years Studied	Quality	Patients (N)				Mortality (%)				
						Total	TAC	LI	Partial Colectomy	Overall	TAC	LI	Partial Colectomy	P-value
2017	Ferrada et al.	Retrospective	Multicenter	2011–2014	Low	98	77 (79%)	21 (21%)	–	32%	40%	17%	–	0.002
2017	Fashandi et al	Retrospective	Single center	2011–2015	Very low	27	13 (57%)	10 (43%)	–	26%	23%	30%	–	1.0
2018	Hall et al.	Retrospective	Database (ACS-NSQIP)	2011–2016	Low	457	410 (90%)	47 (10%)	–	–	31%	36%	–	0.45
2019	Juo et al.	Retrospective	Database (NIS)	2011–2015	Low	3021	2408 (80%)	613 (20%)	–	30.1%	31%	26%	–	0.28
2019	Peprah et al.	Retrospective	Database (ACS-NSQIP)	2007–2015	Low	733	582 (79%)	–	151 (21%)		35%	–	37%	0.58

LI loop ileostomy, *TAC* Total abdominal colectomy, *CDI Clostrioides difficile* infection

(12.9–26.5%). There was no significant difference in in-hospital mortality between LI and TAC (26% vs. 31%, $p = 0.28$). However, those who underwent LI were significantly younger (60.4 vs. 68.2, $p < 0.01$), had fewer comorbidities (Elixhauser index, >5; 9.6% vs 13.3%, $p = 0.03$), and occurred more often in hospitals with large bed sizes (76.3% vs 65.4%, $p < 0.01$) and urban teaching hospitals (84.0% vs. 66.3%, $p < 0.01$) [14]. Interestingly, Juo et al. also found that significantly more patients underwent LI compared to TAC on hospital day 0 (23% vs 12%, $p < 0.01$). The authors suggest a bias towards less severe cases of CDI on patients who underwent LI, which may affect mortality in subsequent studies and should be considered.

Finally, Peprah et al. queried the ACS NSQIP (2007–2015) database for patients with a diagnosis of *C. difficile* colitis who underwent a TAC or partial colectomy [15]. This was the only study comparing these two surgical approaches. The authors found no significant difference in mortality between TAC or partial colectomy (34.7% vs. 37.1%, $p = 0.58$). After controlling for patient factors, there was no difference for partial colectomy in complication rate (OR 0.92, 95% CI 0.51–1.62) compared with TAC.

Recommendations Based on the Data

As stated above, the overall grade of evidence on this subject is low due to the retrospective nature of this data and heterogeneous populations of patients studied. Additionally, only a small number of articles were identified comparing surgical procedures in the management of severe CDI. Overall, the mortality rates following surgical intervention for severe CDI remain high. The surgical management chosen is often patient specific and heavily reliant on individual surgeon's bias or judgement. None of the new data presented here should change the recommendations suggested in the ASCRS Clinical Practice Guidelines. (1) "Surgery for *C. difficile* colitis should be typically reserved for patients with colonic perforation or severe colitis who do not improve with medical therapy." (2) "Subtotal colectomy with end ileostomy is typically the operative procedure recommended for severe complicated fulminant *C. difficile* colitis." [3]

Personal View of the Data

The art of being a surgeon lies in selecting the correct operation for a patient and intervening at the correct time. Surgery for *C. difficile* is no different. As a patient progresses to severe colitis, a surgical team should be consulted to help make these difficult decisions. Though vancomycin and fidaxomicin have shown promising results, a small proportion of patients will fail medical management. Surgery should be reserved for the most severe, fulminant cases that are progressing towards organ dysfunction. The standard operation in this rare setting is still total abdominal colectomy with end ileostomy. This operation has historically been shown to be superior to any type of segmental colectomy. The concept of a diverting loop ileostomy is intriguing and though the original study by Neal did include critically ill patients in the loop ileostomy group, the remaining literature on this topic is subject to selection bias [9]. Many patients with less severe illness were offered diverting ileostomy, leaving the reader to wonder whether they would have recovered with no surgical intervention at all. This is similar to laparoscopic lavage for diverticulitis, where many patients who likely did not need any surgical intervention at all were treated with laparoscopic lavage. Their positive outcomes likely skewed the literature in favor of lavage. The recent EAST study on LI vs. Colectomy was criticized because LI offered no advantage in postoperative sepsis, renal failure, acute lung injury, or overall mortality [10]. More information is needed, ideally in the form of a well-powered randomized trial to make LI the standard practice.

References

1. Mada PK AM *Clostridioides Difficile*. 2022.
2. Control CfD. C. diff (Clostridioides difficile). Available at: https://www.cdc.gov/cdiff/what-is.html. July 3, 2022.
3. Poylin V, Hawkins AT, Bhama AR, Boutros M, Lightner AL, Khanna S, et al. The American Society of Colon and Rectal Surgeons clinical practice guidelines for the Management of Clostridioides difficile infection. Dis Colon Rectum. 2021;64:650–68.
4. Paquette IM, Stwart DB. *Clostridium Difficile* infection. In: ASCRS textbook of colon and Rectal surgery. Springer; 2022.
5. Stewart DB. Loop ileostomy for Clostridium difficile infection: know thy enemy. J Trauma Acute Care Surg. 2017;83:1214–5.
6. Bhangu A, Nepogodiev D, Gupta A, Torrance A, Singh P, West Midlands Research C. Systematic review and meta-analysis of outcomes following emergency surgery for Clostridium difficile colitis. Br J Surg. 2012;99:1501–13.
7. Steele SR, McCormick J, Melton GB, Paquette I, Rivadeneira DE, Stewart D, et al. Practice parameters for the management of Clostridium difficile infection. Dis Colon Rectum. 2015;58:10–24.
8. Lee DY, Chung EL, Guend H, Whelan RL, Wedderburn RV, Rose KM. Predictors of mortality after emergency colectomy for Clostridium difficile colitis: an analysis of ACS-NSQIP. Ann Surg. 2014;259:148–56.
9. Neal MD, Alverdy JC, Hall DE, Simmons RL, Zuckerbraun BS. Diverting loop ileostomy and colonic lavage: an alternative to total abdominal colectomy for the treatment of severe, complicated Clostridium difficile associated disease. Ann Surg. 2011;254:423–7; discussion 427-9.
10. Ferrada P, Callcut R, Zielinski MD, Bruns B, Yeh DD, Zakrison TL, et al. Loop ileostomy versus total colectomy as surgical treatment for Clostridium difficile-associated disease: an Eastern Association for the Surgery of Trauma multicenter trial. J Trauma Acute Care Surg. 2017;83:36–40.
11. Felsenreich DM, Gachabayov M, Rojas A, Latifi R, Bergamaschi R. Meta-analysis of postoperative mortality and morbidity after total abdominal colectomy versus loop ileostomy with colonic lavage for fulminant clostridium difficile colitis. Dis Colon Rectum. 2020;63:1317–26.
12. Hall BR, Leinicke JA, Armijo PR, Smith LM, Langenfeld SJ, Oleynikov D. No survival advantage exists for patients undergoing loop ileostomy for clostridium difficile colitis. Am J Surg. 2019;217:34–9.
13. Fashandi AZ, Martin AN, Wang PT, Hedrick TL, Friel CM, Smith PW, et al. An institutional comparison of total abdominal colectomy and diverting loop ileostomy and colonic lavage in the treatment of severe, complicated Clostridium difficile infections. Am J Surg. 2017;213:507–11.

14. Juo YY, Sanaiha Y, Jabaji Z, Benharash P. Trends in diverting loop ileostomy vs total abdominal colectomy as surgical management for Clostridium difficile Colitis. JAMA Surg. 2019;154:899–906.
15. Peprah D, Chiu AS, Jean RA, Pei KY. Comparison of outcomes between total abdominal and partial colectomy for the management of severe, complicated clostridium difficile infection. J Am Coll Surg. 2019;228:925–30.

33 Are Antibiotics Needed for the Management of Uncomplicated Diverticulitis?

Nathan Kohrman and Glenn T. Ault

Introduction

As colorectal surgeons we are familiar with diverticulitis, its complications, its epidemiology, and its burden on our health system. We are also familiar with the new hypothesis about its etiology: inflammation and changes in the colonic microbiome cause micro-perforations, which in turn cause infection [1–7]. Two major randomized control trials, DIABOLO [8] and AVOD [9], offer compelling evidence for this new hypothesis. Both trials showed that patients with acute uncomplicated diverticulitis (AUD) who receive conservative management have clinical outcomes similar to patients who receive antibiotics, long the standard of care.

The DIABOLO Trial was conducted at 22 clinical sites across the Netherlands and included patients over 18 years old who met the Hinchey classification of 1a or 1b or the Ambrosetti classification of 'mild.' All diagnoses were confirmed with a CT within 24 h of admission. The AVOD trial was conducted across 10 surgical departments in Sweden and one in Iceland. It included patients over 18 years old based on clinical criteria such as lower abdominal pain with tenderness, temperature >38 °C, elevated WC, and signs of diverticulitis on CT. The trials used different inclusion criteria because there are several ways to diagnose AUD, which is a source of heterogeneity in the way colorectal surgeons approach the disease. Patients in both trials were randomly assigned treatment with antibiotics or conservative

N. Kohrman
Keck School of Medicine of USC, Los Angeles, CA, USA

G. T. Ault (✉)
Keck School of Medicine of USC, Los Angeles, CA, USA

Division of Colon and Rectal Surgery, Keck School of Medicine, Los Angeles, CA, USA
e-mail: ault@med.usc.edu

K. Umanskiy, N. Hyman (eds.), *Difficult Decisions in Colorectal Surgery*, Difficult Decisions in Surgery: An Evidence-Based Approach,
https://doi.org/10.1007/978-3-031-42303-1_33

management, and then followed upon discharge to track complications, readmission, or other adverse events.

The trials found no statistically significant difference in clinical outcomes, and subsequent meta-analyses and retrospective studies supported the findings reported by the AVOD and DIABOLO trials. Two noteworthy studies, by Bolkenstein et al. [10] and Emile et Al [11], evaluated potential causes of conservative management failure, and found associations with two factors: elevated inflammatory markers and comorbidities. As such, there are still instances where antibiotics are appropriate.

Many colorectal surgeons still prescribe oral and IV antibiotics for all cases of AUD, in line with decades of personal experience, as well as the ASCRS clinical practice guidelines published 2014 [12]. However, current ASCRS clinical practice guidelines published in 2020 state that in majority of cases of AUD, antibiotics are not indicated [13]. As for those of us who treat less healthy patients, choosing between conservative management or prescribing antibiotics is not so straightforward.

Search Strategy

A comprehensive literature search of Cochrane Database of Collected Research [14], EMBASE, MEDLINE, and PubMed was performed to identify all the English-language publications related to acute uncomplicated diverticulitis, antibiotic use, conservative management, and rates of treatment failure from 2010 to 2020. Key search terms included "diverticulitis," "diverticulosis," "diverticular," "colonic," "colon diverticulosis," "surgery," "medical therapy," and "antibiotics," in line with the search performed in the 2020 ASCRS clinical practice guidelines on the topic [13]. Studies were excluded if they did not refer specifically to uncomplicated diverticulitis. Complicated diverticulitis was defined as diverticular disease resulting in an uncontained perforation, fistula, stricture, or abscess formation. Table 33.1 summarizes the population, intervention, comparator and key outcomes (PICO) for the patient population.

Table 33.1 PICO table

Patients	Intervention	Comparator	Outcome
Patients with acute uncomplicated diverticulitis	Conservative management with NSAIDs	Antibiotics (oral or IV) with NSAIDs	Resolution of symptoms, treatment failure, subsequent surgery, cost, subsequent antibiotics, hospitalization

Results

In the past decade, DIABOLO and AVOD, two randomized controlled trials (RCTs) conducted across several institutions in Northern Europe, showed there was no difference in outcomes between patients with AUD who received NSAIDs and antibiotics (oral and IV) and those treated conservatively with just NSAIDs [8, 9]. The measured outcomes included recurrence of diverticulitis, development of complicated diverticulitis, subsequent surgery, readmission, or other complications [15–19]. There was no statistically significant difference in these findings in the long or short term. Of note, van Dijk et al. [20] found that patients who received observational treatment had a higher rate of sigmoid colon resection at 2 years (9.0% compared to 5.0%), but those findings were not statistically significant (p = 0.085). As the authors noted, this may be because the study sample was under powered. However, van Dijk's meta-analyses of patient records two years after the initial episode of AUD found no difference in the rates of diverticulitis recurrence, complications, or surgical intervention [20]. After more than 10 year follow up of patients in the AVOD trial, there was no difference in rates of recurrent diverticulitis or quality of life between patients who received antibiotics and those who did not [21]. Table 33.2 summarizes these key studies.

Table 33.2 Results summary table

Study	Patients (N) observation v. antibiotics	Outcome measure	Results observation v. antibiotics	Quality of evidence
Megge [16]	1394 v 927	Treatment failure Emergency surgery Recurrence	Comparable Comparable Comparable	Moderate
Daniels [8]	262 v. 266	Median time to recovery Complications Recurrence Sigmoid resection Readmission Adverse events Mortality	Comparable Comparable Comparable Comparable Comparable Comparable Comparable	High
Chabok [9]	309 v. 314	Complications Recurrence within 1 year Readmission Length of hospital stay	Comparable Comparable Comparable Comparable	High
Desai [15]	1346 v. 895	Length of hospital stay Recurrence Complications Readmission Treatment failure Sigmoid resection Mortality	Comparable Comparable Comparable Comparable Comparable Comparable Comparable	Moderate

(continued)

Table 33.2 (continued)

Study	Patients (N) observation v. antibiotics	Outcome measure	Results observation v. antibiotics	Quality of evidence
Au [17]	1663 v. 842	Length of hospital stay Additional treatment Recurrence Complications	−0.68; $p = 0.04$ Comparable Comparable Comparable	Moderate
Van Dijk [18]	545 v. 564	Ongoing diverticulitis at 1 year Recurrence Sigmoid resection	Comparable Comparable Comparable	Moderate
Mocanu [19]	1626 v. 843	Recurrence within 1 month Treatment failure Complications Elective or emergent surgery	Comparable Comparable Comparable Comparable	Moderate
Isacson [21]	275 v. 281	Recurrence rate at 10 years Complication rate at 10 years Surgery rate at 10 years Cancer rate at 10 years Quality of life at 10 years	Comparable Comparable Comparable Comparable Comparable	Moderate
Van Dijk [20]	262 v. 266	Recurrence at 2 years Complications at 2 years Sigmoid resection at 2 years	Comparable Comparable Comparable	Moderate

Other meta-analyses, by Bolkenstein et al. and Emile et al. found associations between conservative treatment failure and a CRP of >170 [10], and between conservative treatment failure and comorbidities, especially immunosuppressive comorbidities such as diabetes [11]. The study by Emile et al. did not address specific comorbidities that may have put patients at elevated risk, or the risk posed by non-immunosuppressive conditions such as heart failure. While Bolkenstein et al. [10] did find a statistically significant relationship between elevated CRP and conservative treatment failure, Emile et al. [11] failed to find one. Both meta-analyses are sufficiently powered to support their contradictory conclusions. While it seems intuitive that elevated CRP would correlate with an increased rate of conservative treatment failure, other measures of inflammation and infection such as white blood cell count and temperature had no relationship with treatment failure in any of the meta-analyses we reviewed.

Among the studies looking at the consequences of antibiotic use, Au et al. [17] found an association between antibiotics and a prolonged hospital stay, while Megge et al. [16] found that for AUD patients treated with antibiotics, a short course of oral antibiotics had similar outcomes compared to a longer course of IV antibiotics. These findings were consistent with a randomized prospective trial performed by Schug-Pass et al. [22] which found that a 4-day dose of ertapenem was as effective as a 7-day course. The DIVER trial performed by Biondo et al., [23] found that AUD can be safely treated in an outpatient setting at a third of the cost of treating AUD in the hospital setting. Estrada Ferrer et al. [24] found that 88% of patients with AUD who received conservative treatment in an outpatient setting successfully completed their treatment. They also found that many patients who did require antibiotics for acute diverticulitis could be managed outpatient as well.

Recommendations

- Patients with AUD who have no comorbidities can be safely treated with observation and NSAIDs. (Evidence: strong; Recommendation: strong)
- Patients with AUD who are immunosuppressed or have comorbidities affecting their immune function can receive oral antibiotics and can be safely treated outpatient. (Evidence: moderate; Recommendation: moderate)
- Patients with AUD and other poorly controlled comorbidities should be seriously considered for inpatient antibiotics.
- (Evidence: moderate; Recommendation; moderate)

Personal View

Most colorectal surgeons have been taught to prescribe antibiotics for AUD. Despite available evidence, surgeons may be reluctant to change the treatment approaches they have relied on over the course of their career. However, the evidence is overwhelming that immunocompetent patients can be treated effectively with conservative management. While the outcomes are similar, the benefits of observational management are substantial. Many patients are spared the discomfort and logistical difficulty of taking another drug and are spared the potential side effects of antibiotics. While not specifally addressed by this chapter, avoiding antibiotics will result in decreasing healthcare costs. The patient will face less risk from antibiotic resistance and C. Difficile infection. For physicians who treat AUD in healthy patient populations, this will streamline care. The patients can be followed on an outpatient basis with phone calls, electronic messaging or video visits. The timeframe for follow up can be left to individual provider's clinical judgment.

The recommendations are not as clear-cut for management patients with AUD who have comorbidities. Emile et al. [11], a metanalysis of 2565 patients, found that comorbidities were the only variable significantly associated with treatment failure in the non-antibiotic group. While this group was small—85 patients out of 1671—it makes sense that immunosuppressive conditions such as diabetes could impede the healing process. Since Bolkenstein et al. and Emile et al. had different findings on the relationship between elevated CRP and treatment failure, we defer to individual provider's judgment whether to use this value in managing of AUD. In our opinion, because it is a non-specific marker, elevated CRP value alone should not inform the decision for or against an antibiotic treatment.

Would we discharge a patient with AUD without antibiotics if they have pre-diabetes or take low-dose steroids? What if they have a serious but non-immunosuppressive disease like congestive heart disease? Additional research is necessary to answer these questions. In the meantime, we will have to use our individualized clinical judgment.

The AVOD and DIABOLO studies were conducted in European countries with patient populations that are healthier than the patients we serve at LAC+USC Medical Center, which is a large public safety net hospital. Our patients often have low health literacy and comorbidities, both diagnosed and undiagnosed. Many are low-income and Latino, which according to the CDC means between one in four and one in five of our patients have diabetes [25]. These rates likely grow as patients get older—which is also when AUD is more likely to present. Many patients also have cirrhosis and inflammatory conditions for which they must take steroids. These patients need antibiotics when they present with AUD. Treating our patient population on an outpation basis would be challenging. Even with coaching, patients with low health literacy often struggle to fill prescriptions and take their medications as prescribed.

So where does this leave us? We would feel comfortable using conservative management to treat a patient with AUD and DM with an A1c below 7.0, the threshold above which patients develop an increased risk of infection [26]. As for patients with AUD and non-immunosuppressive comorbidities, we would use conservative management if the comorbid condition is well controlled, such as asymptomatic heart failure. For patients with AUD and uncontrolled comorbidities, we would, despite the findings of Schug-Pas et al. [22] and Estrada Ferrer et al. [24] admit the patient for a 4-day course of antibiotics to reduce the risk of treatment failure or non-adherence. Each surgeon will likely have a different approach based on his or her patient population. Treating acute uncomplicated diverticulitis is, well, complicated.

References

1. Strate LL, Modi R, Cohen E, Spiegel BM. Diverticular disease as a chronic illness: evolving epidemiologic and clinical insights. Am J Gastroenterol. 2012 Oct;107(10):1486–93. https://doi.org/10.1038/ajg.2012.194. Epub 2012 Jul 10. PMID: 22777341.
2. Espín F, Rofes L, Ortega O, Clavé P, Gallego D. Nitrergic neuro-muscular transmission is up-regulated in patients with diverticulosis. Neurogastroenterol Motil 2014 Oct;26(10):1458–1468. https://doi.org/10.1111/nmo.12407. Epub 2014 Aug 11. PMID: 25109425.
3. Floch MH. A hypothesis: is diverticulitis a type of inflammatory bowel disease? J Clin Gastroenterol 2006 Aug;40 Suppl 3:S121–S125. https://doi.org/10.1097/01.mcg.0000225502.29498.ba. PMID: 16885694.
4. Simpson J, Sundler F, Humes DJ, Jenkins D, Scholefield JH, Spiller RC. Post inflammatory damage to the enteric nervous system in diverticular disease and its relationship to symptoms. Neurogastroenterol Motil 2009 Aug;21(8):847-e58. https://doi.org/10.1111/j.1365-2982.2009.01308.x. Epub 2009 May 14. PMID: 19453515.
5. Humes DJ, Simpson J, Smith J, Sutton P, Zaitoun A, Bush D, Bennett A, Scholefield JH, Spiller RC. Visceral hypersensitivity in symptomatic diverticular disease and the role of neu-

ropeptides and low grade inflammation. Neurogastroenterol Motil 2012 Apr;24(4):318-e163. https://doi.org/10.1111/j.1365-2982.2011.01863.x. Epub 2012 Jan 25. PMID: 22276853.
6. Tursi A, Elisei W, Brandimarte G, Giorgetti GM, Inchingolo CD, Nenna R, Picchio M, Giorgio F, Ierardi E. Musosal tumour necrosis factor α in diverticular disease of the colon is overexpressed with disease severity. Color Dis 2012 May;14(5):e258–e263. https://doi.org/10.1111/j.1463-1318.2012.02926.x. PMID: 22469482.
7. Jeganathan NA, Davenport ER, Yochum GS, Koltun WA. The microbiome of diverticulitis. Curr Opin Physiol. 2021;22:100452, ISSN 2468–8673. https://doi.org/10.1016/j.cophys.2021.06.006.
8. Daniels L, Ünlü Ç, de Korte N, van Dieren S, Stockmann HB, Vrouenraets BC, Consten EC, van der Hoeven JA, Eijsbouts QA, Faneyte IF, Bemelman WA, Dijkgraaf MG, Boermeester MA; Dutch Diverticular Disease (3D) Collaborative Study Group. Randomized clinical trial of observational versus antibiotic treatment for a first episode of CT-proven uncomplicated acute diverticulitis. Br J Surg 2017 Jan;104(1):52–61. https://doi.org/10.1002/bjs.10309. Epub 2016 Sep 30. PMID: 27686365.
9. Chabok A, Påhlman L, Hjern F, Haapaniemi S, Smedh K; AVOD Study Group. Randomized clinical trial of antibiotics in acute uncomplicated diverticulitis. Br J Surg 2012 Apr;99(4):532–539. https://doi.org/10.1002/bjs.8688. Epub 2012 Jan 30. PMID: 22290281.
10. Bolkenstein HE, Draaisma WA, van de Wall B, Consten E, Broeders I. Treatment of acute uncomplicated diverticulitis without antibiotics: risk factors for treatment failure. Int J Colorectal Dis. 2018 Jul;33(7):863–869. https://doi.org/10.1007/s00384-018-3055-1. Epub 2018 Apr 21. PMID: 29679152; PMCID: PMC6002463.
11. Emile SH, Elfeki H, Sakr A, Shalaby M. Management of acute uncomplicated diverticulitis without antibiotics: a systematic review, meta-analysis, and meta-regression of predictors of treatment failure. Tech Coloproctol 2018 Jul;22(7):499–509. https://doi.org/10.1007/s10151-018-1817-y. Epub 2018 Jul 6. PMID: 29980885.
12. Feingold D, Steele SR, Lee S, Kaiser A, Boushey R, Buie WD, Rafferty JF. Practice parameters for the treatment of sigmoid diverticulitis. Dis Colon Rectum 2014 Mar;57(3):284–294. https://doi.org/10.1097/DCR.0000000000000075. PMID: 24509449.
13. Hall J, Hardiman K, Lee S, Lightner A, Stocchi L, Paquette IM, Steele SR, Feingold DL; Prepared on behalf of the clinical practice guidelines Committee of the American Society of colon and Rectal surgeons. The American Society of Colon and Rectal Surgeons clinical practice guidelines for the treatment of left-sided colonic diverticulitis. Dis Colon Rectum 2020 Jun;63(6):728–747. https://doi.org/10.1097/DCR.0000000000001679. PMID: 32384404.
14. Shabanzadeh DM, Wille-Jørgensen P. Antibiotics for uncomplicated diverticulitis. Cochrane Database Syst Rev. 2012 Nov 14;11:CD009092. https://doi.org/10.1002/14651858.CD009092.pub2. Update in: Cochrane Database Syst Rev. 2022 Jun 22;6:CD009092. PMID: 23152268.
15. Desai M, Fathallah J, Nutalapati V, Saligram S. Antibiotics versus no antibiotics for acute uncomplicated diverticulitis: a systematic review and meta-analysis. Dis Colon Rectum 2019 Aug;62(8):1005–1012. https://doi.org/10.1097/DCR.0000000000001324. PMID: 30664553.
16. Mege D, Yeo H. Meta-analyses of current strategies to treat uncomplicated diverticulitis. Dis Colon Rectum 2019 Mar;62(3):371–378. https://doi.org/10.1097/DCR.0000000000001295. PMID: 30570549.
17. Au S, Aly EH. Treatment of uncomplicated acute diverticulitis without antibiotics: a systematic review and meta-analysis. Dis Colon Rectum 2019 Dec;62(12):1533–1547. https://doi.org/10.1097/DCR.0000000000001330. PMID: 30663999.
18. van Dijk ST, Chabok A, Dijkgraaf MG, Boermeester MA, Smedh K. Observational versus antibiotic treatment for uncomplicated diverticulitis: an individual-patient data meta-analysis. Br J Surg. 2020 Jul;107(8):1062–1069. https://doi.org/10.1002/bjs.11465. Epub 2020 Feb 19. PMID: 32073652; PMCID: PMC7318319.
19. Mocanu V, Dang JT, Switzer N, Tavakoli I, Tian C, de Gara C, Birch DW, Karmali S. The role of antibiotics in acute uncomplicated diverticulitis: a systematic review and meta-analysis. Am J Surg 2018 Sep;216(3):604–609. https://doi.org/10.1016/j.amjsurg.2018.01.039. Epub 2018 Feb 2. PMID: 29454479.

20. van Dijk ST, Daniels L, Ünlü Ç, de Korte N, van Dieren S, Stockmann HB, Vrouenraets BC, Consten EC, van der Hoeven JA, Eijsbouts QA, Faneyte IF, Bemelman WA, Dijkgraaf MG, Boermeester MA; Dutch diverticular disease (3D) collaborative study group. Long-term effects of omitting antibiotics in uncomplicated acute diverticulitis. Am J Gastroenterol 2018 Jul;113(7):1045–1052. https://doi.org/10.1038/s41395-018-0030-y. Epub 2018 May 11. PMID: 29700480.
21. Isacson D, Smedh K, Nikberg M, Chabok A. Long-term follow-up of the AVOD randomized trial of antibiotic avoidance in uncomplicated diverticulitis. Br J Surg 2019 Oct;106(11):1542–1548. https://doi.org/10.1002/bjs.11239. Epub 2019 Aug 6. PMID: 31386199.
22. Schug-Pass C, Geers P, Hügel O, Lippert H, Köckerling F. Prospective randomized trial comparing short-term antibiotic therapy versus standard therapy for acute uncomplicated sigmoid diverticulitis. Int J Colorectal Dis. 2010 Jun;25(6):751–759. https://doi.org/10.1007/s00384-010-0899-4. Epub 2010 Feb 6. Erratum in: Int J Colorectal Dis. 2010 Jun;25(6):785. PMID: 20140619.
23. Biondo S, Golda T, Kreisler E, Espin E, Vallribera F, Oteiza F, Codina-Cazador A, Pujadas M, Flor B. Outpatient versus hospitalization management for uncomplicated diverticulitis: a prospective, multicenter randomized clinical trial (DIVER trial). Ann Surg 2014 Jan;259(1):38–44. doi: https://doi.org/10.1097/SLA.0b013e3182965a11. PMID: 23732265.
24. Estrada Ferrer O, Ruiz Edo N, Hidalgo Grau LA, Abadal Prades M, Del Bas Rubia M, Garcia Torralbo EM, Heredia Budo A, Suñol Sala X. Selective non-antibiotic treatment in sigmoid diverticulitis: is it time to change the traditional approach? Tech Coloproctol 2016 May;20(5):309–315. https://doi.org/10.1007/s10151-016-1464-0. Epub 2016 Apr 6. PMID: 27053254.
25. Cheng YJ, Kanaya AM, Araneta MRG, et al. Prevalence of diabetes by race and ethnicity in the United States, 2011-2016. JAMA. 2019;322(24):2389–98. https://doi.org/10.1001/jama.2019.19365.
26. Critchley JA, Carey IM, Harris T, DeWilde S, Hosking FJ, Cook DG. Glycemic control and risk of infections among people with Type 1 or Type 2 diabetes in a large primary care cohort study. Diabetes Care. 2018 October 1;41(10):2127–35. https://doi.org/10.2337/dc18-0287.

34 Do We Need to Operate on Patients After Successful Percutaneous Drainage of a Diverticular Abscess?

Tobi J. Reidy and Scott C. Dolejs

Introduction

Diverticulitis with abscess (modified Hinchey Ib and II) accounts for approximately 15% of all diverticular abdominal pain presentations in the United States [1]. The acute management of these patients has become streamlined with the ability to clear most infections through combined use of percutaneous drainage, antibiotics and bowel rest. After the resolution of the acute infection, colectomy was recommended in the past [2]. However, this paradigm has been challenged with the most recent practice guidelines either not recommending routine colectomy or recommending consideration of colectomy after successful nonoperative treatment of a diverticular abscess [3, 4]. This chapter will provide the evidence basis for these recent changes to help guide clinicians to make evidence-based decisions of this common problem.

Search Strategy

A comprehensive literature search of PubMed and MEDLINE from 2002 to 2022 was performed to identify English language publications related to diverticulitis with abscess, percutaneous drainage procedures for diverticular abscess and surgical interventions in diverticulitis with abscess to answer the Patient, Intervention, Comparator, Outcome (PICO) question as outlined in Table 34.1. Key search words included, "perforated diverticulitis", "percutaneous drain", "Hinchey Ib and II", and "diverticulitis with abscess". Systematic reviews and full text articles were also reviewed for additional studies that may meet inclusion criteria. Studies were excluded if they only looked at short term outcomes (defined as surgery within

T. J. Reidy (✉) · S. C. Dolejs
Indiana Colon and Rectal Specialists, Indianapolis, IN, USA

K. Umanskiy, N. Hyman (eds.), *Difficult Decisions in Colorectal Surgery*, Difficult Decisions in Surgery: An Evidence-Based Approach,
https://doi.org/10.1007/978-3-031-42303-1_34

Table 34.1 Patient, Intervention, Comparator, Outcome (PICO) question

Patient	Intervention	Comparator	Outcome
Patients with diverticulitis who underwent successful drainage of a diverticular abscess	Colon resection	Observation	Complications/need for urgent surgery due to persistent or worsening symptoms, development of new complication such as fistula formation or peritonitis

30 days of presentation or drainage) or did not include patients who underwent percutaneous drainage. Only the most recent studies were included if similar studies were released from the same group.

Results

Over the past 2 decades, there have been numerous retrospective series written (Table 34.2). There is a large degree of heterogeneity in the data. There are different definitions of recurrence. Some studies specify radiographic recurrence, some are based solely on readmission which may miss outpatient recurrence, and others employed telephone follow-up. The reason for eventual colectomy is usually poorly defined owing to the frequent retrospective design. Thus, it is often unclear if a surgery was planned and elective secondary to an initial episode, due to recurrent or unresolving disease, or emergent. Finally, the number of patients who had percutaneous drains and did not pursue operative management is small in most studies ranging from 7 to 81 patients except for a few larger database studies, which have their own methodological challenges [5, 6]. The differing and at times unclear definitions of recurrence and rational for surgery result in substantial heterogeneity between studies with recurrence rates varying from 0% to 74% and eventual need for operation in patients in whom elective colectomy was not pursued between 0% and 56% [7–10].

Overall, the rate of recurrence in patients undergoing a percutaneous drain had a wide variability from 0% to 74% with most studies noting a recurrence rate between 15% and 35% (Table 34.2). These recurrences were complicated between 0% and 100% of the time with most of the studies demonstrating complicated recurrences about 40–60% of the time (Table 34.2). Most of these recurrences were able to be managed non-operatively. The rate of operation in patients who had percutaneous drainage and then planned non-operative management ranged between 0% and 56% with the bulk of the studies having an operative rate of 0–25% (Table 34.2).

Only one study directly compared patients who underwent elective colectomy versus observation following successful percutaneous drainage [11]. In this study, the rate of stoma was higher in patients who underwent elective colectomy (13% in elective colectomy versus 9% in patients with planned non-operative management, $p < 0.05$) [11]. Elective colectomy in this study was also associated with increased inpatient days and increased cost [11]. This was a population-based study based on statewide data from New York and thus granular detail about what drove these

Table 34.2 Outcomes of non-operative management after successful percutaneous drainage of a diverticular abscess

Article	Study design	Number of patients with drain	Recurrence rate, %	Percent of recurrences that were complicated, %	Operative rate amongst patients initially planned for non-op management, %	Follow-up, months
Aquina [11]	Observational cohort database	1137	27%	14%	22%[a]	60
Brandt [19]	Retrospective, case-control	34	18%	Unknown	18%	
Bridoux [9]	Retrospective with telephone follow-up	9	7%[b]	Unknown	0%	32
Broderick-Villa [20]	Retrospective, cohort	44	13%	Unknown, all recurrences were treated non-operatively	0%	107
Buchwald [21]	Retrospective	22	27%	No end colostomy required for recurrences	19%	110
Devaraj [7]	Retrospective	65	74%	71%	56%	14
Elagili [16]	Retrospective	18	39%	43%	17%	90
Felder [8]	Retrospective	7	0%	0%	0%	47
Gaertner [10]	Retrospective	32	42%	44%	0%	89
Garfinkle [14]	Retrospective with telephone follow-up	33	30%	10%	12%	62
Gregersen [13]	Retrospective database	490	24%	66%	16%[c]	38
Jalouta [6]	Retrospective with telephone follow-up	81	23%	21%	26%[d]	

(continued)

Table 34.2 (continued)

Article	Study design	Number of patients with drain	Recurrence rate, %	Percent of recurrences that were complicated, %	Operative rate amongst patients initially planned for non-op management, %	Follow-up, months
Kaiser [5]	Retrospective	16	42%	Unknown	42%	
Lambricht [15]	Retrospective	115	25%	Unknown	Unknown[e]	72
Li [31]	Retrospective database	409	15%[f]	Unknown	7%	47
Macias [22]	Retrospective	10	30%	67%	19%[g]	
Nelson [23]	Retrospective	11	46%[h]	21%[h]	10%	76
Singh [24]	Retrospective	16	11%	Unknown	50%[d]	35
Trenti [12]	Retrospective	9	15%[i]	Unknown	0%	67
Van de Waal [25]	Retrospective	7	33%[j]	44%[j]	41%[j]	28
You [26]	Randomized control trial	30	32%	100%	2%	24

[a] Unclear how many of these operations were planned elective operation. Had an 11% rate of non-elective surgery
[b] This was recurrence rate in 105 patients with complicated disease. Did not have this stratified by patients with drain
[c] Rate reflects operative rate in all patients with complicated disease, not just those drained. Some of these operations were elective, but this rate was not specified
[d] Unclear why operative rate is higher than rate of recurrence if all patients were initially intended to be managed non-operatively
[e] 68% of patients with drain underwent surgery, but it is unclear how many of these were planned elective operations versus need for surgery secondary to recurrence as the recurrence rate in those with a drain was only 25%
[f] This is the rate of readmission and may not reflect the true rate of recurrence
[g] This reflects a cohort of 70 patients with complicated disease and not just those with a drain
[h] Rate reflects a cohort of 99 patients with complicated disease and not just those with a drain
[i] Rate reflects a cohort of 560 patients with complicated disease and not just those with a drain
[j] Rate reflects cohort of 59 patients with complicated disease and not just those with a drain

differences was not available and it is possible that recurrences were missed that would have biased the study towards non-operative management.

Recommendations

After successful percutaneous drainage and resolution of complicated diverticulitis, the decision to pursue elective surgical resection versus observation only should be individualized and made in a shared decision-making framework that weighs the patient comorbidities, surgical risks, and risk of recurrence.

Strong recommendation based on low-quality evidence.

The current literature points to around a 15–35% risk of recurrence after successful percutaneous drainage in complicated diverticulitis, of which about half will be complicated. The majority of these recurrences can be managed non-operatively. Certain patient populations, such as those on chronic steroids, may additionally have a higher rate of recurrence and greater impact of recurrence and are likely better steered to definitive resection [12, 13]. Prior episodes of diverticulitis preceding the need for a drain are also associated with higher risks of recurrence [14]. Pursuing elective surgical resection in patients with diverticulitis and abscess after successful percutaneous drainage may have a paradoxically higher rate of ostomy than a trial of non-operative management, and thus, the primary aim of elective resection should not be to prevent a stoma [11]. With this data in mind, care of these patients should be individualized considering patient perspectives and preferences.

Personal View

Patients presenting with complicated diverticulitis with a localized abscess need to be assessed and cared for individually. Initial management of these patients should include control of sepsis with percutaneous drainage and antibiotics. These patients should undergo colonoscopy after symptom resolution to rule out malignancy as a source of their disease. Following this, patients with ongoing complication of their diverticulitis such as stricture, fistula, or ongoing impairment to their quality of life should be managed operatively. The decision to pursue elective resection if the initial episode has completely resolved should be individualized.

Of particular interest to me are patients with quality-of-life decline after percutaneous drainage of diverticular abscess. These patients have become the most nuanced group to manage in my practice. Their clinical symptoms are subtle and often impossible to quantify on imaging or examination. Despite clearing their disease radiographically, they complain of chronic abdominal pain, pelvic pain, and often have food fear. They repetitively visit the emergency room, primary care physicians, and surgeons with concern of repeat infection even when radiographically and chemically there is no sign of recurrence. They do not respond to probiotics, antispasmodics or dietary changes and they live with anxiety of possibly requiring an ostomy at some point in their lives. In these situations, the surgeon must parse out patients who are likely to have remarkable symptom reduction from resection such as in those with post-diverticular hyperalgesia due to phlegmonous diverticulitis versus those where benefit from resection is controversial such as those with psychosomatic effects resulting from the index disease state and underlying irritable bowel syndrome complicating the initial flare [17, 18].

When quality of life is negatively impacted and resection is deemed appropriate, extensive counseling is required to assure all patients understand that there is not a guarantee symptoms will resolve if there is substantial overlap with a functional bowel disorder. I find that most patients do have remarkable improvement overall when expectations are defined.

In patients without diverticular complications (fistula or stricture) or quality of life impairment, my practice is to individualize recommendations for surgery versus observation based on the patient in front of me. A young and healthy patient with no surgical history and two prior episodes of diverticulitis before the complicated attack is likely best treated with definitive resection after successful percutaneous drainage. In this patient, the risk of recurrence and complicated recurrence is high while the expected postoperative morbidity is low. In contrast, the data highlighted in this chapter could be used to steer a very obese elderly patient with multiple comorbidities and multiple prior abdominal operations away from surgery. In this patient, the risks of surgery likely outweigh the potential benefits.

Until we have prospective trials with well-defined inclusion criteria and end points which include quality of life measurements to study the evolving role of elective surgery in patients who have undergone successful percutaneous drainage of diverticular abscesses, the role of surgery in these patients need to be individualized.

Recommendations

After successful percutaneous drainage and resolution of complicated diverticulitis, the decision to pursue elective surgical resection versus observation only should be individualized and made in a shared decision-making framework that weighs the patient comorbidities, surgical risks, and risk of recurrence.

Strong recommendation based on low-quality evidence.

Disclaimers Dr.'s Reidy and Dolejs have no conflicts of interest to disclose.

Funding There is no funding for this book chapter.

References

1. Strate LL, Morris AM. Epidemiology, pathophysiology, and treatment of diverticulitis. Gastroenterology. 2019;156(5):1282–98.e1281.
2. Feingold D, Steele SR, Lee S, et al. Practice parameters for the treatment of sigmoid diverticulitis. Dis Colon Rectum. 2014;57(3):284–94.

3. Francis NK, Sylla P, Abou-Khalil M, et al. EAES and SAGES 2018 consensus conference on acute diverticulitis management: evidence-based recommendations for clinical practice. Surg Endosc. 2019;33:2726–41.
4. Hall J, Hardiman K, Lee S, et al. The American Society of Colon and Rectal Surgeons clinical practice guidelines for the treatment of left-sided colonic diverticulitis. Dis Colon Rectum. 2020;63(6):728–47.
5. Kaiser AM, Jiang JK, Lake JP, et al. The management of complicated diverticulitis and the role of computed tomography. Am J Gastroenterol. 2005;100(4):910–7.
6. Jalouta T, Jrebi N, Luchtefeld M, Ogilvie JW Jr. Diverticulitis recurrence after percutaneous abscess drainage. Int J Color Dis. 2017;32(10):1367–73.
7. Devaraj B, Liu W, Tatum J, Cologne K, Kaiser AM. Medically treated diverticular abscess associated with high risk of recurrence and disease complications. Dis Colon Rectum. 2016;59(3):208–15.
8. Felder SI, Barmparas G, Lynn J, Murrell Z, Margulies DR, Fleshner P. Can the need for colectomy after computed tomography-guided percutaneous drainage for diverticular abscess be predicted? Am Surg. 2013;79(10):1013–6.
9. Bridoux V, Antor M, Schwarz L, et al. Elective operation after acute complicated diverticulitis: is it still mandatory? World J Gastroenterol WJG. 2014;20(25):8166–72.
10. Gaertner WB, Willis DJ, Madoff RD, et al. Percutaneous drainage of colonic diverticular abscess: is colon resection necessary? Dis Colon Rectum. 2013;56(5):622–6.
11. Aquina CT, Becerra AZ, Xu Z, et al. Population-based study of outcomes following an initial acute diverticular abscess. Br J Surg. 2019;106(4):467–76.
12. Trenti L, Kreisler E, Galvez A, Golda T, Frago R, Biondo S. Long-term evolution of acute colonic diverticulitis after successful medical treatment. World J Surg. 2015;39(1):266–74.
13. Gregersen R, Andresen K, Burcharth J, Pommergaard HC, Rosenberg J. Long-term mortality and recurrence in patients treated for colonic diverticulitis with abscess formation: a nationwide register-based cohort study. Int J Color Dis. 2018;33(4):431–40.
14. Garfinkle R, Kugler A, Pelsser V, et al. Diverticular abscess managed with long-term definitive nonoperative intent is safe. Dis Colon Rectum. 2016;59(7):648–55.
15. Lambrichts DPV, Bolkenstein HE, van der Does D, et al. Multicentre study of non-surgical management of diverticulitis with abscess formation. Br J Surg. 2019;106(4):458–66.
16. Elagili F, Stocchi L, Ozuner G, Dietz DW, Kiran RP. Outcomes of percutaneous drainage without surgery for patients with diverticular abscess. Dis Colon Rectum. 2014;57(3):331–6.
17. Lamb MN, Kaiser AM. Elective resection versus observation after nonoperative management of complicated diverticulitis with abscess: a systematic review and meta-analysis. Dis Colon Rectum. 2014;57(12):1430–40.
18. Cohen E, Fuller G, Bolus R, et al. Increased risk for irritable bowel syndrome after acute diverticulitis. Clin Gastroenterol Hepatol Off Clin Pract J Am Gastroenterol Assoc. 2013;11(12):1614–9.
19. Brandt D, Gervaz P, Durmishi Y, Platon A, Morel P, Poletti PA. Percutaneous CT scan-guided drainage vs. antibiotherapy alone for Hinchey II diverticulitis: a case-control study. Dis Colon Rectum. 2006;49(10):1533–8.
20. Broderick-Villa G, Burchette RJ, Collins JC, Abbas MA, Haigh PI. Hospitalization for acute diverticulitis does not mandate routine elective colectomy. Arch Surg (Chicago, Ill : 1960). 2005;140(6):576–81; discussion 581–573.
21. Buchwald P, Dixon L, Wakeman CJ, Eglinton TW, Frizelle FA. Hinchey I and II diverticular abscesses: long-term outcome of conservative treatment. ANZ J Surg. 2017;87(12):1011–4.
22. Macias LH, Haukoos JS, Dixon MR, et al. Diverticulitis: truly minimally invasive management. Am Surg. 2004;70(10):932–5.
23. Nelson RS, Ewing BM, Wengert TJ, Thorson AG. Clinical outcomes of complicated diverticulitis managed nonoperatively. Am J Surg. 2008;196(6):969–72; discussion 973–964.
24. Singh B, May K, Coltart I, Moore NR, Cunningham C. The long-term results of percutaneous drainage of diverticular abscess. Ann R Coll Surg Engl. 2008;90(4):297–301.

25. van de Wall BJ, Draaisma WA, Consten EC, van der Kaaij RT, Wiezer MJ, Broeders IA. Does the presence of abscesses in diverticular disease prelude surgery? J Gastrointest Surg Off J Soc Surg Aliment Tract. 2013;17(3):540–7.
26. You K, Bendl R, Taut C, Sullivan R, Gachabayov M, Bergamaschi R. Randomized clinical trial of elective resection versus observation in diverticulitis with extraluminal air or abscess initially managed conservatively. Br J Surg. 2018;105(8):971–9.

35 How to Manage Diverticular Abscess Not Amenable to Percutaneous Drainage?

Bhuwan Giri and Gustavo A. Rubio

Introduction

Patients with acute left sided colonic diverticulitis complicated by abscess can be managed either medically or surgically depending on presentation and severity of disease. Abscesses 3 cm or greater in patients without generalized peritonitis are managed with percutaneous drainage, if feasible, in conjunction with antibiotics [1, 2]. In patients who fail medical management, or those that are not amenable to percutaneous drainage, management options include colonic primary resection and anastomosis (PRA) with or without a diverting loop ileostomy (DLI) or a Hartmann procedure [1]. Additionally, laparoscopic peritoneal lavage (LPL) with or without fecal diversion followed by staged colon resection has also been reported [3, 4]. In patients with Hinchey II diverticulitis treated medically, treatment failure and abscess recurrence rate is as high as 25% with long term follow up showing lower recurrence rate with percutaneous drainage compared to antibiotics alone [2, 5]. This is mostly because smaller abscesses are treated medically whereas larger abscesses tend to be treated with percutaneous drainage. Therefore, percutaneous drainage is the intervention of choice for simple abscesses with a success rate of more than 80%. Complex abscesses (loculations, fistulas, infected fluid collections with drainage route through viscera) have higher failure rates [6]. Optimal treatment

B. Giri (✉)
DeWitt Daughtry Family Department of Surgery, University of Miami Leondard M. Miller School of Medicine, Miami, FL, USA

Jackson Health System, Miami, FL, USA
e-mail: bhuwan.giri@med.miami.edu

G. A. Rubio
Jackson Health System, Miami, FL, USA
e-mail: grubio87@med.miami.edu

K. Umanskiy, N. Hyman (eds.), *Difficult Decisions in Colorectal Surgery*, Difficult Decisions in Surgery: An Evidence-Based Approach,
https://doi.org/10.1007/978-3-031-42303-1_35

strategy for diverticular abscesses not amenable to percutaneous drainage remains debated. In this chapter, we evaluate the various strategies used to treat diverticular abscesses not amenable to percutaneous drainage in Hinchey Ib/II acute diverticulitis.

Patients	Intervention	Comparator	Outcomes
Patients with diverticular abscess not amenable to percutaneous drainage	Antibiotics alone, laparoscopic peritoneal lavage, or fecal diversion followed by colon resection	Colon resection	Complications, recurrence, functional outcomes, need for permanent ostomy

Search Strategy

A Pubmed, EMBASE and Cochrane database search using the terms "Diverticulitis", "Diverticular abscess" + "colectomy" "Hinchey I/1", "Hinchey 2/II" and "ostomy" was performed. Relevant articles were selected for review. Articles whose main text was not in English, and articles published more than 20 years ago were excluded from review.

Studies were excluded if they did not specify if patients with Hinchey <2 were included. Studies that included surgical treatment after failure of medical or percutaneous management were included. Only the most recent study was included if similar studies from the same institution were encountered. References of the included studies and the related articles were reviewed to identify additional studies that were incorporated as appropriate.

Results

Few studies have directly evaluated the best treatment strategy for patients with acute left sided colonic diverticulitis complicated by abscess not amenable to percutaneous drainage. Only observational studies have been published on this specific topic. Majority of studies did not specifically compare different interventions (e.g. laparoscopic lavage vs sigmoid resection). Of the studies listed below, majority only had a subset of patients with Hinchey Ib/II diverticular abscesses. Medical management with antibiotics alone was typically the initial intervention in stable patients with inaccessible or small (<3 cm) diverticular abscesses. Across studies, failure of nonoperative management with antibiotics alone was 20–25% [2, 7, 8]. In one study, all patients with abscesses 5 cm or greater required either percutaneous drainage or surgery [7]. Of stable patients treated with surgery, indications usually included failure of non-operative management (either antibiotics alone or percutaneous drainage). Studies also included patients with abscesses treated with surgery due to generalized purulent peritonitis (Hinchey III). Operations included laparoscopic/open sigmoid resection with primary anastomosis +/– diverting ostomy, laparoscopic/open Hartmann procedure, or laparoscopic lavage +/− diverting ostomy. Tartaglia et al. [4] compared laparoscopic lavage (LPL) versus laparoscopic sigmoid (LS) colectomy in patients with diverticular abscesses failing medical management. Study population included 29% of patients with Hinchey II presentation. In the LPL group, 18% required reoperation and there was increased rate of long term recurrence compared with LS group. LS group included 37% Hartmann procedure, 50% primary anastomosis without DLI, and 13% primary anastomosis with DLI. LS group had an 18% morbidity rate and 74% rate of ostomy reversal [4]. Therefore, authors concluded that laparoscopic lavage carried higher risk of treatment failure, recurrence, and morbidity compared to laparoscopic sigmoid resection. Rosen et al. [7] also reported lower recurrence rate 7% (vs 21%) in patients who underwent sigmoid resection during index hospitalization. Finally, a single institution study evaluated management with initial laparoscopic diverting loop ileostomy followed by staged sigmoid resection and subsequent ileostomy closure in patients failing medical management or at high operative risk [3]. 6/19 patients included in the study had evidence of diverticular abscess. There were no initial treatment failures and majority (84%) of patients had ostomies reversed (Table 35.1).

Table 35.1 Summary of results

Study	Patients	Outcome classification	Typical risk for therapy A	Relative risk for therapy B	Quality of evidence
Tartaglia, 2019 [4] Prospective multi center study $n = 66$	66 patients were enrolled with pelvic abscess not amenable to conservative management and Hinchey 3 acute diverticulitis 29% of patients had Hinchey II disease (46% underwent laparoscopic lavage and 42% underwent laparoscopic sigmoidectomy)	Laparoscopic peritoneal lavage (LPL) vs laparoscopic sigmoidectomy (LS) in patients with modified Hinchey II, not responding to medical therapy	LPL: 6/22 patients who had complete recovery from the procedure presented one or more episodes of recurrent diverticulitis. 18.5% rate of reoperation	LS: No recurrence for LS group $p = 0.003$. 74% (14/19) had their ostomies reversed and remaining 4 had end colostomy (HA). No significant differences were found in overall morbidity, mean length of postoperative stay, or stoma closure rate. Incisional hernia rate was significantly higher in the HA group (12.5% vs 42.8%; $p = 0.034$)	Level IV
Brandt, 2006 [8] Case control study in patients with Hinchey II diverticulitis. Single institution study comparing patients who underwent abscess drainage under CT guidance vs treated with antibiotics alone.	34 patients underwent abscess drainage under CT scan guidance and 32 patients were treated with antibiotic therapy (mostly because CT scan guided abscess drainage was considered not technically feasible by interventional radiology team)	Primary outcome of failure of conservative management (emergency surgery, signs of worsening sepsis, or abscess recurrence with 4 weeks of drainage	CT drainage 33% failure in CT guidance group 29% underwent emergency surgery 12 patients (35%) subsequently underwent an elective sigmoid resection Four postoperative deaths (26.6%) Median size of abscess was 6 (3–18) cm	Antibiotics alone 19% failed antibiotics alone. ($p = 0.26$) 16% underwent emergency surgery ($P = 0.24$) 16 patients (50%) subsequently underwent an elective sigmoid resection ($P = 0.31$). 0 post op deaths in antibiotics alone group Median size of abscess was 4 (3–10) cm ($P = 0.002$)	Level IV

Katsuno 2011 [11] Single institution Japanese retrospective review of laparoscopic one stage resection vs open sigmoid resection in Hinchey I and II acute diverticulitis. Laparoscopic surgery was performed for all patients with recurrent episodes. No preoperative percutaneous drainage of abscess	58 patients total 36 patients underwent laparoscopic resection and 16 patients underwent open colon resection	Overall complication rate, wound infection, hospital stay compared between two groups.	Laparoscopic resection Wound infection: 4/36 (11%) Overall complications: 6/136 16.7% Major complications (leakage, obstructions, bleeding and mortality and recurrence similar between two groups)	Open resection Wound infection: 6/16 (37.5%), $p < 0.05$ Overall complications 9/16 43.8% $P < -.05$	Level V
Rosen, 2019 [7] Single institution retrospective study	134 patients with Hinchey Ib/II diverticulitis. 78% treated non-operatively (including 62% with antibiotics alone). 22% underwent sigmoid resection +/− ostomy	Primary outcome was failure of conservative management (need for surgery), LOS, recurrence rates, rate of stoma formation	113/134 (84%) not amenable to percutaneous drainage 85/113 (75%) managed non-operatively during index hospitalization 21% recurrence rate All abscesses >5 cm required IR drainage or surgery	28/113 (25%) not amenable to percutaneous drainage required surgery during index hospitalization 3% done laparoscopically 50% had diverting stoma 7% recurrence rate	Level V

(continued)

Table 35.1 (continued)

Study	Patients	Outcome classification	Typical risk for therapy A	Relative risk for therapy B	Quality of evidence
Gregensen, 2016 [2] Systematic review, 42 studies (all observational) including Hinchey I/II patients with abscess	*N* = 8766 patients Management options included antibiotics alone, percutaneous drainage, or surgery	Treatment failure, short term mortality, recurrence.	20% failure of non-operative management Abscesses <3 cm typically treated adequately with antibiotics alone 25% recurrence 16% recurrence after percutaneous drainage	Acute surgery associated with 12.1% mortality rate	Level III
Graham, 2022 [3] Single institution retrospective study (published abstract)	19 patients with acute diverticulitis underwent DLI without initial resection	Need for sigmoid resection for failure to improve	6 of 19 patients had abscess pre-operatively No patient needed resection during index admission 84% underwent ostomy reversal		Level V

Recommendations Based on the Data

For stable patients with Hinchey Ib/II diverticulitis and small (<3 cm) abscesses, initial nonoperative management with antibiotics alone is treatment of choice (Quality of evidence: moderate; Strong recommendation)

For stable patients with diverticular abscesses >3 cm not amenable to percutaneous drainage, initial nonoperative management with antibiotics alone can be considered (Quality of evidence: Low; Strong recommendation)

Patients with diverticular abscesses that fail non-operative management with antibiotics alone should undergo sigmoid colectomy (primary anastomosis +/− diverting loop ileostomy or Hartmann procedure) (Quality of evidence: Low; Strong recommendation)

Minimally-invasive approach to sigmoid resection is preferred (Quality of evidence: Moderate; Strong recommendation)

Laparoscopic lavage is associated with higher treatment failure and recurrence rates for patients with diverticular abscess and is generally not recommended (Quality of evidence: Low; Weak recommendation)

In high operative risk patients, a staged approach with initial laparoscopic diverting loop ileostomy with interval sigmoid resection and ileostomy closure can be considered (Quality of evidence: Low, Weak recommendation).

A Personal View of the Data

Patients presenting with left-sided colonic diverticulitis complicated by abscesses not amenable to percutaneous drainage present a clinical challenge. There are several treatment strategies described for this complex and heterogenous patient population. These include a trial of antibiotics alone, laparoscopic lavage, staged fecal diversion followed by interval colectomy, and sigmoid resection (laparoscopic/open Hartmann procedure or primary anastomosis with/without a protective diverting ostomy). Unlike for patients who present with an indication for immediate operation such as peritonitis, the timing and choice of surgical intervention is not well studied for stable patients with diverticular abscesses (Hinchey Ib/II). Patients with small abscesses <3 cm are generally successfully managed with antibiotics alone. Those with larger abscesses not amenable to percutaneous drainage can also be managed with antibiotics alone initially if they are clinically stable. Clinicians should be aware of the relatively high failure rate and recurrence rate in this patient population treated with antibiotics alone [2, 7, 8]. Repeat cross sectional imaging should be considered in patients treated initially with antibiotics who remain clinically stable but fail to improve after a few days (inability to tolerate enteral feeds, persistent localized pain). In such instances, percutaneous drainage may become feasible if abscesses enlarge or a safe window becomes evident.

For patients who fail to improve after a trial of antibiotics alone, surgical intervention is required. Procedure of choice remains unclear and may depend on multiple patient factors and surgical expertise available. There is more robust data on surgical management of patients with Hinchey III diverticulitis that may be extrapolated to those with Hinchey Ib/II [1]. In general, there has been a shift recently towards utilization of both minimally invasive techniques and of primary anastomosis with/without protective stoma. Primary anastomosis with/without protective stoma offers several advantages including lower overall morbidity and significantly higher long term stoma free rates [9, 10]. In these settings, minimally invasive approaches have been shown to be safe and offer additional advantages with lower overall morbidity [11]. In the setting of stable Hinchey Ib/II patients that failed antibiotic therapy and require surgery, laparoscopic sigmoid resection with primary anastomosis should be strongly considered when feasible and expertise is available. Hartmann procedure also remains a safe and effective operation for patients with left sided colonic diverticulitis, particularly in hemodynamically unstable patients or those otherwise high risk for anastomotic failure such as those that are immunocompromised. Surgical expertise plays an important role in decision to perform a Hartmann procedure versus primary anastomosis. Another option that has been studied in patients with Hinchey II and Hinchey III diverticulitis is laparoscopic lavage. Enthusiasm for this approach has recently waned with recent studies primarily including Hinchey III patients showing higher rates of treatment failure, recurrence, and need for secondary procedures compared to sigmoid resection [12]. Similar results were reported in one study that included a subset of patients with Hinchey II diverticulitis [4]. Therefore, there is insufficient evidence currently to widely recommend laparoscopic lavage for patients with diverticular abscess not amenable to percutaneous drainage. There may be a role for this less invasive approach in a subset of patients that needs to be further elucidated with additional studies.

There is also insufficient data to support staged resections in patients with Hinchey II diverticulitis consisting of initial diverting loop ileostomy followed by interval sigmoid resection and subsequent ileostomy closure. Although these three staged resections were commonly done in the past for more severe fulminant diverticulitis, perioperative mortality was found to be higher in these patients [13]. However, recently this approach has been reported to be safe and associated with favorable long term outcomes including high rates of stoma closure [3]. There may be a subset of patients that may benefit from this approach, such as those with significant perioperative risk factors during index hospitalization. Future studies are needed to determine which patients, if any, would most benefit from this approach.

In summary, there is limited, low quality, evidence evaluating optimal management of patients with diverticular abscess not amenable to percutaneous drainage. Based on these data, we recommend sigmoid resection and primary anastomosis with/without protective ileostomy or a Hartman procedure, depending on local expertise and patient factors. The role of laparoscopic lavage or initial fecal diversion alone in these patients requires further study.

References

1. Hall J, Hardiman K, Lee S, Lightner A, Stocchi L, Paquette IM, et al. The American Society of Colon and Rectal Surgeons clinical practice guidelines for the treatment of left-sided colonic diverticulitis. Dis Colon Rectum. 2020 Jun;63(6):728–47.

2. Gregersen R, Mortensen LQ, Burcharth J, Pommergaard HC, Rosenberg J. Treatment of patients with acute colonic diverticulitis complicated by abscess formation: a systematic review. Int J Surg. 2016 Nov;35:201–8.
3. Graham A, Umanskiy K, Hurst R, Shogan B, Hyman N, Olortegui K. Back to the FUTURE-is diversion without resection a safe option for complicated diverticulitis? Dis Colon Rectum. 2022:73–4.
4. Tartaglia D, Di Saverio S, Stupalkowska W, Giannessi S, Robustelli V, Coccolini F, et al. Laparoscopic peritoneal lavage versus laparoscopic sigmoidectomy in complicated acute diverticulitis: a multicenter prospective observational study. Int J Color Dis. 2019 Dec;34(12):2111–20.
5. Buchwald P, Dixon L, Wakeman CJ, Eglinton TW, Frizelle FA. Hinchey I and II diverticular abscesses: long-term outcome of conservative treatment. ANZ J Surg. 2017 Dec;87(12):1011–4.
6. Golfieri R, Cappelli A. Computed tomography-guided percutaneous abscess drainage in coloproctology: review of the literature. Tech Coloproctol. 2007 Sep;11(3):197–208.
7. Rosen DR, Pott EG, Cologne KG, Lee SW, Ault GT, Grabo DJ, et al. Percutaneous drainage for hinchey Ib and II acute diverticulitis with abscess improves outcomes. Turk J Gastroenterol. 2019 Nov;30(11):976–83.
8. Brandt D, Gervaz P, Durmishi Y, Platon A, Morel P, Poletti PA. Percutaneous CT Scan-guided drainage vs. antibiotherapy alone for Hinchey II diverticulitis: a case-control study. Dis Colon Rectum 2006 Oct;49(10):1533–1538.
9. Binda GA, Karas JR, Serventi A, Sokmen S, Amato A, Hydo L, et al. Primary anastomosis vs nonrestorative resection for perforated diverticulitis with peritonitis: a prematurely terminated randomized controlled trial. Color Dis. 2012 Nov;14(11):1403–10.
10. Oberkofler CE, Rickenbacher A, Raptis DA, Lehmann K, Villiger P, Buchli C, et al. A multicenter randomized clinical trial of primary anastomosis or Hartmann's procedure for perforated left colonic diverticulitis with purulent or fecal peritonitis. Ann Surg 2012 Nov;256(5):819–826; discussion 826-827.
11. Katsuno G, Fukunaga M, Nagakari K, Yoshikawa S. Laparoscopic one-stage resection of right and left colon complicated diverticulitis equivalent to Hinchey stage I-II. Surg Today. 2011 May;41(5):647–54.
12. Penna M, Markar SR, Mackenzie H, Hompes R, Cunningham C. Laparoscopic lavage versus primary resection for acute perforated diverticulitis: review and meta-analysis. Ann Surg. 2018 Feb;267(2):252–8.
13. Krukowski ZH, Matheson NA. Emergency surgery for diverticular disease complicated by generalized and faecal peritonitis: a review. Br J Surg. 1984 Dec;71(12):921–7.

36 Hartmann Procedure vs Primary Anastomosis for Acute Complicated Diverticulitis

Susanna S. Hill and Aneel Damle

Introduction

The prevalence of acute diverticulitis has been increasing in Western nations. A recent 2016 prospective study found 42% of patients on screening colonoscopy had diverticulosis [1, 2] and progression to diverticulitis has been estimated at 10–25% [3]. Historically, surgical management options for patients presenting with acute complicated diverticulitis have included a 3-stage operative approach proposed by Rankin and Brown (diverting colostomy with drainage, segmental colectomy, colostomy reversal) [4], the 2-stage Hartmann's procedure (segmental colectomy with end colostomy, colostomy reversal) [5], segmental colectomy (with consideration for diverting loop ileostomy, on-table colonic lavage, and laparoscopic lavage) [6].

The current practice has shifted to more frequently performing segmental colectomy with diverting loop ileostomy over the more traditional Hartmann's procedure. The primary reasons for this culture shift include higher reversal rates and less technically challenging ostomy reversal with primary anastomosis with proximal diversion. The most recent set of American Society of Colon and Rectal Surgery guidelines for treatment of left-sided diverticulitis discuss emergency surgery for acute diverticulitis. They recommend urgent sigmoid colectomy for patients who have diffuse peritonitis and that restoration of bowel continuity

S. S. Hill
Division of Colon and Rectal Surgery, Department of Surgery, University of Minnesota School of Medicine, Minneapolis, MN, USA

A. Damle (✉)
Colon and Rectal Surgery Associates, University of Minnesota School of Medicine, Minneapolis, MN, USA

K. Umanskiy, N. Hyman (eds.), *Difficult Decisions in Colorectal Surgery*, Difficult Decisions in Surgery: An Evidence-Based Approach, https://doi.org/10.1007/978-3-031-42303-1_36

should weigh "patient factors, intraoperative factors, and surgeon preference." This chapter explores the most recent literature published over the last 20 years regarding operative approach (i.e. Hartmann's procedure vs. primary anastomosis) should be chosen for patient management in the setting of acute complicated diverticulitis.

Search Strategy

A comprehensive search of PubMed and MedLINE databases were performed using the following MeSH terms: "diverticulitis, colonic," "anastomosis, surgical," "ileostomy," "colectomy," and "colostomy." The search was limited to the last 20 years (January 2002 – August 2022) and non-English studies were excluded. Only the most recent study was used if it was a continuation of the same study from the same institution. All article abstracts were reviewed as well as full text when a study potentially satisfied the inclusion criteria. The reference lists of included studies were manually reviewed to identify additional studies to incorporate as appropriate. Systematic reviews and meta-analyses were reviewed for their references but data were not used primarily. Studies using databases were excluded if they featured data from overlapping years and the studies with the most inclusive dates were chosen. The primary outcome evaluated was mortality (Table 36.1). Secondary outcomes included major morbidity, stoma reversal rates, and morbidity associated with reversal. Each study was evaluated for its level of quality of evidence based on the GRADE approach [7].

Table 36.1 PICO Table

P (Patients)	I (Intervention)	C (Comparator)	O (Outcomes)
Patients with acute complicated diverticulitis	Hartmann procedure	Primary anastomosis	Primary: 30-day mortality Secondary: 30-day morbidity, stoma reversal rate, reversal morbidity

Results

The initial search revealed 72 hits for "diverticulitis" AND "ileostomy" or "colostomy" and 165 hits for "diverticulitis" and "surgical anastomosis." All abstracts were reviewed for studies that compared Hartmann's procedure to primary anastomosis (with and without diverting ileostomy). Studies were removed according to above exclusion criteria. A total of 21 studies were used in the final analysis. There were four prospective multi-center randomized control trials, four prospective non-randomized series, nine retrospective series, and four retrospective database studies (Table 36.2).

Table 36.2 Outcomes after index procedure of the analyzed studies

Author (Year)	Study type	Patients (n) Hartmann's vs PA	Mortality (%) after index procedure	p-value	Post-operative major morbidity (%) after index procedure	p-value	Quality of Evidence
Blair NP, Germann E (2002) [12]	RS	64 vs. 33	20 vs. 9	0.26	NR	n/a	Very low
Mäkelä J et al. (2002) [13]	RS	75 vs. 45	13 vs. 4	0.12	32 vs. 36	0.69*	Low
Zorcolo L et al. (2003) [14]	RS	140 vs. 176	20 vs. 6	<0.001	24 vs. 14$^{\vartheta}$	0.02*	Low
Regenet N et al. (2003) [15]	PS	33 vs. 27	12 vs. 11	NS	NR	n/a	Moderate
Constantinides VA et al. (2006) [16]	PS	167 vs. 248	23 vs. 4	<0.001	22 vs. 19	0.46	Moderate
Richter S et al. (2006) [17]	PS	36 vs. 5	60 vs. 11	0.007*	NR	n/a	Very low
Breitenstein S et al. (2007) [18]	PS	30 vs. 30	17 vs. 10	0.69	37 vs. 30	0.58*	Moderate
Stumpf MJ et al. (2007) [19]	RS	30 vs. 36	17 vs. 0	0.03	33 vs. 14^	0.20	Very low
Vermeulen J et al. (2007) [20]	RS	139 vs. 61	34 vs. 11	<0.01	33 vs. 13	<0.01	Low
Zingg U et al. (2010) [21]	RS	64 vs. 46	29 vs. 17	0.18	51 vs. 44$^{\vartheta}$	0.56	Low

(continued)

Table 36.2 (continued)

Author (Year)	Study type	Patients (n) Hartmann's vs PA	Mortality (%) after index procedure	p-value	Post-operative major morbidity (%) after index procedure	p-value	Quality of Evidence
Trenti L et al. (2011) [22]	RS	60 vs. 27	45 vs. 7	0.001	NR	n/a	Low
Mueller MH et al. (2011) [23]	RS	26 vs. 47	27 vs. 4	0.008	46 vs. 30	0.16*	Low
Binda GA et al. (2012) [8]	PM - RCT	56 vs. 34	11 vs. 3	0.25	46 vs. 35^	0.38	Moderate
Gawlick U, Nirula R (2012) [24]	RS - NSQIP	1678 vs. 340	6 vs. 8	NS	NR	n/a	Low
Masoomi H et al. (2012) [25]	RS - NIS	56,866 vs. 3361	5 vs 4	0.03	41 vs. 39^	0.04	Low
Oberkofler CE et al. (2012) [11]	PM - RCT	30 vs. 32	13 vs. 9	0.67	40 vs. 44	0.80	High
Alizai PH et al. (2013) [26]	RS	72 vs. 26	25 vs. 12	0.18	NR	n/a	Low
Bridoux V et al. (2017) [9]	PM - RCT	52 vs. 50	4 vs. 4	0.97*	14 vs. 14^	0.93	High
Cauley CE et al. (2018) [27]	RS - NIS	65,084 vs. 2637	6 vs. 16	<0.001	23 vs. 32	<0.001	Low
Lambrichts DPV et al. (2019) [10]	PM - RCT	66 vs. 64	3 vs. 6	0.44	12 vs. 14	0.60	High
Lee JM et al. (2019) [28]	RS - NSQIP	2915 vs. 239	8 vs. 3	0.01	55 vs. 49^	0.06	Low

All outcomes are provided as % of patients in the Hartmann's procedure vs. % of patients in the primary anastomosis (p-value). NR = not reported. NS = non-significant. Retrospective series (RS), Prospective non-randomized series (PS), Prospective multi-center randomized control trial (PM-RCT), Prospective single-center randomized control trial (PS-RCT). The * symbol denotes instances where p-value for comparisons were not reported; these were calculated using a two-tailed two-population z-test based on reported *n* in each cohort. When complications were reported by Clavien-Dindo scoring, those that were class IIIb-IV were considered major morbidities. Otherwise, a composite any-morbidity percentage is reported by the ^ symbol and composite surgical morbidity percentage is reported by the ⁸ symbol.

It is important to note that quality of evidence for these studies varies from very low to moderate on the GRADE criteria. The randomized control trials [8–11] were all terminated early prior to meeting their *a priori* sample size calculations, ranging from 30%–56% of recruitment targets. Furthermore, there was wide variation in primary anastomosis technique in the randomized control trials with 66% - 100% of patients receiving diverting loop ileostomies. Then, the rest of the studies are retrospective studies at institutional, multi-institutional, or large database levels and are subject to the inherent biases related to retrospective studies, especially those of patient selection.

Mortality

For the primary outcome of post-operative mortality, none of the randomized controlled trials showed a statistical difference. Two of four prospective series [16, 17], five of nine retrospective series [14, 19, 20, 22, 23], and two retrospective database studies [25, 28] found higher mortality rates in the Hartmann's group. However, using the National Inpatient Sample, Cauley CE et al. [27] found higher rate of mortality in their primary anastomosis group (16% vs. 6% in the Hartmann's group, $p < 0.001$), which could be partially due to the primary anastomosis cohort being older, having higher Charlson Comorbidity Index scores, and have more patients belonging to Medicaid insurance status. The remaining eleven studies found no significant difference in mortality rates.

Post-operative Morbidity

All four of the multicenter randomized controlled trials reported on the secondary outcomes. There were no significant differences in post-operative morbidity after index procedure. Two of the four prospective series looked at post-operative morbidity and both failed to find a significant difference. Six of nine retrospective studies reported data regarding post-operative morbidity and two studies observed less morbidity in the primary anastomosis group (24% in Hartmann's vs. 14% in primary anastomosis, $p = 0.02$, [14] and 33% in Hartmann's vs. 13% in primary anastomosis, $p < 0.01$ [20]). Two of three retrospective database studies that reported morbidity data found differences in post-operative morbidity but in differing directions; Cauley CE with 23% in the Hartmann's cohort vs. 32% in the primary anastomosis cohort ($p < 0.001$) using the NIS database but from 1998–2011 [27], while Masoomi H et al. observed 41% vs. 39% ($p = 0.04$) also using the NIS database but from 2002–2007 [25].

Stoma Reversal

Stoma reversal rates and post-operative morbidity are summarized in Table 36.3. Two multicenter randomized controlled trials showed higher rates of stoma reversal in the primary anastomosis cohorts (90% for ileostomy reversal vs. 58% for colostomy reversal [11] and 96% vs 58% [9]). Only Oberkofler et al. [11] found a significant difference in rates of complications following stoma reversal (20% following colostomy reversal vs. 0% following ileostomy reversal). Of the prospective studies, only Breitenstein S. reported both colostomy and ileostomy reversal rates, finding 60% vs. 96% ($p = 0.001$), respectively, but no significant difference in post-operative morbidity following reversal. Only two retrospective series reported both reversal rates [22, 26], and the latter showed a significant difference in rates (58% in Hartmann's vs. 85% in primary anastomosis, $p = 0.046$). No retrospective series reported both colostomy and ileostomy reversal post-operative morbidity. Only five studies reported data on combined morbidity from both procedures (index resection and stoma reversal; Table 36.3). All of the studies showed that primary anastomosis had lower overall morbidity rates but all failed to achieve statistical significance.

In recent years, multiple meta-analyses and systematic reviews on these studies have been published. Cirrochi et al. included three randomized controlled trials and found no statistically significant permanent stoma rate, anastomotic leaks, but found lower rates of intra-abdominal abscess after primary anastomosis [29]. Gachabayov M et al. combined seventeen studies and found patients with primary anastomosis had lower mortality in patients (OR 0.38, $p < 0.001$), organ/space surgical site infections (OR 0.25, $p = 0.003$), reoperation (OR 0.48, $p = 0.02$), and ostomy non-reversal rates (OR 0.27, $p = 0.02$) [30]. Ryan OK et al. analyzed twelve studies and found patients with primary anastomosis had lower rate of permanent stoma (RR 0.43, $p = 0.001$), but no significant differences in mortality or morbidity [31]. Lambrichts et al. evaluated eleven studies, including four randomized control trials, of patients with Hinchey III/IV diverticulitis comparing Hartmann procedure vs primary anastomosis and found no differences in mortality, morbidity, or re-intervention after index procedure but improved stoma reversal rates with primary anastomosis (OR 2.62, 95% CI 1.29–5.31) [32].

Table 36.3 Stoma reversal rates procedure of the analyzed studies

Author (Year)	Study type	Patients (n) HP vs. PA	Stoma reversal rate (%) (HP vs. PA)	p-value	30-day major morbidity (%) after reversal (HP vs. PA)	p-value	Combined major morbidity (%) after both procedures	p-value
Mäkelä J et al. (2002) [13]	RS	75 vs. 45	45 vs. NR	n/a	NR	n/a	NR	n/a
Zorcolo L et al. (2003) [14]	RS	140 vs. 176	39 vs. NR	n/a	20 vs. NR	n/a	NR	n/a
Regenet N et al. (2003) [15]	PS	33 vs. 27	69 vs. NA	n/a	24 vs. NR	n/a	NR	n/a
Richter S et al. (2006) [17]	PS	36 vs. 5	50 vs. 100	0.17*	NR	n/a	NR	n/a
Breitenstein S et al. (2007) [18]	PS	30 vs. 30	60 vs. 96	0.001	27 vs. 8	0.10	33 vs. 20	0.12*
Trenti L et al. (2011) [22]	RS	60 vs. 27	27 vs. 60	0.14*	NR	n/a	NR	n/a
Binda GA et al. (2012) [8]	PM - RCT	56 vs. 34	60 vs. 65	0.66	24 vs. 5	0.06	25 vs. 38	0.11*
Oberkofler CE et al. (2012) [11]	PM - RCT	30 vs. 32	58 vs. 90	0.01	20 vs. 0	0.046	50 vs. 44	0.80
Alizai PH et al. (2013) [26]	RS	72 vs. 26	58 vs. 85	0.046	NR	n/a	NR	n/a
Bridoux V et al. (2017) [9]	PM - RCT	52 vs. 50	65 vs. 96	<0.001*	9 vs. 3	0.32*	17 vs. 16	0.42
Lambrichts DPV et al. (2019) [10]	PM - RCT	66 vs. 64	68 vs. 83	0.09	16 vs 3	0.06	48 vs. 36	0.29

All outcomes are provided as % of patients in the Hartmann's procedure vs. % of patients in the primary anastomosis (p-value). NR = not reported. NS = non-significant. Retrospective series (RS), Prospective non-randomized series (PS), Prospective multi-center randomized control trial (PM-RCT), Prospective single-center randomized control trial (PS-RCT). The * symbol denotes instances where p-value for comparisons were not reported; these were calculated using a two-tailed two-population z-test based on reported n in each cohort. When complications were reported by Clavien-Dindo scoring, those that were class IIIb-IV were considered major morbidities.

Recommendations Based on the Data

Primary anastomosis and diverting loop ileostomy in the setting of acute complicated diverticulitis is a safe procedure. There is no high-level evidence that there are differences in mortality or immediate post-operative morbidity between patients undergoing Hartmann's procedure vs. primary anastomosis with diversion. Outcomes of meta-analyses have inconsistently demonstrated findings of decreased mortality, intra-abdominal abscess, surgical site infection, and re-operation – all in favor of primary anastomosis. However, the key difference between the two cohorts lies in stoma reversal rates. Half of the randomized controlled trials showed a difference with 90–96% of ileostomies being reversed vs. 58–65% of colostomies. Only one study showed a statistically significant difference in major morbidity following reversal. Ultimately, decision making regarding Hartmann's vs. primary anastomosis should be influenced by patient comorbidities such as poorly controlled diabetes, immunosuppression, their ability to tolerate a potential leak, and overall patient presentation (e.g. septic shock, hemodynamic instability, vasopressor requirement, etc.).

- Acute complicated diverticulitis patients with appropriate operative risk should be considered for a primary anastomosis. (**Grade of recommendation**: moderate; **Quality of evidence**: moderate).

The benefit of diverting loop ileostomy in the setting of primary anastomosis has been more difficult to quantify. There are no randomized control trials comparing primary anastomosis with or without ileostomy in the setting of complicated diverticulitis. This stems from a fundamental lack of equipoise between the interventions given the published data regarding the consequences of anastomotic leak with and without the presence of a diverting stoma. For instance, a patient in septic shock with multiple severe medical co-morbidities would not be appropriate to randomize to a primary and unprotected anastomosis. Likely for these reasons, diverting loop ileostomy rates in the evaluated randomized control trials ranged from 66–100%. Ultimately, surgeons must balance the risk of anastomotic leak and its consequences with the morbidity of an ileostomy and second procedure for takedown on an individualized patient level.

- When performing a primary anastomosis for complicated diverticulitis, consideration should be given to a diverting loop ileostomy. (**Grade of recommendation**: moderate; **Quality of evidence**: low).

Personal View

The decision to perform a Hartmann procedure vs primary anastomosis is does not neatly fit into a "one size fits all" strategy. My primary considerations to operative approach include:

How long can the patient tolerate being in the operating room?

Severe hemodynamic instability, escalating vasopressor requirement, hypothermia, acidosis, and coagulopathy are indications for damage control surgery. In these patients, the primary goal is source control and subsequent resuscitation in the intensive care unit without consideration of anastomosis. However, in patients that respond to resuscitation and require minimal use of vasopressors, anastomosis should be considered.

What is the extent of contamination?

The level of contamination within Hinchey III and IV diverticulitis can vary widely. Often, in the setting of an acute perforation, a thorough washout is adequate to provide an appropriate environment from anastomosis. This can be more difficult when the perforation presents in a delayed fashion which may be associated with an abscess/phlegmon and less pliability of the otherwise healthy rectum to accept an anastomosis.

Will the patient be able to tolerate a leak? Will they tolerate an undiverted leak? Will they be able to tolerate an ileostomy? Will medical optimization make them a better candidate for an anastomosis in the future? Is a stoma technically possible?

In the situation of a stable patient with a reasonably clean operative field, the single most important question I ask myself is whether the patient can tolerate an anastomotic leak. Several scoring systems including the sequential organ failure assessment (SOFA) and acute physiology and chronic health evaluation II (APACHE II) can be utilized to estimate the risk of morbidity and mortality in the setting of sepsis. In a patient where a leak and subsequent sepsis would be associated with very high rates of serious morbidity and mortality, I am more likely to perform a Hartmann's procedure. This is particularly true if the patient has modifiable risk factors that would significantly lower their risk of complications if optimized. Conversely, consideration also has to be given to whether the patient will tolerate a stoma or if it is technically feasible. Patients with significant prior small bowel resections or chronic kidney disease may suffer serious consequences from an ileostomy including dehydration, readmission, and worsening of their kidney disease. In these patients, consideration can be given to a diverting colostomy or a primary unprotected anastomosis. Finally, consideration has to be given as to whether a stoma can be performed at all. It is not infrequent to operate on patients with BMIs in the 50 s, 60 s, and 70 s. In the severely obese patient, it may not be possible for an ostomy to reach the skin surface. In these patients, I am more likely to attempt a primary anastomosis, even if unprotected.

Overall, my goal is to perform a primary anastomosis whenever possible as long as the above-mentioned criteria are met. I often create a diverting loop ileostomy to mitigate the effects of a possible leak. I rarely, if ever, use a diverting colostomy due to the increased complexity of reversal as well associated reach issues with the conduit. Typically, I will perform an on-table antegrade colonic irrigation though the enterotomy that I will subsequently use for the ileostomy. However, it is important not to get trapped into a pre-operative plan to perform a primary anastomosis if the situation is not appropriate. As in every other operation, there is no substitute for sound surgical judgement.

References

1. Peery AF, Keku TO, Martin CF, et al. Distribution and characteristics of colonic diverticula in a United States screening population. Clin Gastroenterol Hepatol. 2016 Jul;14(7):980–5 e1.
2. Hall J, Hardiman K, Lee S, et al. The American Society of Colon and Rectal Surgeons clinical practice guidelines for the treatment of left-sided colonic diverticulitis. Dis Colon Rectum. 2020 Jun;63(6):728–47.
3. Hughes LE. Postmortem survey of diverticular disease of the colon. II. The muscular abnormality of the sigmoid colon. Gut. 1969 May;10(5):344–51.
4. Rankin FWB, P. W. Diverticulitis of the colon. Surg Gynecol Obstet. 1930;50(05):836–47.
5. Sanderson ER. Henri Hartmann and the Hartmann operation. Arch Surg. 1980 Jun;115(6):792–3.
6. Hawkins AT, Wise PE, Chan T, et al. Diverticulitis: an update from the age old paradigm. Curr Probl Surg. 2020 Oct;57(10):100862.
7. Wilson JM, Holzgrefe RE, Staley CA, Schenker ML, Meals CG. Use of a 5-item modified frailty index for risk stratification in patients undergoing surgical Management of Distal Radius Fractures. J Hand Surg Am. 2018 Aug;43(8):701–9.
8. Binda GA, Karas JR, Serventi A, et al. Primary anastomosis vs nonrestorative resection for perforated diverticulitis with peritonitis: a prematurely terminated randomized controlled trial. Color Dis. 2012 Nov;14(11):1403–10.
9. Bridoux V, Regimbeau JM, Ouaissi M, et al. Hartmann's procedure or primary anastomosis for generalized peritonitis due to perforated diverticulitis: a prospective multicenter randomized trial (DIVERTI). J Am Coll Surg. 2017 Dec;225(6):798–805.
10. Lambrichts DPV, Vennix S, Musters GD, et al. Hartmann's procedure versus sigmoidectomy with primary anastomosis for perforated diverticulitis with purulent or faecal peritonitis (LADIES): a multicentre, parallel-group, randomised, open-label, superiority trial. Lancet Gastroenterol Hepatol. 2019 Aug;4(8):599–610.
11. Oberkofler CE, Rickenbacher A, Raptis DA, et al. A multicenter randomized clinical trial of primary anastomosis or Hartmann's procedure for perforated left colonic diverticulitis with purulent or fecal peritonitis. Ann Surg 2012 Nov;256(5):819–26; discussion 26–7.
12. Blair NP, Germann E. Surgical management of acute sigmoid diverticulitis. Am J Surg. 2002 May;183(5):525–8.
13. Makela J, Kiviniemi H, Laitinen S. Prevalence of perforated sigmoid diverticulitis is increasing. Dis Colon Rectum. 2002 Jul;45(7):955–61.
14. Zorcolo L, Covotta L, Carlomagno N, Bartolo DC. Safety of primary anastomosis in emergency Colo-rectal surgery. Color Dis. 2003 May;5(3):262–9.
15. Regenet N, Pessaux P, Hennekinne S, et al. Primary anastomosis after intraoperative colonic lavage vs. Hartmann's procedure in generalized peritonitis complicating diverticular disease of the colon. Int J Color Dis. 2003 Nov;18(6):503–7.
16. Constantinides VA, Tekkis PP, Senapati A. Association of Coloproctology of Great Britain I. prospective multicentre evaluation of adverse outcomes following treatment for complicated diverticular disease. Br J Surg. 2006 Dec;93(12):1503–13.
17. Richter S, Lindemann W, Kollmar O, Pistorius GA, Maurer CA, Schilling MK. One-stage sigmoid colon resection for perforated sigmoid diverticulitis (Hinchey stages III and IV). World J Surg. 2006 Jun;30(6):1027–32.

18. Breitenstein S, Kraus A, Hahnloser D, Decurtins M, Clavien PA, Demartines N. Emergency left colon resection for acute perforation: primary anastomosis or Hartmann's procedure? A case-matched control study. World J Surg. 2007 Nov;31(11):2117–24.
19. Stumpf MJ, Vinces FY, Edwards J. Is primary anastomosis safe in the surgical management of complications of acute diverticulitis? Am Surg 2007 Aug;73(8):787–90; discussion 90–1.
20. Vermeulen J, Akkersdijk GP, Gosselink MP, et al. Outcome after emergency surgery for acute perforated diverticulitis in 200 cases. Dig Surg. 2007;24(5):361–6.
21. Zingg U, Pasternak I, Dietrich M, Seifert B, Oertli D, Metzger U. Primary anastomosis vs Hartmann's procedure in patients undergoing emergency left colectomy for perforated diverticulitis. Color Dis. 2010 Jan;12(1):54–60.
22. Trenti L, Biondo S, Golda T, et al. Generalized peritonitis due to perforated diverticulitis: Hartmann's procedure or primary anastomosis? Int J Color Dis. 2011 Mar;26(3):377–84.
23. Mueller MH, Karpitschka M, Renz B, et al. Co-morbidity and postsurgical outcome in patients with perforated sigmoid diverticulitis. Int J Color Dis. 2011 Feb;26(2):227–34.
24. Gawlick U, Nirula R. Resection and primary anastomosis with proximal diversion instead of Hartmann's: evolving the management of diverticulitis using NSQIP data. J Trauma Acute Care Surg 2012 Apr;72(4):807–814; quiz 1124.
25. Masoomi H, Stamos MJ, Carmichael JC, Nguyen B, Buchberg B, Mills S. Does primary anastomosis with diversion have any advantages over Hartmann's procedure in acute diverticulitis? Dig Surg. 2012;29(4):315–20.
26. Alizai PH, Schulze-Hagen M, Klink CD, et al. Primary anastomosis with a defunctioning stoma versus Hartmann's procedure for perforated diverticulitis--a comparison of stoma reversal rates. Int J Color Dis 2013 Dec 28(12):1681–1688.
27. Cauley CE, Patel R, Bordeianou L. Use of primary anastomosis with diverting ileostomy in patients with acute diverticulitis requiring urgent operative intervention. Dis Colon Rectum. 2018 May;61(5):586–92.
28. Lee JM, Bai PCJ, El Hechi M, et al. Hartmann's procedure vs primary anastomosis with diverting loop ileostomy for acute diverticulitis: Nationwide analysis of 2,729 emergency surgery patients. J Am Coll Surg. 2019 Jul;229(1):48–55.
29. Cirocchi R, Afshar S, Shaban F, et al. Perforated sigmoid diverticulitis: Hartmann's procedure or resection with primary anastomosis-a systematic review and meta-analysis of randomised control trials. Tech Coloproctol. 2018 Oct;22(10):743–53.
30. Gachabayov M, Oberkofler CE, Tuech JJ, Hahnloser D, Bergamaschi R. Resection with primary anastomosis vs nonrestorative resection for perforated diverticulitis with peritonitis: a systematic review and meta-analysis. Color Dis. 2018 Sep;20(9):753–70.
31. Ryan OK, Ryan EJ, Creavin B, Boland MR, Kelly ME, Winter DC. Systematic review and meta-analysis comparing primary resection and anastomosis versus Hartmann's procedure for the management of acute perforated diverticulitis with generalised peritonitis. Tech Coloproctol. 2020 Jun;24(6):527–43.
32. Lambrichts DP, Edomskis PP, van der Bogt RD, Kleinrensink GJ, Bemelman WA, Lange JF. Sigmoid resection with primary anastomosis versus the Hartmann's procedure for perforated diverticulitis with purulent or fecal peritonitis: a systematic review and meta-analysis. Int J Color Dis. 2020 Aug;35(8):1371–86.

Deciding on an IRA vs. IPAA for FAP

37

Samuel H. Lai and Jon D. Vogel

Introduction

Familial adenomatous polyposis (FAP) is an inherited colorectal cancer syndrome that results from a germline mutation of the *adenomatous polyposis coli (APC)* gene. Transmission of this mutation occurs in an autosomal dominant manner. However, in up to 25% of cases [1, 2], vertical transmission of the *APC* mutation cannot be clearly determined and is considered to be sporadic or *de novo* in origin. The precise APC mutation is quite variable and results in significant differences in the phenotype, or clinical manifestations, of the mutation. For example, certain APC mutations will result in hundreds of colorectal adenomatous polyps and others in thousands. Other APC mutations are associated with desmoid tumor formation or advanced periampullary adenoma [3]. In some cases, the APC mutation may result in an "attenuated" phenotype with scores, rather than hundreds or thousands, of colorectal polyps.

A primary concern in patients with FAP is that one of or more of the colorectal adenomas will progress to adenocarcinoma [4]. Endoscopic surveillance is used to assess polyp (i.e. adenoma) burden and perform biopsies, as needed, to exclude high-grade dysplasia or cancer. Colectomy is generally indicated when either high-grade dysplasia or cancer is detected, when endoscopic management is hindered by polyp number or density, or when technical or logistical challenges make endoscopic surveillance impractical. The surgical options for FAP include proctocolectomy with ileostomy or ileal pouch anal anastomosis (IPAA) or total abdominal colectomy with ileorectal anastomosis (IRA). When IRA is performed, endoscopic surveillance of the remnant rectum is required. Determination of the best surgical

S. H. Lai · J. D. Vogel (✉)
University of Colorado Surgery, Aurora, CO, USA
e-mail: samuel.lai@cuanschutz.edu; jon.vogel@cuanschutz.edu

K. Umanskiy, N. Hyman (eds.), *Difficult Decisions in Colorectal Surgery*, Difficult Decisions in Surgery: An Evidence-Based Approach,
https://doi.org/10.1007/978-3-031-42303-1_37

option for FAP requires consideration of multiple variables including oncological and functional outcomes, operative, and postoperative complications. Other considerations include postoperative desmoid formation and fertility impairment. This chapter aims to provide a summary of the current literature with evidence-based recommendations in selecting the appropriate procedure for patients with FAP.

Search Strategy

Patients	Intervention	Comparator	Outcomes
Patients with familial adenomatous Polyposis	Ileorectal anastomosis	Ileal pouch-anal anastomosis	Health-related quality of life; operative complications; functional outcomes; surgical outcomes

We performed a systematic literature search through June 2022 with the aims of answering the following PICO (Patients, Intervention, Comparator, Outcome) question: *"In patients with familial adenomatous polyposis (FAP), who should undergo ileorectal anastomosis (IRA) versus ileal pouch-anal anastomosis (IPAA)?"*. A targeted search of published literature in English up to 2022 was performed in PubMed, MEDLINE, Google Scholar, and Cochrane Database of Collected Review. Search terms utilized included: "familial adenomatous polyposis", "ileorectal anastomosis", "ileal-pouch anal anastomosis", and "restorative proctocolectomy". Studies were excluded if there were no direct comparisons between IRA and IPAA, unable to differentiate the outcomes between IPAA, IRA, total colectomy with end ileostomy or other procedures, or were not specific to patients with FAP (e.g., included patients with ulcerative colitis). Reference lists of included studies, systematic reviews, and meta-analyses were then reviewed to identify and incorporate additional relevant studies.

Results

Currently, there are no randomized control trials directly comparing IRA to IPAA in patients with FAP. The majority of studies are retrospective and include FAP registries or single center series Tables 37.1 and 37.2 summarizes the major findings in postoperative [5–14] and functional outcomes [7, 9–12, 14–17] from the available studies. Few studies published in the last 10 years include only FAP patients. More often, both FAP and ulcerative colitis patients are analyzed together. However, as FAP and ulcerative colitis (UC) are distinct diseases, studies incorporating both UC and FAP without separated subgroup analyses have been excluded. As a result, the grade of evidence in current literature remains low to moderate regarding this topic.

Table 37.1 Surgical outcomes after IRA vs IPAA

Study Range	Authors	Study Design	Grade of Evidence	Cohort Size, n(%)	Overall Survival		Metachronous Cancer in pouch or rectum, n(%)			Secondary proctectomy or pouch excision		Desmoid Tumor	Overall Complications	
					IRA	IPAA	IRA	IPAA	IRA	IPAA	IRA	IPAA	IRA	IPAA
1947–2015	Ardoino et al.	Retrospective review	Low quality	IRA = 585 (63) IPAA = 340 (37)	0.82 (survival risk)	0.75 (survival rsk)	52 (9)	1 (0.3)	IRA greater risk HR 14.9, CI 1.8–121		5 (1)	2 (1)	–	–
1950–2006	Bulow et al.	Retrospective review	Low quality	IRA = 776 (62) IPAA = 471 (38)	–	–	60 (8)	0 (0)	18% risk at 10 years	–	–	–	–	–
1963–2012	Koskenvuo et al.	Retrospective review	Low quality	IRA = 140 (61) IPAA = 88 (39)	77%	96%	18 (13)	0 (0)	39 (28)	–	–	–	28 (21)	26 (30)
1980–1997	Soravia et al.	Retrospective review	Low quality	IRA = 60 (55) IPAA = 50 (45)	–	–	–	–	–	–	10 (17)	3 (6)	13 (23)	13 (26)
1977–2006	Campos et al.	Retrospective review	Low quality	IRA = 42 (49) IPAA = 27 (31)	–	–	6 (17)	1 (4)	3 (7)	–	–	–	8 (19)	13 (48)
1978–1988	Ambroze et al.	Retrospective review	Low quality	IRA = 21 (12) IPAA = 94 (82)	–	–	2 (11)	0 (0)	–	–	–	–	4 (17)	24 (26)

(continued)

Table 37.1 (continued)

Study Range	Authors	Study Design	Grade of Evidence	Cohort Size, n(%)	Overall Survival		Metachronous Cancer in pouch or rectum, n(%)			Secondary proctectomy or pouch excision		Desmoid Tumor	Overall Complications	
					IRA	IPAA	IRA	IPAA	IRA	IPAA	IRA	IPAA	IRA	IPAA
1984–1995	Tonelli et al.	Prospective cohort	Low quality	IRA = 14 (37) IPAA = 24 (63)	–	–	–	0 (0)	0 (0)	0 (0)	4 (29)	5 (15)	3 (21)	6 (25)
1961–1996	Duijvendijk et al.	Retrospective review	Low quality	IRA = 183 (57) IPAA = 140 (43)	–	–	4 (3)	–	32 (20)	4 (3)	10 (6)	6 (5)	–	–
1984–1996	Bjork et al.	Retrospective review	Low quality	IRA=43 (42) IPAA = 59 (64)	86%	100%	12 (28)	–	12 (28)	0 (0)	0 (0)	2 (3)	11 (26)	39 (51)
2008–2012	Mozafar et al.	Retrospective review	Low quality	IRA = 6 (24) IPAA = 19 (76)	–	–	–	–	–	–	–	–	4 (66)	3 (16)
2000–2012	Konishi et al.	Retrospective review	Low quality	Open IRA = 33 (39) Lap IRA = 52 (61) Open IPAA = 97 (57) Lap IPAA = 74 (43)	Open = 100% Lap = 96%	Open = 98% Lap = 98%	–	–	–	–	Open = (13) Lap = (4.8)	Open = (22) Lap = (19)	–	–

IRA ileorectal anastomosis, *IPAA* ileal pouch-anal anastomosis, *Lap* laparoscopic surgery, *Open* open surgery

Table 37.2 Functional outcomes after IRA vs IPAA

Study Range	Authors	Study Design	Grade of Evidence	Cohort Size, n(%)	Number of stools/ day		Incontinence episodes, n(%)	Urgency, n(%)			Antidiarrheal Use, n(%)		Sexual dysfunction, (%)	
					IRA	IPAA	IRA	IPAA	IRA	IPAA	IRA	IPAA	IRA	IPAA
1980–1997	Soravia et al.	Retrospective review	Low quality	IRA = 60 (55) IPAA = 50 (45)	<6/day = 30 (75) > 6/day = 10 (25)	<6/day = 30 (70) > 6/day = 13 (30)	Daytime = 4(6) Night time = 5(13)	Daytime = 10(23) Night time = 21(49)	16(40)	12(28)	8(20)	7(16)	–	–
1978–1988	Ambroze et al.	Retrospective review	Low quality	IRA = 21 (12) IPAA = 94 (82)	Daytime = 4 Night time = 1	Daytime = 5 Night time = 1	Daytime = 4 (17) Night time = 3 (11)	Daytime = 12 (13) Night time = 28 (30)	–	–	0 (0)	16 (17)	Male = (10) Female = (13)	Male = (2) Female = (8)
1984–1996	Bjork et al.	Retrospective review	Low quality	IRA = 43 (42) IPAA = 59 (64)	>5/day = 5 (17)	>5/day = 14 (24)	Daytime = 0 (0) Night time = 0 (0)	Daytime = 6 (11) Night time = 20 (37)	15 (50)	17 (32)	1 (3)	13 (24)	Male = 0 (0) Female = 2 (18)	Male = 2 (7) Female = 3 (11)
1961–1996	Duijvendijk et al.	Retrospective review	Low quality	IRA = 183 (57) IPAA = 140 (43)	Daytime = 4.7 Night time = 1.5	Daytime = 6 Night time = 2	Daytime = (14) Night time = (3)	Daytime = (6) Night time = (26)	–	–	(15)	(28)	–	–
1981–1998	Hassan et al.	Retrospective review	Low quality	IRA = 21 (18) IPAA = 94 (82)	Daytime = 5 Night time = 1	Daytime = 6 Night time = 2	Daytime = 7(33) Night time = 5(24)	Daytime = 23(24) Night time = 36(38)	6(29)	6(6)	3(14)	13(14)	–	–
1980–1998	Ko et al.	Retrospective review	Low quality	IRA = 14 (32) IPAA = 30 (68)	5	8	0 (0)	13 (43)	–	–	–	–	–	–

(continued)

Table 37.2 (continued)

Study Range	Authors	Study Design	Grade of Evidence	Cohort Size, n(%)	Number of stools/day		Incontinence episodes, n(%)	Urgency, n(%)			Antidiarrheal Use, n(%)		Sexual dysfunction, (%)	
					IRA	IPAA	IRA	IPAA	IRA	IPAA	IRA	IPAA	IRA	IPAA
1977–1989	Madden et al.	Retrospective review	Low quality	IRA = 62 (75) IPAA = 20 (25)	3	5	17 (28)	8 (40)	31 (50)	3 (15)	10 (17)	7 (35)	–	–
2008–2012	Mozafar et al.	Retrospective review	Low quality	IRA = 6 (24) IPAA = 19 (76)	–	–	(50)	(21)	–	–	(50)	(26)	–	–
1984–1995	Tonelli et al.	Prospective cohort	Low quality	IRA = 1 4 (37) IPAA = 24 (63)	Night time = 0.9	Night time = 0.5	Daytime = 0 (0) Night time = 0 (0)	Daytime = 2 (8) Night time = 6 (25)	3 (21)	2 (8)	3 (19)	4 (17)	–	–

IRA ileorectal anastomosis, *IPAA* ileal pouch-anal anastomosis

Surgical Outcomes

The technical challenges and complexity of IPAA raise the concern for significantly greater risks for morbidities compared to IRA. Indeed, Bjork et al. demonstrated a significantly higher overall complication rates in patients who underwent IPAA compared to patients with IRA at 51% vs 26%, respectively (p = 0.04; OR3, CI 1.3–7.1) [12]. Similarly, in a retrospective series of 39 patients, Tonelli et al. showed more frequent early postoperative complications in patients with IPAA (21%) compared to IRA (0%) [10]. Additional studies likewise suggest higher complication rates after IPAA than IRA [9, 17]. On the contrary, other studies have not shown a higher rate of complication with IPAA. In a meta-analysis of 12 comparative studies between IRA and IPAA, Aziz et al. found no significant differences in rates of bowel obstruction, bleeding, anastomotic leak, surgical site infection, or intra-abdominal sepsis. However, the 30-day re-operation rate was found to be higher in patients who underwent IPAA (23.4%) than IRA (11.6%) (OR 2.11, CI 1.21–3.70) [18].

Risk of Desmoid Tumor Development

Desmoid tumor is a significant contributor to mortality in FAP and can affect up to 31% of FAP patients [19]. Risk factors for desmoid tumor in FAP patients includes family history of desmoid disease, APC mutation location, and colorectal surgery [20, 21]. Because surgical trauma is a significant trigger in desmoid development, substantial interest exists in establishing the optimal surgical operation in FAP patients who are more prone to desmoid disease.

Multiple strategies have been advocated, including the recommendation to perform IPAA for all patients or those who may be more prone to desmoid development [22]. This approach is based on the concern of the potential inability to perform a secondary proctectomy and ileoanal pouch after initial IRA since mesenteric desmoid development after initial IPAA may cause mesenteric shortening or hinder the ability to perform proctectomy [23]. Alternatively, another approach recommends the avoidance of a primary IPAA due to concern that restorative proctocolectomy may actually be associated with an increased risk of desmoid development [24–26]. In addition, with proper screening and selection of patients based on disease severity (e.g. polyp number and amenability to endoscopic surveillance) and the precise APC mutation, proctectomy may not be necessary [27]. In one of the largest studies to date, Sommovilla et al. showed that in FAP patients who underwent either IPAA (n = 172) or IRA (n = 173), IPAA was the single greatest independent risk factor for desmoid formation [21]. Additional independent risk factors for desmoid disease included family medical history (FMH) of desmoids, desmoid risk factor score (based on patient gender, APC mutation location, extra-intestinal manifestations of FAP, and FMH desmoids), and increasing patient height. However, the increased association of IPAA with desmoid development is not universally accepted. In a retrospective cohort analysis of 387 patients from 5 European polyposis registries, no significant differences were found in risk of desmoid development between IRA ww(11.1%) and IPAA (10.1%) ($p = 0.53$) [20]. Similarly, a meta-analysis of 12 retrospective studies on incidence of desmoid tumor showed no significant difference in desmoid development between the two procedures (11.8% vs. 9.5%, OR 0.95, $p = 0.85$) [28].

Notwithstanding the conflicting data, Burgess et al. showed that in patients who develop intraabdominal desmoid disease after initial prophylactic surgery, there is no differences in complication rates after IRA (69.4%) or IPAA (70.3%) [22]. This data suggests that in patients who may be more prone to desmoid tumor development, the notion of increased post-surgical morbidity related to desmoid tumors, including bowel obstructions, fistulas, reoperations, and need for permanent stoma, may not be true. Thus, selecting the optimal treatment selection may be based more heavily on considerations of functional and oncological outcomes rather than concerns about desmoid formation and its complications.

Risk of Metachronous Rectal Cancer

Perhaps the most important factor in deciding which operation to perform is the oncological outcome. IPAA will reduce the risk of developing rectal cancer as it involves removal of all (mucosectomy with sutured IPAA) or most (stapled IPAA) of the rectal mucosa. In contrast, with IRA, the rectum remains and with it the risk of rectal cancer. In the pre-pouch era, rates of metachronous rectal cancer in FAP patients who underwent IRA ranged from 10–30% [29, 30]. However, since the introduction of IPAA, in late 1970s, along with the accumulation of knowledge about this disease, the risk of rectal cancer after IRA has decreased to less than 10% [29] along with a 30% decrease in rate of secondary proctectomy [30]. In a study that compared FAP patients with IRA, pre- and post-1983, Moreira et al. showed a significantly lower rate of rectal cancer in the post-1983 cohort [27]. Nevertheless, it is important to note that in some patients, the need for secondary proctectomy after IRA is not due to development of rectal cancer. Other reasons include progressive and unmanageable rectal polyposis [31, 32], functional Iroblems such as incontinence [5], patient preference, or other reasons [33].

The improvement in rectal cancer risk after IRA can be attributed to a more appropriate patient selection for IRA or IPAA. Factors associated with worse oncological outcomes should be carefully assessed, including number and size of colonic and rectal adenomas. Patients with severe polyposis (>1000 polyps) have a 2.3 times greater predicted risk for development of colorectal cancer than patients with <1000 polyps [34]. Thus, in patients with >1000 colorectal adenomas, IPAA or proctocolectomy with end ileostomy is generally preferred [35]. Similarly, patients with >20 rectal polyps should also be considered for IPAA or proctocolectomy with end ileostomy given the significantly higher risk of rectal failure and secondary proctectomy compared to mild (<5) rectal polyposis (HR 25.5, 95% CI 11.1–58.8, $p < 0.001$) [31, 36].

The use of genotype and mutational analyses to select the appropriate surgery in patients with FAP has been suggested. Although there is considerable variability between phenotypic presentations among patients with identical APC mutations, some mutations at certain *APC* codons, including 1250, 1309, and 1382, have been shown to be associated with a more severe disease presentation [37]. Nieuwenhuis et al. retrospectively categorized 475 patients with FAP into attenuated, intermediate, and severe genotype groups and determined the risk of rectal cancer and secondary proctectomy at 20 years after IRA to be 6% and 10% in attenuated polyposis genotype, 3% and 43% in intermediate genotype, and 8% and 74% in patients with severe genotype [38]. This data suggest that IRA is an appropriate choice in patients with attenuated genotype while removal of the rectum, with IPAA or ileostomy creation, should be more strongly considered in patients with an intermediate or severe polyposis genotype. However, the utility of genotype in surgical selection has been overshadowed by the more generally accepted use of phenotype (i.e. polyp number) as a severity indicator [39].

Finally, it is worth noting that while the risk of cancer is significantly lower with IPAA than IRA, retained mucosa in the anal transition zone (ATZ), even after rectal mucosectomy and sutured IPAA, is still at risk for neoplasia [39]. Debate continues to exist regarding whether a sutured or stapled ileal anal anastomosis is optimal for IPAA in patients with FAP. While this topic is outside the scope of this chapter, a separate discussion of the benefits, risks, and other nuisances of each technique is warranted. In general, stapled IPAA is considered to be a technically easier operation with better functional outcomes, and fewer postoperative complications, while mucosectomy and sutured anastomosis may have a more favorable oncological outcome [4, 29, 40].

Functional Outcomes and Quality of Life

Functional outcomes and quality of life are important considerations in selecting the optimal surgical approach for FAP patients. In general, IRA results in better functional outcomes due to the preserved rectum, with reduced stool frequency, less watery stool, less stool seepage, or need for antidiarrheal medication when compared to patients with IPAA [41]. Results from a meta-analysis of 12 studies of functional outcomes after IRA or IPAA, suggest that majority of functional outcomes were better in patients who underwent IRA than IPAA [18].

In addition, IRA may pose a lower risk to female fecundity than IPAA. In a survey of 162 female patients on reproductive history and length of time to pregnancies, there was a significant 54% decrease in fecundity after IPAA compared to IRA [42]. Similarly, in a meta-analysis of the impact of IPAA on female fecundity in ulcerative colitis and FAP patients, IPAA still posed a significantly higher relative risk for infertility (HR 3.91; 95% CI 2.06—7.44).43 In the appropriate young female patients, these findings have led to some surgeons advocating for IRA or a staged approach to IPAA with initial IRA followed by secondary proctectomy and IPAA after childbearing.42

However, differences in functional outcomes after surgery does not necessarily translate to worse quality of life. Ko et al. showed that despite having worse functional outcomes in patients who underwent IPAA, quality of life was not different between IPAA and IRA patients.16 Other studies have similarly found no significant differences in patients' self-perceived quality of life in various areas of daily activities including social, sexual, travel, or recreation.7, 11, 15 Conversely, a decision analysis Markov modeling of possible outcomes after IRA or IPAA suggested that when taking quality of life into account, patients with IRA performed better compared to those with IPAA.44 Inherent to modeling studies, however, is the study limitation of exclusion of variables including desmoid tumor development and risk of infertility. Interestingly, in a study of colorectal surgeons' preferences and assessment of patients' quality of life after postoperatively, IRA was found to have the highest "postoperative health state utilities" through the time trade-off method.45 This method represents preferences for a given state of health compared to normal life and death and has previously been used to determine value of prophylactic surgery in cancer prevention. Thus, previous quality of life surveys may not be sensitive enough to fully capture the differences in preferences and values placed on quality of life postoperatively by FAP patients.

While this chapter is focused mainly on the creation of an IPAA or IRA in patients with FAP, it is important to note that patients, who choose or require an end ileostomy after proctocolectomy, may have similar overall quality of life as patients with an ileal pouch anal anastomosis. Even though no current studies have focused specifically on FAP patients in this context, several authors have reported similar quality of life outcomes in ulcerative colitis patients after IPAA versus end ileostomy 46, 47. In particular, Seidel et al., showed similar outcomes in work, social and family life, and relationships in ulcerative colitis and FAP patients who underwent IPAA or end ileostomy 48.

Data Based Recommendations

1. In general, patients with mild or attenuated polyposis are best suited for total abdominal colectomy with IRA, while those with severe polyposis (>1000 colonic polyps) are more appropriate for proctocolectomy with IPAA or end ileostomy *(evidence quality low to moderate; weak recommendation).*
2. Patients with less than 20 rectal polyps are generally good candidates for IRA, while patients with more than 20 rectal polyps are better suited for an operation that includes proctectomy *(evidence quality low; weak recommendation).*
3. In general, patients with a diagnosis of colon or rectal cancer should undergo proctocolectomy *(evidence quality low; weak recommendation).*
4. In female patients of childbearing age, the association of a diminished ability to get pregnant and IPAA surgery should be discussed when surgery is being planned *(evidence quality low; moderate recommendation).*

Personal View of the Data

When patients with FAP need an operation, the decision for proctocolectomy with IPAA or end ileostomy, or preservation of the rectum with IRA, is guided largely by the anticipated oncological and functional outcomes related to each operation. It is important that the surgeon and patient to recognize that one operation does not fit all FAP patients: some need more (IPAA or end ileostomy) and others will do better with less (IRA).

FAP patients with <1000 colorectal adenomas, <20 rectal adenomas, and no colon or rectal cancer, should do well with an IRA. This is a relatively simple operation, without need for a diverting ileostomy, less postoperative complications, and more favorable functional outcomes compared to IPAA. Alternatively, in patients with >1000 colorectal adenomas, or more than 20 rectal adenomas, or colon or (particularly) rectal cancer, or high-risk for desmoid tumor formation, proctocolectomy with IPAA or end ileostomy are often better surgical options.

The decision on IPAA or end ileostomy involves consideration of the patients' base-line anal sphincter function (e.g., their ability to defer defecation), their preference for one operation versus another, and an assessment of the anticipated complexity of the planned surgical procedure. For example, in the obese, male FAP patient, with distal rectal high-grade dysplasia or cancer, for whom mucosectomy with sutured IPAA may be the ideal cancer-preventing operation, it may be technically impossible to perform due to the inability of an ileal pouch to reach to the mid anal canal. The decision on stapled or hand sewn IPAA (with distal rectal mucosectomy) also warrants consideration of the outcomes of each approach as more favorable functional outcomes are expected with a stapled IPAA and no guarantee against rectal remnant cancer development even after mucosectomy.

When proctocolectomy is indicated, the option of a permanent end ileostomy may be preferable for some patients who have considered the pros and cons of each operation. For example, with an IPAA, 5–7 bowel movements per day and 1–2 that awaken the patient from sleep, should be expected. This frequency of bowel movements may be unacceptable to some patients who may then choose an end ileostomy. Finally, in the young female patient, with say hundreds of colon adenomas or 20–30 rectal adenomas without high-grade dysplasia or cancer, a staged approach, starting with IRA, then annual rectal endoscopic surveillance, and eventual proctectomy, as needed, may be the best strategy to prevent cancer while also limiting interference with pregnancy and childbirth.

References

1. Aretz S, Uhlhaas S, Caspari R, et al. Frequency and parental origin of de novo APC mutations in familial adenomatous polyposis. Eur J Hum Genet. 2004;12(1):52–8. https://doi.org/10.1038/sj.ejhg.5201088.
2. Olkinuora AP, Peltomäki PT, Aaltonen LA, Rajamäki K. From APC to the genetics of hereditary and familial colon cancer syndromes. Hum Mol Genet. 2021;30(R2):R206–24. https://doi.org/10.1093/hmg/ddab208.

3. Björk J, Åkerbrant H, Iselius L, et al. Periampullary adenomas and adenocarcinomas in familial adenomatous polyposis: cumulative risks and APC gene mutations. Gastroenterology. 2001;121(5):1127–35. https://doi.org/10.1053/gast.2001.28707.
4. Herzig D, Hardimann K, Weiser M, et al. The American Society of Colon and Rectal Surgeons clinical practice guidelines for the management of inherited polyposis syndromes. Dis Colon Rectum. 2017;60(9):881–94. https://doi.org/10.1097/DCR.0000000000000912.
5. Bülow S, Bülow C, Vasen H, Järvinen H, Björk J, Christensen IJ. Colectomy and ileorectal anastomosis is still an option for selected patients with familial adenomatous polyposis. Dis Colon Rectum. 2008;51(9):1318–23. https://doi.org/10.1007/s10350-008-9307-3.
6. Koskenvuo L, Mustonen H, Renkonen-Sinisalo L, Järvinen HJ, Lepistö A. Comparison of proctocolectomy and ileal pouch-anal anastomosis to colectomy and ileorectal anastomosis in familial adenomatous polyposis. Familial Cancer. 2015;14(2):221–7. https://doi.org/10.1007/s10689-014-9773-9.
7. Soravia C, Klein L, Berk T, O'Connor B, Cohen Z, McLeod RS. Comparison of ileal pouch-anal anastomosis and ileorectal anastomosis in patients with familial adenomatous polyposis. Dis Colon Rectum. 1999;42(8):1028–33.
8. Campos FG, Perez RO, Imperiale AR, Seid VE, Nahas SC, Cecconello I. Surgical treatment of familial adenomatous polyposis: Ileoretal anastomosis or restorative proctolectomy? Arq Gastroenterol. 2009;46(4):294–9. https://doi.org/10.1590/S0004-28032009000400009.
9. Ambroze WL, Dozois RR, Pemberton JH, Beart RW, Ilstrup DM. Familial adenomatous polyposis: results following ileal pouch-anal anastomosis and ileorectostomy. Dis Colon Rectum. 1992;35(1):12–5. https://doi.org/10.1007/BF02053332.
10. Tonelli F, Valanzano R, Monaci I, Mazzoni P, Anastasi A, Ficari F. Restorative proctocolectomy or rectum-preserving surgery in patients with familial adenomatous polyposis: results of a prospective study. World J Surg. 1997;21(6):653–9. https://doi.org/10.1007/s002689900289.
11. Van Duijvendijk P, Slors JFM, Taat CW, et al. Quality of life after total colectomy with ileorectal anastomosis or proctocolectomy and ileal pouch-anal anastomosis for familial adenomatous polyposis. Br J Surg. 2000;87(5):590–6. https://doi.org/10.1046/j.1365-2168.2000.01442.x.
12. Björk J, Åkerbrant H, Iselius L, et al. Outcome of primary and secondary ileal pouch-anal anastomosis and ileorectal anastomosis in patients with familial adenomatous polyposis. Dis Colon Rectum. 2001;44(7):984–92. https://doi.org/10.1007/BF02235487.
13. Konishi T, Ishida H, Ueno H, et al. Feasibility of laparoscopic total proctocolectomy with ileal pouch–anal anastomosis and total colectomy with ileorectal anastomosis for familial adenomatous polyposis: results of a nationwide multicenter study. Int J Clin Oncol. 2016;21(5):953–61. https://doi.org/10.1007/s10147-016-0977-x.
14. Mozafar M, Shateri K, Tabatabaey A, Lotfollahzadeh S, Atqiaee K. Familial adenomatous polyposis: Ileo-anal pouch versus ileo-rectal anastomosis. Gastroenterol Hepatol Bed Bench. 2014;7(4):206–10.
15. Hassan I, Chua HK, Wolff BG, et al. Quality of life after ileal pouch-anal anastomosis and ileorectal anastomosis in patients with familial adenomatous polyposis. Dis Colon Rectum. 2005;48(11):2032–7. https://doi.org/10.1007/s10350-005-0169-7.
16. Ko CY, Rusin LC, Schoetz DJ, et al. Does better functional result equate with better quality of life? Implications for surgical treatment in familial adenomatous polyposis. Dis Colon Rectum. 2000;43(6):829–37. https://doi.org/10.1007/bf02238022.
17. Madden MV, Neale KF, Nicholls RJ, et al. Comparison of morbidity and function after colectomy with ileorectal anastomosis or restorative proctocolectomy for familial adenomatous polyposis. Br J Surg. 2005;78(7):789–92.
18. Aziz O, Athanasiou T, Fazio VW, et al. Meta-analysis of observational studies of ileorectal versus ileal pouch-anal anastomosis for familial adenomatous polyposis. Br J Surg. 2006;93(4):407–17. https://doi.org/10.1002/bjs.5276.
19. Hartley JE, Church JM, Gupta S, McGannon E, Fazio VW, Phillips RKS. Significance of incidental desmoids identified during surgery for familial adenomatous polyposis. Dis Colon Rectum. 2004;47(3):334–40. https://doi.org/10.1007/s10350-003-0063-0.

20. Nieuwenhuis MH, Lefevre JH, Bülow S, et al. Family history, surgery, and APC mutation are risk factors for desmoid tumors in familial adenomatous polyposis: an international cohort study. Dis Colon Rectum. 2011;54(10):1229–34. https://doi.org/10.1097/DCR.0b013e318227e4e8.
21. Sommovilla J, Liska D, Jia X, et al. Ileal Pouch anal anastomosis is more "Desmoidogenic" than ileorectal anastomosis in familial adenomatous polyposis. Dis Colon Rectum. 2021; Publish Ah:1351–1361. https://doi.org/10.1097/dcr.0000000000002172.
22. Burgess A, Xhaja X, Church J. Does intra-abdominal desmoid disease affect patients with an ileal pouch differently than those with an ileorectal anastomosis? Dis Colon Rectum. 2011;54(11):1388–91. https://doi.org/10.1097/DCR.0b013e31822f8d91.
23. Vasen HFA, Möslein G, Alonso A, et al. Guidelines for the clinical management of familial adenomatous polyposis (FAP). Gut. 2008;57(5):704–13. https://doi.org/10.1136/gut.2007.136127.
24. Vogel J, Church JMLL. Minimally invasive pouch surgery predisposes to desmoid tumor formation in patients with familial adenomatous polyposis. Dis Colon Rectum. 2005;48:662.
25. Saito Y, Hinoi T, Ueno H, et al. Risk factors for the development of Desmoid tumor after colectomy in patients with familial adenomatous polyposis: multicenter retrospective cohort study in Japan. Ann Surg Oncol. 2016;23:559–65. https://doi.org/10.1245/s10434-016-5380-3.
26. Walter T, Zhenzhen Wang C, Guillaud O, et al. Management of desmoid tumours: a large national database of familial adenomatous patients shows a link to colectomy modalities and low efficacy of medical treatments. United Eur Gastroenterol J. 2017;5(5):735–41. https://doi.org/10.1177/2050640616678150.
27. Da Luz MA, Church JM, Burke CA. The evolution of prophylactic colorectal surgery for familial adenomatous polyposis. Dis Colon Rectum. 2009;52(8):1481–6. https://doi.org/10.1007/DCR.0b013e3181ab58fb.
28. Xie M, Chen Y, Wei W, et al. Does ileoanal pouch surgery increase the risk of desmoid in patients with familial adenomatous polyposis? Int J Color Dis. 2020;35(8):1599–605. https://doi.org/10.1007/s00384-020-03578-y.
29. Fábio GC. Surgical treatment of familial adenomatous polyposis: dilemmas and current recommendations. World J Gastroenterol. 2014;20(44):16620–9. https://doi.org/10.3748/wjg.v20.i44.16620.
30. Church J, Burke C, McGannon E, Pastean O, Clark B. Risk of rectal cancer in patients after colectomy and ileorectal anastomosis for familial adenomatous polyposis: a function of available surgical options. Dis Colon Rectum. 2003;46(9):1175–81. https://doi.org/10.1007/s10350-004-6710-2.
31. Sinha A, Tekkis PP, Rashid S, Phillips RKS, Clark SK. Risk factors for secondary proctectomy in patients with familial adenomatous polyposis. Br J Surg. 2010;97(11):1710–5. https://doi.org/10.1002/bjs.7202.
32. Bülow C, Vasen H, Järvinen H, Björk J, Bisgaard ML, Bülow S. Ileorectal anastomosis is appropriate for a subset of patients with familial adenomatous polyposis. Gastroenterology. 2000;119(6):1454–60. https://doi.org/10.1053/gast.2000.20180.
33. Koskenvuo L, Renkonen-Sinisalo L, Järvinen HJ, Lepistö A. Risk of cancer and secondary proctectomy after colectomy and ileorectal anastomosis in familial adenomatous polyposis. Int J Color Dis. 2014;29(2):225–30. https://doi.org/10.1007/s00384-013-1796-4.
34. Debinski HS, Love S, Spigelman AD, Phillips RKS. Colorectal polyp counts and cancer risk in familial adenomatous polyposis. Gastroenterology. 1996;110(4):1028–30. https://doi.org/10.1053/gast.1996.v110.pm8612989.
35. Wu JS, Paul P, McGannon EA, Church JM. APC genotype, polyp number, and surgical options in familial adenomatous polyposis. Ann Surg. 1998;227(1):57–62. https://doi.org/10.1097/00000658-199801000-00009.
36. Church J, Burke C, McGannon E, Pastean O, Clark B, Cohen Z. Predicting polyposis severity by proctoscopy: how reliable is it? Dis Colon Rectum. 2001;44(9):1249–52. https://doi.org/10.1007/bf02234779.
37. Talseth-Palmer BA. The genetic basis of colonic adenomatous polyposis syndromes. Hered Cancer Clin Pract. 2017;15(1):1–7. https://doi.org/10.1186/s13053-017-0065-x.

38. Nieuwenhuis MH, Mathus-Vliegen LM, Slors FJ, et al. Genotype-phenotype correlations as a guide in the management of familial adenomatous polyposis. Clin Gastroenterol Hepatol. 2007;5(3):374–8. https://doi.org/10.1016/j.cgh.2006.12.014.
39. Church JM. Controversies in the surgery of patients with familial adenomatous polyposis and lynch syndrome. Familial Cancer. 2016;15(3):447–51. https://doi.org/10.1007/s10689-016-9886-4.
40. Möslein G. Surgical considerations in FAP-related pouch surgery: could we do better? Familial Cancer. 2016;15(3):457–66. https://doi.org/10.1007/s10689-016-9904-6.
41. Van Duijvendijk P, JFM S, Taat CW, Oosterveld P. Functional outcome after colectomy and ileorectal anastomosis compared with proctocolectomy and ileal pouch anal anastomosis in familial adenomatous polyposis. Ann Surg. 1999;230(5):648–54.
42. Olsen K, Juul S, Bülow S, et al. Female fecundity before and after operation for familial adenomatous polyposis. Br J Surg. 2003;90(2):227–31. https://doi.org/10.1002/bjs.4082.
43. Rajaratnam SG, Eglinton TW, Hider P, Fearnhead NS. Impact of ileal pouch-anal anastomosis on female fertility: meta-analysis and systematic review. Int J Color Dis. 2011;26(11):1365–74. https://doi.org/10.1007/s00384-011-1274-9.
44. Melnitchouk N, Saadat LV, Bleday R, Goldberg JE. A decision analysis for rectal-sparing familial adenomatous polyposis: total colectomy with Ileorectal anastomosis versus proctocolectomy with IPAA. Dis Colon Rectum. 2019;62(1):27–32. https://doi.org/10.1097/DCR.0000000000001186.
45. Dossa F, Morris AM, Wilson AR, Baxter NN. Life after surgery: surgeon assessments of quality of life among patients with familial adenomatous polyposis. Dis Colon Rectum. 2018;61(10):1217–22. https://doi.org/10.1097/DCR.0000000000001146.
46. Kuruvilla K, Osler T, Hyman NH. A comparison of the quality of life of ulcerative colitis patients after IPAA vs ileostomy. Dis Colon Rectum. 2012;55(11):1131–7. https://doi.org/10.1097/DCR.0b013e3182690870.
47. Murphy PB, Khot Z, Vogt KN, Ott M, Dubois L. Quality of life after total proctocolectomy with ileostomy or IPAA: a systematic review. Dis Colon Rectum. 2015;58(9):899–908. https://doi.org/10.1097/DCR.0000000000000418.
48. Seidel S, Newman M, Sharp K. Ileoanal pouch versus ileostomy: is there a difference in quality of life? Am Surg. 2000;66(6):540–6.

Rectal Prolapse: Rectopexy vs Perineal Proctosigmoidectomy

38

Sarah A. Vogler and Kristen A. Ban

Introduction

Surgical options to treat rectal prolapse include abdominal and perineal approaches. Abdominal approaches include resection, suture, and mesh rectopexy. Suture rectopexy can be performed with or without resection of the sigmoid colon and employs an anterior, posterior, or circumferential mobilization of the rectum. Mesh rectopexy is typically performed with a ventral or anterior dissection. Increasingly, abdominal repairs are performed with a minimally invasive laparoscopic or robotic approach. Perineal approaches to treat rectal prolapse include perineal proctosigmoidectomy, also known as the Altemeier procedure, as well as the Delorme procedure.

Historically, the abdominal approach was favored due to the lower risk of recurrence, with the perineal approach reserved for high-risk surgical candidates including the elderly or those with significant comorbidities. In recent decades, the incidence of abdominal surgeries has increased, while the number of perineal surgeries has decreased. This is reflective of minimally invasive surgical (MIS) techniques offering ease of tolerance, acceptable outcomes, and rapid recovery even for high-risk surgical candidates. Numerous factors impact procedure choice, including overall health of the patient, gender, prior surgical history, symptoms, and presence of concomitant prolapse in other pelvic compartments.

S. A. Vogler (✉)
Cleveland Clinic Florida, Martin Health, Port St Lucie, FL, USA
e-mail: voglers@ccf.org

K. A. Ban
Cleveland Clinic Foundation, Cleveland, OH, USA
e-mail: bank4@ccf.org

K. Umanskiy, N. Hyman (eds.), *Difficult Decisions in Colorectal Surgery*, Difficult Decisions in Surgery: An Evidence-Based Approach,
https://doi.org/10.1007/978-3-031-42303-1_38

One challenge in assessing the surgical literature on rectal prolapse repair is the paucity of adequately powered level 1 data. Additionally, there is heterogeneity among studies comparing the abdominal versus perineal approach as within each category there are multiple surgical options. Kim et al. note that "the myriad of methods available to correct the underlying anatomic defects in complete rectal prolapse poses a perplexing question for the surgeon, *i.e.* the choice of an ideal operation." [1] The objective of this review is to compare the various rectal prolapse repair surgeries and outcomes including morbidity, recurrence, functional, and quality of life.

Search Strategy

A search was performed using search terms defined by the PICO model outlined in Table 38.1. The population of interest was patients with rectal prolapse undergoing rectopexy and the comparator was patients undergoing perineal proctosigmoidectomy. Outcomes of interest included recurrence of rectal prolapse, functional outcomes, quality of life, morbidity, and mortality.

PubMed was searched for relevant studies including systematic reviews (SR) and meta-analyses (MA). The following keywords were employed: "rectal prolapse", "procidentia", "rectopexy", "perineal proctosigmoidectomy", "perineal proctectomy", "Altemeier", "Delorme". All articles identified during the initial search were screened. The references of relevant articles were reviewed to identify additional studies. Inclusion criteria for consideration included publication in English, adult (> age 18) human subjects, and a study population of more than 20 patients.

Table 38.1 PICO model

Patient Population	Intervention	Comparator	Outcomes
Patients with rectal prolapse	Rectopexy	Perineal proctosigmoidectomy	Recurrence
			Functional outcomes
			Quality of life
			Morbidity
			Mortality

Results

Abdominal Versus Perineal Approach

Data comparing outcomes after abdominal compared to perineal rectal prolapse repair come from four recent randomized trials and retrospective reviews of single-institution experiences.

The PROSPER trial was an international, multicenter, pragmatic, factorial study that randomized 293 patients to abdominal (suture vs. resection rectopexy) vs. perineal (Altemeier vs. Delorme) rectal prolapse procedures and controlled for age, ASA status and preoperative bowel function [2]. Median follow-up was 3 years. A more recent multicenter, factorial randomized trial reported by Smedberg et al. recruited 134 patients who underwent the same four procedures [3]. Recurrence was determined at 3 years. Both studies were underpowered and neither study included ventral mesh rectopexy (VMR). Deen et al. reported a randomized trial allocating 20 total patients to abdominal resection rectopexy and pelvic floor repair versus perineal proctosigmoidectomy with median follow-up of 17 months [4]. Emile et al. randomized 50 patients to laparoscopic ventral mesh rectopexy versus Delorme with a median follow-up of 18 months [5]. A high percentage of patients were male (38%).

Kim et al. at the University of Minnesota reported one of the largest retrospective reviews over 19 years of rectal prolapse repairs performed on 372 patients [1]. 183 underwent perineal proctosigmoidectomy, 161 underwent resection rectopexy, 11 underwent Delorme, and the remaining underwent partial colectomies or anterior resections. Patients who underwent perineal procedures were significantly older and sicker and had shorter recurrence-free survival. A long-term retrospective review by Ng et al. in Australia evaluated 157 patients undergoing surgical prolapse repair, including 44 patients who underwent resection rectopexy, 38 who underwent rectopexy, 55 who underwent Delorme, and 20 who underwent Altemeier with median follow-up of 4.5 years [6]. Patients who underwent perineal procedures were significantly older with a mean age of 80 compared to 67 years in the abdominal cohort ($p = 0.001$). Hu et al. compared laparoscopic ventral mesh rectopexy and perineal repair specifically in men with a median follow-up of 48.5 months [7].

Morbidity

The PROSPER trial reported higher morbidity in the perineal group compared to the abdominal group [2]. Four mortalities were reported following perineal procedures, and one mortality was reported following an abdominal procedure. Four serious morbidities were reported in the perineal group, all anastomotic leakages following Altemeier operations, and no serious morbidities were reported in the abdominal group. The 4-arm randomized trial reported by Smedberg described higher complications in the perineal group than the abdominal group (3 total versus none), but this difference was not significant ($p = 0.314$) [3]. Hospital stay was significantly longer in the abdominal versus perineal cohort (mean 8 days versus 5 days, p = 0.022). Deen et al. reported higher morbidity in the resection rectopexy group with 2 ileus, one wound infection, and one anastomotic stricture [4]. Emile et al. reported no major morbidity or mortality in either group [5].

Kim et al. reported similar overall complication rates in the abdominal and perineal cohorts, though the complications differed in the two groups [1]. Small bowel obstruction was the most common complication after an abdominal procedure (21/176 patients), but was not reported in any patient undergoing a perineal procedure. Patients undergoing perineal procedures reported higher numbers of urinary, cardiac, and anastomotic complications than in the abdominal cohort. Ng et al. found that morbidity was higher in the perineal cohort (17.1%) compared to abdominal (10.7%), though the difference was not significant [6]. The Altemeier procedure carried the highest morbidity (20%) followed by resection rectopexy (18%), rectopexy alone (16%), and Delorme (7%). In the male study population described by Hu et al., no mortalities were reported, and complication rates were significantly lower after ventral mesh rectopexy (0%) compared to perineal repair (20.7%) (p=0.031) [7].

Recurrence

The PROSPER trial did not report any significant differences in recurrence rates between abdominal versus perineal approaches or between different procedures in the same approach category [2]. Reported recurrence among randomized patients was 20% in the perineal group compared to 26% in the abdominal group (p = 0.8). Reported recurrence for all patients, including those who did not undergo intended procedure, was 24% after Altemeier, 31% after Delorme, 13% after resection rectopexy, and 26% after suture rectopexy. Smedberg et al. reported 3-year recurrence rates favoring the abdominal approach that were not significant [3]. Recurrence after suture rectopexy was 21%, after resection rectopexy 10%, after Delorme 58%, and after Altemeier 50%. Deen et al. reported no recurrence after resection rectopexy and one recurrence after Altemeier, which was not statistically significant [4]. Emile et al. reported higher recurrence following Delorme (16%) compared to ventral mesh rectopexy (8%), but the difference was not significant (p = 0.66) [5]. None of the studies reported above were adequately powered to detect differences in recurrence.

Kim et al. reported significantly lower recurrence after abdominal (5%) versus perineal (16%) procedures (p = 0.002) [1]. Ng et al. reported significantly lower recurrence rates in their abdominal operation cohort and found that perineal versus abdominal surgical approach independently predicted recurrence in Cox regression analysis [6]. 5-year recurrence was highest after Delorme (52%), followed by Altemeier (30%), rectopexy (5%), and lowest after resection rectopexy (3%). Hu et al. reported significantly lower recurrence in men following ventral mesh rectopexy (9.5%) versus perineal repair (41.7%) (p = 0.018) with median follow-up of 48.5 months [7].

Function and Quality of Life

The PROSPER trial reported similar significant functional and quality of life improvements following all procedures evaluated that were maintained at 3-year follow-up without significant differences between groups [2]. Fecal incontinence measured by the Vaizey score, bowel function measured by the bowel thermometer, and quality of life measured by the EQ-5D all improved after surgery. Smedberg et al. reported improvements in Wexner and RAND-36 scores after all procedures without significant differences between procedures [3]. In the perineal procedure cohort, Deen et al. reported significantly higher residual fecal incontinence (FI) (OR 13.5) and significantly lower maximum resting and squeeze pressures on manometry ($p = 0.003$) [4]. Constipation and global quality of life scores were not reported. Emile et al. reported similar postoperative improvement in bleeding, fecal incontinence, constipation, Wexner constipation and incontinence scores, Gastrointestinal Quality of Life Index (GIQoL), and Fecal Incontinence Quality of Life (FIQL) scores after both Delorme and ventral mesh rectopexy [5]. Improvements in anal manometry measurements were also similar in both groups.

Kim et al. reported similar improvement in fecal incontinence, constipation, and overall satisfaction following both abdominal and perineal procedures [1]. In a male population, Hu et al. reported only perineal repair significantly improved constipation ($p = 0.001$) with an improvement from 72% preop to 25% postop [7]. No sexual dysfunction was reported in either group.

Robotic Versus Laparoscopic Abdominal Approach

The highest volume of literature comparing minimally invasive surgical approaches pertains to ventral mesh rectopexy. Four recent SRs and three MAs compare robotic and laparoscopic ventral mesh rectopexy outcomes. Bao et al. found 14 observational studies with over 750 patients assessing the safety and efficacy of laparoscopic and robotic ventral mesh rectopexy [8]. Follow-up was variable, from 1 months to 5 years. Operative time was longer in the robotic population, but hospital length of stay was shorter. All studies captured in the SR by Albayati et al. were included in the larger analysis by Bao and colleagues [9]. Emile et al. performed SR and MA of outcomes following laparoscopic ventral mesh rectopexy and performed meta-regression analysis of predictors of recurrence [10]. The MA included 17 studies and 1242 patients with a median follow-up of 23 months. Flynn et al. found six studies meeting inclusion criteria [11], all of which were also included in the Bao SR and MA. In total, the studies included 382 patients with follow-up ranging from 1 month to almost 5 years.

Morbidity

Bao et al. in their MA reported fewer conversions to open in the robotic compared to laparoscopic populations, though this difference was not statistically significant [8]. The robotic approach had a significantly lower mean intraoperative blood loss (weighted mean difference −20.69, 95% CI −35.74 to −5.63, p = 0.007). Robotic ventral mesh rectopexy had significantly lower post-operative complications (OR 0.45, 95% CI 0.24–0.83, p = 0.009). The review by Emile et al. reported pooled outcomes after laparoscopic VMR, including a conversion to open rate of 1.8% and a complication rate of 12.4%, primarily driven by urinary tract infection, urinary retention, with rare reports of urethral injury, bladder injury, and vas deferens injury in male patients [10]. Mesh-related complications were reported in less than 1% of patients.

Flynn et al. reported no significant difference in complications (pooled OR in favor of robotic surgery 0.74, 95% CI 0.35–1.56) or conversion to open (pooled OR 1.09, 95% CI 0.28–4.20) [11]. Robotic VMR had a trend toward longer operative times (pooled SMD 0.39 favoring laparoscopic, 95% CI −0.43–1.22) and significantly shorter length of stay (pooled SMD −0.42, 95% CI −0.67–0.17).

Recurrence

Bao et al. reported no statistically significant difference recurrence between the robotic and laparoscopic populations, including after sensitivity analysis [8]. Follow-up in included studies ranged from 1 month to 5 years and in many cases was inadequate to capture recurrence except in cases of early technical failure. Emile et al. reported a weighted mean rate of recurrence of full thickness prolapse following laparoscopic VMR of 2.8% at a median follow-up of 23 months [10]. Meta-regression analysis of factors significantly associated with prolapse recurrence included male gender (SE = 0.018, 95% CI 0.008–0.044, p = 0.008) and length of mesh (SE = −0.007, 95% CI −0.01 to −0.001, p = 0.025), with shorter mesh associated with recurrence.

Flynn et al. did not pool or compare recurrence rates for MA, however, a summary of recurrence rates was similar between the two procedures and was overall very low, less than 10% after both procedures with follow-up ranging from 1 month to 5 years [11].

Function and Quality of Life

In their MA, Bao et al. reported no statistically significant difference in pre- and post-operative mean Wexner scores (weight mean difference 0.09, 95% CI −0.63-0.82, p = 0.79) [8]. The pooled laparoscopic cohort had a higher unadjusted rate of post-operative FI, but this difference was not significant. In their SR, Emile et al. reported significant improvement in pre- versus post-operative FI in majority of patients undergoing laparoscopic VMR [10]. The weighted mean rate of improvement in FI was 79.3% (95% CI 69.4–89.1, $I^2 = 87.8\%$), and the weighted mean rate of improvement in constipation was 71% (95% CI 55.2–86.9, $I^2 = 91.2\%$).

Flynn et al. noted that heterogeneity of functional outcome assessment scores prevented pooling of results [11]. Overall, both groups showed improvements in functional outcomes including constipation, FI, and global quality of life measures regardless of the surgical approach, though differences seemed to favor the robotic platform.

Anterior Versus Posterior Rectopexy

Data comparing rectopexy techniques has been updated with two SR/MAs, long-term results from a randomized controlled trial (RCT), and a retrospective review including a large number of male patients.

A SR and MA by Lobb et al. evaluated anterior suture rectopexy versus VMR from 22 studies including 976 patients. Subgroup analysis was performed to compare VMR with biologic versus synthetic mesh [12]. Included were randomized and non-randomized studies of open or laparoscopic techniques with follow-up of at least 12 months. Hajibandeh et al. performed SR and MA of laparoscopic mesh rectopexy (anterior or posterior) versus posterior suture rectopexy, including 5 comparative studies and 307 patients [13]. Follow-up ranged from 1 to 6 years.

Hidaka et al. reported long-term outcomes of an RCT comparing outcomes following laparoscopic ventral mesh rectopexy and laparoscopic posterior suture rectopexy [14]. The studies randomized 75 patients in total and assessed outcomes with median follow-up of 6.1 years. Previously, 1-year outcomes from this study including complications were reported by Lundby et al. [15]. Madbouly et al. compared laparoscopic VMR to posterior rectopexy and included 74 patients, 19% of which were male [16]. All ventral rectopexy cases incorporated mesh. The minimum follow-up was 2 years with a range of 2–7 years.

Morbidity

Lobb et al. reported an overall complication rate following anterior suture rectopexy of 8.8% and following VMR of 7.9% ($p = 0.509$) [12]. The most common postoperative complication following suture rectopexy was surgical site infection (1.9%) and following VMR was urinary tract infection (2.4%). Hajibandeh reported no significant difference between laparoscopic mesh rectopexy (anterior or posterior) and laparoscopic posterior suture rectopexy in complications including surgical site infection (OR 1.48, $p = 0.71$) [13]. There was no significant difference in length of stay (MD: −1.54, $p = 0.47$). No mesh erosion was reported in any of the studies at maximum follow-up.

Lundby et al. reported a similar rate of overall complications in their RCT, with 1/37 following posterior suture rectopexy and 1/38 following VMR [15]. Madbouly et al. reported similar morbidity in the 2 cohorts, 3/41 in VMR and 2/33 in laparoscopic posterior rectopexy ($p = 0.99$) [16]. The most common complications of VMR were urinary tract infection and prolonged ileus, and 1 patient experienced mesh erosion into the vagina. The most common complication after posterior suture rectopexy was wound infection. Conversion to open was necessary in 2/41 VMR patients and in no posterior suture rectopexy patients (p = 0.001). Operative time was significantly longer for VMR (122 min) compared to posterior suture rectopexy (105 min) (p = 0.001). Length of stay was significantly longer for VMR (4.5 days) versus posterior suture rectopexy (3.7 days) (p = 0.04).

Recurrence

In their SR, Lobb et al. reported a recurrence rate of 8.6% after suture rectopexy compared to 3.7% for VMR (p < 0.001) [12]. Results from the MA showed high heterogeneity, and the difference in recurrence rates was not found to be statistically significant (p = 0.76). On subgroup analysis, there was no difference in recurrence rate comparing VMR with biologic versus synthetic mesh (4.1% versus 3.6%, respectively, p = 0.789). Hajibandeh et al. reported significantly lower recurrence after laparoscopic rectopexy with mesh (anterior or posterior approach) compared to laparoscopic posterior suture rectopexy (OR 0.28, p = 0.009) [13].

In their RCT, Lundby et al. reported early recurrence within one year in 5% of patients undergoing posterior suture rectopexy and in no patients undergoing VMR (p = 0.305) [15]. Long-term recurrence rates from the same RCT at a median of 6.1 years were reported by Hidaka et al. as 23% following posterior suture rectopexy and 9% following VMR [14]. Authors note the study was not powered to assess recurrence, and this difference was not significant. Madbouly et al. reported similar recurrence after laparoscopic VMR (1/41) compared to laparoscopic posterior suture rectopexy (1/33) (p = 0.93) [16].

Function and Quality of Life

Lobb et al. reported variable findings in the comparison of functional outcomes after anterior suture rectopexy versus VMR [12]. Of five studies comparing outcomes, two found no statistical difference in FI, and one reported a significant difference favoring VMR. Regarding constipation, two studies reported a significant difference favoring VMR. Hajibandeh et al. reported no significant difference in Cleveland Clinic Incontinence Score (CCIS) (MD: −1.02, p = 0.50) or Cleveland Clinic Constipation Score (CCCS) (MD: −1.54, p = 0.47) between laparoscopic mesh rectopexy (anterior or posterior) versus laparoscopic posterior suture rectopexy [13].

Lundby et al. reported short-term outcomes of their RCT [15]. Patients who underwent laparoscopic VMR had a significant pre- to post-operative improvement in obstructive defecation syndrome (ODS) score (1.97, 95% CI 0.01–3.93), and a non-significant improvement following laparoscopic posterior suture rectopexy (2.18, 95% CI −0.14–4.49). The difference between the two groups was not significant. Long-term outcomes from this RCT reported by Hidaka et al. found total Patient Assessment of Constipation Quality of Life Questionnaire (PAC-QoL) score was significantly lower in the VMR cohort (0.26, 0.14–0.83) compared to posterior suture rectopexy (0.93, 0.32–1.61) (p = 0.008). The total constipation symptom score measured by Patient Assessment of Constipation-Symptoms (PAC-SYM) was significantly lower in the VMR cohort (0.5, 0.21–0.87) compared to posterior suture rectopexy (1.0, 0.5–1.5) (p = 0.031). Except for the CCIS, other scores including the ODS and the CCCS significantly favored the VMR group (p = 0.011 and p = 0.017, respectively). Madbouly et al. found significant improvement in incontinence (measured by Wexner incontinence scale) and obstructed defecation (measured by Wexner constipation scale) after both laparoscopic VMR and laparoscopic posterior suture rectopexy [16]. After 1 year, GIQoL improved significantly in all patients in both cohorts but was significantly higher after VMR (p = 0.05). After VMR, 50% of patients reported improvement in pre-existing constipation compared to 23% of patients after posterior suture rectopexy, which was significant (p = 0.04). There was no significant difference in fecal incontinence between the two procedures.

Altemeier Versus Delorme Procedure

Two factorial randomized trials, PROSPER and the more recent trial reported by Smedberg et al., performed additional comparison of outcomes after Altemeier vs. Delorme procedures [2, 3].

Morbidity

The PROSPER trial did not compare postoperative complications but described outcomes in both cohorts [2]. Four mortalities were reported following perineal procedures, 2 following Altemeier and 2 following Delorme. Other serious complications included 4 anastomotic leakages in the Altemeier group, though one of the patients had been randomized to receive Delorme. Three of these patients were men and were demographically distinct from most of the study population. Overall morbidity was similar in the randomized trial reported by Smedberg et al. [3]. Most complications were Clavien-Dindo Grade I or II, with 5 total complications reported in the Delorme cohort and 10 total complications reported in the Altemeier cohort (p = 0.331) including one mortality 11 days after discharge deemed unrelated to the surgery.

Recurrence

The PROSPER trial found fewer recurrences after Altemeier compared to Delorme (25% versus 31%), but this difference was not significant (p = 0.4) [2]. Smedberg et al. reported recurrence rates favoring Altemeier over Delorme, but at no time point were these differences significant [3]. Authors reported recurrence rates at 3 months, 1 year, 3 years, and in longer-term follow-up. Recurrence at 1 year was 50% following Delorme and 32% following Altemeier (p = 0.203). Recurrence at more than 3 years was 58% following Delorme and 47% following Altemeier (p = 0.345).

Function and Quality of Life

The PROSPER trial reported no significant differences in bowel function and quality of life scores following Delorme versus Altemeier procedures as measured by the Vaizey score, the Bowel thermometer, and the EQ-5D [2]. In both cases, scores improved from baseline to 6 weeks, and were maintained at 1 and 3 years postoperatively. Smedberg et al. had higher baseline Wexner incontinence scores in patients randomized to Delorme (14.9) versus Altemeier (10.7) ($p = 0.005$), but reported similar scores at 3 months, 1 and 3 years with long-term scores of 8.6 in both groups ($p = 0.995$) [3].

Recommendations

Surgical treatment options for rectal prolapse continue to expand and evolve. There is not a single gold-standard approach. There are numerous factors that influence a surgeon's recommended surgical approach.

Abdominal prolapse repairs continue to have a lower recurrence rate compared to perineal approaches (evidence quality strong). As minimally invasive abdominal approaches continue to mature with shorter operative time, minimal postoperative pain and faster return to normal activity, this approach can be performed on high-risk patients with minimal morbidity (evidence quality moderate; weak recommendation). Perineal proctosigmoidectomy (Altemeier) confers greater advantage over Delorme repair with lower recurrence rate as well as improved function and quality of life (evidence quality moderate; weak recommendation). There is insubstantial evidence to guide the choice of perineal repair versus ventral mesh rectopexy. There is no advantage proven in surgical approach (laparoscopic versus robotic) for rectopexy (evidence quality moderate; weak recommendation). Ventral rectopexy consistently improves functional outcomes relating to constipation, mechanical outlet obstruction, and fecal incontinence (evidence quality moderate, weak recommendation). Ventral mesh rectopexy is favored over posterior suture rectopexy in functional outcome improvement (evidence quality moderate, weak recommendation). The risk of mesh related complications after ventral mesh rectopexy is <1%. However, the risk of recurrent after ventral mesh rectopexy is lower than suture rectopexy. The risks and benefits of prolapse repair using mesh should be specifically discussed with patients preoperatively (evidence quality moderate, strong recommendation).

Personal View

The evaluation and treatment approach to rectal prolapse has evolved rapidly over the last 5 years as the surgical treatment for pelvic floor related disorders and symptoms has improved. The fact that all surgical treatment options continue to carry a risk of recurrent prolapse indicates that there is still more to learn and better techniques and approaches that can be performed. Minimally invasive abdominal approaches for repair of rectal prolapse are safe for high-risk patients and continue to have a lower risk of recurrence. Thus, the appeal of perineal approaches has faded rapidly. In fact, we reserve Altemeier repairs for young men with full thickness rectal prolapse who have low anal tone. Perineal repairs have the lowest risk of injury to nerves of sexual function. Additionally, this population of patients tends to have a significant behavioral component of habitually straining which is less likely to result in deterioration of repair after Altemeier compared to all of the "pexy" procedures.

Women in the fifth to seventh decade of life are most afflicted by rectal prolapse. This patient population is also the most likely to experience symptoms of urinary incontinence and urgency, pelvic pressure, fecal urgency, bowel habit irregularity, and incomplete defecation. This constellation of symptoms is commonly associated with multicompartment pelvic organ prolapse. Occasionally, pelvic organ prolapse will include laxity in one or more compartments that is frankly visible on resting exam. But commonly, laxity in one or more pelvic compartments is not visible on exam, and pelvic floor testing is the only means of identifying the extent of pelvic floor laxity. Studies such as defecography, anal manometry, and urodynamics can be used to identify points of weakness that contribute to a patient's constellation of symptoms. Identifying all points of dysfunctional laxity may require multidisciplinary collaboration for evaluation and treatment. Neglecting to address dysfunctional laxity in one compartment while fixing another compartment may compromise the repair or exacerbate dysfunction in the untreated compartment. The growing enthusiasm to evaluate and treat pelvic organ prolapse in a multidisciplinary fashion has likely been instrumental in the increased frequency of robotic approach utilization since port site layout and instruments can more easily be shared between specialists compared to the laparoscopic approach.

VMR has earned a spot amongst the most commonly performed and most effective surgeries for treatment of rectal prolapse. This approach targets strengthening of the tissue in the rectovaginal septum. The anterior rectum and posterior vagina are incredibly dynamic in women during defecation. Conversely, men have inherent stability along the anterior rectal wall due to the prostate. In women with normal pelvic floor coordination, ballooning of the anterior rectal wall into a large rectocele during defecation can be the initial structural laxity that results in internal intussusception of the anterior rectal wall and subsequent prolapse. Similarly, loss of support of the uterus can result in exaggerated posterior and inferior positioning of the uterus, cervix and/or bladder. This exaggerated posterior positioning results in increased pressure and stress to the anterior rectal wall, which can also contribute to rectal intussusception and prolapse. Ultimately, the only female pelvic structures that are uniformly sturdy with age are the pubic bone and tailbone. Pelvic organ laxity and loss of connective tissue strength with age require surgical repairs that provide new strength and structure to the most susceptible areas. VMR is ideal for providing support to the anterior rectal wall and posterior vagina. When combined with sacrocolpopexy, this surgery can provide even greater support in the pelvis.

Unfortunately, the constellation of symptoms typical of pelvic organ prolapse are non-specific and can also be secondary to other pelvic floor disorders. Thus, it is imperative to confirm the underlying cause of symptoms with examination and testing. Failure to accurately identify the underlying cause of symptoms and inappropriate patient selection for surgery will result in poor outcomes and even complications. For example, obstructive defecation caused by pelvic floor tension and failure of appropriate muscle coordination results in poor relaxation with Valsalva and symptoms of incomplete defecation, overflow seepage, and urgency. All of these symptoms mimic internal prolapse. However, treating a patient that has significant pelvic tension and poor coordination with placement of mesh will *worsen* the stiffness and lack of pelvic movement. Again, caution and a systematic approach to the diagnosis of pelvic floor disorder symptoms is imperative.

In conclusion, we fully expect that the data presented in this chapter will continue to evolve as our understanding of rectal prolapse and associated pelvic organ prolapse improves. Longstanding perineal approaches will continue to be a safe option for repair, yet the patients who will benefit most from this approach may change over time. We think the most exciting advance in rectal prolapse treatment is the recognition that this problem rarely occurs in isolation of other pelvic compartment laxity. This recognition has led to new operative approaches, new surgical techniques, and multidisciplinary collaboration.

References

1. Kim DS, et al. Complete rectal prolapse: evolution of management and results. Dis Colon Rectum. 1999;42(4):460–6; discussion 466–9.
2. Senapati A, et al. PROSPER: a randomised comparison of surgical treatments for rectal prolapse. Color Dis. 2013;15(7):858–68.
3. Smedberg J, Graf W, Pekkari K, Hjern F. Comparison of four surgical approaches for rectal prolapse: multicentre randomized clinical trial. BJS Open. 2022 Jan 6;6(1):zrab140.
4. Deen KI, et al. Abdominal resection rectopexy with pelvic floor repair vs. perineal rectosigmoidectomy and pelvic floor repair for full-thickness rectal prolapse. Br J Surg. 1994;81(2):302–4.
5. Emile SH, Elbanna H, Youssef M, Thabet W, Omar W, Elshobaky A, Abd El-Hamed TM, Farid M. Laparoscopic ventral mesh rectopexy vs Delorme's operation in management of complete rectal prolapse: a prospective randomized study. Color Dis. 2017 Jan;19(1):50–7.
6. Ng ZQ, et al. Long-term outcomes of surgical management of rectal prolapse. ANZ J Surg. 2019;89(6):E231–5.
7. Hu B, Zou Q, Xian Z, Su D, Liu C, Lu L, Luo M, Chen Z, Cai K, Gao H, Peng H, Cao W, Ren D. External rectal prolapse: abdominal or perineal repair for men? A retrospective cohort study. Gastroenterol Rep (Oxf). 2022 Feb 21;10(1):goac007.
8. Bao X, Wang H, Song W, Chen Y, Luo Y. Meta-analysis on current status, efficacy, and safety of laparoscopic and robotic ventral mesh rectopexy for rectal prolapse treatment: can robotic surgery become the gold standard? Int J Color Dis. 2021 Aug;36(8):1685–94.
9. Albayati S, Chen P, Morgan MJ, Toh JWT. Robotic vs. laparoscopic ventral mesh rectopexy for external rectal prolapse and rectal intussusception: a systematic review. Tech Coloproctol. 2019 Jun;23(6):529–35.
10. Emile SH, Elfeki H, Shalaby M, Sakr A, Sileri P, Wexner SD. Outcome of laparoscopic ventral mesh rectopexy for full-thickness external rectal prolapse: a systematic review,

meta-analysis, and meta-regression analysis of the predictors for recurrence. Surg Endosc. 2019 Aug;33(8):2444–55.

11. Flynn J, Larach JT, Kong JCH, Warrier SK, Heriot A. Robotic versus laparoscopic ventral mesh rectopexy: a systematic review and meta-analysis. Int J Colorectal Dis. 2021 Aug;36(8):1621–31.
12. Lobb HS, Kearsey CC, Ahmed S, Rajaganeshan R. Suture rectopexy versus ventral mesh rectopexy for complete full-thickness rectal prolapse and intussusception: systematic review and meta-analysis. BJS Open. 2021 Jan 8;5(1):zraa037.
13. Hajibandeh S, Hajibandeh S, Arun C, Adeyemo A, McIlroy B, Peravali R. Meta-analysis of laparoscopic mesh rectopexy versus posterior sutured rectopexy for management of complete rectal prolapse. Int J Color Dis. 2021 Jul;36(7):1357–66.
14. Hidaka J, Elfeki H, Duelund-Jakobsen J, Laurberg S, Lundby L. Functional outcome after laparoscopic posterior sutured rectopexy versus ventral mesh rectopexy for rectal prolapse: six-year follow-up of a double-blind, randomized single-center study. eClinicalMedicine. 2019;16:18–22.
15. Lundby L, Iversen LH, Buntzen S, Wara P, Hoyer K, Laurberg S. Bowel function after laparoscopic posterior sutured rectopexy versus ventral mesh rectopexy for rectal prolapse: a double-blind, randomized single-centre study. Gastroenterol Hepatol. 2016 Dec;1(4):291–7.
16. Madbouly KM, Youssef M. Laparoscopic ventral rectopexy versus laparoscopic wells rectopexy for complete rectal prolapse: long-term results. J Laparoendosc Adv Surg Tech A. 2018 Jan;28(1):1–6.

Optimal Management of the Transsphincteric Anal Fistula

39

Shahrose Rahman and Vassiliki Liana Tsikitis

Introduction

The management of complex anal fistulas can be quite challenging for the surgeon and frustrating for the patient. These fistulas arise as an abnormal epithelial-line tract which connects the anal canal to the perianal skin and are mainly caused by cryptoglandular disease followed by inflammatory bowel disease. Up to 50% of anorectal abscesses will eventually develop into a fistula-in-ano. They are characterized using the Park's classification, established in 1976, which separates anal fistulas into four types based on its relation to the sphincter muscle: intersphincteric, transsphincteric, suprasphincteric, and extrasphincteric. The goals for the surgical management of fistulas are to (1) control sepsis, (2) define the anatomy, (3) preserve sphincter function, and (4) minimize the risk of recurrence. Over the years, a number "sphincter sparing" procedures have been developed to improve healing and reduce the risk of incontinence. The goal of this chapter is to review the literature pertaining specifically to transsphincteric fistulas and offer our opinion on best management options.

S. Rahman
Department of Surgery, Oregon Health & Science University, Portland, OR, USA
e-mail: Rahmasha@ohsu.edu

V. L. Tsikitis (✉)
Division of Gastrointestinal and General Surgery, School of Medicine, Oregon Health & Science University, Portland, OR, USA
e-mail: Tsikitis@ohsu.edu

K. Umanskiy, N. Hyman (eds.), *Difficult Decisions in Colorectal Surgery*, Difficult Decisions in Surgery: An Evidence-Based Approach,
https://doi.org/10.1007/978-3-031-42303-1_39

Search Strategy

In this chapter, we review the data behind the use of fistulotomy, seton placement, fibrin glue, fibrin plug, endorectal advancement flap (ERAF), ligation of intersphincteric fistula tract (LIFT), fistula laser closure (FiLaC), and video assisted anal fistula treatment (VAAFT). Table 39.1 summarizes the clinical results from the studies reviewed and analyzed.

We performed a literature search in the MEDLINE database (using PUBMED) under the search titles "transsphincteric fistula" (TSF) or "fistula-in-ano". Emphasis was placed on more recent studies published with in the last 7-years. Some older studies were included given absence of more recent data of some of the techniques that were evaluated. Table 39.2 outlines our search strategy.

Table 39.1 Summary of evidence reviewed

Author (year)	Procedure	Population	Number of subjects	Median follow-up (months)	Healing rate	Recurrence Rate	Incontinence rate
Abramowitz (2015)	Seton & Fistulotomy (2-stage)	High transsphincteric	62	12			Wexner score <5 pre vs post-intervention: 86 vs 66%
	Fistulotomy (1-stage)	Low transsphincteric	133				Wexner score <5 pre vs post-intervention: 88 vs 86%
Papaconstantinou (2017)	Fistulotomy	Low/mid-transsphincteric in Crohn's	29	18	96%	4%	20%
Wang (2016)	Serial seton followed by fistulotomy	Low transsphincteric fistula	21	11.9	100%	0%	0%
Rosen (2016)	Cutting seton (vessel loop)	Transsphincteric	121	5.1	97%		7%
Emile (2017)	Loose seton (silk #1)	High transsphincteric	251	16	89.6%	10.3%	3.2%
Ali (2022)	Cutting seton (silk #2)	High transsphincteric	72	12	97.2%	2.8%	1.4%
Diaz (2021)	ERAF, with fistulectomy	Transsphincteric low & medium: 83.4% High: 16.5%	115	155.5	76.2%	23.8%	16.9%

(continued)

Table 39.1 (continued)

Author (year)	Procedure	Population	Number of subjects	Median follow-up (months)	Healing rate	Recurrence Rate	Incontinence rate
Stellingwerf (2018)	ERAF	High perianal fistula	797	3–84	74.6%	25.6%	7.8%
	LIFT		498		69.1%	21.9%	1.6%
Seifarth (2021)	ERAF	Crohn's fistula	55	6.3	47%		
		Cryptoglandular fistula	100		60%		
Han (2016)	LIFT	High TSF	118	6	83.9%	0	0
	LIFT-plug		117		94%	0	0
Wexner (2020)	LIFT	Transsphincteric fistula	22		59%	41%	
Rojanasakul (2017)	LIFT	High TSF		71	60%		
		Low TSF			92%		
Altomare (2009)	Fibrin glue	TSF	39	12	39.5%		Wexner scores pre vs post-treatment: 0.67, 0.49
	Seton (majority cutting seton)	TSF	25		87.5%		1.79, 5.1
Oca (2011)	2-stage: (1) Fistulectomy with seton followed by (2) Fibrin glue	Mid and High TSF	28	20.6	68%	32%	

FIAT Trial (2021)	Plug	TSF	146	12	54%		
	Surgeons preference		146		55%		
Hansen (2019)	Plug	TSF	36	18	39%	26.3%	0%
Wilhelm (2017)	FiLaC	TSF	90	25.4	61.1%		0%
Marref (2019)	FiLaC	High TSF	45	6.3	60%		0%
		Low TSF	10		20%		0%
Elfekl (2020)	FiLaC	Fistula-in-ano 69% with TSF	454	23.7	67.3%		1%
Meinero (2011)	VAAFT	Fistula-in-ano 75.5% with high TSF	98	13	73.5%		
Meinero (2020)	VAAFT	Fistula-in-ano	96	36	83.3%		
Emile (2017)	VAAFT	Fistula-in-ano 66.5% with high TSF	788	9	85.8%	14.2%	

[a]transsphincteric fistula (TSF)

Table 39.2 Comparison of available approaches for management of transsphincteric fistulas

Patient population	Intervention	Comparator	Outcomes studied
Patients with transsphincteric fistulas	Fistulotomy	Sphincter-saving approaches	Healing rate, continence

Results

Fistulotomy

After the anatomy of a fistula is determined, a fistulotomy is performed by cannulating the fistula and dividing the overlying tissue with electrocautery. The wound is then left to heal by secondary intention after either fulguration, electrocautery, or marsupilizing the fistulous tract. Historically, a fistulotomy is appropriate for fistulas below the dentate line, including superficial, intersphincteric, and low transsphincteric fistulas. Success rates are generally high, however fecal incontinence rates are elevated in fistulotomies performed for complex or high transsphincteric fistulas.

Abramowitz in 2015 performed a prospective multi-center trial and performed seton placement and 2-stage fistulotomy for patients with high transsphincteric fistulas. They found a statistically significant increase in both the Wexner score (median score 1 pre-procedure and 4 at 1-year follow-up) and an increase in the Vaizey score (1.5 pre-procedure vs 4 at 1-year follow-up). The median scores in the 1-stage fistulotomy group were not statistically significant (Wexner 1 vs 2 at one-year follow-up; Vaizey 2 vs 3 at one-year follow-up) [1]. Papaconstantinou 2017 study found a fistulotomy an effective way to manage a low or mid-transsphincteric fistula in patients with Crohn's disease. However, 20% of these patients demonstrated incontinence which was defined as uncontrolled passage of flatus or <1 teaspoon passage of mucus in a 24-h period [2]. Wang et al's report is concurrent with the existing literature as they had no fistula recurrence following seton then fistulotomy for low transsphincteric fistulas. They also reported 0% incontinence rates however no validated questionnaires and scoring systems were utilized [3]. Overall, fistulotomy in one-stage, two-stage, or followed by seton placement is appropriate for patients with short tract fistulas and overall should be avoided in complex or high-transsphincteric fistulas given the increased risk of incontinence.

Seton

Two types of setons have been described to date. The first is a loose, non-cutting seton whose goal is to promote drainage, control sepsis, and allow for tract fibrosis. In higher risk patients, they can be left for years and used as definitive treatment; while for others it can be used in preparation for a secondary procedure. Loose setons are well tolerated with minimal risk. A cutting seton is serially tightened over time to bring the fistulous tract closer to the skin. The goal is to create a fibrous tract under the skin in an effort to preserve sphincter-function, although incontinence rates are reported to be increased compared to non-cutting setons.

Setons continue to be used with good success rates, even for high transsphincteric fistulas. The reported healing rate at 12-months was reported to be 97.2% in a series of 72 patients when a cutting seton (silk size 2) was used with only 2 patients (2.8%) recurring at 6-months. Of the 72 patients, 66.7% required two additional procedures for seton tightening and 33.3% required three procedures for tightening. Flatus incontinence occurred in 1 patient (1.4%) however no standardized questionnaires were used. Additionally, pruritus with perianal discharge was noted in 4 patients (6.9%) and was not considered to be incontinence [4]. This is in contrast to a large series review of 1460 patients that underwent a cutting seton. The authors report an overall incontinence rate of 12% and signify that an increased rate of incontinence was shown when location of the internal fistula opening was more proximal in the anal canal [5]. Alternatively, the use of a loose seton in a series of 251 patients with a high TSF had a near 90% healing rate with 10.3% recurring, however, half the subjects in their study had undergone previous surgery for fistula-in-ano [6].

Endorectal Advancement Flap

The endorectal advancement flap (ERAF) is typically used as a second-stage procedure following either seton placement or fistulectomy. With this procedure, a trapezoidal-shaped flap is created which includes the mucosa, submucosa, and a few fibers of the internal sphincter muscle. The internal opening of the fistula tract is then sutured closed and covered with the flap.

Perhaps one of the best long-term studies to recently be published on the use of ERAF was in a series of 115 patients with a transsphincteric fistula with a mean follow-up of 13 years. They reported a recurrence rate of 23.8%, with 90% of the recurrences occurring within the first year. Recurrence was defined as recurrent fistula tract, but also included presence of an abscess which may partially explain this higher recurrence rate. Taking this into account, the overall success rate was 76.2%. When assessing incontinence using the Wexner score, overall continence worsened in 16.9% of cases with a mean score of 0.78 pre-procedure compared to 1.16 >10 years at the conclusion of the study. When specifically assessing patients with normal continence pre-procedure, overall incontinence was documented in 10.5% of cases after ERAF [7]. This data is similar to a recent meta-analysis of 30 studies which included ERAF for the treatment of high perianal fistulas in 797 patients. They reported an overall success of 74.6%, recurrence in 25.6%, and an incontinence rate of 7.8%. The pooled data had a variation in follow-up which ranged from 3–84 months; however, a subgroup analysis of 12 studies with a minimum follow-up of 12-months demonstrated an overall success rate of 73.6% [8]. Other reported data continue to demonstrate the poor healing rates with ERAF in patients whose etiology for their fistula is due to Crohn's disease with 47% healed, compared to 60% in non-Crohn's patients, although this did not reach statistical significance ($p = 0.088$) [9].

Ligation of Intersphincteric Fistula Tract

The ligation of intersphincteric fistula tract (LIFT) procedure was designed as a total sphincter-preserving technique first described in 2007. It is used as a second stage procedure after the fistula tract has matured, either with or without a seton. In this procedure, the fistula tract is cannulated with a probe, then an incision is made over the intersphincteric groove and dissected down to the level of the fistula tract. Once the tract is circumferentially isolated, it is suture ligated and divided sharply without dividing the sphincter complex. Historically, LIFT is not used for very high fistula tracts due to the difficulty in isolating the intersphincteric plane.

In a 2016 study, Han et al. performed a randomized prospective study comparing LIFT vs LIFT with addition of a porcine plug placed into the curetted fistula tract. The healing rate was 83.9% healing in the LIFT group and 94% in the LIFT-plug group. There was no significant difference in the Wexner scores pre- and post-operatively and they ranged from 0 to 1 at 6-months post-op. They concluded that LIFT is an effective surgical technique with low impact on fecal incontinence [10]. However, these remarkable results were not replicated by Wexner's group who reported a 41% recurrence rate. Of 40 patients who had a pre-operative MRI, they stratified this data into laterality of the fistula tract and concluded that posterior transsphincteric fistula tracts carried the highest recurrence rates (5/7, 71%) compared to an anterior track (1/9, 11.1%) [11]. A more recent study by the creator of the LIFT procedure reported their ten-year experience of using the procedure. Of the 251 patients included, 56% had a low transsphincteric fistula and 6% had a high TSF. Of these, the primary healing rate was excellent in the low TSF at 92% and only 60% in high TSF. Of the 31 patients with an unhealed fistula regardless of classification, following either one or two repeat procedures (re-LIFT, fistulotomy, curettage, or spontaneous healing), only 2 of the 251 patients remained unhealed. The overall healing rate after primary surgery and reoperation was 99.2% [12].

Fibrin Sealant

Fibrin sealants were approved for use by the FDA in 1998 for the treatment of perianal fistula. Its primary benefit serves as having a minimal risk to profile given that there is no manipulation to the sphincter complex with fibrin administration. However, many insurance companies will not cover these expensive products given their reported low success rates. Fibrin sealants are not recommended as a first-line therapy, however given their low risk profile, they may be suitable when other surgical options are not achievable.

A 2009 randomized crossover trial was performed comparing setons to fibrin glue. This study was terminated early based on interim analysis given the high failure rates seen with fibrin administration. At 3-months, 87.5% of patients with a TSF who had a seton placed were healed compared to 38% in the fibrin arm. Of those who failed in the fibrin arm, 8 of the 23 went on to receive a second fibrin injection and 4/8 (50%) healed. The remaining 18/23 went on to have a seton placed and

10/23 (60%) healed. This study did include anal manometry results and found a poorer score in the seton compared to the fibrin group. However, a majority of the setons used in this group were cutting setons. They concluded that the higher success rate with seton is counterbalanced by the higher incontinence rate and fibrin should be considered for patients at higher risk for fecal incontinence [13].

Higher success rates with fibrin are seen when it is not used as the primary treatment modality. A 2011 study performed a fistulectomy with seton in 28 consecutive patients followed by seton removal and fibrin administration 12.5 months after the first procedure. By 21 months, 19/28 (68%) patients healed, of which 9 recurred. They demonstrate that fibrin may serve a complimentary role in the long-term treatment of TSF [14].

Plugs

Biosynthetic fistula plugs are inserted into the fistula tract and encourage tissue ingrowth and healing to close the tract. They have wide rates of healing however do not alter incontinence given no disruption of the sphincter occurs.

The Fistula-in-ano trial (FIAT) in 2009 was commissioned to perform a randomized control trial evaluating plug use versus surgeon preference. The results of the FIAT trial were reported in 2021. 304 subjects were recruited from 45 centers and randomized in a 1:1 ratio to plug versus surgeon's preference. At 12-months, 54% of fistulas in the plug arm were healed compared to 55% in the surgeon's preference arm. A 12-month MRI was also performed in 86% of patients and the healing rate judged by MRI was 49% for plug and 57% for surgeon's preference, though this was not statistically significant. There was also no difference in the incontinence scores between the two groups at 12-months. These comparable results with a higher cost procedure led to the FIAT trials conclusion that plugs are not a cost-effective treatment for anal fistulas in the UK NHS [15]. These results were similar to a prior study which reported outcomes of 36 patients who had a plug inserted. The initial healing rate was 52.8%, however by 18-months when adjusting for recurrence rate, the overall success rate was 39% [16]. These data demonstrate that plugs should not be the treatment of choice for TSF.

Fistula Laser Closure

Fistula laser closure (FiLaC) is a new sphincter-preserving technique developed in 2011 by Wilhelm et al. to be used in patients who were at high risk of incontinence after fistulotomy [17]. The technique utilizes a radial laser probe to burn the fistula tract. This circumferential heating works by obliterating and sealing the fistula tract.

After developing the procedure, Wilhelm reported his five-year experience with FiLaC in a series of 117 patients, 90 of whom had a TSF. They achieved a 61% primary healing rate, and a secondary healing rate of 88.9%, although only 5/31 secondary procedures were repeat FiLaC [18]. A separate 2019 prospective study reported that the only predictive factor for success with FiLaC is for high TSF's. The rate of healing in low TSF's were low at 20% compared to 60% for high TSF. A 2020 meta-analysis on 7 articles encompassing 454 patients was also performed to evaluate the efficacy of FiLaC [19]. 314/454 patients had a TSF. At a median follow-up of 23.7 months, 65% of patients achieved healing after primary FiLaC for all types of fistulas. They did not stratify healing rates based on fistula type. Notably, of the 158 patients who failed in the study, 97% did not achieve primary healing while only 3% had recurrence [20].

Video-Assisted Anal Fistula Treatment

Video-assisted anal fistula treatment (VAAFT) is a novel technique first described in 2006 [21]. The technique is performed by inserting a fistuloscope into the external opening. The internal opening and secondary tracts are then identified. These tracts are disrupted using electrocautery and the necrotic debris is removed using continuous irrigation and an endobrush. Finally, the internal opening is closed using either suture, an advancement flap, or an endostapler.

The outcomes of VAAFT were first published by Meinero and Mori in 2011 who reported their outcomes on a series of 98 patients, where 76% of the patient population had a high trans-sphincteric fistula. These patients achieved a primary healing rate of 73.5% by 6-months [21]. Meinero also recently published 3-year outcomes on patients undergoing VAAFT in 2020. This was a different patient population from their original study, and they again had convincing results. By 3-years, 80/96 (83.3%) of patients achieved healing of their fistula [22]. These results were corroborated by a meta-analysis performed in 788 patients, 66.5% of whom had a high or complex FIA. At a median follow-up of 9-months, 14.2% of patients had a recurrence with a heal rate of 85.8%. Interestingly, when stratified by type of closure used for the internal opening, the highest recurrence rate occurred after advancement flap (25%), followed by suture-closure (17.7%), then stapler (15.3%) [23]. This data demonstrates VAAFT as being a promising management option for the treatment of fistulas in the future.

Conclusion and Personal View

One of the difficulties in evaluating studies related to the treatment of TSFs are that many of the patients have had one or more prior surgical procedures prior to study enrollment. Additionally, outcomes are not all defined the same. For example, patients' outcomes will be reported as "primary healing" based on the study intervention rather than accounting for the prior fistula procedures they have received. The definition of fecal or stool incontinence also vary among studies, although the use of the Wexner and Vaizey scores provide an objective measure that help alleviate this issue.

In our practice, the approach to TSF depends on the length of the fistula tract and patients' current anatomy and sphincter function. Overall, after control of the initial infection and possible sepsis, our goal for subsequent procedures is to balance the risk of fecal incontinence with the risk of recurrence while addressing the patients' needs. Our initial approach includes either an MRI of the pelvis or an exam under anesthesia to delineate the fistula tract. During an exam under anesthesia, after delineation of the fistula tract, we may concurrently proceed with either a simple fistulotomy if the tract is short and superficial or with a placement of a draining seton if the fistula tract is long and complex. A draining seton may stay for a period of 8–12 weeks and then we will proceed with either a LIFT or ERAF procedure. Our preference is ERAF over LIFT when the fistula tract is long and complex; however, studies demonstrate that results are equivalent between the two procedures.

At this juncture, complex TSF still poses a challenge to the colorectal surgeon; it is fundamental that the patient understands the anatomical limitations and the technical complexities associated with each approach and shared decision-making may be entertained addressing the patients' needs and preferences.

References

1. Abramowitz L, Soudan D, Souffran M, Bouchard D, Castinel A, Suduca JM, Staumont G, Devulder F, Pigot F, Ganansia R, Varastet M; Groupe de Recherche en Proctologie de la Société Nationale Française de Colo-Proctologie and the Club de Réflexion des cabinets et Groupe d'Hépato-Gastroentérologie. The outcome of fistulotomy for anal fistula at 1 year: a prospective multicentre French study. Color Dis 2016 Mar;18(3):279–285. https://doi.org/10.1111/codi.13121. PMID: 26382623.
2. Papaconstantinou I, Kontis E, Koutoulidis V, Mantzaris G, Vassiliou I. Surgical Management of Fistula-in-ano among Patients with Crohn's disease: analysis of outcomes after Fistulotomy or Seton placement-single-center experience. Scand J Surg 2017 Sep;106(3):211–215. https://doi.org/10.1177/1457496916665763. Epub 2016 Aug 22. PMID: 27550245.
3. Wang C, Rosen L. Management of low transsphincteric anal fistula with serial setons and interval muscle-cutting fistulotomy. J Integr Med 2016 Mar;14(2):154–158. https://doi.org/10.1016/S2095-4964(16)60229-7. PMID: 26988437.
4. Elnaim Ali ALK, Wong MP, Sagap I. The value of cutting seton for high Transsphincteric anal Fistula in the era of its misery. Malays J Med Sci. 2022 Feb;29(1):55–61. https://doi.org/10.21315/mjms2022.29.1.6. Epub 2022 Feb 23. PMID: 35283682; PMCID: PMC8887976.
5. Ritchie RD, Sackier JM, Hodde JP. Incontinence rates after cutting seton treatment for anal fistula. Color Dis 2009 Jul;11(6):564–571. https://doi.org/10.1111/j.1463-1318.2008.01713.x. Epub 2008 Oct 17. PMID: 19175623.
6. Emile SH, Elfeki H, Thabet W, Sakr A, Magdy A, El-Hamed TMA, Omar W, Khafagy W. Predictive factors for recurrence of high transsphincteric anal fistula after placement of seton. J Surg Res 2017 Jun 1;213:261–268. https://doi.org/10.1016/j.jss.2017.02.053. Epub 2017 Mar 6. PMID: 28601324.
7. Chaveli Diaz C, Esquiroz Lizaur I, Marzo Virto J, Oteiza Martínez F, Gonzalez Álvarez G, de Miguel Velasco M, Ciga Lozano MÁ. Fistulectomy and endorectal advancement flap repair for cryptoglandular anal fistula: recurrence and functional outcome over 10 years of follow-up. Int J Color Dis 2021 Apr;36(4):841–846. https://doi.org/10.1007/s00384-021-03867-0. Epub 2021 Feb 12. PMID: 33580275.
8. Stellingwerf ME, van Praag EM, Tozer PJ, Bemelman WA, Buskens CJ. Systematic review and meta-analysis of endorectal advancement flap and ligation of the intersphincteric fistula tract

for cryptoglandular and Crohn's high perianal fistulas. BJS Open. 2019 Jan 21;3(3):231–241. https://doi.org/10.1002/bjs5.50129. Erratum in: BJS Open. 2020 Feb;4(1):166–167. PMID: 31183438; PMCID: PMC6551488.

9. Seifarth C, Lehmann KS, Holmer C, Pozios I. Healing of rectal advancement flaps for anal fistulas in patients with and without Crohn's disease: a retrospective cohort analysis. BMC Surg. 2021 Jun 5;21(1):283. https://doi.org/10.1186/s12893-021-01282-4. PMID: 34088303; PMCID: PMC8178918.
10. Han JG, Wang ZJ, Zheng Y, Chen CW, Wang XQ, Che XM, Song WL, Cui JJ. Ligation of Intersphincteric fistula tract vs ligation of the Intersphincteric fistula tract plus a bioprosthetic anal fistula plug procedure in patients with Transsphincteric anal fistula: early results of a multicenter prospective randomized trial. Ann Surg 2016 Dec;264(6):917–922. https://doi.org/10.1097/SLA.0000000000001562. PMID: 26606429.
11. Sarmiento-Cobos M, Rosen L, Wasser E, Yang F, Wexner SD. High failure rates following ligation of the intersphincteric fistula tract for transsphincteric anal fistulas: are preoperative MRI measurements of the fistula tract predictive of outcome? Color Dis 2021 Apr;23(4):932–936. https://doi.org/10.1111/codi.15452. Epub 2020 Dec 4. PMID: 33222365.
12. Malakorn S, Sammour T, Khomvilai S, Chowchankit I, Gunarasa S, Kanjanasilp P, Thiptanakij C, Rojanasakul A. Ligation of Intersphincteric fistula tract for fistula in Ano: lessons learned from a decade of experience. Dis Colon Rectum 2017 Oct;60(10):1065–1070. https://doi.org/10.1097/DCR.0000000000000880. PMID: 28891850.
13. Altomare DF, Greco VJ, Tricomi N, Arcanà F, Mancini S, Rinaldi M, Pulvirenti d'Urso A, La Torre F. Seton or glue for trans-sphincteric anal fistulae: a prospective randomized crossover clinical trial. Color Dis 2011 Jan;13(1):82–86. https://doi.org/10.1111/j.1463-1318.2009.02056.x. PMID: 19832873.
14. de Oca J, Millán M, Jiménez A, Golda T, Biondo S. Long-term results of surgery plus fibrin sealant for anal fistula. Color Dis 2012 Jan;14(1):e12–e15. https://doi.org/10.1111/j.1463-1318.2011.02747.x. PMID: 21819522.
15. Jayne DG, Scholefield J, Tolan D, Gray R, Senapati A, Hulme CT, Sutton AJ, Handley K, Hewitt CA, Kaur M, Magill L; FIAT Trial Collaborative Group. A multicenter randomized controlled trial comparing safety, efficacy, and cost-effectiveness of the Surgisis anal fistula plug versus Surgeon's preference for Transsphincteric fistula-in-Ano: the FIAT trial. Ann Surg 2021 Mar 1;273(3):433–441. https://doi.org/10.1097/SLA.0000000000003981. PMID: 32516229.
16. Hansen MS, Kjær ML, Andersen J. Efficacy of plug treatment for complex Anorectal Fistulae: long-term Danish results. Ann Coloproctol. 2019 Mar 20;35(3):123–128. https://doi.org/10.3393/ac.2018.07.14. Epub ahead of print. PMID: 30889947; PMCID: PMC6625774.
17. Wilhelm A. A new technique for sphincter-preserving anal fistula repair using a novel radial emitting laser probe. Tech Coloproctol 2011 Dec;15(4):445–449. https://doi.org/10.1007/s10151-011-0726-0. Epub 2011 Aug 16. PMID: 21845480.
18. Wilhelm A, Fiebig A, Krawczak M. Five years of experience with the FiLaC™ laser for fistula-in-ano management: long-term follow-up from a single institution. Tech Coloproctol. 2017 Apr;21(4):269–276. https://doi.org/10.1007/s10151-017-1599-7. Epub 2017 Mar 7. PMID: 28271331; PMCID: PMC5423928.
19. Marref I, Spindler L, Aubert M, Lemarchand N, Fathallah N, Pommaret E, Soudan D, Pillant-le Moult H, Safa Far E, Fellous K, Crochet E, Mory B, Benfredj P, de Parades V. The optimal indication for FiLaC® is high trans-sphincteric fistula-in-ano: a prospective cohort of 69 consecutive patients. Tech Coloproctol 2019 Sep;23(9):893–897. https://doi.org/10.1007/s10151-019-02077-9. Epub 2019 Sep 26. PMID: 31559547.
20. Elfeki H, Shalaby M, Emile SH, Sakr A, Mikael M, Lundby L. A systematic review and meta-analysis of the safety and efficacy of fistula laser closure. Tech Coloproctol 2020 Apr;24(4):265–274. https://doi.org/10.1007/s10151-020-02165-1. Epub 2020 Feb 17. PMID: 32065306.

21. Meinero P, Mori L. Video-assisted anal fistula treatment (VAAFT): a novel sphincter-saving procedure for treating complex anal fistulas. Tech Coloproctol. 2011 Dec;15(4):417–422. https://doi.org/10.1007/s10151-011-0769-2. Epub 2011 Oct 15. Erratum in: Tech Coloproctol. 2012 Feb;16(1):111. PMID: 22002535; PMCID: PMC3226694.
22. Regusci L, Fasolini F, Meinero P, Caccia G, Ruggeri G, Serati M, Braga A. Video-assisted anal fistula treatment (VAAFT) for complex anorectal fistula: efficacy and risk factors for failure at 3-year follow-up. Tech Coloproctol 2020 Jul;24(7):741–746. https://doi.org/10.1007/s10151-020-02213-w. Epub 2020 Apr 21. PMID: 32318991.
23. Emile SH, Elfeki H, Shalaby M, Sakr A. A systematic review and meta-analysis of the efficacy and safety of video-assisted anal fistula treatment (VAAFT). Surg Endosc 2018 Apr;32(4):2084–2093. https://doi.org/10.1007/s00464-017-5905-2. Epub 2017 Oct 19. PMID: 29052068.

Chronic and Refractory Anal Fissure: What Are the Treatment Options?

40

Ga-ram Han and Nitin Mishra

Introduction

Anal fissures are one of the most common causes of perianal pain with a cumulative lifetime risk of 11% [1]. Most acute anal fissures resolve with conservative management using stool softeners and fiber supplements to ensure bulky, soft and regular bowel movements. The regimen can also include sitz baths, and topical analgesics such as lidocaine gel [2]. In a small but significant number of patients, symptoms persist for longer than 4 to 8 weeks, at which time it is categorized as a chronic anal fissure (CAF). The underlying pathophysiology leading to a tear in the anoderm is not fully understood, but it is thought that they may result from local trauma caused by a hard bowel movement or explosive diarrhea further exacerbated by chronic ischemia from a hypertonic anal sphincter.

Multiple non-operative and operative treatments for CAF have been studied with varying degrees of healing, recurrence, and side effects. The goal of most of these treatments is to reduce sphincter tone or spasm which in turn improves the blood supply to the anal mucosa to allow for wound healing. Some operative methods such as mucosal advancement flaps are focused on wound coverage, and therefore, may be more appropriate for patients without high anal sphincter tone. Medical therapies are typically employed initially but have a lower rate of healing and higher rate of recurrence when compared to surgical procedures. Internal sphincterotomy

G.-r. Han
Department of General Surgery, Division of Colon and Rectal Surgery, Mayo Clinic, Phoenix, AZ, USA
e-mail: Han.Ga-ram@mayo.edu

N. Mishra (✉)
Department of Colon and Rectal Surgery, Mayo Clinic, Phoenix, AZ, USA
e-mail: Mishra.Nitin@mayo.edu

K. Umanskiy, N. Hyman (eds.), *Difficult Decisions in Colorectal Surgery*, Difficult Decisions in Surgery: An Evidence-Based Approach,
https://doi.org/10.1007/978-3-031-42303-1_40

Table 40.1 PICO table

P (Patients)	I (Intervention)	C (Comparator)	O (Outcomes)
Patients with chronic or recurrent anal fissure	Surgical management	Non-operative management (Medical therapy, Botulinum toxin injection)	Cure, Recurrence, Postoperative incontinence, Side-effects

is the most effective treatment but may lead to transient or permanent anal incontinence. Given these nuances, choosing the most appropriate treatment for patients with chronic or recurrent anal fissures can be challenging.

Search Strategy

A comprehensive literature search of PubMed, MEDLINE, and the Cochrane Database of Systematic Reviews and Central Register of Controlled Trials was performed from 2012 to 2022 to identify all English-language publications in adult patients related to treatment outcomes for chronic or refractory anal fissure (Table 40.1). A combination of keywords and subject headings included "fissure in ano" or "chronic and refractory anal fissure" or "chronic anal fissure" or "refractory anal fissure" or "anal fissure" and "surgical flaps" or "sphincterotomy" or "fissurectomy" or "surgical procedures" or "surgery" or "drug therapy" or "topical nitrate" or "botulinum toxin injection" or "nifedipine" or "diltiazem" or "topical calcium channel blocker" or "calcium channel blockers" and "treatment outcome" or "outcome" or "recurrence" or "cure" or "incontinence" or "pain" or "bleeding" or "infection" or "pelvic sepsis" or "complications." A total of 149 papers were identified in the searches. After Endnote de-duplication, there were 128 remaining papers. Exclusion criteria consisted of results that were out of scope or did not address treatment options for chronic or refractory anal fissures. The results were further filtered to include only systematic reviews, meta-analyses, and randomized controlled trials (RCT). Publications that contained inconsistent results between the body of the text and the tables or figures were also excluded. Ultimately, our search strategy produced 29 studies for inclusion – 18 RCTs (Table 40.2) and 11 systematic reviews or meta-analyses (Table 40.3).

Results

Treatment options that have been investigated for management of CAF include medical therapy with topical nitrates or topical calcium channel blockers (CCB), botulinum toxin injection (BT), operative interventions such as lateral internal sphincterotomy (LIS), anal advancement flaps (AAF), fissurectomy, or anal dilation, and a combination of these various treatments. With each of these treatment options, patients are encouraged to continue the conservative therapies for anal

Table 40.2 Randomized controlled trials studying the treatment of chronic and refractory anal fissures

First Author	Yr	F/U	Pt, n	Intervention: n	Rate of healing	Resolution of pain	Recurrence rate	Incontinence rate	A/E	Conclusions
Comparing topical medications										
Ala	2012	Review q2 wk	61	0.2% GTN: 25	60%	100%	NR	NR	100% HA; 48% Constipation; 40% Pruritis	**DTZ** is more effective with fewer A/E
				2% DTZ: 36	91.7%	100%	NR	NR	No HA; 5.6% Constipation; 8.3% Pruritis	
Bulus	2013	Review at 1 wk for complications Review after 8 wk	55	0.2% Isosorbide 5 mononitrate: 18	77.8%	55.6%	NR	0%	22.2% HA; 11.1% Pruritis	These agents are not significantly superior to each other
				2% DTZ: 18	72.2%	27.8%	NR	0%	5.6% HA; 11.1% Pruritis; 5.6% Perianal dermatitis	
				2% DTZ + 0.1% Isosorbide 5 mononitrate: 19	73.7%	42.1%	NR	0%	15.8% HA; 26.3% Pruritis; 5.3% ED	
Ala	2015	Review q10 days for 60 days	50	0.5% Captopril: 24	NR	NR. No significant difference in reduction of pain scores.	NR	NR	45.8% Pruritis	**DTZ** is recommended over captopril due to pruritis with captopril. They are equally effective in managing symptoms of CAF.
				2% DTZ: 26	NR		NR	NR	No pruritis. 7% Mild HA. 3.8% Vertigo. 3.8% Constipation.	

(continued)

Table 40.2 (continued)

First Author	Yr	F/U	Pt, n	Intervention: n	Rate of healing	Resolution of pain	Recurrence rate	Incontinence rate	A/E	Conclusions
Shrestha	2017	Review q2 wk for 2 mo for healing. Review q2 mo for 6 mo for recurrence	90	2% GTN: 45	60%	NR	23.8%	NR	16.6% (HA, flushing)	**Nifedipine** has a higher healing rate and fewer recurrences and A/E.
				0.5% Nifedipine: 45	82.5%	NR	18.1%	NR	6.9%	
Khan	2017	Review at 1 mo	184	0.2% GTN: 92	62%	63%	NR	NR	NR	**DTZ** has better outcomes in healing and reduction of symptoms
				2% DTZ: 92	80.4%	72.8%	NR	NR	NR	
Emile	2020	Review q1 wk for 1 mo, then q2 wk for another mo	62	5% Minoxidil: 30	76.5% (shorter duration to healing)	NR. Both had a significant decrease in pain scores with a significantly lower score with GTN.	NR	None	6.6% Pruritis	Minoxidil had greater and quicker healing with fewer adverse effects, but post-treatment pain scores were lower with GTN.
				0.2% GTN: 32	46.9%		NR	None	40.6% (21.9% HA, 15.6% Postural hypotension, 3.1% Palpitations)	
Ruiz-Tovar	2022	Review at 2, 8 and 24 wk	160	100% Tocopherol acetate: 80	86.3%	87.5%	2.9%	NR	None	**Tocopherol acetate** had lower pain scores, higher healing rate and a lower recurrence rate.
				0.4% GTN: 80	66.3%	70%	13.2%	NR	27.5% Mild-moderate HA, 17.5% Severe HA	

Comparing BT alone to BT + Topical medications										
Asim	2014	Review at 6 and 12 wk	41	20U BT: 21	57%	No difference in pain scores after treatment.	NR	14.3%	1 pt with severe HA (reported to have these at baseline)	No significant differences in healing rates. **BT alone** was better tolerated.
				20U BT + 0.1% GTN: 20	50%		NR	None	79% HA (58% Moderate-severe)	
Comparing LIS to Topical medications										
Arslan	2012	Review at 1, 2, 3, 6 and 12 mo	207	LIS: 102	97.1%	NR	1%	5.9% (Moderate; all improved by 6 mo)	3.9% Ecchymosis. 6.9% Bleeding. 3.9% Urinary retention. 1% Perianal wetness.	Medical treatment should be the first line treatment. With the high success rate, few side-effects and easy application, **isosorbide dinitrate may be the first choice** for medical treatment. **LIS remains the gold standard.**
				0.25-0.5% Isosorbide dintrate: 105 (Dose increased from 0.25% to 0.5% if not healed after 1 mo)	77.1%	NR	4.8%	0%	6.7% HA	

(continued)

Table 40.2 (continued)

First Author	Yr	F/U	Pt, n	Intervention: n	Rate of healing	Resolution of pain	Recurrence rate	Incontinence rate	A/E	Conclusions
De Rosa	2013	Review at 2, 4 and 8 wk	142	LIS: 68	88.2%	86.8% after 7d	NR	2.9% (Gas)	No HA. 1.5% Anal irritation. 1.5% Anal abscess.	**LIS** is an effective, less painful, fast recovery treatment with an often-overestimated incontinence rate. Topical nifedipine is effective but side-effects can sometimes compromise compliance.
				Warm anal dilator with 0.3% Nifedipine + 1.5% Lidocaine: 74	68.9%	52.7% after 7d	NR	None	1.4% HA causing non-compliance and withdrawal. 2.7% Anal irritation.	
Butt	2017	Review at 8 wk	60	LIS: 30	100%	NR	NR	3.3% (n=1; Incontinence to flatus)	None (other than incontinence)	**LIS** is better than GTN and is the **gold standard** treatment.
				2% GTN: 30	73.3%	NR	NR	None	100% HA (20% discontinued Tx due to severe HA)	

Acar	2020	Review at 1, 2, 4 and 8 wk.	550	LIS: 200	93%	91%	4%	2% (1% Gas – resolved in 4 mo; 1% fluid)	1% Perianal abscess. 1% Thrombosed hemorrhoids.	**LIS** is the **gold standard** when clinicians would like to avoid recurrence and obtain the best pain relief. **pLIS** can be considered as an **effective alternative with a lower risk of incontinence. Medical** treatment may be tried as the **first step**.
				pLIS: 50	86%	84%	12%	2% (gas – resolved in 6 mo)	None	
				2% DTZ: 150	68.7%	68%	NR	None	2% Nausea. 1.3% Arrhythmia.	
				0.2% GTN: 150	62.7%	74%	NR	None	14.7% HA (4% severe HA).	
Comparing LIS to BT										
Valizadeh	2012	Review at 1 and 2 wk, and at 2, 3, 6, and 12 mo.	50	LIS: 25	92%	NR	12%	48% (4% Persistent intermittent incontinence to gas/fluid at 12 mo)	4% Hematoma. 8% Bleeding.	Treatment should be **individualized**. BT has a higher recurrence rate. LIS provides rapid and permanent recovery with a higher risk of incontinence.
				50U BT: 25	80%	NR	48%	12% (No incontinence at 3 mo)	NR	

(continued)

Table 40.2 (continued)

First Author	Yr	F/U	Pt, n	Intervention: n	Rate of healing	Resolution of pain	Recurrence rate	Incontinence rate	A/E	Conclusions
Nour	2020	Review at 1 wk, and at 1, 2, 3, 6, 9 and 12 mo.	96	LIS: 48	91.7%	Significantly higher pain scores after 1 wk in LIS than BT group	13.5%	10.4% (4.2% Persistent gas incontinence)	4.2% Bleeding.	**BT is safer** but with **less efficacy** and its **dose needs to be adjusted**. **LIS** is **more effective** but **anal sphincter tone** needs to be assessed preoperatively.
				80U BT: 48	77.1%		2.3%	16.6% (Transient)	2.1% Ecchymosis.	
Comparing pLIS to BT + Topical medications										
Gandomkar	2015	Review at 1 wk, and at 1, 2, 6 and 12 mo.	99	pLIS: 50	94%	Reduction of ≥50% pain score: - pLIS: 94% - BT + DTZ: 67.3%	None	16% (2% Persistent)	44% Urinary retention. 8% Pruritis.	**BT + DTZ can be as effective** as pLIS in pt **with sx ≤12 mo**. In CAF of **longer duration, pLIS** has a significantly higher cure rate.
				150U BT + DTZ: 49	65.3% (Sx ≤12 mo = no difference. Sx >12 mo = pLIS significantly higher)		10%	4.1% (Resolved after a few days)	6.2% Urinary retention. 4.1% Ecchymosis. 36.7% Pruritis.	
Comparing LIS to TENS										
Youssef	2015	Review at 1 day, 1 wk, and at 1 and 3 mo, and then q3 mo x 1 yr.	73	LIS: 37	89.1%	100% with improved pain at 1 mo and 97.3% at 1 yr.	2.7%	8.1% (2.7% Persistent intermittent gas incontinence)	8.1% Hematoma.	**LIS** remains the gold standard. TENS is non-invasive and without complications. It may be reserved for pt who deny surgical intervention.
		Review at 1 and 3 mo, and then q3 mo x1 yr.		TENS: 36	72.2%	75% with improved pain at 1 mo and 44.4% at 1 yr	40.7%	None	None	

Comparing surgical procedures										
Magdy	2012	Review at 1 wk, and then 3, 6, and 12 mo. Seen in clinic if sx developed.	150	LIS: 50	88%	Significantly higher rate of pain relief with combined Tailored LIS + V-Y advancement flap group	4%	14%	4% Ecchymosis.	**Tailored LIS with V-Y advancement flap** has the greatest healing rate, lowest recurrence rate, greatest patient satisfaction and highest improvements in quality of life with few complications.
				V-Y advancement flap: 50	70%		22%	None	6% Flap ischemia. 4% Partial flap breakdown. 2% Sepsis.	
				Tailored LIS + V-Y advancement flap: 50	96%		2%	2%	4% Flap ischemia. 2% Partial flap breakdown. 2% Sepsis. 2% Ecchymosis.	
Bara	2021	Review at 2 wk, and then 1 and 2 mo, and then telephone conversation for the next 6 mo.	80	LIS: 40	NR	NR	5%	17.5% Gas incontinence. 12.5% Liquid incontinence. 2.5% Solid incontinence.	10% Urinary retention.	**LIS** is a better treatment option than fissurectomy. There are **less postoperative complications but higher recurrence rate** with LIS.
				Anal dilatation + Fissurectomy: 40	NR	NR	None	40% Gas incontinence. 32.5% Liquid incontinence. 17.5% Solid incontinence.	30% Urinary retention.	

Abbreviations: *Yr* Year, *F/U* Follow-up, *A/E* Adverse events, *NR* Not reported, *GTN* Glyceryl trinitrate, *DTZ* Diltiazem, *HA* Headache, *ED* Erectile dysfunction, *Pt* Patients, *Wk* Weeks, *Mo* Months, *Yr* Years, *BT* Botulinum toxin injection, *U* Units, *Tx* Treatment, *LIS* Lateral internal sphincterotomy, *pLIS* Partial lateral internal sphincterotomy, *Sx* Symptoms, *TENS* Transcutaneous electrical posterior tibial nerve stimulation

Table 40.3 Systematic reviews and meta-analyses studying the treatment of chronic and refractory anal fissures

First Author	Yr	Databases used; time period	Studies, n & Study Type	Pt, n	Intervention: n	Conclusions
Sajid	2012	CCCG, Cochrane, Medline, EMBASE; Inception to 4/2011	7 RCTs	481	DTZ: 238 GTN: 243	DTZ and GTN are equally effective, but DTZ has fewer overall side-effects, HA, and recurrences; Therefore, **DTZ** is the preferred first line.
Chen	2014	MEDLINE, PubMed, Web of Science, Cochrane; 1996 – 8/31/13	7 RCTs	489	BT: 248 LIS: 241	**LIS** was superior to BT in terms of **healing** and **recurrence rates**. There was no significant difference between total complications, but **BT caused less incontinence.**
Nelson	2014	Medline; 1966 – 1/2014. EMBASE; 1980 – 1/2014. Cochrane; 1966 – 1/2014. DARE, HTA; NR.	9 RCTs	NR	NR	**LIS** is more **effective** than medical therapy or BT with a 90% chance of permanent cure. The incontinence risk with LIS is higher than with BT but lower than with anal stretch. **Open pLIS may be equivalent to closed pLIS** in healing rates. **Longer** sphincter division may be **more effective** at fissure healing. GTN has a higher risk of HA. More evidence is needed to compare AAF to LIS. LIS may be offered as a first-line treatment for CAF, or it may be offered as back-up for those who fail other treatments.
Sahebally	2017	PubMed, EMBASE, Cochrane; Inception to 3/2017	6 RCTs	393	GTN: 199 BT: 194	There was **no difference in rates of healing or recurrence**, but **BT** had **improved incidences** of both and a **better side effect** profile. There was a **higher incidence of transient incontinence** with BT.

Ebinger	2017	Medline (PubMed); 1/1975 – 10/7/2015	44 RCTs	3268	NR	LIS is the most effective treatment (highest healing rate and lowest no-success rate) but has an incontinence risk over 9%. A **stepwise** approach is recommended. **Firstly**, **medical treatment** is safe with few side effects. In persistent CAF, **fissurectomy and/or BT** may be used to address both fissure scarring and sphincter hypertonicity. In patients with treatment failure, **LIS** may be used but patients should be **selected carefully** to minimize risk of postoperative incontinence. **Anoplasty and/or fissurectomy and BT may be good alternatives**. Anal dilatation had the highest incontinence risk exceeding 18% and should be abandoned in clinical practice.
Nelson	2017	Cochrane; Issue 3, 2017. Medline; 1950 – 1/18/2017. EMBASE; 1/17/2017. ClinicalTrials.gov and ICTRP; up to 3/7/2017.	Surgical: 31 RCTs. Non-surgical: 117 RCTs.	12,062	Surgical: 2606. Non-surgical: 9456.	**LIS** is superior to non-operative management in achieving a sustained cure. The incontinence risk with LIS is 3.4 – 4.4%. **Open and closed LIS are equally efficacious** with a moderate quality of evidence. **CCBs are more effective than GTN** with lower rates of HA, but with **low quality** of evidence, especially due to short follow-up times in prior studies.
Sahebally	2018	PubMed/Medline, CINAHL, EMBASE, Cochrane; Inception to 1/2017	2 RCTs, 2 retrospective studies	300	AAF: 150 LIS: 150	**AAF** is associated with **similar** rates of wound complications and unhealed fissure as LIS, but **with lower incontinence rates**.

(continued)

Table 40.3 (continued)

First Author	Yr	Databases used; time period	Studies, n & Study Type	Pt, n	Intervention: n	Conclusions
Nevins	2020	Medline, Embase, PubMed, Scopus, Google Scholar; Since 1/2000	9 RCTs	756	DTZ: 385 GTN: 371	**DTZ** should be considered as the **first line** non-operative treatment for CAF. DTZ and GTN have comparable healing rates, but DTZ is superior in regards to HA and late recurrence rates.
Boland	2020	PubMed, Cochrane, Scopus; 1/2000 – 2/8/2020	9 RCTs	775	Nitrates: 206 DTZ: 44 Minoxidil 44 BT: 132 LIS: 349	**LIS** has the **highest healing rate** at 8 weeks but with a small risk of causing permanent incontinence. Topical nitrates and BT also have reasonable results. Ultimately, management of CAF should be **tailored** to the patient. As a **generalization**, **topical therapies** should be tried **first**, followed by **fissurectomy with/without BT and/or AAF**, before **LIS**.
Jin	2022	Medline, EMBASE, Scopus, Cochrane; NR	37 RCTs	2888	NR	There is **low certainty** evidence that **topical nitrates** are an **effective** treatment for anal fissure in terms of healing and pain reduction compared to placebo, but it has a significant risk of **HA**. **DTZ is marginally better than GTN** for healing; however, the **certainty of evidence is very low**. CCBs are less likely to cause HA compared to topical nitrates. Further studies are required to establish the effectiveness of CCBs compared to placebo.

Jin	2022	Medline, EMBASE, Cochrane; 1/1/1990 – 2/15/2021	69 RCTs	6242	Med: 1935. BT + Med: 84. BT: 714. Self-massage: 25. Anal dilation: 158. Anal dilation + Med: 16. Sphincterolysis: 41. AAF: 70. AAF + LIS: 50. Fissurectomy: 30. pLIS: 93. LIS: 2989.	**LIS** had the highest healing rates and should be considered as the **definitive treatment after failed initial therapy** with BT or medical therapies. **BT was equally effective compared to medical treatment. AAF** shows **similar effectiveness** compared to LIS, but **more studies are needed** to evaluate its efficacy.

Abbreviations: *Yr* Year, *NR* Not reported, *Pt* Patients, *RCT* Randomized controlled trial, *DTZ* Diltiazem, *GTN* Glyceryl trinitrate, *HA* Headache, *BT* Botulinum toxin injection, *LIS* Lateral internal sphincterotomy, *AAF* Anal advancement flap, *CAF* Chronic anal fissure, *DARE* Database of Abstracts of Reviews of Effects, *HTA* Health Technology Assessment, *CCCG* The Cochrane Colorectal Cancer Group Controlled Trials Register, *Cochrane* The Cochrane Central Register of Controlled Trials, *ICTRP* World Health Organization's Internet clinical trial portal, *Med* Medical therapy, *pLIS* Partial lateral internal sphincterotomy fissure, including fiber supplementation with appropriate water intake and stool softeners to ensure regular bowel movements and sitz baths for symptomatic relief.

Initial management of CAF is usually with medical therapy as this approach is safe with few side effects, especially given the concern for anal incontinence with sphincterotomy. A systematic review and meta-analysis including 37 studies with 2888 patients to evaluate the efficacy of topical treatments for anal fissures found that topical diltiazem and topical nifedipine are both better at achieving fissure healing than topical glyceryl trinitrate (GTN). In addition, there was a significantly higher risk of headaches with GTN compared to placebo or topical CCB. There have been more studies comparing GTN to placebo than for CCB to placebo; these studies have demonstrated that GTN is more effective at healing anal fissures and reducing pain compared to placebo, but this was not found in the three studies that compared topical CCB to placebo. Of note, this systematic review and meta-analysis did include patients with both acute and chronic anal fissures, and the studies were noted to have high heterogeneity and significant publication bias [3]. A 2017 systematic review including 117 RCTs studying non-surgical therapies with 9456 patients had similar results. This study demonstrated that topical CCB are more effective than GTN with decreased risk of headaches, but with a low grade of evidence, mainly due to limited follow-up times in the included studies [4].

An RCT by Khan et al. studying 184 patients with CAF randomized half the patients to treatment with 0.2% topical GTN and the other half to 2% topical diltiazem. After 1 month of treatment, 80% of patients treated with diltiazem achieved fissure healing which was significantly greater than the 62% who achieved healing with GTN. There was a higher incidence of patients who had resolution of perianal pain with diltiazem at 73% compared to GTN at 63%, but this did not reach statistical significance [5].

These results are similar to the RCT by Shrestha et al. studying 90 patients randomized evenly to treatment with 2% GTN and 0.5% nifedipine [6]. This study found an 83% healing rate with nifedipine use at 8 weeks which was significantly higher than the 60% of patients who had fissure healing using GTN. There was also a significantly lower rate of fissure recurrence in 6 months with nifedipine compared to GTN (24% and 18%, respectively). 17% of patients with GTN complained of headache compared to 7% in the nifedipine group, which led to poor compliance among the GTN users [6].

Alternative topical treatment that have not yet been extensively studied include minoxidil. A 2020 study by Emile et al. looking at 30 patients treated with 5% minoxidil and 32 patients treated with 0.2% GTN showed a significantly higher rate of healing with minoxidil at 77% compared to 47% with GTN, as well as a shorter duration to healing and fewer adverse effects. However, the patients treated with GTN had a significantly lower perianal pain score compared to those using minoxidil [7].

Another topical therapy that has not been proposed, but not widely studied for the management of CAF is topical tocopherol acetate. Ruiz-Tovar et al. studied 160 patients evenly divided into two groups treated with 100% tocopherol acetate and 0.4% GTN. Compared to the group treated with GTN, those managed with tocopherol acetate had a significantly higher cure rate (87% vs 66%), higher resolution of pain (88% vs. 70%), and lower recurrence rate at 16 weeks after completing the treatment course (3% vs. 13%). In the GTN arm, there were 28% of patients who had mild to moderate headaches and 18% with severe, incapacitating headaches while none of the patients in the tocopherol acetate group reported this side-effect [8]. Due to the limited number of studies evaluating the safety and efficacy of topical tocopherol acetate, it is not yet an accepted treatment for CAF, but it remains a promising area for future research.

Although GTN has been more extensively studied than CCB, it appears that topical CCB are superior at treating CAF with fewer intolerable side-effects and lower recurrence rates. However, medical treatment of CAF is limited by a significant risk of symptom recurrence compared to other therapies such as BT or surgical procedures [9].

BT injection represents a step between management with topical agents and surgical treatment, but the dosage and the injection protocol has not yet been well-established, and it is debatable if it offers any significant benefit over medical therapy. The dosages of BT injected according to various studies range from 20 IU to 150 IU [10, 11]. The protocol for internal sphincter BT injection is quite variable with some surgeons infiltrating BT at the 3 and 9 o'clock positions, other surgeons doing so on each side of the anterior midline or posterior midline, and still others injecting it at the four perianal quadrants [10, 12, 13]. Some surgeons inject BT in the intersphincteric groove whereas others inject it in the internal sphincter muscles. Therefore, the technique and dosage for BT injection is quite heterogeneous which makes it difficult to interpret prior studies.

A meta-analysis including six RCTs with 393 patients comparing BT to topical nitrates for the treatment of CAF showed lower incidences for incomplete fissure healing and fissure recurrence with BT compared to topical nitrates, but these rates did not reach statistical significance [14]. There was a higher rate of total side effects with topical nitrates but patients who underwent BT injection had an increased risk of transient anal incontinence [14]. A 2022 systematic review with network meta-analysis by Jin et al. including 69 RCTs also failed to demonstrate a significant difference in fissure healing between BT and topical medications [9].

A 2020 RCT by Nour et al. compared 48 patients undergoing BT injection to 48 patients undergoing partial or tailored lateral internal sphincterotomy (pLIS) [13]. The BT group had 80 IU infiltrated in the internal anal sphincter at the 1:00, 5:00, 7:00 and 11:00 positions. In the BT group, postoperative pain was lower, but the pLIS group had a higher rate of healing (92% vs. 77%) and a lower rate of recurrence (2% vs. 14%). The BT group had a higher rate of early postoperative incontinence at 17%, but symptoms had all resolved by 6 months post-treatment. In the pLIS group, there were 10% who developed incontinence, but 4% unfortunately had persistent gas incontinence after 6 months. The authors concluded that BT is safer than pLIS but is less effective and its dose needs to be adjusted. pLIS is more effective but preoperative assessment of anal sphincter tone is essential [13]. Unlike this study, a systematic review and meta-analysis published in 2017 found lower rates of anal incontinence with both LIS and BT at up to 4.4% and 2.3%, respectively [4].

It is possible that the duration of CAF symptoms may also play a factor in the effectiveness of different treatment modalities. A study by Gandomkar et al. randomized 99 patients with CAF to undergoing pLIS or receiving combination therapy with BT injection and topical diltiazem ointment for 6 weeks [11]. The overall healing rate in the 1-year follow-up period was significantly higher for the pLIS group at 94% vs. 65% in the BT with diltiazem group. The overall recurrence rate was 10% in the combination therapy group while none who had pLIS had recurrence. Incontinence was higher in the pLIS group. By the end of the study period, all the patients with incontinence in the combination therapy group had resolution of their symptoms, but 2% in the pLIS group had persistent incontinence. The authors performed an interesting subanalysis based on duration of CAF symptoms. Patients with symptoms for ≤12 months were found to have a 100% healing rate in both treatment arms, and none of these patients suffered a recurrent fissure. Patients with CAF for >12 months had significantly greater success with undergoing pLIS. Therefore, the authors suggested that BT with diltiazem may be just as effective as pLIS in patients with CAF symptoms for ≤12 months. Patients with CAF for a longer duration should consider pLIS instead due to its higher rate of healing.

Surgical options for CAF include LIS, AAF, anal dilatation, and fissurectomy. LIS remains the gold standard for CAF treatment with the highest rates of cure (88% – 100%) and the lowest rates of recurrence [15, 16]. A meta-analysis by Acar et al. including 550 patients who underwent treatment with LIS, pLIS, 2% diltiazem and 0.2% GTN showed the highest rates of healing with sphincterotomy (93%, 86%, 69% and 63%, respectively) [17]. The results for achieving resolution of perianal pain were similar. The recurrence rates were only available for those who underwent sphincterotomy and was 4% for LIS and 12% for pLIS. Both sphincterotomy groups had a 2% rate of incontinence but all the patients in the pLIS group had resolution of the incontinence by 6 months. The authors concluded that medical therapy may be tried as the first step and that pLIS could be considered as an effective alternative therapy due to the decreased risk of incontinence compared to a standard LIS [17].

These results are similar to the findings of a 2017 systematic review by Nelson et al. which actually studied all the treatment modalities for CAF and included 31 publications on surgical techniques and 117 on non-operative methods. They found that LIS is the most effective method of achieving sustained cure of CAF. Anal incontinence which is a feared side-effect with sphincterotomy was found to occur in up to 4.4% of patients. In addition, they found equivalent results with the open and closed techniques of performing an LIS. Manual anal dilation was found to have a lower rate of healing and higher rate of incontinence as 12% compared to LIS [4]. A 2021 RCT by Bara et al. comparing patients undergoing LIS with those undergoing anal dilatation and fissurectomy also noted significantly higher rates of incontinence with the anal dilatation and fissurectomy [18]. When aiming to guarantee the highest chances of perianal pain relief with the lowest risk of recurrence, LIS remains the gold standard [4].

pLIS can be combined with AAF for the treatment of CAF as shown in a 2012 RCT by Magdy et al. which studied 150 patients with CAF randomized to treatment with LIS, V-Y advancement flap, or combined pLIS with V-Y advancement flap. The highest healing rate was achieved with the combined technique at 94% with the lowest rate of recurrence at 2% and a low rate of postoperative incontinence at 2% [15].

The current literature is limited in guiding management of atypical or recurrent anal fissures, as almost all the studies exclude patients with these characteristics. Recurrences after sphincterotomy may be due to incomplete division of the sphincter muscle, so a repeat examination under anesthesia with completion of the sphincterotomy to the dentate line or repeat pLIS could be trialed in patients with normal or high anal sphincter tone [19]. An interesting retrospective study including 57 patients with recurrent anal fissures underwent repeat pLIS at the opposite side to the original sphincterotomy. The authors found that 98% of these patients achieved cure of their fissure with high patient satisfaction scores, and only 4% had postoperative incontinence [20].

Patients who are inappropriate surgical candidates and have failed other therapies could be considered for transcutaneous electrical nerve stimulation (TENS) based on a 2015 RCT by Youssef et al. including 73 patients randomized to LIS and TENS [21]. In this study, 75% of patients in the TENS arm had improvement of their symptoms within one month of treatment compared to 100% in the LIS arm. However, the recurrence rate with TENS was significantly higher at 41% compared to 3% in the LIS group [21].

Another option for patients who develop recurrent anal fissures after prior sphincterotomy, or for those with poor baseline anal sphincter tone or risk factors for postoperative incontinence, would be performing an AAF. Sahebally et al's 2018 meta-analysis including 2 RCTs and 2 retrospective studies showed similar rates of fissure healing and wound complications between LIS and AAF. In addition, AAF was associated with lower rates of incontinence. The included studies lacked enough data to analyze recurrence rates; therefore, the authors were unable to comment on the sustainability of fissure healing [22]. However, a prior RCT comparing LIS with AAF noted a significantly higher rate of recurrence at 22% with AAF compared to 4% with LIS [15]. Since AAF does not address the contribution of anal sphincter hypertonia to the development of fissures and with previous studies suggesting that there is a higher recurrence rate than with sphincterotomy, this technique may be more suitable for those without baseline increased anal sphincter tone or those who are at increased risk of developing postoperative issues with continence.

Further studies are needed to determine the dosing and injection protocol for BT, the order in which treatments should be performed for those with CAF, and the best treatment modalities for those with atypical, refractory, or recurrent fissures.

Recommendations

1. *Medical therapy is usually considered as the first line step. Topical CCBs may be a better medical treatment option than topical nitric oxide donors, especially because of the decreased patient compliance due to a significant incidence of headaches with the latter.*
   - Moderate level of evidence; Weak recommendation
2. *Surgical intervention with sphincterotomy offers the best healing rate and may be used when anal fissures do not respond to nonoperative therapy. Anal sphincter tone and risk factors for developing incontinence should be carefully assessed prior to consideration of sphincterotomy.*
   - High level of evidence; Strong recommendation.

Personal View

Chronic anal fissures can be quite debilitating for patients as they cause pain and bleeding. Moreover, many patients worry about cancer when they see bleeding associated with bowel movements. It is important for the treating physician to reassure the patient that the likelihood of a typical anal fissure harboring cancer is very low. It is also important to make sure that the patients are up to date with their screening colonoscopies depending on their age and colon cancer risk stratification when we evaluate the patient for an anal fissure.

Treatment of atypical CAFs is directed towards the etiology; we start with a biopsy of the fissure and the results guide the treatment. Treatment of typical fissures is directed towards reduction of the tone of the internal anal sphincter. For typical CAFs, our practice is geared towards symptomatic relief of anal fissures and not towards healing, per se. We set this expectation up-front when we meet with the patient, and most often the patient shares this goal. Ideally, we want both bleeding and pain to resolve; however, if we can relieve the pain and the patient notices on and off anal outlet bleeding, we consider that as a success and as an acceptable endpoint in treatment of CAFs. We offer LIS as the initial treatment for patients (especially men) who are in severe pain and have failed conservative treatment at an outside facility. For all other typical CAFs we start treatment with sitz baths, fiber supplementation, adequate water intake and topical CCBs (2% Nifedipine 3 times a day) for 2 months. If this does not cause substantial improvement or complete resolution of symptoms, then we offer the patients BT injection. If the patient has had partial improvement and is not in distress, then continuing CCBs for another 2 months is an excellent option. For those patients who need BT injection, we inject a total of 100 units of BT: 30 units are injected on either sides of the fissure into the internal anal sphincter muscle and 40 units are injected into the internal anal sphincter muscle opposite the anal fissure (i.e. if it is a posterior midline anal fissure, then we inject 30 units into the internal anal sphincter muscle on either side of it and 40 units are injected in the anterior midline). After injecting BT, we advise the patient to continue using the topical CCBs and reassess them in 2 months. If the patient has had partial improvement from the BT injection and is not in distress, then repeating BT injection is a reasonable option. If the symptoms have not substantially improved or there has not been complete resolution of symptoms, then we discuss LIS; in our practice, we quote a 98% success rate with a 2% rate of incontinence to flatus in the long term. In our practice, we perform LIS using a closed technique and tailor the length of the sphincterotomy to the length of the fissure. Any patient with a fissure-fistula is best served with a fissure fistulotomy with marsupialization of the fistula tract, as most often that is curative.

Rarely, some patients have atypical CAFs without increase in anal tone. Our initial approach of to treat these patients remains the same. We start with Sitz baths, fiber supplementation, adequate water intake and topical CCB (2% Nifedipine 3 times a day) for 2 months. However, if they fail to improve and are in pain, then we offer them an AAF as the surgical option.

References

1. Ebinger SM, Hardt J, Warschkow R, Schmied BM, Herold A, Post S, et al. Operative and medical treatment of chronic anal fissures-a review and network meta-analysis of randomized controlled trials. J Gastroenterol. 2017;52(6):663–76.
2. Arslan K, Erenoğlu B, Doğru O, Turan E, Eryilmaz MA, Atay A, et al. Lateral internal sphincterotomy versus 0.25% isosorbide dinitrate ointment for chronic anal fissures: a prospective randomized controlled trial. Surg Today. 2013;43(5):500–5.
3. Jin JZ, Hardy MO, Unasa H, Mauiliu-Wallis M, Weston M, Connolly A, et al. A systematic review and meta-analysis of the efficacy of topical sphincterotomy treatments for anal fissure. Int J Color Dis. 2022;37(1):1–15. https://doi.org/10.1007/s00384-021-04040-3.
4. Nelson RL, Manuel D, Gumienny C, Spencer B, Patel K, Schmitt K, et al. A systematic review and meta-analysis of the treatment of anal fissure. Tech Coloproctol. 2017;21(8):605–25. https://doi.org/10.1007/s10151-017-1664-2.
5. Khan MS, Akbar I, Zeb J, Ahmad S, Khan A. Outcome of 0.2% Glyceryltrinitrate cream versus 2% diltiazem cream in the treatment of chronic anal fissure. J Ayub Med Coll Abbottabad. 2017;29(2):280–4p.
6. Shrestha SK, Thapa PB, Maharjan DK, Tamang TY. Effectiveness of 0.2% glyceryl Trinitrate and 0.5% Nifedipine in the treatment of chronic anal fissure. JNMA J Nepal Med Assoc. 2017;56(205):149–52p.
7. Emile SH, Abdel-Razik MA, Elshobaky A, Elbaz SA, Khafagy W, Shalaby M. Topical 5% minoxidil versus topical 0.2% glyceryl trinitrate in treatment of chronic anal fissure: a randomized clinical trial. Int J Surg. 2020;75:152–8. https://doi.org/10.1016/j.ijsu.2020.01.143.
8. Ruiz-Tovar J, Llavero C. Perianal application of glyceryl Trinitrate ointment versus tocopherol acetate ointment in the treatment of chronic anal fissure: a randomized clinical trial. Dis Colon Rectum. 2022;65(3):406–12. https://doi.org/10.1097/dcr.0000000000002120.
9. Jin JZ, Bhat S, Park B, Hardy MO, Unasa H, Mauiliu-Wallis M, et al. A systematic review and network meta-analysis comparing treatments for anal fissure. Surgery. 2022;172(1):41–52. https://doi.org/10.1016/j.surg.2021.11.030.
10. Asim M, Lowrie N, Stewart J, Lolohea S, Van Dalen R. Botulinum toxin versus botulinum toxin with low-dose glyceryltrinitrate for healing of chronic anal fissure: a prospective, randomised trial. NZ Med J. 2014;127(1393):80–6.
11. Gandomkar H, Zeinoddini A, Heidari R, Amoli HA. Partial lateral internal sphincterotomy versus combined botulinum toxin A injection and topical diltiazem in the treatment of chronic anal fissure: a randomized clinical trial. Dis Colon Rectum. 2015;58(2):228–34.

12. Valizadeh N, Jalaly NY, Hassanzadeh M, Kamani F, Dadvar Z, Azizi S, et al. Botulinum toxin injection versus lateral internal sphincterotomy for the treatment of chronic anal fissure: randomized prospective controlled trial. Langenbeck's Arch Surg. 2012;397(7):1093–8.
13. Nour H, Bari AA, Ibrahim A. Treatment of chronic anal fissure; lateral internal sphincterotomy versus local injection of high dose botulinum toxin. A randomized clinical trial. Res J Pharm, Biol Chem Sci. 2020;11(1):68–74p. https://doi.org/10.33887/rjpbcs/2020.11.1.11.
14. Sahebally SM, Meshkat B, Walsh SR, Beddy D. Botulinum toxin injection vs topical nitrates for chronic anal fissure: an updated systematic review and meta-analysis of randomized controlled trials. Color Dis. 2018;20(1):6–15. https://doi.org/10.1111/codi.13969.
15. Magdy A, El Nakeeb A, Fouda EY, Youssef M, Farid M. Comparative study of conventional lateral internal sphincterotomy, VY anoplasty, and tailored lateral internal sphincterotomy with VY anoplasty in the treatment of chronic anal fissure. J Gastrointest Surg. 2012;16(10):1955–62.
16. Butt F, Aslam MN, Nadeem N. Comparison of lateral internal sphincterotomy and GTN gel for management of chronic anal fissure: a randomized controlled trial. Pak J Med Health Sci. 2017;11(2):695–7p.
17. Acar T, Acar N, Güngör F, Kamer E, Genç H, Atahan K, et al. Comparative efficacy of medical treatment versus surgical sphincterotomy in the treatment of chronic anal fissure. Niger J Clin Pract. 2020;23(4):539–44. https://doi.org/10.4103/njcp.njcp_383_19.
18. Bara BK, Mohanty SK, Behera SN, Sahoo AK, Swain SK. Fissurectomy versus lateral internal Sphincterotomy in the treatment of chronic anal fissure: a randomized control trial. Cureus. 2021;13(9):e18363. https://doi.org/10.7759/cureus.18363.
19. Nelson RL. Anal fissure (chronic). BMJ Clin Evid. 2014;2014:0407.
20. Liang J, Church JM. Lateral internal sphincterotomy for surgically recurrent chronic anal fissure. Am J Surg. 2015;210(4):715–9.
21. Youssef T, Youssef M, Thabet W, Lotfy A, Shaat R, Abd-Elrazek E, et al. Randomized clinical trial of transcutaneous electrical posterior tibial nerve stimulation versus lateral internal sphincterotomy for treatment of chronic anal fissure. Int J Surg. 2015;22:143–8.
22. Sahebally SM, Walsh SR, Mahmood W, Aherne TM, Joyce MR. Anal advancement flap versus lateral internal sphincterotomy for chronic anal fissure- a systematic review and meta-analysis. Int J Surg. 2018;49:16–21. https://doi.org/10.1016/j.ijsu.2017.12.002.

Benign Anal Disease: Third Degree Hemorrhoids—Who Really Needs Surgery?

41

Ernie Soto and Jonathan Laryea

Introduction

Hemorrhoidal disease is one of the most common anorectal disorders, with a prevalence of 39% [8]. Although quite common, the pathophysiology is not fully understood. The current theory is the sliding anal canal lining. From this theory, hemorrhoids are defined as the symptomatic enlargement and downward displacement of anal cushions. Anal cushions are folds of tissue which aid in continence and sense of urgency. They descend from their normal position due to deterioration of the supporting tissues. Pathologic evaluation of these tissues demonstrate venous dilation, thrombosis, degeneration of collagen and fibroelastic tissues along with a severe inflammatory reaction [28]. There have been studies finding dysregulation of the vascular tone from the superior rectal artery leading to a larger diameter of terminal branches to the hemorrhoidal tissue [28]. Patients with hemorrhoids tend to have a higher resting anal pressure on anal manometry. In sum, the supporting tissues undergo degeneration leading to the sliding of the anal canal and its associated anal cushions [28]. Constipation, passage of hard stool and increased intraabdominal pressure are thought to lead to this degeneration, although there is some dispute [28].

Surgeons possess a wide variety of therapeutic options to treat hemorrhoids. According to the ASCRS clinical practice guidelines for hemorrhoidal disease, management of symptomatic grade I/II hemorrhoidal disease starts with adequate fluid and fiber intake and proper bowel habits, such as avoidance of straining and

E. Soto · J. Laryea (✉)
Division of Colon and Rectal Surgery, Department of Surgery, University of Arkansas for Medical Sciences, Little Rock, AR, USA
e-mail: efsoto@uams.edu; jalaryea@uams.edu

K. Umanskiy, N. Hyman (eds.), *Difficult Decisions in Colorectal Surgery*, Difficult Decisions in Surgery: An Evidence-Based Approach,
https://doi.org/10.1007/978-3-031-42303-1_41

limiting time on the commode, along with medical therapy with phlebotonics to help increase venous tone [29].

After failing medical management, office-based procedures are then considered to help decrease the size or vascularity of the hemorrhoidal tissue [29]. These therapies include rubber band ligation, sclerotherapy and infrared coagulation. The benefits of these in-office procedures are the low major complication rate and ability to perform the procedure multiple times. Although pain and bleeding are some of the more common complications, perianal sepsis is a life-threatening major complication that can develop with signs such as worsening pain, fever and urinary dysfunction [29].

These therapies are effective for grade I/II whereas grade IV hemorrhoids commonly require surgery. However, there are no clear-cut guidelines for the optimal treatment of grade III hemorrhoids. According to ASCRS clinical practice guidelines, select patients with grade III internal hemorrhoids who have failed medical therapy may undergo office-based treatments. However, select patients are not defined. Furthermore, Goligher's grading system for hemorrhoids does not address the size or whether the hemorrhoids are isolated or circumferential, or include an external component, which are drivers of decision-making [1].

The choice between operative procedures versus office-based procedures must be made by the surgeon, balancing the success and durability of excisional hemorrhoidectomy with its associated cost, postoperative pain and disability [2, 3]. Though associated with less postoperative pain, newer techniques such as the procedure for prolapse and hemorrhoids (PPH) and Doppler-guided hemorrhoidal artery ligation (DGHAL), are associated with higher recurrence rates. Office based techniques offer a relatively safe and simple approach for many patients, although long-term durability remains a concern. RBL is relatively contraindicated in patients using clopidogrel, warfarin, or heparin due to the significant incidence of post-procedure bleeding [4]. However, of the available office-based procedures, RBL is typically the most effective option and has been used as the comparison group to surgical hemorrhoidectomy [5].

Complications may result from any technique and can range from minor to life-threatening. They include bleeding, urinary retention, wound infection, incontinence, anal-stricture, ectropion, and local sepsis [3]. To appropriately answer the question of who should have surgery for grade III hemorrhoids, we must evaluate the ability of a treatment to control symptoms, the re-treatment rate, postoperative pain, complication rates, disability, and patient satisfaction (Table 41.1).

Table 41.1 Identification of patient population, intervention, comparison and outcomes

Patient population	Intervention	Comparator	Outcomes studied
Patients with 3rd degree haemorrhoids	Hemorrhoidectomy	Rubber Band Ligation	Symptom control and morbidity

Search Strategy/Methods

A literature search of MEDLINE, PubMed, the Cochrane Database of Collected Reviews, and Google Scholar was performed using English language articles from January 2000 to present. Search terms included hemorrhoids, internal and external hemorrhoids, hemorrhoid disease, rubber band ligation, hemorrhoidectomy, hemorrhoidopexy and Doppler-guided hemorrhoidectomy. Selected references from articles identified in the primary literature search were used when relevant. Literature was evaluated using the GRADE evidence quality classification system [6]. Post-hoc data analysis was conducted using Fisher's exact test.

Results

Although high quality evidence comparing office techniques to surgical hemorrhoidectomy for grade III hemorrhoids had been lacking previously, several meta-analyses have been published in the past few years. Most data demonstrates EH to be superior to RBL in the control of hemorrhoidal symptoms at the expense of increased pain and complication rate. There are several different forms of EH including open and closed, with or without the use of energy sealing devices that may improve pain and recurrence rate.

The following discussion includes the results of available studies (Table 41.2).

Control of Hemorrhoidal Symptoms

Excisional hemorrhoidectomy is often referred to as the "gold standard" for the treatment of hemorrhoids when it comes to control of symptoms [8]. A large retrospective case series of 693 patients who underwent EH (Ferguson closed technique) for grade III and IV hemorrhoids reported a recurrence rate of 1% and 3% at 1 and 2 years [9].

RBL has also been shown to control symptoms for many individuals, but to a lesser extent. A retrospective study of 701 patients showed an overall success rate (alleviation of symptoms) of 70% [13]. When only patients with grade III hemorrhoids were included, the success rate decreased to 59%. (only Grade II 73.1%)

Three studies were identified that compared outcomes of EH directly to RBL. Murie et al. evaluated 100 patients with either grade II or III hemorrhoids and randomized them to EH or RBL [14]. Of the 56 patients with grade III hemorrhoids, 97% of patients undergoing EH had no symptoms of prolapse at 1 year compared to 70% in the RBL group ($p = 0.04$). When adding in the patients with grade II hemorrhoids, 86% of EH patients had no bleeding at 1 year compared to 74% in the RBL group ($p = 0.28$).

A systematic review in 2021 by Dekker et al. evaluated 8 RCTs comparing RBL and EH in grade II/III hemorrhoids [31]. This study found that EH was superior in the control of hemorrhoidal symptoms at the expense of increased pain and

Table 41.2 Results of studies comparing surgery to office management of grade III hemorrhoids

Study	Group	No. of patients (Grade 3/total)	Results	Quality of evidence
Murie et al. [14]	EH vs RBL	56/88	RR 0.12 for prolapse for grade III (95% CI, 0.02–0.87, p = 0.04) RR 0.55 for bleeding for all patients (95% CI, 0.2–1.3, p = 0.2) RR 1.50 for pain > 48 h for all patients (95% CI, 1.2–1.9, p < 0.01) WMD + 29 days off work for all patients (95% CI, 21–36, p < 0.01)	Low
Lewis et al. [15]	EH vs RBL	56[a]	RR 0.44 for short-term symptom recurrence (95% CI, 0.2–0.7, p < 0.01) RR 0.18 for long-term symptom recurrence (95% CI, 0.1–0.4, p < 0.01) RR 3.8 for pain requiring systemic analgesia (95% CI, 2.1–6.8, p < 0.01)	Low
Gagloo et al. [17]	EH vs RBL	38/100	RR 0.25 for prolapsed for grade III (95% CI, 0.1–0.8, p = 0.2) RR 5.0 for requiring post-operative analgesia for all patients (95% CI, 2.8–8.7, p < 0.01)	Low
Peng et al. [19]	PPH vs RBL	55/65	RR 0.21 for bleeding symptoms 2 weeks post op (95% CI. 0.1–0.4, p < 0.01)	Moderate
Dekker et al. [31]	EH vs RBL	671/1208	RR 0.2 for recurrence (95% CI, 0.10–0.38, p < 0.0001), H = 0% RR 6.4 for postoperative pain (95% CI, 5.2–8.1, p < 0.0001), H = 76% (p < 0.001) RR 3.8 for postoperative bleeding (95% CI, 2.44–6.05, p < 0.0001), H = 48% (p < 0.001) RR 25.9 for anal stenosis (95% CI, 3.5–190, p = 0.0014) RR 7.3 for urinary retention (95% 4.3–12, p < 0.0001)	Moderate
Shukla et al. [30]	EH vs PPH	52/100	Operative time 50 vs 35 mins, p < 0.05 Day 7 VAS 3.3 vs 2.2, p < 0.05 Return to work 16.2 vs 8.08, p = 0.001 RR 0.33 for recurrence (95% CI, 0.07–1.6, p = 0.1652)	Low
Brown et al. [31]	RBL vs HAL	128/337	aOR 2.23 for recurrence (95%, CI 1.42–3.51, p = 0.0005)	Moderate

RR relative risk, *WMD* weighted mean difference, *aOR* adjusted odds ratio

[a]A total of 112 patients were in the study, but patients who had anal dilation or cryotherapy were excluded from ad-hoc analysis

complication rate. In this study, RBL was found to have a higher recurrence rate with a RR 4.77 (95% CI 2.60–8.76); $p < 0.001$) compared to EH. Inversely, RBL scored less on post procedural pain surveys with a RR 0.17 (95% CI 0.11–0.28); $p < 0.001$), post procedural bleeding with a RR 0.31 (95% CI 0.15–0.66), anal incontinence RR 0.16 [95% CI 0.02–1.28] $p = 0.080$), and urinary retention RR 0.15 [95% CI 0.09–0.25]; $p < 0.001$). Importantly, these studies did not comment on the number of RBLs used in the treatment arm, as this is a major advantage of these office-based procedures. A Cochrane Database Systematic Review of three randomized studies comparing EH to RBL was published in 2005 [7]. EH was found to be superior to RBL for grade III hemorrhoids in terms a of symptom control in two trials with 116 patients with a RR 1.23 (95% CI 1.04-1.45; $p = 0.01$). There was, however, no difference between the two procedures in grade II hemorrhoids in one trial with 32 patients, RR 1.07 (95% CI 0.94-1.21; $p=0.32$). Patients undergoing EH had significantly more pain, higher complication rate and more time off work. Despite these outcomes, patient satisfaction and acceptance was similar between the two procedures.

Comparing EH to other surgical techniques such as PPH, a meta-analysis in 2004 demonstrated that patients undergoing EH were significantly less likely to complain of ongoing hemorrhoidal symptoms than those who underwent PPH (6 trials, 388 patients, OR 0.52, 95% CI, 0.3–0.91; $p = 0.02$) [10]. However, this study also found an earlier return to normal activities in the PPH group (standardized mean difference, −4.03 days; 95% CI −6.95 to −1.10; $p = 0.007$). A larger meta-analysis from 2007 [40] reviewing 25 RCTs encompassing 1918 procedures also demonstrated similar results. Postoperative complications seem to not favor PPH or EH with a similar overall complication rate (20.5% vs 25.2%; $P = 0.06$) [40]. These results seem to have held true over the years as a more recent randomized control trial (100 patients with grade II/III) in 2018 again showed similar findings [30].

DGHAL has also been shown to have a high recurrence rate with 31% of patients having symptoms within the subsequent 5 years [11]. Conversely, a clinical trial comparing EH to DGHAL with mucopexy demonstrated no difference in symptoms including pain and bleeding at 2 years post-procedure [12].

The HubBLe trial was a multi-center randomized controlled trial comparing DGHAL to RBL for grade II/III hemorrhoids. This study found a 30% recurrence rate for DGHAL compared to a 49% in RBL with adjusted OR of 2.23 (95%, CI 1.42–3.51, $p = 0.0005$). When including multiple treatments with RBL, recurrence dropped to 37% [32].

Lewis et al. compared EH with anal dilatation, RBL and cryotherapy [15]. Of the 26 patients undergoing EH, 100% had fewer symptoms and 65% had no symptoms at 1 year, as opposed to 67% and 13% for RBL. In the long-term (6 months–5 years) 100% of EH patients had fewer symptoms and 86% had no symptoms. Only 40% of RBL patients had fewer symptoms and 23% were symptom free. No patients in the EH group required further treatment compared to 80% in the RBL group.

A systematic review of the two aforementioned trials demonstrated greater efficacy for EH over RBL for the treatment of grade III hemorrhoids (2 trials, 116 patients, RR 1.23, 95% CI 1.0–1.5, $p = 0.01$). However, this difference was not seen with grade II hemorrhoids (1 trial, 32 patients, RR 1.07, 95% CI 0.9–1.2, $p = 0.32$) [16]. When combining grade II and III hemorrhoids, there was no significant difference between RBL and EH with respect to control of bleeding or prolapse (123 patients; RR 1.12 (95% CI 0.97 to 1.29); $P = 0.120$) (109 patients; RR 1.05 (95% CI 0.98 to 1.12); $P = 0.160$).

A 2011 study randomized 100 patients with grade II/III hemorrhoids to EH or RBL [17]. Of the grade III patients (38 patients), 12.5% of the EH group experienced recurrent prolapse symptoms after 6 months compared to 50% in the RBL group. Although no statistical analysis was included in the study, post-hoc analysis reveals this is a statistically significant finding ($p = 0.03$). Consistent with the systematic review is the finding that RBL leads to better results with grade II hemorrhoids compared to grade III (77% vs. 50% without prolapse at 6 months, respectively).

In a comparison of PPH with RBL, there was a significant decrease in the percentage of patients experiencing the symptoms of bleeding from hemorrhoids at 2-weeks post-procedure in the PPH group (27% vs. 68%, $p < 0.005$). This difference was not seen for prolapse, pruritus, or wound discharge [18]. By 2 months, there was no difference in symptoms experienced in either group. A multicenter randomized control trial (The Napoleon Trial) has been recently opened in Europe to evaluate the effectiveness and cost-effectiveness of RBL versus sutured mucopexy versus EH in patients with recurrent hemorrhoidal disease (ClinicalTrials.gov identifier: NCT04101773) [41]. This trial may shed more light on the most effective/cost-effective treatment for patients with recurrent hemorrhoidal disease.

Post-treatment Pain and Complications

A systematic review of trials comparing EH to RBL for grade II/III hemorrhoids (including Murie and Lewis, et al.) demonstrated significantly more patients that underwent EH experienced postoperative pain (3 trials, 212 patients, RR 1.94, 95% CI 1.62–2.33, $p < 0.001$) [16]. There was no statistically significant difference in other postoperative complications such as urinary retention, hemorrhage, or anal stenosis. A meta-analysis of the same three trials revealed similar results [5]. The more recent systematic review by Dekker et al. confirmed some of these findings. Patients experienced less post procedural pain after RBL (7 studies, 1110 patients, RR 0.17 (95% CI 0.11–0.28); $p < 0.001$). Patients experienced less bleeding following RBL (RR 0.31 (95% CI 0.15–0.66); $p = 0.002$), less urinary retention (6 studies, 1054 patients, random effects; RR 0.15 [95% CI 0.09–0.25]; $p < 0.001$), less anal incontinence (RR 0.16 [95% CI 0.02–1.28] $p = 0.080$). Gagloo et al. found 100% of patients undergoing EH required postoperative analgesia compared to 20% of patients after RBL [17]. Severe pain from RBL may result from placement of the band below the dentate line, which precludes the banding of external hemorrhoids [3].

While EH has been repeatedly shown to be associated with more postoperative pain than RBL, a recent Cochrane Review has demonstrated a significant decrease in pain when hemorrhoidectomy is performed with an energy sealing device [20]. Pain scores on the first postoperative day showed a WMD of −2.07 (10 studies, 835 patients, CI −2.77 − 1.38). There was no relevant difference in other postoperative complications. A study comparing "DGHAL with mucopexy to EH demonstrated no significant difference in post-operative pain scores up to 2 weeks [12]. A meta-analysis in 2022 by Zhang et al. comparing energy sealing device hemorrhoidectomy vs PPH found that the energy sealing group also had no difference in postoperative pain (mean difference = 0.55, 95% CI: −0.15 to 1.25, P = .12) and also had a decreased recurrence rate in the energy sealing device group (RR = 0.21, 95% confidence interval (CI): 0.06 to 0.72, P = .01) [34].

In a comparison of PPH with RBL, PPH was associated with a higher maximal pain score at discharge (5 vs 2, $p < 0.001$) and at 2 weeks (5 vs 0, $p < 0.001$). However, by 2 months, no patient in either group complained of pain. There was no difference in other complications such as urinary retention, bleeding, anal stenosis, or change in continence. However, his study was not sufficiently powered for these endpoints [18].

There are new studies evaluating bipolar or harmonic hemorrhoidectomy in search of reduction of pain. Balcisueta et al. published a systematic review and network meta-analysis of randomized trials in 2021. Twenty-nine studies were included (3309 patients). None of the procedures were associated with severe pain. Open hemorrhoidectomy was associated with the most pain on postoperative days 1 and 7. Hemorrhoidopexy was the least painful. Additionally, closed hemorrhoidectomy and use of bipolar energy or Harmonic scalpel was associated with decreased pain [35]. Moreover, a RCT by Wang et al. found decreased operating times, blood loss, postoperative pain, parenteral analgesic use and length of stay in patients undergoing hemorrhoidectomy with Ligasure compared to conventional Ferguson hemorrhoidectomy [38]. Aibuedefe et al. in 2021 published a systematic review and meta-analysis of 26 RCTs including 3137 patients with grade III/IV hemorrhoids. They showed less pain with laser (OR 0.34, CI 0.01–6.51), and infrared photocoagulation (OR 0.38, CI 0.02–5.61) compared to EH. Notably, they found less recurrence with Starion (OR 0.01, CI 0.00–0.46) and harmonic scalpel (OR 0.00, CI 0.00–0.49), compared to infrared photocoagulation and DGHAL. There were fewer postoperative clinical complications with infrared photocoagulation (OR 0.04, CI 0.00–2.54) and LigaSure (OR 0.16, CI 0.03–0.79), compared to suture ligation and open hemorrhoidectomy. Patients undergoing DGHAL (OR 0.26, CI 0.05–1.51) and stapled (OR 0.36, CI 0.15–0.84) techniques, returned to work earlier when compared to open hemorrhoidectomy and laser [36].

A systematic review of 9 RCTs including over 523 patients found that patients receiving metronidazole either topical or oral had decreased pain scores without increased complication rates. [33]

Lifestyle (Return to Work and Patient Satisfaction)

Murie et al. reported that 100% of working patients undergoing EH lost time from work with a mean of 32 days compared to 44% of the RBL group with an average time away from work of 3 days (SD 7 days-$p < 0.01$) [14]. However, the newer techniques of hemorrhoid surgery have considerably improved return to work times.

A Cochrane review comparing LigaSure hemorrhoidectomy to standard EH demonstrated a return to work 4.88 days earlier (4 studies, 451 patients, CI 2.18–7.59). When comparing DGHAL to EH, DGHAL patients returned to work after 10 days compared to 22 days in the EH group (p = 0.09) [12].

A systematic review demonstrated similar overall patient satisfaction in both EH and RBL patients (RR 1.02, 2 studies, 148 patients, 95% CI, 0.94–1.10) [16]. Gagloo, et al. reported 70% of patients considered EH an "excellent" modality compared to 64% for RBL [17]. There was no difference noted between PPH and RBL in terms of patient satisfaction at discharge, 2 weeks, 2 or 6 months [18].

Cost

None of the identified studies comparing EH to RBL evaluated cost. However, in the current healthcare climate, cost of therapy must be a consideration. Factors that may impact cost include operative time, equipment, and need for further treatment. In addition, the time of convalescence financially impacts patients, and the economy as a whole.

There is considerable variation of operative time based on surgical technique. Multiple studies have demonstrated EH to have longer operative times than other techniques such as PPH [21]. However, when accounting for equipment costs, EH was demonstrated to be less expensive than PPH ($252 vs. $504) [22]. The addition of disposable LigaSure diathermy forceps adds an additional $225 per operation to EH [23].

RBL does not require operating room time and the cost of equipment is minimal. However, a long-term study of over 700 patients demonstrated that 30% of patients require re-treatment with a median 2 bandings per patient and a range of 1–17 bands placed [13]. Also, as previous studies have demonstrated increased pain with multiple bandings in a single session, patients often need to be brought back for several sessions [13, 24, 25]. However, as stated above, RBL does allow a considerably earlier return to work, reducing lost wages.

Recommendations

There are insufficient randomized controlled trials to make a strong recommendation based on high-quality evidence. However, there are trends in the literature sufficient for recommendations.

1. Most patients with uncomplicated grade III internal hemorrhoids may be effectively treated with office procedures as first line treatment after appropriate medical therapy. Strong recommendation based on moderate quality evidence.

   Due to the relatively low complication rate, decreased pain, faster return to work and reasonable efficacy, office techniques such as rubber band ligation may be an appropriate first option for many patients. While not as efficacious as surgical hemorrhoidectomy, many patients may succeed without a trip to the operating room. This technique does not burn any bridges and therapy may always be escalated to surgical management.

2. Patients with large multi-column grade III hemorrhoids with mixed internal/external component should undergo surgical hemorrhoidectomy. Strong recommendation based on moderate quality evidence.

   Large hemorrhoids may not be treated as effectively with office-based procedures. This may be due to the small size of the ligation barrel limiting the size of the hemorrhoid banded [26]. In these cases, surgical hemorrhoidectomy is the better choice to remove all affected tissue. In addition, as multi-column disease may require multiple banding episodes, these patients may be good candidates for surgery. Finally, as rubber band ligation should not be applied below the dentate line, patients who seek treatment for mixed component hemorrhoids should preferably undergo surgery.
3. Patients who are unable to tolerate or have failed office-based techniques should undergo surgical hemorrhoidectomy. Strong recommendation based on moderate quality evidence.

   While office based procedures such as rubber band ligation may have the advantages of decreased invasiveness, many patients require repeat therapy. In addition, while the risk of late bleeding after RBL is similar in patients who take no antithrombotic therapy and those who hold antithrombotic therapy, not all patients are able to do so [27]. Patient preference may play a large role in how many times this is done. In patients who continue to be symptomatic from their hemorrhoids or no longer wish to have repeat procedures, surgical therapy is appropriate.
4. For patients undergoing surgical hemorrhoidectomy, the type of procedure performed should be driven by surgeon expertise. Moderate recommendation based on moderate quality evidence.

   There are some benefits to new techniques including energy sealing devices or stapling devices that may be beneficial in regard to operating time and post-operative pain, but can have similar complications, such as blood loss, anal incontinence, stenosis, or urinary retention with an increase to operating cost [39].

Expert Opinion

Most patients with symptomatic grade III hemorrhoids present with tissue prolapse, bleeding, mucous drainage, and pruritus ani. Some patients present with difficulty with anal hygiene and a minority with pain from engorgement with the prolapse. Non-operative measures alone are inadequate for grade III hemorrhoidal prolapse. When the symptoms are mainly related to bleeding or the prolapse, office-based RBL is offered. I routinely use the Saeed Shortshot Multi-Band Ligator kit, which also contains a trislot anoscope. The anoscope is fashioned such that when it is inserted to limit, it covers the dentate line and ensures that the bands will not be placed below the dentate line. The use of the trislot anoscope also ensures a single positioning of the anoscope without a need to reposition it. This system, with the use of suction, allows the use of one hand to deploy the bands. I typically band 1–3 columns in one session, depending on the size of the columns. Banding more than one column in one session is safe and not associated with increased risk of complications. I warn patients to expect a gush of blood in 4–5 days post procedure, however, it may be mixed with stool and may not be easily recognized. I also warn patients that some slight bleeding with wiping is expected once the hemorrhoids slough off. Additional complications discussed include urinary retention and sepsis. I typically see the patients back in 8 weeks to allow the resulting ulcers from the banding to heal. Patients with extremely large hemorrhoids may require repeat banding. I routinely caution patients on expectations of rectal 'spasms' or 'pressure' which may last up to 48 hours. I counsel patients to do warm Sitz baths to help with this. I do not typically prescribe any analgesics other than Acetaminophen for discomfort. I warn patients that severe pain is a sign of a serious complication that requires a phone call and immediate evaluation.

When patients are anticoagulated on medications beyond aspirin, we hold the anticoagulation prior to RBL due to the risk of hematoma and bleeding. For patients who cannot hold their anticoagulation for elevated risk of thromboembolic complications, excisional hemorrhoidectomy is recommended.

For patients presenting with symptomatic, circumferential grade III hemorrhoids, I offer them PPH. This offers a durable resolution of symptoms in one setting as opposed to serial RBL. When patients present with mixed symptomatic internal/external hemorrhoids or when they do not tolerate in-office anoscopy and/or RBL, I offer EH. I typically excise 1–3 columns depending on the situation. I use the Harmonic Focus bipolar device for excisional hemorrhoidectomy. This is associated with less blood loss (in most cases no blood loss) and less postoperative pain. I typically do the Ferguson (closed) technique, however, in some cases, I do not close all the incisions to avoid anal stenosis. I routinely use Liposomal Bupivacaine to help with postoperative pain. Doppler-guided hemorrhoid artery ligation remains an alternative, however, I do not typically use this technique. It is associated with an increased rate of recurrence. The addition of mucopexy improves outcomes and long term success. However, I find mucopexy to be antithetical to the principles of surgery. No wonder the enthusiasm for this procedure has waned significantly after an initial strong acceptance.

References

1. Goligher JC, Leacock AG, Brossy JJ. The surgical anatomy of the anal canal. Br J Surg. 1955;43(177):51–61.. CrossrefPubMed
2. Acheson AG, Scholefield JH. Management of haemorrhoids. BMJ. 2008;336:380–3. CrossrefPubMedPubMedCentral
3. Sneider EB, Maykel JA. Diagnosis and management of symptomatic hemorrhoids. Surg Clin North Am. 2010;90:17–32.
4. Rivadeneira DE, Steele SR, Ternent C, et al. Practice parameters for the management of hemorrhoids (revised 2010). Dis colon rectum. 2011;54:1059–64. CrossrefPubMed.
5. MacRae HM, McLeod RS. Comparison of hemorrhoidal treatment modalities. Dis Colon Rectum. 1995;38(7):687–94.

6. Brozek JL, Akl EA, Alonso-Coello P, et al. Grading quality of evidence and strength of recommendations in clinical practice guidelines. Allergy. 2009;64:669–77. CrossrefPubMed
7. Shanmugam V, Hakeem A, Campbell KL, et al. Rubber band ligation versus excisional haemorrhoidectomy for haemorhoids (review). Cochrane Database Syst Rev. 2005;2005(3):CD005034.
8. Yeo D, Tan KY. Hemorrhoidectomy-making sense of the surgical options. World J Gastroenterol. 2014;20(45):16976–83. CrossrefPubMedPubMedCentral
9. Milone M, Maietta P, Leongito M, et al. Ferguson hemorrhoidectomy: is it still the gold standard treatment? Updates Surg. 2012;64:191–4. CrossrefPubMed
10. Nisar PJ, Acheson AG, Neal RK, et al. Stapled hemorrhoidopexy compared with conventional hemorrhoidectomy: systematic review of randomized, controlled trials. Dis Colon Rectum. 2007;50(9):1297–305. Crossref
11. Avital S, Inbar R, Karin E, et al. Five-year follow-up of Doppler-guided hemorrhoidal artery ligation. Tech Coloproctol. 2012;16:61–5. CrossrefPubMed
12. De Nardi P, Capretti G, Corsaro A, et al. A prospective, randomized trial comparing the short- and long-term results of Doppler-guided transanal hemorrhoid dearterialization with mucopexy versus excision hemorrhoidectomy for grade III hemorrhoids. Dis Colon Rectum. 2014;57:348–53. CrossrefPubMed.
13. Iyer VS, Shrier I, Gordon PH. Long-term outcome of rubber band ligation for symptomatic primary and recurrent internal hemorrhoids. Dis Colon Rectum. 2004;47:1364–70. CrossrefPubMed
14. Murie JA, Mackenzie I, Sim AJ. Comparison of rubber band ligation and haemorrhoidectomy for second and third degree haemorrhoids: a prospective clinical trial. Br J Surg. 1980;67:786–8. CrossrefPubMed
15. Lewis AAM, Rogers HS, Leighton M. Trial of maximal anal dilatation, cryotherapy and elastic band ligation as alternatives to haemorrhoidectomy in the treatment of large prolapsing haemorrhoids. Br J Surg. 1983;70:54–6. CrossrefPubMed
16. Shanmugam V, Thaha MA, Rabindranath KS, et al. Systematic review of randomized trials comparing rubber band ligation with excisional haemorrhoidectomy. Br J Surg. 2005;92(12):1481–7. CrossrefPubMed
17. Gagloo MA, Hijaz SW, Nasir SA, et al. Comparitive study of hemorrhoidectomy and rubber band ligation in treatment of second and third degree hemorrhoids in Kashmir. Indian J Surg. 2013;75(5):356–60.
18. Peng BC, Jayne DG, Ho YK. Randomized trial of rubber band ligation vs. stapled hemorrhoidectomy for prolapsed piles. Dis Colon Rectum. 2003;46(3):291–7; discussion 296–7. CrossrefPubMed
19. Tiernan J, Hind D, Watson A. The HubBLe trial: haemorrhoidal artery ligation (HAL) versus rubber band ligation (RBL) for haemorrhoids. BMC Gastroenterol. 2012;12:53. Crossref
20. Nienhuijs SW, de Hingh IHJT. Conventional versus LigaSure hemorrhoidectomy for patients with symptomatic hemorrhoids (review). Cochrane Database Syst Rev. 2009;21(1):CD006761.
21. Singer M, Abcarian H. Stapled hemorrhoidopexy: the argument for usage. Clin Colon Rectal Surg. 2004;17(2):131–42. CrossrefPubMedPubMedCentral
22. Wilson MS, Pope V, Doran HE, et al. Objective comparison of stapled anopexy and open hemorrhoidectomy: a randomized, controlled trial. Dis Colon Rectum. 2002;45(11):1437–44. CrossrefPubMed
23. Jayne DG, Botterill I, Ambrose NS, et al. Randomized clinical trial of LigasureTM versus conventional diathermy for day-case haemorrhoidectomy. Br J Surg. 2002;89:428–32. CrossrefPubMed
24. Kombrorozos VA, Skrekas GJ, Pissiotis CD. Rubber band ligation of symptomatic internal hemorhoids: results of 500 cases. Dig Surg. 2000;17:71–6. Crossref
25. Lee HH, Spencer RJ, Beart RW. Multiple hemorrhoidal bandings in a single session. Dis Colon Rectum. 1994;37:37–41. CrossrefPubMed
26. Cintron J, Abcarian H. Benign anorectal: hemorrhoids. In: Wolff BG, Fleshman JW, Beck DE, et al., editors. The ASCRS textbook of colon and rectal surgery. New York: Springer; 2007. p. 156–77.

27. Nelson RS, Ewing BM, Ternent C, et al. Risk of late bleeding following hemorrhoidal banding in patients on antithrombotic prophylaxis. Am J Surg. 2008;196(6):994–9. CrossrefPubMed
28. Lohsiriwat V. Hemorrhoids: from basic pathophysiology to clinical management. World J Gastroenterol. 2012;18(17):2009–17. https://doi.org/10.3748/wjg.v18.i17.2009.
29. Davis BR et al. The American Society of Colon and Rectal Surgeons Clinical practice guidelines for the management of hemorrhoids. American Society of Colon and Rectal Surgeons Clinical Practice Guidelines, ASCRS, 2018, https://fascrs.org/ascrs/media/files/downloads/Clinical%20Practice%20Guidelines/cpg_management_of_hemorrhoids.pdf.
30. Shukla S, Maheshwari A, Tiwari B. Randomized trial of open hemorrhoidectomy versus stapled hemorrhoidectomy for grade II/III hemorrhoids. Indian J Surg. 2018;80:574–9. https://doi.org/10.1007/s12262-017-1670-7.
31. Dekker L, Han-Geurts IJM, Rørvik HD, et al. Rubber band ligation versus haemorrhoidectomy for the treatment of grade II–III haemorrhoids: a systematic review and meta-analysis of randomised controlled trials. Tech Coloproctol. 2021;25:663–74. https://doi.org/10.1007/s10151-021-02430-x.
32. Brown SR, Tiernan JP, Watson AJM, Biggs K, Shephard N, Wailoo AJ, Bradburn M, Alshreef A, Hind D. Haemorrhoidal artery ligation versus rubber band ligation for the management of symptomatic second-degree and third-degree haemorrhoids (HubBLe): a multicentre, open-label, randomised controlled trial. The Lancet. 2016;388(10042):356–64. https://doi.org/10.1016/S0140-6736(16)30584-0. ISSN 0140-6736, https://www.sciencedirect.com/science/article/pii/S0140673616305840
33. Xia W, Manning JPR, Barazanchi AWH, Su'a B, Hill AG. Metronidazole following excisional haemorrhoidectomy: a systematic review and meta-analysis. ANZ J Surg. 2018;88:408–14.
34. Zhang L, Xie Y, Huang D, Ma X, Wang W, Xiao H, Zhong W. LigaSure hemorrhoidectomy versus the procedure for prolapse and hemorrhoids: a meta-analysis of randomized controlled trials. Medicine (Baltimore). 2022;101(3):e28514. https://doi.org/10.1097/MD.0000000000028514. PMID: 35060505; PMCID: PMC8772652
35. Balciscueta Z, Balciscueta I, Uribe N. Post-hemorrhoidectomy pain: can surgeons reduce it? A systematic review and network meta-analysis of randomized trials. Int J Color Dis. 2021;36:2553–66. https://doi.org/10.1007/s00384-021-04013-6.
36. Aibuedefe B, Kling SM, Philp MM, et al. An update on surgical treatment of hemorrhoidal disease: a systematic review and meta-analysis. Int J Color Dis. 2021;36:2041–9. https://doi.org/10.1007/s00384-021-03953-3.
37. Kuiper SZ, Dirksen CD, Kimman ML, Van Kuijk SMJ, Van Tol RR, Muris JWM, et al. Effectiveness and cost-effectiveness of rubber band ligation versus sutured mucopexy versus haemorrhoidectomy in patients with recurrent haemorrhoidal disease (Napoleon trial): study protocol for a multicentre randomized controlled trial. Contemp Clin Trials. 2020;99:106177.
38. Wang JY, Lu CY, Tsai HL, Chen FM, Huang CJ, Huang YS, Huang TJ, Hsieh JS. Randomized controlled trial of LigaSure with submucosal dissection versus Ferguson hemorrhoidectomy for prolapsed hemorrhoids. World J Surg. 2006;30(3):462–6. https://doi.org/10.1007/s00268-005-0297-1. PMID: 16479346
39. Tan EK, Cornish J, Darzi AW, Papagrigoriadis S, Tekkis PP. Meta-analysis of short-term outcomes of randomized controlled trials of LigaSure vs conventional hemorrhoidectomy. Arch Surg. 2007;142(12):1209–18. https://doi.org/10.1001/archsurg.142.12.1209.
40. Tjandra JJ, Chan MKY. Systematic review on the procedure for prolapse and hemorrhoids (stapled Hemorrhoidopexy). Dis Colon Rectum. 2007;50:878–92. https://doi.org/10.1007/s10350-006-0852-3.
41. Kuiper SZ, Dirksen CD, Kimman ML, Van Kuijk SMJ, Van Tol RR, Muris JWM, Watson AJM, Maessen JMC, Melenhorst J, Breukink SO; Napoleon Trial Study Group. Effectiveness and cost-effectiveness of rubber band ligation versus sutured mucopexy versus haemorrhoidectomy in patients with recurrent haemorrhoidal disease (Napoleon trial): Study protocol for a multicentre randomized controlled trial. Contemp Clin Trials. 2020;99:106177. https://doi.org/10.1016/j.cct.2020.106177. Epub 2020 Oct 17. PMID: 33080380.

Management Options for Bleeding Hemorrhoids in Patients on Anticoagulation

42

John Konen and Karim Alavi

PICO table

Patients	Intervention	Comparator	Outcome
Patients with bleeding hemorrhoids in anticoagulation	Office-based procedures	Surgical procedures	Cessation of bleeding, recurrence, complications

Hemorrhoids are part of the normal anatomy of the anal canal and are comprised of arterio-venous connections and fibroelastic connective tissue within the submucosa. They are important for maintaining continence as well as reducing the trauma from passage of stool. Hemorrhoids typically occur at three locations—left lateral, right anterolateral, and right posterolateral. Most patients, however, have variations of this 'classic' distribution pattern. Hemorrhoids are classified in relation to the dentate line. Mucosa proximal to the dentate is endodermal in origin and is lined with columnar epithelium, while mucosa distal to the dentate is from the ectoderm, and is lined with squamous epithelium. Appreciation of this demarcation is critical, as innervation proximal to the dentate is by the autonomic nervous system, while mucosa distal to the dentate is somatically innervated and sensitive to pain. Internal hemorrhoids, which are proximal to the dentate line, are further subclassified into four grades based on the degree of prolapse, while external hemorrhoids are distal

J. Konen (✉)
Rush University Medical College, Department of Surgery, Division of Colon & Rectal Surgery, Chicago, IL, USA
e-mail: John_Konen@rush.edu

K. Alavi (✉)
UMass Chan Medical School, Department of Surgery, Division of Colon & Rectal Surgery, Worcester, MA, USA
e-mail: Karim.Alavi@umassmemorial.org

K. Umanskiy, N. Hyman (eds.), *Difficult Decisions in Colorectal Surgery*, Difficult Decisions in Surgery: An Evidence-Based Approach,
https://doi.org/10.1007/978-3-031-42303-1_42

to the dentate. "Mixed"-type hemorrhoids straddle the dentate line and contain both components. Chronic straining and irregular bowel movements leads to engorgement of the arterio-venous connections and development of symptomatic hemorrhoids characterized by bleeding, prolapse, pain, and/or itching.

Patients with symptomatic hemorrhoids comprise a significant percentage of annual office visits in the United States. Recent data estimate three million visits at an annual cost of over 770 million dollars [1]. However, this cost may be a gross under-estimation as many patients self-medicate or seek alternative treatment options on the internet [2]. In fact, the top trending health issue in the United States in 2012 was "hemorrhoids" according to Google's annual roundup of the world's search trends [3]. Unfortunately, the quality of online information on hemorrhoids is variable, and nearly 50% of websites are graded as poor quality [4]. This makes it imperative that physicians treat patients with hemorrhoids using evidence-based medicine.

Medical Treatment

Treatment options of hemorrhoids are generally guided by the severity of the chief complaints of the patient, which are usually a combination of the following four symptoms: pruritus and/or discomfort, bleeding, pain (thrombosis), or prolapse. In general, the higher the grade of internal hemorrhoids, the more likely it is that banding and/or surgery will play a significant role, and the less likely that a conservative treatment paradigm will be successful. Regardless, *all* patients should be counseled on dietary and lifestyle modifications as a first-line approach to treatment and prevention of recurrence. Conservative measures include ingestion of 20–30 g of fiber daily, which has been shown in several studies to reduce bleeding events in patients with hemorrhoids [5, 6]. A recent Cochrane meta-analysis, examined 378 patients who were enrolled in randomized controlled trials (RCTs) and showed that fiber supplementation resulted in a significant risk reduction in bleeding (RR 0.50, 95% CI 0.28 to 0.89) [7]. Additionally, it is also important to counsel patients to avoid straining and to limit time on the toilet, as these habits have been shown to be more frequent among patients with symptomatic hemorrhoids [8]. Regular physical activity and increased water intake promote stool regularity, although the exact efficacy of these recommendations have not been scientifically validated.

In terms of topical therapies, high-quality evidence supporting their use is lacking. The one exception are phlebotonics—a class of venoactive medications thought to increase venous tone, strengthen vascular wall integrity, improve capillary permeability, facilitate lymphatic drainage, and have anti-inflammatory properties. A 2012 Cochrane review examined twenty RCTs with a total of 2334 patients, of which two trials and a total of 99 patients examined bleeding as an outcome measure. Pooled analysis demonstrated a statistically significant beneficial effect of phlebotonics in treating symptomatic bleeding hemorrhoids compared to controls (OR 0.12; 95% CI 0.04 to 0.37, P = 0.0002) [9]. They also showed similar significant benefit of phlebotonics over controls for pruritus (OR, 0.23; 95% CI, 0.07–0.79) and for prevention of drainage/leakage (OR, 0.12; 95% CI, 0.04–0.42). Unfortunately, routine use and availability of phlebotonics for hemorrhoids in the U.S. is limited compared to Asia and Europe. In general, if patients are receiving symptomatic relief from topical agents, it is reasonable to continue their use, for at least a brief period with the caveat that these products have not been rigorously tested for efficacy. Steroid-containing products should be discontinued beyond 7 days, as they can lead to thinning and subsequent erosion of the anoderm. Lastly, sitz baths using hot tap water soaks, or application of moist heat to the perianal area have been shown to provide relaxation of the anal sphincters and symptomatic relief [10].

Office-Based Procedures

Office-based procedures should be considered for patients with recalcitrant disease after a trial of conservative treatments. Patients with mixed-type hemorrhoids refractory to medical treatment should proceed directly to surgery as office-based procedures will not address their symptoms. Office-based procedures include: rubber band ligation, sclerotherapy, and infrared coagulation. Rubber band ligation (RBL) is the most commonly utilized method and has been shown to be more effective, require fewer treatment sessions, and have better patient outcomes compared to sclerotherapy and infrared coagulation [11, 12] The most recent Clinical Practice Guidelines on hemorrhoid management published by the American Society of Colorectal Surgeons, considers RBL in the setting of anticoagulation or antiplatelet therapy a contraindication [13]. This recommendation is based on the theoretical increased risk of bleeding at the 5–7 post-procedure day range, at which the hemorrhoidal tissue necroses and the rubber band falls off. A large retrospective review of 805 patients demonstrated that 25% of patients on warfarin had post-procedure bleeding, statistically higher compared to 7.5% taking aspirin or NSAIDs, compared to only 2.9% in patients not taking these medications [14]. The overall number of bleeding complications was small (only 8 patients taking warfarin and 40 taking ASA/NSAIDs) and the authors did not comment on the clinical significance of the bleeding and if intervention was necessary. Marshman et al. examined 241 patients who underwent RBL, of which only two had had bleeding, both of whom required hospitalization and clot evacuation. Both patients were on oral anticoagulation [15]. Conversely, a recent retrospective case-control study of 82 patients showed no difference in bleeding for patients on clopidogrel versus controls (3.75% vs 2.78%, $p = 0.74$) [16].

The greatest risk of bleeding is 5–7 days post-banding, thus holding antithrombotic medication such as aspirin, clopidogrel, and coumadin at the time of banding allows for a reduction in their potency at the most critical time [17]. Additionally, time off these medications will be reduced by not stopping the medication for a predetermined amount of time before the procedure, limiting complications such as stroke, acute myocardial infarction (AMI), or DVT/PE. Nelson et al. reviewed their experience with this approach in 364 patients who had RBL while on antithrombotic medication (NSAIDs, aspirin, clopidogrel, and warfarin) and stopping the medication at the time of banding for 7–10 days [18]. They instructed patients to hold NSAIDs, aspirin, and clopidogrel for 10 days, and warfarin for 7 days post-procedure before restarting. Only 3.7% (23 patients) of patients had a bleeding episode, the majority of whom were considered insignificant (i.e. requiring no further therapy), and only 0.9% (6 patients) required emergency evaluation, admission, or transfusion. The authors concluded that these rates were not different compared to rates reported in the literature of post-procedural bleeding from RBL in patients not taking antithrombotic therapy (1.7–2.9%) [14, 19, 20]. They also reported average post-band bleeding occurred on day 6.5, whereas patients taking clopidogrel bled later, on post-band day 9.5 [18].

Several studies examined the risk of stroke and AMI following abrupt discontinuation of antithrombotic medications. In a study examining frequency of stroke occurring after discontinuation of antiplatelet medication in neurology wards, 4.49% of all strokes were related to stopping antiplatelet drugs, with events happening between 6–10 days after stopping the medications [19]. The authors also postulated this was an underestimate, as patients who developed a post-operative stroke were not likely to be referred to a neurology ward. Another study looking at cessation of clopidogrel following treatment of AMI with either medical management or with percutaneous coronary intervention identified that AMI occurred in 17.1% and 7.9% of patients, respectively, and there was a significant rebound effect with events occurring more frequently in the first 90 days following cessation [20]. These findings suggest that the risk of potential bleeding following placement of a hemorrhoidal band should be carefully weighed against potential risk of stroke, AMI, or other thrombotic issue.

An alternative office-based procedure for patients on anticoagulation is sclerotherapy. This involves injecting 1–1.5 mL of a sclerosing agent into the base of the hemorrhoid in the submucosal layer using a 21-gauge spinal needle, causing fibrosis and fixating the hemorrhoid. Anesthesia is not necessary. Injection into the submucosa is crucial, as superficial injection can cause mucosal necrosis, and deep injection can cause pain, abscess/fistula, or sepsis, although this is exceedingly rare [21–23]. Commonly used sclerosants include: hypertonic saline and 5% phenol in vegetable oil, or polidocanol foam, and sodium tetradecyl sulfate (Sotradecol), among others. While there are no randomized data to support use in anticoagulated patients, the American Society of Colorectal Surgeons' (ASCRS) Clinical Practice Guidelines and the ASCRS textbook both assert its safety in these patients. A Japanese case-matched study of 37 patients who underwent sclerotherapy on antiplatelet therapy (aspirin, ticlopidine, clopidogrel, and cilostazol), anticoagulant therapy (warfarin), or both, showed no difference in efficacy to improve bleeding symptoms or post-procedure bleeding rates between patients on antithrombic medication versus case-matched controls. The authors concluded that this provided evidence supporting its use and safety in patients on antithrombotic medications [24]. Efficacy at controlling hemorrhoidal bleeding has been quoted at 75–89% [25, 26], and a recent systematic review found resolution of bleeding in 69–88% of first degree hemorrhoids and prolapse resolution in 90–100% of second degree hemorrhoids, with subjective 'excellent improvement' rating in 80% of first degree hemorrhoid patients [27]. Recurrent bleeding was low (1.5–29%), and 36–49% of patients reported post-procedural pain.

Finally, infrared coagulation (IRC) is considered an alternative to RBL in patients who are on antithrombotic medications given the lower bleeding risk. IRC involves using a tungsten-halogen lamp as an energy source to deliver light converted to heat energy at the apex of an internal hemorrhoid to cause tissue coagulation, though high initial investment costs may be a barrier to use. A small prospective randomized crossover study of 94 patients comparing IRC to RBL demonstrated less pain and bleeding in the IRC group compared to the RBL group in the first 24 hours following the procedure (6.8% vs. 10.2%, respectively; $p < 0.01$) [28]. A systematic review of IRC found one RCT identified improvement in bleeding symptoms in 78%, 51%, and 22% for grade I, II, and III hemorrhoids, respectively, while two other RCTs reported 81% to 93% 'moderate improvement' rates [27]. An RCT of RBL vs IRC demonstrated equal efficacy of the two treatments, but higher pain reports after RBL, but slightly more patients required additional procedures after IRC [29], and the exact same trends were found in a meta-analysis [11]. While no office-based procedure has been consistently shown to be superior, it is important to note that there are no studies examining the safety and efficacy of IRC in patients on antithrombotic medications.

Surgical Management

Surgical hemorrhoidectomy may be necessary for patients who are on anticoagulation and continue to bleed despite all conservative measures. Hemorrhoidectomy eliminates the potential need for repeat office-based procedures and the risk of bleeding associated with each of those procedures. Additionally, patients with grade III-IV hemorrhoids or "mixed-type" hemorrhoids will be undertreated or inappropriately treated with an office procedure and should be considered for hemorrhoidectomy. This needs to be balanced with the increased risk of pain and higher complication rates in surgical approaches, especially in the setting of chronic anticoagulation [11]. Hemorrhoid artery ligation (HAL) may also be an alternative to traditional hemorrhoidectomy. This approach involves specialized equipment including a doppler probe-integrated anoscope followed by suture mucopexy to both ablate the inflow hemorrhoidal arteriole and pexy the hemorrhoid column. Studies have shown favorable short-term results with a recent systematic review showing an overall bleeding rate reported at 5% and an overall reintervention rate was 6% [30]. Although there is limited long-term follow-up data, HAL has increased residual disease and symptom recurrence rates compared to hemorrhoidectomy. Studies of HAL have reported recurrence rates between 6% and 22%, and especially higher rates in advanced disease grades, with a range as high as 50–60% in grade IV hemorrhoids [30–33]. Atallah et al. examined their experience with HAL in patients on anticoagulation and found no difference in post-operative bleeding between patients who were continued on anticoagulants before and after the procedure (except for the day Surgical hemorrhoidectomy may be necessary for patients who are on anticoagulation and continue to bleed despite all conservative measures. Hemorrhoidectomy eliminates the potential need for repeat office-based procedures and the risk of bleeding associated with each of those procedures . Additionally, patients with grade III-IV hemorrhoids or "mixed-type" hemorrhoids will be undertreated or inappropriately treated with an office procedure and should be considered for hemorrhoidectomy. This needs to be balanced with the increased risk of pain and higher complication rates in surgical approaches, especially in the setting of chronic anticoagulation [11]. Hemorrhoid artery ligation (HAL) may also be an alternative to traditional hemorrhoidectomy. This approach involves specialized equipment including a doppler probe-integrated anoscope followed by suture mucopexy to both ablate the inflow hemorrhoidal arteriole and pexy the hemorrhoid column. Studies have shown favorable short-term results with a recent systematic review showing an overall bleeding rate reported at 5% and an overall reintervention rate was 6% [30]. Although there is limited long-term follow-up data, HAL has increased residual disease and symptom recurrence rates compared to hemorrhoidectomy. Studies of HAL have reported recurrence rates between 6% and 22%, and of surgery) and those not on any anticoagulation. Patients on anticoagulation included: aspirin, clopidogrel, warfarin, apixaban, fondaparinux, enoxaparin, and dipyridamole. The study was limited by small sample size (106 patients), and the majority of the anticoagulated cohort (55.6%) were on monotherapy low-dose aspirin alone. Additionally, complications from stopping anticoagulation in these patients were not reported [34].

A final consideration is management of antithrombotic medications surrounding surgical hemorrhoidectomy. In the only prospective study of hemorrhoidal surgery on patients with antithrombotic medication, evaluation of 980 patients undergoing hemorrhoid surgery without interruption of antithrombotic medication (aspirin, clopidogrel, oral anticoagulants, or patients "bridged" to low molecular weight heparin (LMWH) peri-operatively) revealed the overall rate of post-operative bleeding to be 6.5% [35]. On multivariate analysis, patients who stopped warfarin and were bridged with LMWH had the highest rate of bleeding (57%, RR = 42), compared to those who remained fully anticoagulated during their hemorrhoidectomy (23%, RR = 5.8). Patients on clopidogrel also had a significantly higher rate of bleeding (15%, RR = 10). No difference was detected in post-operative bleeding in patients taking aspirin compared to those not on aspirin (5.6% vs 3.5%, P = 0.373). This data suggests that for patients undergoing hemorrhoidectomy, it is safe to continue aspirin perioperatively, and that continuing antithrombotic medications may be an appropriate alternative strategy to bridging, which seems to increase bleeding risk to an unacceptably high level. In addition, clopidogrel seems to significantly increase risk of bleeding, and if the patient's condition allows, stopping it perioperatively should be seriously considered. In general, studies investigating the impact of antithrombic agents following hemorrhoid procedures are limited by small sample size, lack of generalizability, and poor study quality. Based on the lack of available high quality evidence guiding physicians, management of patients on antiplatelet or anticoagulant medications who undergo hemorrhoidectomy should be individualized with early involvement of physicians managing these medications to help weigh the risk of bleeding versus the cardiovascular benefit of these medications.

References

1. Yang JY, Peery AF, Lund JL, Pate V, Sandler RS. Burden and cost of outpatient hemorrhoids in the United States employer-insured population, 2014. Am J Gastroenterol. 2019;114(5):798.
2. Johanson JF, Sonnenberg A. The prevalence of hemorrhoids and chronic constipation: an epidemiologic study. Gastroenterology. 1990;98(2):380–6.
3. Lupkin S. Patients who Google hemorrhoids may want to avoid doctor. https://abcnews.go.com/Health/biggest-google-health-trend-2012-hemorrhoids/story?id=17973862 (2012). Accessed..
4. Yeung T, D'Souza N. Quality analysis of patient information on surgical treatment of haemorrhoids on the internet. Ann R Coll Surg Engl. 2013;95(5):341–4.
5. Moesgaard F, Nielsen L, Hansen JB, Knudsen JT. High-fiber diet reduces bleeding and pain in patients with hemorrhoids. Dis Colon Rectum. 1982;25(5):454–6.
6. Perez-Miranda M, Gomez-Cedenilla A, Leon-Colombo T, Pajares J, Mate-Jimenez J. Effect of fiber supplements on internal bleeding hemorrhoids. Hepato-Gastroenterology. 1996;43(12):1504–7.
7. Alonso-Coello P, Guyatt GH, Heels-Ansdell D, Johanson JF, Lopez-Yarto M, Mills E, et al. Laxatives for the treatment of hemorrhoids. Cochrane Database Syst Rev. 2005;4:CD004649.
8. Johannsson HÖ, Graf W, Påhlman L. Bowel habits in hemorrhoid patients and normal subjects. Am J Gastroenterol. 2005;100:401–6.
9. Perera N, Liolitsa D, Iype S, Croxford A, Yassin M, Lang P, et al. Phlebotonics for haemorrhoids. Cochrane Database Syst Rev. 2012;8:CD004322.
10. Dodi G, Bogoni F, Infantino A, Pianon P, Mortellaro L, Lise M. Hot or cold in anal pain? Dis Colon Rectum. 1986;29(4):248–51.
11. MacRae HM, McLeod RS. Comparison of hemorrhoidal treatment modalities. Dis Colon Rectum. 1995;38(7):687–94.
12. Nasir MA, Masroor R, Arafat Y, Butt Q, Sarwar S. Injection sclerotherapy versus rubber band ligation for second degree hemorrhoids. Pak Armed Forces Med J. 2017;6:996–1002.
13. Davis BR, Lee-Kong SA, Migaly J, Feingold DL, Steele SR. The American Society of Colon and Rectal Surgeons clinical practice guidelines for the management of hemorrhoids. Dis Colon Rectum. 2018;61(3):284–92.
14. Iyer V, Shrier I, Gordon P. Long-term outcome of rubber band ligation for symptomatic primary and recurrent internal hemorrhoids. Dis Colon Rectum. 2004;47(9):1364–70.
15. Marshman D, Huber PJ, Timmerman W, Simonton CT, Odom FC, Kaplan ER. Hemorrhoidal ligation. Dis Colon Rectum. 1989;32(5):369–71.
16. Hite N, Klinger AL, Miller P, Beck DE, Whitlow CB, Hicks TC, et al. Clopidogrel bisulfate (Plavix) does not increase bleeding complications in patients undergoing rubber band ligation for symptomatic hemorrhoids. J Surg Res. 2018;229:230–3.
17. Steele SR, Davids JS, Ridolfi TJ. The ASCRS textbook of colon and rectal surgery. Hemorrhoids: Springer Nature; 2021.
18. Nelson RS, Ewing BM, Ternent C, Shashidharan M, Blatchford GJ, Thorson AG. Risk of late bleeding following hemorrhoidal banding in patients on antithrombotic prophylaxis. Am J Surg. 2008;196(6):994–9.
19. Sibon I, Orgogozo J-M. Antiplatelet drug discontinuation is a risk factor for ischemic stroke. Neurology. 2004;62(7):1187–9.
20. Ho PM, Peterson ED, Wang L, Magid DJ, Fihn SD, Larsen GC, et al. Incidence of death and acute myocardial infarction associated with stopping clopidogrel after acute coronary syndrome. JAMA. 2008;299(5):532–9.
21. Kaman L, Aggarwal S, Kumar R, Behera A, Katariya RN. Necrotizing fascitis after injection sclerotherapy for hemorrhoids. Dis Colon Rectum. 1999;42(3):419–20.
22. Barwell J, Watkins R, Lloyd-Davies E, Wilkins D. Life-threatening retroperitoneal sepsis after hemorrhoid injection sclerotherapy: report of a case. Dis Colon Rectum. 1999;42(3):421–3.

23. Schulte T, Fändrich F, Kahlke V. Life-threatening rectal necrosis after injection sclerotherapy for haemorrhoids. Int J Color Dis. 2008;23(7):725–6.
24. Yano T, Nogaki T, Asano M, Tanaka S, Kawakami K, Matsuda Y. Outcomes of case-matched injection sclerotherapy with a new agent for hemorrhoids in patients treated with or without blood thinners. Surg Today. 2013;43:854–8.
25. Khoury G, Lake S, Lewis MC, Lewis A. A randomized trial to compare single with multiple phenol injection treatment for haemorrhoids. Br J Surg. 1985;72(9):741–2.
26. Mann C, Motson R, Clifton M. The immediate response to injection therapy for first-degree haemorrhoids. J R Soc Med. 1988;81(3):146–8.
27. Cocorullo G, Tutino R, Falco N, Licari L, Orlando G, Fontana T, et al. The non-surgical management for hemorrhoidal disease. A systematic review. G Chir. 2017;38(1):5.
28. Marques C, Nahas S, Nahas C, Sobrado C, Habr-Gama A, Kiss D. Early results of the treatment of internal hemorrhoid disease by infrared coagulation and elastic banding: a prospective randomized cross-over trial. Tech Coloproctol. 2006;10(4):312–7.
29. Poen A, Felt-Bersma R, Cuesta M, Deville W, Meuwissen S. A randomized controlled trial of rubber band ligation versus infra-red coagulation in the treatment of internal haemorrhoids. Eur J Gastroenterol Hepatol. 2000;12(5):535–40.
30. Pucher P, Sodergren M, Lord A, Darzi A, Ziprin P. Clinical outcome following D oppler-guided haemorrhoidal artery ligation: a systematic review. Color Dis. 2013;15(6):e284–e94.
31. Lehur PA, Didnée AS, Faucheron J-L, Meurette G, Zerbib P, Siproudhis L, et al. Cost-effectiveness of new surgical treatments for Hemorrhoidal disease. Ann Surg. 2016;264(5):710–6.
32. Festen S, Van Hoogstraten M, Van Geloven A, Gerhards M. Treatment of grade III and IV haemorrhoidal disease with PPH or THD. A randomized trial on postoperative complications and short-term results. Int J Color Dis. 2009;24:1401–5.
33. De Nardi P, Capretti G, Corsaro A, Staudacher C. A prospective, randomized trial comparing the short-and long-term results of doppler-guided transanal hemorrhoid dearterialization with mucopexy versus excision hemorrhoidectomy for grade III hemorrhoids. Dis Colon Rectum. 2014;57(3):348–53.
34. Atallah S, Maharaja G, Martin-Perez B, Burke J, Albert M, Larach S. Transanal hemorrhoidal dearterialization (THD): a safe procedure for the anticoagulated patient? Tech Coloproctol. 2016;20(7):461–6.
35. Pigot F, Juguet F, Bouchard D, Castinel A. Do we have to stop anticoagulant and platelet-inhibitor treatments during proctological surgery? Color Dis. 2012;14(12):1516–20.

Sacral Nerve Stimulation: Choices vs Non-surgical Care for Fecal Incontinence

43

William Allen, Alexandra Jones, Hillary Simon, and Russ Farmer

Executive Summary

Sacral nerve stimulation (SNS) has revolutionized the surgical treatment of fecal incontinence (FI). Patients that previously were treated only with medication to minimal benefit or colostomy can now get significant symptom relief from fecal (and urinary) incontinence with this procedure. The surgery is technically relatively simple and has a low complication rate. However, once implanted, the need for reoperation is high as is the cost of both entry to therapy and ongoing therapy. Patients need to be counselled extensively and their long-term expectations managed prior to SNS implantation. While SNS is not the metaphorical "silver bullet" for the FI, it can go a long way to improving the quality of life for a huge number of well-selected patients.

PICO table

Patients	Intervention	Comparator	Outcome
Patients with fecal incontinence	Sacral nerve stimulation	Medical management	Symptom improvement, quality of life

W. Allen · A. Jones
Department of Surgery, University of Louisville, Louisville, KY, USA
e-mail: william.allen.4@louisville.edu; alexandra.jones.1@louisville.edu

H. Simon · R. Farmer (✉)
Division of Colon and Rectal Surgery, Department of Surgery, University of Louisville, Louisville, KY, USA
e-mail: hillary.simon@louisville.edu; russell.farmer@louisville.edu

K. Umanskiy, N. Hyman (eds.), *Difficult Decisions in Colorectal Surgery*, Difficult Decisions in Surgery: An Evidence-Based Approach,
https://doi.org/10.1007/978-3-031-42303-1_43

Epidemiology/Incidence of Fecal Incontinence

Fecal incontinence is increasingly more prevalent with potentially debilitating social, economic, and health consequences. FI has been estimated to occur in up to 50% of elderly people living within care homes and up to 18% in the general population from a UK population-based survey via the 2010 National Audit of Continence Care [1]. In the United States a large population-based survey revealed that 1 in 7 people experienced fecal incontinence in their lifetime with an increased prevalence among those with inflammatory bowel disease, celiac disease, or irritable bowel syndrome [2]. One of the most common risk factors for fecal incontinence is increasing age. As the average life expectancy continues to increase, the incidence of FI will continue to increase concomitantly. One study revealed FI to be the second most common cause of an individual being placed in a nursing facility [3]. This is partly due to the increased time in care the individual requires as well as the emotional distress experienced by the caregiver. FI has been shown to have a strong association with both the incidence and severity of sacral decubitus ulcers [4]. FI is associated with an overall decrease in health and increase in frailty with the inability to adequately, and independently, complete activities of daily living. Given its correlation with deconditioning, FI has been used as a measure of functional impairment with evidence of an increased likelihood of death (hazard ratio 1.28) [5].

Diagnostic Criteria

The diagnosis of FI is made based upon a thorough history of the patient's symptomatology. The Rome IV criteria, often modified for use in research, requires the patient to have had recurrent, uncontrolled passage of feces for at least 3 months and the patient must have a developmental age of at least 4 years [6]. A second commonly used diagnostic criteria is the Cleveland Clinic Fecal Incontinence score (Wexner Score) which is a scoring system with a total value between 1 and 20, 0 is complete continence and 20 is complete incontinence. The Wexner Score is calculated using the patient's responses in regards to incontinence of gas, liquid, or solid stool, and the necessity for lifestyle modifications [7].

Causes of FI

FI can result from a variety of etiologies including loose stool caused by infection, diet, intestinal pathology, or functional abnormalities caused by sphincter injury, radiation, central or peripheral neuropathy, and myopathy. Women have a higher incidence of primary pelvic floor dysfunction compared to men, often related to pregnancy. It has been shown that pelvic floor dysfunction was significantly increased in women who underwent caesarean section, spontaneous vaginal delivery, or instrumental delivery when compared with nulliparous women [8]. Obstetric trauma remains one of the most common causes of FI due to the risk of mechanical tears of the sphincter occurring in 0.6–9% of vaginal deliveries. The innervations of the pelvic floor and the pudendal nerve are at risk of being damaged during prolonged or instrumented delivery.

It is projected that the number of women in the United States affected by pelvic floor disorders will continue to increase and a similar increase will be seen in those with FI from 10.6 million to an estimated 16.8 million by 2050 [9]. Although pelvic floor dysfunction is more common in women, the rates of fecal incontinence in the general population remains similar in women (8.9%) and men (7.7%) [10]. FI is a potential complication of numerous common conditions ranging from hemorrhoidal disease, rectal prolapse, and iatrogenic injuries from surgical procedures. Other causes include any condition the predisposes the patient to rectal hyposensitivity due to nerve damage, including diabetes, spinal cord injuries, and a subset of patients with irritable bowel syndrome.

Non-surgical Management of Fecal Incontinence

Traditionally, medical therapy and biofeedback are used in the management of FI prior to surgery. The purpose of medical therapy focuses on increasing the solidity of the stool and decreasing the frequency of bowel movements. Methylcellulose or psyllium are common sources of fiber which absorb liquid within the intestines and increase the bulk of the stool, decreasing leakage of liquid feces and providing sensory feedback regarding the need to defecate. Antimotility agents such as Loperamide act directly on the mu receptors of the longitudinal and circular muscles of the intestines to inhibit contraction as well as peristalsis. The decrease in peristalsis acts to increase the uptake of the liquid within the stool, increasing its bulk. Anticholinergic agents, such as hyoscyamine, are muscarinic antagonists to the smooth muscle within the gastrointestinal tract and decrease the rate of peristalsis allowing for similar effects seen with other antimotility agents. If the patient does not respond to loperamide or antimuscarinics then liquid narcotics such as codeine are then used to assist in decreasing the transit time of stool, although their systemic effects require thorough consideration before prescribing.

Nonmedication-based treatment for FI may include pelvic floor physiotherapy and biofeedback. Currently, the most common form of pelvic floor rehabilitation includes electromyographic (EMG) biofeedback-guided pelvic floor muscle training (PFMT). PFMT encompasses numerous methods by which an individual increases the coordination of the pelvic floor and anal sphincters. Patients undergo training of the core muscles, particularly the transversus abdominis, as well as the pelvic floor by performing Kegel contractions [11]. Biofeedback may be conducted using a balloon placed within the rectum at the time of the PFMT to assist in instructing the patient as well as coordinating the exercises with the sensation of stool within the rectum. The presence of the balloon serves as the sensation of the rectum gradually filling in order to mimic increasing stool within the rectal vault [11]. The most common type of biofeedback uses EMG. An anal plug with surface electrodes is placed within the rectum and the muscle contractions are recorded so that the patient is able to visualize the effects of performing Kegel exercises (squeezing of the pelvic floor muscles) [12]. EMG guided biofeedback therapy has been reported to have a significant effect on FI with up to 92% of patients in one study experiencing improvement in symptoms [13].

Sacral Nerve Stimulation

Sacral nerve stimulation (SNS) is a safe and efficacious way to treat fecal incontinence (FI) in patient's refractory to behavioral and pharmacological therapies [14]. Originally described in 1982 for its role in urinary incontinence, SNS was developed by Tanegho and Schmidt [15] with official FDA approval in 1997 [16]. It was then introduced by Matzel et al. in the Lancet in 1995 for its use in FI [17]. However, it did not gain FDA approval for this use until 2011 [18].

The underlying mechanism of action for sacral neuromodulation, or SNS, remains unknown. Recent publications theorize results are more related to central nervous system stimulation via afferent nervous system pathways versus previously held beliefs that it worked via peripheral motor neurostimulation [19]. A widely accepted theory is that SNS delivers low dose, frequent electrical pulses to the pudendal nerve to increase both afferent and efferent effects of that central nervous distribution resulting in reflex augmentation [20].

Prior to development of SNS for use in FI, sphincteroplasty had been the mainstay of surgical treatment for fecal incontinence. A recent comparative study performed in 2017 by Rodriques et all demonstrated improvement in the Cleveland Clinic Florida Fecal Incontinence Score (CCF-FIS) (15.9–8.4; P = 0.003) compared to sphincteroplasty (16.9–12.9; P = 0.078) [21]. In 2010 another comparative study performed by Ratto et al. [22], showed similar outcomes in incontinence scores and QOL. Long term effects of SNS placement are still being studied. There has been some speculation that SNS will contribute to long-term neuroplasticity via its central nervous afferent conduction. This is bolstered by the continued improvement in the function of patients following removal of the SNS device after prolonged implantation [1].

Placement of an SNS device is performed in a two-stage process. Patients should initially be marked with plans for placement at the junction of the back and buttocks with some deference of side based on patient preference, sleep and other hygiene habits. The first stage includes placement of temporary percutaneous leads positioned near the S3 nerve root via the S3 foramen for 1–4 weeks. If the patient notes improvement in incontinence symptoms, a more permanent neurostimulator device is placed. A successful trial would be a reduction of incontinence symptoms by >50%. During Stage 1, the patient is placed in prone position with exposure of buttocks and the gluteal crease. Using fluoroscopic guidance, a needle is inserted into the S3 foramen and placement is then verified using external stimulator. Correct positioning elicits motor responses from the pelvic floor and ipsilateral great toe plantar flexion. Once positioning is verified a wire is passed through the needle and the Seldinger technique is used to implant the temporary leads. A pocket is made, and the leads are tunneled to the pocket which will serve as site for permeant stimulator during the next stage of implantation. The temporary external stimulator is attached and enclosed within the pocket. If the temporary leads are successful, Stage 2 is performed with placement of a permanent neurostimulator device. The previous incision is opened, and electrodes exposed. The permeant stimulator, which constitutes a combination battery pack and computer to drive delivery of electricity, is connected and replaced back in the pocket.

Contraindications to placement however still exist. Drawbacks to using older SNS devices include frequency of replacing the battery, inability to recharge, size and MRI incompatibility. In certain neurogenic groups such as chronic back pain, MS or even patients with a history of low anterior resections, the placement of an SNS has been a relative contraindication given the high likelihood of requiring an MRI during their lifetime. The newest generation of products from Medtronic and Axonics have addressed this issue with the development of MRI compatible stimulators. Devices have moved from a large battery to a smaller, rechargeable battery. Newer products such as the Interstim Micro device (2.8 cm^3) is 80% smaller than its recharge free Interstim II neurostimulator (14 cm^3) [23]. In a multicenter prospective trial of 262 patients, the smaller size has also been shown to reduce amount of subjective pain patients experience from implantation of the stimulator from 7% with the Interstim II versus 2% in the Interstim Micro [24].

Work Up

Initial work-up should include a Stool Diary. A Stool (Bowel) Diary may be kept for a single week up to several weeks, and is often recorded on paper; However, Smartphone applications have recently been developed and allow improved recording of incontinence [25]. Non-operative management has been found to benefit approximately only 25% of patients presenting with FI, highlighting the importance of understanding operative strategies to treat FI [26]. Once baseline bowel function has been established via a Stool Diary, surgical intervention options for FI escalate in invasiveness and should be approached as such. The two main surgical options for FI include SNS and anal sphincter repair.

Clinical Practice Guideline Summary

The Clinical Practice Guidelines Committee of the American Society of Colon and Rectal Surgeons (ASCRS) have composed societal Clinical Practice Guidelines for the treatment of FI. The guidelines are created based on the best available evidence [27].

The ASCRS strongly recommends performing thorough history, physical exam, laboratory, and supplementary testing to rule out underlying infectious or pathologic etiologies. Anorectal physiology testing (manometry, anorectal sensation, volume tolerance, compliance), endorectal ultrasound, and pudendal nerve terminal motor latency can be considered to help define the elements of dysfunction and guide management. Validated measures that assess the nature, severity, and impact of incontinence on quality of life should be part of the assessment for FI. The use of a scoring index, such as the Fecal Incontinence Severity Index, St. Marks Incontinence Score, Cleveland Clinic Florida Fecal Incontinence Score (CCF), or other validated tool, is helpful in selecting patients for therapies and for measuring response to treatment over time. Dietary and medical management are recommended as first-line therapy. Biofeedback/pelvic floor physical therapy should be considered as an adjunct to medical management of FI. Patients with more severe symptoms, or for symptoms severely affecting quality of life, may be more appropriate for invasive therapies up to and including colostomy.

Injection of bulking agents, sphincter plication, and radiofrequency application (Secca procedure) are less studied and poorly validated, making them a weak recommendation. Sphincter repair is highly recommended for patients with defined external sphincter defects and can be repeated with success if necessary. Implantation of an artificial bowel sphincter remains an option for severe FI, but with low quality evidence supporting its use. Colostomy creation is a highly recommended and supported surgical option for patients who have failed or do not wish to pursue other therapies for FI. New and emerging technologies, such as percutaneous tibial nerve stimulation and magnetic anal sphincter exist, however data remains insufficient to make recommendations currently. Overall, sacral neuromodulation (SNS) should be considered as a first-line surgical option for incontinent patients with and without sphincter defects. Ultimately, due to etiology variability, treatment can be challenging and should be individualized.

SNS Candidate Selection

Prior works have compared non-operative and operative management. In a single-center, randomized control trial comparing groups with similar baseline characteristics, SNS implantation versus optimal medical management (pelvic floor physical therapy, bulking agent, and dietary modification), SNS was found to significantly improve incontinent episodes by more than 50% in 90% of patients (50/52 patients) [28]. The combined data of two trials showed that the number of people failing to achieve full continence was significantly lower when electrical stimulation was added to biofeedback compared against biofeedback alone (RR 0.60, 95% CI 0.46 to 0.78) [29, 30]. Other prospective studies, while small, have reproduced similar findings, noting SNS improves FI better than conservative management31.While a number of interventions are available for treatment of FI that vary in efficacy and morbidity, SNS comes with validated efficacy and low morbidity. Morbidity surrounding SNS implantation includes pain or infection at the implant site pain, paresthesia, and electrode displacements or breaks requiring revision and battery exchanges [32]

There are few contraindications and relative contraindications to SNS implantation. Bleeding diathesis, pregnancy, or other body habitus or underlying co-morbidities which would not allow prone positioning, as well as limited cognitive function which would interfere with the operation of the SNS device, are contraindications to placement. In the past, many felt the presence of a cardiac pacemaker was a contraindication, but there are case series that demonstrate safety with intraoperative monitoring during placement. Relative contraindications to be considered include psychological instability, unacceptable risk for the consequences of infection, like patient with artificial heart valves, or patients with severe or rapidly progressive neurologic disease. Frail patients, specifically those who are wheelchair bound or with limited life-expectancy, would be more likely to fail SNS trial. However, data demonstrates that patients with disorders such as multiple sclerosis, especially in the earlier stages, have excellent functional outcomes with SNS [33]

Difficult Decisions Surrounding SNS Implantation vs Conservative/Medical Management

Each of the following clinical scenarios are commentaries on specific situations surrounding SNS implantation. Medical therapy is always an option to treat underlying fecal incontinence, with the knowledge that this approach is likely to be less durable and effective long term.

Length of Percutaneous/Test Stimulation

Patients' complaints of incontinence can vary significantly based on their perceptions of their symptoms and the outcomes of these symptoms. Whereas one patient may outline daily episodes of whole bowel incontinence with complete loss of control multiple times a day, other patients may outline fecal incontinence a few times a week or only once a month. It is important in evaluating these patients to be explicit in their complaints. The inclusion of these criteria has likely propagated the adoption of the CCFFIS [7] as the standard for measuring fecal incontinence.

Symptom description and stratification via the CCFFIS or others (of which there are many [34]) allow for appropriate determination if SNS implementation is the appropriate approach. Many patients without fecal incontinence occurring several times a week may indeed see a demonstrable benefit with SNS implantation; however, documenting the ability of SNS to improve symptoms over a longer period may be difficult and create financial problems for patients in whom insurance will not cover a demonstrated improvement in symptoms. Traditionally, most patients undertake a one-to-two-week trial of implantation for symptoms of FI. This time course is also prevalent throughout urologic literature [35]. However, other studies have shown that a prolonged period of percutaneous testing with electrodes does not lead to infection – ultimately, the risk of infection must be weighed against the benefits of a prolonged testing period [36, 37]. Various studies have quoted differing rates of infection for SNS implantation, of around 10 to 12% [38] or 13.5% [39].

(Note: While this is consistent with published data of all kinds, this is not consistent with the authors' anecdotal experience).

Common skin flora produces infections most commonly, with S. aureus being particularly prevalent [38]. One study compared the rates of colonization of removed percutaneous lead extensions after twenty-one days of trial, resulting in a 54% rate of S. aureus colonization deep within the wires of extension [40]. Of particular concern is the tendency for these device infections to present late in the cycle of implantation. In a large study, around 1/3 of all infections seen began presentation at least 1 year following implantation [41]. An excellent review by Lee et al. provides an overall excellent outline for perioperative steps to minimize infection and prevent eventual explantation [35]. The methods so outlined include a significant perioperative oral antibiotic regimen in addition to perioperative IV antibiotics to be used at the surgeon's discretion.

Pertinent Clinical Questions Prior to Choosing SNS

- What is my goal length of percutaneous testing for this patient?
- Will this length of testing put my patient at high risk for infection?
- Do I need to tailor the choice of perioperative antibiotics to include oral medications to minimize risk?
- Though the risk of infection in sacral nerve stimulation is low, can my patient successfully navigate treatment for and healing of an open posterior surgical wound (i.e., immobility, DM, etc.?
- The risk of presacral abscess is very low [42], but would may patient tolerate this?

LARS: Low Anterior Resection Syndrome

SNS can be used as an adjunct to other treatments for those whose fecal incontinence proves refractory to medical management. The fall back for most surgeons treating patients with LARS has been constipating or bulking agents in the past, combined with enemas, pelvic floor physical therapy, and a host of other treatments which may or may not be effective [43]. More has been written in aggregate about SNS as a treatment for LARS than actual published data, with several meta-analyses attempting to collate the same few patients [44–47]. Rather than utilizing LARS scoring systems and assigning treatment modalities based on them, many CRS and other implanting surgeons have been using SNS as a last-ditch effort to avoid a stoma – this is especially true in many patients who often present frustrated with their quality of life.

In essence, SNS is often the last resort for these patients before an ostomy is made permanently. The summary of these series and others [48, 49] shows significant Quality of Life improvement with SNS implantation following failure of other modalities or in combination with them. Of note when treating a patient with LARS and using SNS, one needs to consider the nature of chemotherapeutics used or planned, as most LARS patients have undergone surgery for cancer. If patients are treated with chemotherapeutics that have known neurotoxic or altering effects (i.e., platinum based chemotherapeutic agents), it is possible that SNS may be less effective in this group. It is also important to discuss financial implications with these patients, as many are often at the end of their financial ability to undergo potentially costly surgical treatment that may be fought by their insurance as "outside" the bounds of standard medical care.

Pertinent Clinical Questions Prior to Choosing SNS

- What symptom are you trying to improve with SNS? Be wary of patients with significant non- FI related LARS symptoms like tenesmus, pain, etc.
- Do the patients resources, both social and financial, support SNS implantation in an "edge" case?
- Are you and the patient prepared for the chance this may not work?

Mixed Constipation/Fecal Incontinence

The jury is still out on whether SNS, PTNS, and other neurogenic treatment modalities can result in significant symptom improvement for patients with constipation. Some studies quote improvement of constipation symptoms [50–52], while others outline failure of this treatment [14, 53]. Clearly there is more here than simple neural stimulation as the mixed results seen in adults do not mirror the excellent results seen in pediatric patients with similar complaints [54]. With the seemingly contradictory results, which patients should be getting an SNS with constipation?

There is no clear answer, however, we can impute a few workable premises. Firstly, patients who have mixed FI and Pelvic Outlet Dysfunction related constipation following work up with manometry +/− defecography (classic or MRI) would likely benefit from SNS implantation. The classic presentation for this patient is one who has pelvic outlet dysfunction resulting in constipation which precipitates the consumption of laxatives or cathartics. Most patients will present having tried multiple versions of these medications in combination resulting in severe overflow incontinence of feces without sensation.

SNS implantation is less likely to be effective in patients with slow transit constipation. Some studies have shown promise [55, 56], but often results are mixed. These patients are often better treated with more traditional modalities such as selective colectomy or an ostomy following extensive work up. Patients with idiopathic constipation may derive some benefit, but it is unknown until test stimulation.

Pertinent Clinical Questions Prior to Choosing SNS

- What is the underlying cause of the patients' symptoms? Are they more appropriately treated with another form of surgery or medical management?
- Given that the rate of success is moderate for patients with constipation related symptoms, can the patient afford for this not to work? (Two procedures, potentially significant charges)

Radiation Proctitis/Pelvic Radiation

SNS can be considered an adjunct to treatment for radiation proctitis that occurs frequently following radiotherapy for any number of malignancies. Following radiation, the rectum loses capacitance and plasticity, going from an organ - similar in function and efficacy to the stomach - to a non-dynamic tube for the conveyance of waste. The end result often creates a situation where the rectum show moderate to minimal functionality and continence becomes compromised [57]. The implantation of an SNS type device can potentially assist in the incontinence related to radiation proctitis, but available literature is very limited [58–60] and patients should be counselled that results are not guaranteed / can't be foreseen. Practitioners should also be advised that this will likely be an "off-label" implantation and funding / insurance may be difficult to acquire.

Pertinent Clinical Questions Prior to Choosing SNS

- Have you tried EVERYTHING else?

Congenital Sacral Malformation, Spina Bifida, and Sacral Agenesis

Implantation in patients with sacral malformations can create unique technical challenges for implanting surgeons. According to Povo et al. [61], the rate of the malformations is much higher than would be estimated in the population. In a review of around 1000 imaging studies, they identified malformations of the sacrum at a rate of 24.1% which could impact percutaneous placement and foraminal anatomy.

Much of the literature surrounding implantation in patients with spina bifida originates in the pediatric literature, most being small case series. Size of study notwithstanding, the results of implantation using standard percutaneous, fluoroscopically guided techniques have been good, with many patients moving on to formal implantation for either fecal incontinence, neurogenic bladder, or both [62–64]. Of note is the 2012 study by Lansen-Koch et al. Though the number of patients was low [10], 8 of them were able to undergo successful percutaneous implantation in the setting of spina bifida and the median age was 26.4 years old. This view is challenged directly by others – Michael et al. opining that spina bifida or other sacral malformation is a direct contraindication to percutaneous implantation [65].

Sacral agenesis represents an even more difficult problem for traditional lead implantation techniques. Adjunctive techniques, such as intraoperative CT guidance, have been used for implantation in this highly selected patient group [66]. These malformations are often associated with anal agenesis / imperforate anus. Despite this implantation can be successful [67–69]. In any group of patients, percutaneous implantation is not the only method practiced, as SNS implants were originally undertaken in a cut-down method over the sacrum with directed identification of the pudendal nerve and the S3 foramen; however, technical review of this method is outside the scope of this chapter and likely best left to neurosurgical colleagues with sacral experience. Should traditional implantation techniques fail, other methods do exist [70] for sacral nerve stimulation in these patients, but reports are rare.

Pertinent Clinical Questions Prior to Choosing SNS

- Do you have pertinent imaging prior to implantation to guide you?
- What other procedures has the patient undergone and what were the outcomes?
- Are alternative implantation techniques and other specialist consultations necessary prior to operation?

Previous Implantation

Patient outcomes from SNS are not in doubt. Indeed, those surgeons who have seen successful outcomes from this operation can attest to the patient satisfaction present as a part of this line of treatment. However, patients need to be aware of the lifetime risk of reoperation for non-battery related issues. Many authors present a rate of reoperation for complications from initial implantation somewhere between 15–18% [71–74]. This can be due to changes in body anatomy (i.e. significant weight gain or loss), localized trauma, or other factors.

Some patients will complain that the device has difficulty achieving connection to their personal controller. Others will state they had a fall at home which has led to issues with the device; trauma is a very common reason for reoperation in these patients. Many of them are elderly and have issues with balance – something to consider before implantation – while one general anesthetic might be successful, you might be in more down the road with SNS implantation. Rarely, patients will present with a lead which has become dislodged or shifted because of the above issues. **For a patient presenting with recurrent Fecal Incontinence issues despite reprogramming success, the authors recommend a simple 2-view AP and Lateral pelvic xray mirroring the operative fluoroscopy images to determine shifting or malposition of the device.** Note that this will occur independently from surgical skill or technique.

For patients that have undergone previous SNS implantation and need a new lead placed, the authors recommend using the contralateral S3 foramen for placement rather than the original implantation site. Additionally, if the SNS is to be removed, performing explant of the lead should also be done fluoroscopically to facilitate explantation of the lead and prevent lead breakage during removal. The authors also concur with previous published accounts that efficacy of contralateral implantation is often diminished on follow up following explant of the original SNS device [71]. The mechanism behind this is unknown.

Pertinent Clinical Questions Prior to Choosing SNS

- Are your patients aware the second implant may not work as well as the first?
- Is your patient aware of the long-term need for potential reoperation?

Spinal Cord Injury

Patients with spinal cord injuries who develop neurogenic bowel, bladder, or both can be candidates for successful SNS. Rosen and colleagues [75] report a series of patients with neurogenic bowel of multiple sources, 50% of which had either developed FI as a result of direct spinal cord injury or spinal cord surgery. The remainder of these patients developed FI because of other CNS related diseases (Multiple sclerosis, Friedrich's Ataxia, Meningomyelocele). Of the diverse group of patients, 80% achieved significant improvement of their FI symptoms following implantation of an SNS. Interestingly, Schurch et al. have previously published results of two patients with specifically identified spinal cord segmental injuries that had successful PNE implantation [76]. The authors hypothesize these results to be due to preserved bulbo-spinal loop pathways despite spinal cord injury. SNS has previously been shown efficacious in Urinary Incontinence in this group of patients as well [77].

Pertinent Clinical Questions Prior to Choosing SNS

- What is the level of spinal cord injury and are the lumbo-sacral reflexes intact? If this is true, you have a good case for successful SNS.
- Can you patient be positioned to minimize chance for complications related to wound healing?

Radiculopathy or Other Known Neuropathic Pain

There are two aspects to consider regarding radiculopathy in patients with SNS implantation:

Incidence of Radiculopathy in Patients with SNS Implantation

Radiculopathy in patients status-post SNS implantation is not a commonly reported complication. However, patients will present to the office with radiculopathy style complaints. These symptoms typically mirror the nervous distribution of the stimulated nerves that result in plantarflexion of the great toe (tibial nerve). These complaints are usually resolved with reprogramming. This will take time and potentially multiple office visits. The authors recommend seeing these patients in concert with the device representatives for the implanted SNS as they are invaluable in programming around issues such as this one.

Implantation for Radiculopathy, Chronic Anal or Pelvic Pain

There is a very small amount of literature available regarding implantation of SNS for chronic pelvic pain, anal pain, or lumbosacral radiculopathy. Typically, this type of pain of is best managed by a different form of sacral nerve stimulation utilizing higher nerve roots [78]. Yang et al. have reported implantation for chronic anal pain79. Unfortunately, many providers are not familiar with SNS as a treatment modality and may view it similar to other nerve root stimulation often used in pain situations. They will then refer the patient for possible SNS implantation for non-FI related indications. Given the nature of these complaints, the operation, and the patient expectations, the authors recommend strongly against yielding to the desires of patients and referring physicians outside of approved SNS implantation indications.

Final Notes

The authors view SNS as an excellent option for patients with fecal incontinence provided that the surgeon is invested in the procedure, patients, and follow up. This therapy can be exceptionally effective and rewarding as a means of restoring quality of life to patients who are in the very depths of despair.

References

1. Musa MK, Saga S, Blekken L, Harris R, Goodman C, Norton C. The prevalence, incidence, and correlates of fecal incontinence among older people residing in care homes: a systematic review. J Am Med Dir Assoc. 2019;20:956–962.e8.
2. Menees SB, Almario CV, Spiegel BMR, Chey WD. Prevalence of and factors associated with fecal incontinence: results from a population-based survey. Gastroenterology. 2018;154(6):1672–1681.e3. https://doi.org/10.1053/j.gastro.2018.01.062.
3. Talley NJ, O'Keefe EA, Zinsmeister AR, Melton LJ 3rd. Prevalence of gastrointestinal symptoms in the elderly: a population-based study. Gastroenterology. 1992;102(3):895–901. (0016–5085 (Print))

4. Lachenbruch C, Ribble D, Emmons K, VanGilder C. Pressure ulcer risk in the incontinent patient: analysis of incontinence and hospital-acquired pressure ulcers from the international pressure ulcer prevalence™ survey. J Wound Ostomy Continence Nurs. 2016;43(3):235–41. (1528–3976 (Electronic))
5. Jamieson HA, Schluter PJ, Pyun J, et al. Fecal incontinence is associated with mortality among older adults with complex needs: an observational cohort study. Off J Am Coll Gastroenterol. 2017;112(9):1431–7.
6. Schmulson MJ, Drossman DA. What is new in Rome IV J Neurogastroenterol Motil. 2017;23(2):151–63. (2093–0879 (Print))
7. Jorge JMN, Wexner SD. Etiology and management of fecal incontinence. Dis Colon Rectum. 1993;36(1):77–97. https://doi.org/10.1007/BF02050307.
8. MacLennan AH, Taylor AW, Wilson DH, Wilson D. The prevalence of pelvic floor disorders and their relationship to gender, age, parity and mode of delivery. BJOG. 2000;107(12): 1460–70. (1470-0328 (Print))
9. Wu JM, Hundley AF, Fulton RG, Myers ER. Forecasting the prevalence of pelvic floor disorders in U.S. Women: 2010 to 2050. Obstet Gynecol. 2009;114(6):1278–83. (1873–233X (Electronic))
10. Whitehead WE, Borrud L, Goode PS, Meikle S, et al. Fecal incontinence in US adults: epidemiology and risk factors. Gastroenterology. 2009;137(2):512–7. (1528–0012 (Electronic))
11. Scott KM. Pelvic floor rehabilitation in the treatment of fecal incontinence. Clin Colon Rectal Surg. 2014;27(3):99–105. (1531–0043 (Print))
12. Chiarioni G, Ferri B, Morelli A, Iantorno G, Bassotti G. Bio-feedback treatment of fecal incontinence: where are we, and where are we going? World J Gastroenterol. 2005;11(31):4771–5. (1007–9327 (Print))
13. Ko CY, Tong J, Lehman RE, Shelton AA, Schrock TR, Welton ML. Biofeedback is effective therapy for fecal incontinence and constipation. Arch Surg. 1997;132(8):829–34. https://doi.org/10.1001/archsurg.1997.01430320031004.
14. Thaha MA, Abukar AA, Thin NN, Ramsanahie A, Knowles CH. Sacral nerve stimulation for faecal incontinence and constipation in adults. Cochrane Database Syst Rev. 2015;2015(8):CD004464. https://doi.org/10.1002/14651858.CD004464.pub3.
15. Tanagho EA, Schmidt RA. Electrical stimulation in the clinical management of the neurogenic bladder. J Urol. 1988;140(6):1331–9. https://doi.org/10.1016/s0022-5347(17)42038-6.
16. Fandel T, Tanagho EA. Neuromodulation in voiding dysfunction: a historical overview of neurostimulation and its application. Urol Clin North Am. 2005;32(1):1–10. https://doi.org/10.1016/j.ucl.2004.09.006.
17. Matzel KE, Stadelmaier U, Hohenfellner M, Gall FP. Electrical stimulation of sacral spinal nerves for treatment of faecal incontinence. Lancet. 1995;346(8983):1124–7. https://doi.org/10.1016/s0140-6736(95)91799-3.
18. Steele SS. Sacral nerve stimulation: 50 years in the making. Can Urol Assoc J. 2012;6(4):231–2. https://doi.org/10.5489/cuaj.12194.
19. Carrington EV, Knowles CH. The influence of sacral nerve stimulation on anorectal dysfunction. Color Dis. 2011;13(Suppl 2):5–9. https://doi.org/10.1111/j.1463-1318.2010.02518.x.
20. Tanagho EA, Schmidt RA. Bladder pacemaker: scientific basis and clinical future. Urology. 1982;20(6):614–9.
21. Rodrigues FG, Chadi SA, Cracco AJ, et al. Faecal incontinence in patients with a sphincter defect: comparison of sphincteroplasty and sacral nerve stimulation. Color Dis. 2017;19(5):456–61. https://doi.org/10.1111/codi.13510.
22. Ratto C, Litta F, Parello A, Donisi L, Doglietto GB. Sacral nerve stimulation is a valid approach in fecal incontinence due to sphincter lesions when compared to sphincter repair. Dis Colon Rectum. 2010;53(3):264–72. https://doi.org/10.1007/DCR.0b013e3181c7642c.
23. Jottard K, Van den Broeck S, Komen N, Bruyninx L, De Wachter S. Treatment of fecal incontinence with a rechargeable sacral neuromodulation system: efficacy, clinical outcome, and ease of use-six-month follow-up. Neuromodulation. 2021;24(7):1284–8. https://doi.org/10.1111/ner.13298.

24. Wachter S, McCrery R, Benson K, et al. MP30–02 stimulation output and impedance over 6 months with a constant current sacral neuromodulation system. J Urol. 2020;203(Supplement 4):e438.
25. Zyczynski HM, Richter HE, Sung VW, et al. Performance, acceptability, and validation of a phone application bowel diary. Neurourol Urodyn. 2020;39(8):2480–9. https://doi.org/10.1002/nau.24520.
26. Steele SR, Varma MG, Prichard D, et al. The evolution of evaluation and management of urinary or fecal incontinence and pelvic organ prolapse. Curr Probl Surg. 2015;52(2):17–75. https://doi.org/10.1067/j.cpsurg.2015.01.001.
27. Paquette IM, Varma MG, Kaiser AM, Steele SR, Rafferty JF. The American Society of Colon and Rectal Surgeons' clinical practice guideline for the treatment of fecal incontinence. Dis Colon Rectum. 2015;58(7):623–36.
28. Tjandra JJ, Chan MK, Yeh CH, Murray-Green C. Sacral nerve stimulation is more effective than optimal medical therapy for severe fecal incontinence: a randomized, controlled study. Dis Colon Rectum. 2008;51(5):494–502. https://doi.org/10.1007/s10350-007-9103-5.
29. Norton C, Cody JD. Biofeedback and/or sphincter exercises for the treatment of faecal incontinence in adults. Cochrane Database Syst Rev. 2012;7:Cd002111. https://doi.org/10.1002/14651858.CD002111.pub3.
30. Vonthein R, Heimerl T, Schwandner T, Ziegler A. Electrical stimulation and biofeedback for the treatment of fecal incontinence: a systematic review. Int J Color Dis. 2013;28(11):1567–77.
31. Johnson BL, Abodeely A, Ferguson MA, Davis BR, Rafferty JF, Paquette IM. Is sacral neuromodulation here to stay? Clinical outcomes of a new treatment for fecal incontinence. J Gastrointest Surg. 2015;19(1):15–20.
32. Southwell BR. Electro-neuromodulation for colonic disorders-review of meta-analyses, systematic reviews, and RCTs. Neuromodulation. 2020;23(8):1061–81. https://doi.org/10.1111/ner.13099.
33. Butrick CW. Patient selection for sacral nerve stimulation. Int Urogynecol J. 2010;21(2):447–51.
34. Treatments for Fecal Incontinence (Dept of Health and Human Services) Table E (2016).
35. Lee C, Pizarro-Berdichevsky J, Clifton MM, Vasavada SP. Sacral Neuromodulation Implant Infection: Risk Factors and Prevention. Curr Urol Rep. 2017;18(2):16. https://doi.org/10.1007/s11934-017-0663-1.
36. Huwyler M, Kiss G, Burkhard FC, Madersbacher H, Kessler TM. Microbiological tined-lead examination: does prolonged sacral neuromodulation testing induce infection? BJU Int. 2009;104(5):646–50. https://doi.org/10.1111/j.1464-410X.2009.08501.x.
37. Amend B, Bedke J, Khalil M, Stenzl A, Sievert KD. Prolonged percutaneous SNM testing does not cause infection-related explanation. BJU Int. 2013;111(3):485–91. https://doi.org/10.1111/j.1464-410X.2012.11263.x.
38. Guralnick ML, Benouni S, O'Connor RC, Edmiston C. Characteristics of infections in patients undergoing staged implantation for sacral nerve stimulation. Urology. 2007;69(6):1073–6. https://doi.org/10.1016/j.urology.2007.01.099.
39. Washington BB, Hines BJ. Implant infection after two-stage sacral nerve stimulator placement. Int Urogynecol J. 2007;18(12):1477–80. https://doi.org/10.1007/s00192-007-0386-9.
40. Dudding T, Vaizey C. Bacterial colonization of stimulation electrode wires in patients undergoing temporary sacral nerve stimulation. Color Dis. 2010;12(2):141–3. https://doi.org/10.1111/j.1463-1318.2009.01896.x.
41. Wexner SD, Hull T, Edden Y, et al. Infection rates in a large investigational trial of sacral nerve stimulation for fecal incontinence. J Gastrointest Surg. 2010;14(7):1081–9. https://doi.org/10.1007/s11605-010-1177-z.
42. Gumber A, Ayyar S, Varia H, Pettit S. Presacral abscess as a rare complication of sacral nerve stimulator implantation. Ann R Coll Surg Engl. 2017;99(3):e1–4.
43. Martellucci J. Low anterior resection syndrome: a treatment algorithm. Dis Colon Rectum. 2016;59(1):79–82. https://doi.org/10.1097/dcr.0000000000000495.

44. Ramage L, Qiu S, Kontovounisios C, Tekkis P, Rasheed S, Tan E. A systematic review of sacral nerve stimulation for low anterior resection syndrome. Color Dis. 2015;17(9):762–71. https://doi.org/10.1111/codi.12968.
45. Eftaiha SM, Balachandran B, Marecik SJ, et al. Sacral nerve stimulation can be an effective treatment for low anterior resection syndrome. Color Dis. 2017;19(10):927–33. https://doi.org/10.1111/codi.13701.
46. Huang Y, Koh CE. Sacral nerve stimulation for bowel dysfunction following low anterior resection: a systematic review and meta-analysis. Color Dis. 2019;21(11):1240–8. https://doi.org/10.1111/codi.14690.
47. Croese AD, Whiting S, Vangaveti VN, Ho Y-H. Using sacral nerve modulation to improve continence and quality of life in patients suffering from low anterior resection syndrome. ANZ J Surg. 2018;88(11):E787–91. https://doi.org/10.1111/ans.14871.
48. Mege D, Meurette G, Vitton V, et al. Sacral nerve stimulation can alleviate symptoms of bowel dysfunction after colorectal resections. Color Dis. 2017;19(8):756–63.
49. Schiano di Visconte M, Santoro GA, Cracco N, et al. Effectiveness of sacral nerve stimulation in fecal incontinence after multimodal oncologic treatment for pelvic malignancies: a multicenter study with 2-year follow-up. Tech Coloproctol. 2018;22(2):97–105. https://doi.org/10.1007/s10151-017-1745-2.
50. Malouf AJ, Wiesel PH, Nicholls T, Nicholls RJ, Kamm MA. Short-term effects of sacral nerve stimulation for idiopathic slow transit constipation. World J Surg. 2002;26(2):166.
51. Kamm MA, Dudding TC, Melenhorst J, et al. Sacral nerve stimulation for intractable constipation. Gut. 2010;59(3):333. https://doi.org/10.1136/gut.2009.187989.
52. Holzer B, Rosen HR, Novi G, et al. Sacral nerve stimulation in patients with severe constipation. Dis Colon Rectum. 2008;51(5):524–30. https://doi.org/10.1007/s10350-007-9160-9.
53. Graf W, Sonesson A-C, Lindberg B, Åkerud P, Karlbom U. Results after sacral nerve stimulation for chronic constipation. Neurogastroenterol Motil. 2015;27(5):734–9. https://doi.org/10.1111/nmo.12546.
54. Sulkowski JP, Nacion KM, Deans KJ, et al. Sacral nerve stimulation: a promising therapy for fecal and urinary incontinence and constipation in children. J Pediatr Surg. 2015;50(10):1644–7. https://doi.org/10.1016/j.jpedsurg.2015.03.043.
55. Dinning P, Fuentealba S, Kennedy M, Lubowski D, Cook I. Sacral nerve stimulation induces pan-colonic propagating pressure waves and increases defecation frequency in patients with slow-transit constipation. Color Dis. 2007;9(2):123–32.
56. Sreepati G, James-Stevenson T. Use of sacral nerve stimulation for the treatment of overlapping constipation and fecal incontinence. Am J Case Rep. 2017;18:230–3. https://doi.org/10.12659/ajcr.901821.
57. Cheetham MJ, Malouf AJ, Kamm MA. Fecal incontinence. Gastroenterol Clin N Am. 2001;30(1):115–30.
58. Schiano di Visconte M, Munegato G. The value of sacral nerve stimulation in the treatment of faecal incontinence after pelvic radiotherapy. Int J Color Dis. 2009;24(9):1111–2. https://doi.org/10.1007/s00384-009-0654-x.
59. Thin NN, Carrington EV, Grimmer K, Knowles CH. Advancement anoplasty and sacral nerve stimulation: an effective combination for radiation-induced anal stenosis. Int J Color Dis. 2011;26(2):211–3. https://doi.org/10.1007/s00384-010-1088-1.
60. Maeda Y, Høyer M, Lundby L, Buntzen S, Laurberg S. Temporary sacral nerve stimulation for faecal incontinence following pelvic radiotherapy. Radiother Oncol. 2010;97(1):108–12. https://doi.org/10.1016/j.radonc.2010.04.023.
61. Povo A, Arantes M, Matzel KE, Barbosa J, Ferreira MA. Sacral malformations: use of imaging to optimise sacral nerve stimulation. Int J Color Dis. 2016;31(2):351–7. https://doi.org/10.1007/s00384-015-2417-1.
62. Lansen-Koch SMP, Govaert B, Oerlemans D, et al. Sacral nerve modulation for defaecation and micturition disorders in patients with spina bifida. Color Dis. 2012;14(4):508–14. https://doi.org/10.1111/j.1463-1318.2011.02678.x.

63. Storrs BB. Selective posterior rhizotomy for treatment of progressive spasticity in patients with myelomeningocele. Pediatr Neurosurg. 1987;13(3):135–7.
64. Frimberger D, Cheng E, Kropp BP. The current management of the neurogenic bladder in children with spina bifida. Pediatr Clin N Am. 2012;59(4):757–67. https://doi.org/10.1016/j.pcl.2012.05.006.
65. Michael LM 2nd, Whitworth LA, Feler CA. Spina bifida occulta as a relative contraindication for percutaneous retrograde lead insertion for sacral nerve root stimulation. Neuromodulation. 2002;5(1):38–40. https://doi.org/10.1046/j.1525-1403.2002._2007.x.
66. Castillo J, Cristóbal L, Alonso J, et al. Sacral nerve stimulation lead implantation in partial sacral agenesis using intra-operative computerized tomography. Color Dis. 2016;18(9):O330–3. https://doi.org/10.1111/codi.13437.
67. Brunner M, Cui Z, Matzel KE. Sacral nerve stimulation for faecal incontinence in patients with sacral malformation. Int J Color Dis. 2017;32(6):929–31. https://doi.org/10.1007/s00384-016-2748-6.
68. Thomas GP, Nicholls RJ, Vaizey CJ. Sacral nerve stimulation for faecal incontinence secondary to congenital imperforate anus. Tech Coloproctol. 2013;17(2):227–9. https://doi.org/10.1007/s10151-012-0914-6.
69. Lagares-Tena L, Corbella-Sala C, Navarro-Luna A, Muñoz-Duyos A. Sacral neuromodulation in a patient with faecal incontinence and unknown sacral partial agenesis. Color Dis. 2017;19(5):502–4. https://doi.org/10.1111/codi.13661.
70. Possover M. The laparoscopic implantation of neuroprothesis to the sacral plexus for therapy of neurogenic bladder dysfunctions after failure of percutaneous sacral nerve stimulation. Neuromodulation Technol Neural Interface. 2010;13(2):141–4. https://doi.org/10.1111/j.1525-1403.2009.00230.x.
71. Cracco AJ, Chadi SA, Rodrigues FG, et al. Outcomes of sacral neurostimulation lead reimplantation for fecal incontinence: a cohort study. Dis Colon Rectum. 2016;59(1):48–53. https://doi.org/10.1097/dcr.0000000000000505.
72. Bielefeldt K. Adverse events of sacral neuromodulation for fecal incontinence reported to the federal drug administration. World J Gastrointest Pharmacol Ther. 2016;7(2):294.
73. Force L, da Silva G. Management of complications of sacral neuromodulation. Semin Colon Rectal Surg. 2017;28(4):173–6. https://doi.org/10.1053/j.scrs.2017.07.006.
74. Faucheron J-L, Voirin D, Badic B. Sacral nerve stimulation for fecal incontinence: causes of surgical revision from a series of 87 consecutive patients operated on in a single institution. Dis Colon Rectum. 2010;53(11):1501–7. https://doi.org/10.1007/DCR.0b013e3181f1cf14.
75. Rosen HR, Urbarz C, Holzer B, Novi G, Schiessel R. Sacral nerve stimulation as a treatment for fecal incontinence. Gastroenterology. 2001;121(3):536–41. https://doi.org/10.1053/gast.2001.27120.
76. Schurch B, Reilly I, Reitz A, Curt A. Electrophysiological recordings during the peripheral nerve evaluation (PNE) test in complete spinal cord injury patients. World J Urol. 2003;20(6):319–22. https://doi.org/10.1007/s00345-002-0299-7.
77. Creasey GH, Ho CH, Triolo RJ, et al. Clinical applications of electrical stimulation after spinal cord injury. J Spinal Cord Med. 2004;27(4):365–75. https://doi.org/10.1080/10790268.2004.11753774.
78. Alo KM, Yland MJ, Redko V, Feler C, Naumann C. Lumbar and Sacral Nerve Root Stimulation (NRS) in the treatment of chronic pain: a novel anatomic approach and neuro stimulation technique. Neuromodulation Technol Neural Interface. 1999;2(1):23–31. https://doi.org/10.1046/j.1525-1403.1999.00023.x.
79. Yang KS, Kim YH, Park HJ, Lee MH, Kim DH, Moon DE. Sacral nerve stimulation for treatment of chronic intractable anorectal pain – a case report. Korean J Pain. 2010;23(1):60–4. https://doi.org/10.3344/kjp.2010.23.1.60.

Surgical Management Options for Rectourethral Fistula

44

Jennifer A. Leinicke and Sean J. Langenfeld

Introduction

Acquired rectourethral fistula (RUF) is an uncommon and complex condition, often requiring a multidisciplinary team for successful repair. The majority of RUFs are iatrogenic following medical and/or surgical treatment for prostate cancer, while traumatic pelvic injury, infection, and inflammatory bowel disease are less frequent causes [1, 2]. Multimodal treatment for prostate cancer has become more prevalent over time, and RUFs associated with radiation or other high-energy ablation techniques are increasingly common.

Rivera et al. developed a formal classification system for RUF based on size, distance from the anal verge, and presence or absence of radiation, but this is not universally adopted in the literature [2]. RUFs are usually categorized as either simple or complex [1]. Simple RUF are small (<1 cm), not associated with sepsis, radiation/high-energy ablation, and have not been previously repaired. Complex

Disclosures: the authors have no relevant financial disclosures

J. A. Leinicke
Omaha, USA
e-mail: jennifer.leinicke@unmc.edu

S. J. Langenfeld (✉)
Division of Colon and Rectal Surgery, Department of Surgery, University of Nebraska Medical Center, Omaha, NE, USA
e-mail: sean.langenfeld@unmc.edu

K. Umanskiy, N. Hyman (eds.), *Difficult Decisions in Colorectal Surgery*, Difficult Decisions in Surgery: An Evidence-Based Approach,
https://doi.org/10.1007/978-3-031-42303-1_44

RUFs are >1 cm and have associated complicating factors such as radiation/high energy ablation, urethral or rectal strictures, prior failed repairs, or sepsis.

There is no consensus among experts regarding the surgical management of RUF, and literature on the subject contains significant heterogeneity. The low incidence of RUF eliminates the ability to conduct randomized controlled trials, and the treatment of RUF is instead limited to small retrospective case series with diverse surgical techniques and non-standardized functional outcomes. Thus, the treatment of RUF is often individualized and tailored to patient-dependent variables as well as the experience and preferences of the surgical team and institution.

Multiple surgical approaches to RUF have been described, and the evidence is significantly limited due to retrospective series of diverse patient populations and surgical team biases toward their preferred surgical approach.

Most authors advocate a multidisciplinary team approach for RUF patients, including urologists and colorectal surgeons with plastic surgeons as necessary for creation of muscle interposition flaps. Several treatment algorithms have been proposed [1, 16, 17]. Initial treatment focuses on symptom palliation with urinary and/or fecal diversion, and some patients will heal with diversion alone. Indications for fecal diversion include infection, history of radiation/high-energy ablation, prior failed repair, trial for spontaneous healing, and surgeon preference.

Search Strategy

A comprehensive literature search of MEDLINE, CINAHL, PsycINFO (via EBSCOhost), EMBASE (via embase.com) and the Cochrane Library (via Wiley) was performed. The search utilized keywords for the "RUF" concept, which was not represented by a subject heading in the databases searched, and a combination of the relevant subject heading/subheading combination and keywords for the surgery concept. (Table 44.1: PICO).

Specifically, for the "rectourethral fistula" concept, the search strategy demanded that either title or abstracts or author keywords contained (a) a term for the fistula subconcept located within 3 words of one of two rectourethral terms (rectourethral or rectourinary) or (b) a term for the "fistula" subconcept located within 5 words of a term for the "urethra" subconcept, which, in turn, was located within 5 words of a term for the rectal/anal subconcept. For the surgery concept, the search demanded the presence of either (a) the "fistula" heading with a "surgery"subheading or (b) a surgery keyword likely to indicate fistula surgery (e.g. anorectoplasty or York-Mason) or (c) a "fistula" term located within 4 words of a less fistula-specific

Table 44.1 PICO

Patients	Intervention	Comparator	Outcome
Adult patients with rectourethral fistula	Any surgery	Any comparator	Successful fistula closure, fistula recurrence or persistence, permanent fecal and/or urinary diversion

surgical term (e.g. surgery or excise). The entire record was searched for surgery keywords.

Publication date filters were applied to limit retrieval to items published in 2002 or later. No publication type limits were used in searches for unindexed CINAHL or MEDLINE records or in Cochrane Library searches. Filters were used to limit searches for indexed CINAHL, MEDLINE, and EMBASE records to systematic reviews, meta-analyses, and reports of clinical studies or trials. After a cursory review of the initial result set, the decision was made to limit the literature review to 2012 – present and to full manuscripts. 112 articles designated as needing author review remained.

Results

We identified 14 retrospective case series containing >5 patients [3–16]. Two of the case series, Hanna et al [14] and Hayden et al [16], were from the same institution with study dates that overlapped by 10 years. The Hayden study was excluded from the summarized data. 13 case series with a total of 499 patients were included. One systematic review and meta-analysis by Hechenblekner et al [17] was identified, containing 416 patients from 26 case series published from 1985–2011. The findings of the meta-analysis are similar to the results from these 14 more recent case series. These studies are summarized in Tables 44.2 and 44.3. The quality of the evidence from these observational studies is low to moderate based on the GRADE classification system [Level 5: Evidence from systematic reviews of descriptive and qualitative studies (meta-synthesis)].

Prior to 1997, only 4% of reported RUF were associated with radiation [15, 17]. As the diagnosis and treatment of prostate cancer has increased over recent decades, more patients with RUF have been treated with multimodal therapy. The incidence of RUF associated with radiation (external beam or brachytherapy) or high-energy ablation (e.g. cryoablation or high intensity focused ultrasound) ranged from 14–61%. Most non-radiated RUF were sequalae of prostatectomy. Of the studies which reported radiation exposure, 43% of the RUFs were associated with radiation. Four studies directly compared outcomes of radiation-associated RUF to non-irradiated RUF (Table 44.4). Radiation-associated RUFs have a worse prognosis as compared to non-radiated RUF, with lower rates of fistula healing (50–86% vs 88–100%) and restoration of intestinal continuity (52–55% vs 87–100%). In the 6 studies reporting transphincteric or transanal repairs, 97% of these patients were non-irradiated.

Overall, 472 RUF patients (95%) underwent definitive surgical repair. The remaining 27 patients either healed spontaneously with urinary and/or fecal diversion or declined surgical repair. Initial rates of preoperative urinary diversion, reported in 8/14 studies, were 63–100%. Temporary fecal diversion, reported in 11/14 studies, was performed in 38–100% of patients.

A total of 524 surgeries were performed with a cumulative closure rate of 91%. Permanent urinary diversion and fecal diversion was reported in 8 of 13 studies

Table 44.2 Summary of patient specific data

Study	Publication date	n	Radiation n (%)	Surgical repair n%	No surgical repair n %	Initial urinary diversion %	Initial fecal diversion %	Follow up, mean or median, time
Martins	2021	23	10 (43)	23 (100)	0	23 (100)	23 (100)	18–115 months, 54
Sbizzera	2021	21	3 (14.2)	21 (100)	0	NR	12 (57.1)	8–47 mo, 27
Park	2021	36	22 (61)	36 (100)	0	NR	33 (91.6)	2.8–27 months, 11.3 and 6
Bislenghi	2020	52	30 (57.7)	49 (94.2)	3 (5.8)	35 (67.3)	20 (38.4)	0.5–16.8 years, 10.5
Bergerat	2018	30	0	30	0	NR	NR	2–195, 70 mo
Dafnis	2018	20	2 (10)	20 (100)	0	NR	20 (100)	4.5–185 months, 78.7
Harris	2017	225	104 (49.6)	210 (93.3)	15	NR	155 (73.8)	NR, minimum 6 months
Munoz-Duyos	2017	9	NR	9	0	NR	NR	2–72 54 mo median
Prabha	2017	6	NR	6	0	6 (100)	6 (100)	6–48, mean 27
Hanna	2014	37	21 (56.7)	30 (81)	7 (18.8)	37 (100)	22 (59)	22.6–205 months, 55.1
Voelzke	2013	23	13 (56.5)	23 (100)	0	23 (100)	13 (56)	0.55 and 0.96 years for PO and REA groups
Total		482	205/467 (43.9)	457 (95)	25 (5)	124	384	

Table 44.3 Summary of types of surgical repair and primary outcomes

Study	n patients, n procedures	Transanal repair n%	Transabdominal repair +/− perineal n%	Transsphicnteric repair n%	Transperineal repair n%	Tissue flap n%	Gracillis n%	Omental flap n%	Dartos/ other n%	Cumulative RUF closure n(%)	Permanent FD n%	Permanent UD n%
Martins	23, NR	0	7 (30)	0	16 (70)	7 (30)	4	3		18 (78)	5 (22)	5 (22)
Sbizzera	21, 22	0	0	0	22 (100)	22 (100)	22 (100)	0	0	21 (100)	2 (9.5)	0
Park	36, NR	0	0	0*	24*		24		7	28 (73.6)	NR	NR
Bislenghi	49, 76	14(18.4)	45 (59.2)	0	14(18.4)	13(17.1)	10 (13.1)	0	3 (3.9)	50 (96)	18 (36.7)	18 (36.7)
Bergerat	30, 36	0	0	30 (100)						30 (100)	NR	NR
Dafnis	20, 23	0	0	20 (100)	0	0	0	0	1 (4.3)	18 (90)	7 (35)	2 (10)
Harris	210	0	42 (20)	0	166 (79)	193 (91.9)	NR	NR	0	195 (92.9)	NR	7 (3.3)
Munoz-Duyos	9, 9	0	0	0	9	9	9			9 (100)	1 (11)	0
Prahba	6, 6	0	0	0	6	6	6			6 (100)	0	0
Hanna	37, NR	0	4 (10.8)	10 (27)	16 (43)	11 (29)	11 (100)	0	0	28 (75.6)	6 (27.2)	NR
Voelzke	23	0	0	0	23	7(30.4)	2	0	5	18 (78)	NR	NR
	457, 501	14 (2.8)	98 (19.5)	60 (11.9)	258	253	88	3	16	421 (87.3)		

Table 44.4 Studies comparing non-radiated to radiated patients

Study	Total N	Non radiated, closure rate	Non radiated, ostomy closure	Radiated, closure rate	Ostomy closure R	Cumulative closure rate (%)
Martins	23	13 of 13, 100%		5/10, 50%		78
Voelzke	23	10 of 10, 100%		8/13, 61.5%		78.2
Harris	210	Initial 99 of 106 93.3% eventual 105 of 106, 99%		Initial 84 of 104 80.7%90 of 104, 86.5%		87.1 initial 92.8 eventual
Hanna	37	14 of 16, 88%	10 of 11, 91%	14 of 21, 67%	6 of 11, 55%	75.60%
Hayden	79	32/34, 94%	27/31, 87.1%	45 total, 17/26 65.4% (18 exent)	13/25, 52%	49/60, 81.7%

(0–37% urinary diversion and 10–36% fecal diversion). Surgical approaches included transanal (6%), transabdominal +/− transperineal (TA/TP, 19%), posterior/transsphincteric (12%), and transperineal (TP, 50%). Tissue flaps were used in 72% of transperineal and transabdominal +/− transperineal approaches, with gracilis flap being the most common approach. The study from Harris et al., which provided 53% of the reported flaps, did not report the relative frequency for their use of gracilis, levator, dartos, and ometal flaps [10].

Transsphincteric Repair

The transsphincteric approach to simple RUFs has high reported rates of success. A 2018 case series of 20 patients over 15 years reported a 90% success rate for transsphincteric repair [9]. A 2014 case series reported healing in 100% (8/8) of simple fistulas and 50% (1/2) of complex radiated fistulas [14]. A 2018 series of 30 patients over 20 years with simple non-radiated RUFs reported a 100% cumulative healing rate utilizing a modified York-Mason repair [8]. In this series, healing occurred after 1 procedure in 80% of patients while 2 or 3 procedures were needed for the remaining 20%.

Transanal Repair

While the transanal approach to RUF continues to evolve with emerging technologies, the currently-reported healing rates are low. A 2020 series of 14 patients reported healing in 36% of patients [6]. A 2019 study described a novel technique for transanal rectal advancement flap with adipose lipofilling (RAFAL) in 7 patients with small (0.2–0.5 cm), non-radiated RUF, and they reported a a 71% primary success rate [7]. 2 patients had recurrence, with 1 successful repeat RAFAL and one undergoing York-Mason repair. A 2018 study described a transanal endoscopic approach to RUF using either transanal endoscopic operation (TEO) or transanal endoscopic microsurgery (TEM) equipment with biologic mesh interposition [12]. Repair was successful in 2/8 (25%) of patients, and the 6 patients who recurred were then treated with gracilis muscle interposition via a transperineal approach with an 83% (5/6) success rate.

Transperineal and Combined Transperineal/ Transabdominal Repair

In general, complex RUFs usually require transperineal or combined transperineal/ transabdominal repair, often in combination with fecal diversion. A 2017 study reported on 210 patients who underwent surgical repair of RUF [10], of which 50% had a history of radiation/high-energy ablation. Bowel diversion was performed in 84% of radiated fistulas and 65% of non-radiated fistulas. 79% of patients had a transperineal approach and 20% had a combined TA/TP approach. Interposition flaps were used in 92% of patients. For all patients combined, there was an 87% initial success rate and a 93% eventual success rate. Non-radiation patients had initial and eventual success rates of 93% and 99%, respectively, while radiated patients were 81% and 87% successful, respectively.

A 2020 study reported on 59 patients with RUF who underwent repair (24% TP and 76% combined TP/TA) [6]. The healing rate for the TP approach was 64% overall, but 90% (9/10) when a gracilis flap was employed. The healing rate for the combined TA/TP approach was 57% for patients who underwent restorative procedures versus 94% for patients who underwent non-restorative procedures, including abdominoperineal resection and/or ileal conduit. Similar results were reported in multiple smaller series, where the combined TP/TA approach had lower healing rates than isolated TP approaches, presumably related to fistula complexity. Similarly, the use of flaps, either omental or gracilis, improved healing rates while a history of pelvic radiation reduced healing rates [3–5, 11, 13, 15]. For patients with complex fistulas, permanent or temporary fecal diversion was usually employed, and multiple surgeries were often necessary to achieve healing.

Recommendations Based on the Data

The transperineal repair is the most common approach for RUF repair as it provides excellent exposure for both simple and complex RUF and can be performed in combination with several muscle interposition flaps. A transperineal approach with` interposition flap is associated with high rates of healing, even in radiated patients with complex fistulas.

The posterior/transsphincteric (Kraske, York-Mason) repair was developed prior to the routine use of radiation/high-energy ablation in prostate cancer treatment. Although reported closure rates are similar to the transperineal approach, its current use is restricted to small, simple fistulas due to difficulty with exposure, inability to adequately mobilize fibrotic rectal/urethral tissues for closure of larger defects, limited use of interposition flaps, and risks of fecal incontinence with sphincter division. The traditional transanal approach is also limited to small, low RUF due to significant limitations in exposure for adequate excision and repair of the fistula. Results from modified transanal approaches (TEO, TEM with biologic mesh) are poor. Recent case reports and small case series have demonstrated novel modification of the technique using transanal minimally invasive surgery (TAMIS) or robotic-assisted TAMIS [18–22]. Although promising, these results are inherently biased as unsuccessful case reports are unlikely to be published. There is insufficient evidence to promote the use of these techniques currently.

An abdominoperineal approach (pelvic exenteration, cystectomy with ileal conduit, abdominoperineal resection, or proctectomy with coloanal anastomosis) is most often utilized in patients with complex RUF due to concurrent malignancy, large defects, fibrotic or radiated tissues, or nonfunctional bladder/rectum requiring permanent diversion. Abdominoperineal approaches may also be combined with flap interposition (omentum, gracilis, levator). Hayden et al. advocate for primary pelvic exenteration rather than attempted repair in patients with defects >3 cm, fixed tissue, or non-functional bladder [16].

Simple RUFs which do not heal with a trial of diversion may be repaired by the transperineal approach +/− muscle flap or the posterior/transsphincteric (Kraske, York-Mason) approach, depending on surgeon preference. There is limited evidence to support the use of transanal approaches. (Evidence quality low to moderate; Weak recommendation)

Complex RUF are best repaired with a transperineal or abdominoperineal approach with the use of interposition flaps. (Evidence quality low to moderate; Weak recommendation)

A Personal View of the Data

Thankfully, complex rectourethral fistulas are uncommon, as they are inherently difficult to treat, and provide major problems for the patient and surgeon alike. In general, the goals of care are to prevent pelvic sepsis and improve patient quality of life (QOL). It is important to understand the diverse way in which RUFs present, as the treatment is tailored to the individual patient depending on the fistula's etiology, patient comorbidities (including frailty and malnutrition), tissue quality, previous attempts at repair, availability and expertise of the multidisciplinary team, and patient goals/preferences. Surgery for RUF involves a narrow therapeutic window with high rates of failure and associated patient disability, so referral to high-volume centers is recommended when possible.

In our practice, simple rectourethral fistulas are much less common than complex radiated fistulas. This is likely multifactorial, but is partially due to our status as a quaternary referral center, and also due to technical advancements in radical prostatectomy that improve visualization and reduce the likelihood of rectal injury.

Since our patient population predominantly consists of patients with a history of pelvic radiation as well as previous failed attempts at RUF repair, we find that fecal and urinary diversion are often necessary to initially control symptoms. This allows the patients to improve their clinical status and increase the likelihood of a successful definitive surgical repair in the future.

Repair of complex RUFs requires a multidisciplinary team of surgeons, including plastic surgery, colorectal surgery, and urology. It also requires input from radiology, radiation oncology, nutrition, physical therapy, and often geriatrics as well. Once a patient has been optimized and is ready for surgery, a transperineal approach combined with gracilis flap is associated with high rates of success. If it does fail, a repeat attempt is warranted. Once fistula closure is achieved, stoma reversal can be performed for patients who desire intestinal continuity. As we all know, radiation is a gift that keeps on giving, so patients require longitudinal surveillance even after initial success. This not only allows for identification of evolving problems, but it also gives patients an outlet for discussion and treatment of functional problems related to their pathology and medical/surgical treatment. Overall, there is a high rate of genitourinary, gastrointestinal, and sexual dysfunction after surgery for RUF, and ignoring these symptoms can lead to significant reductions in patient quality of life.

For many patients, the degree of pelvic fibrosis combined with the surgically-altered anatomy prevent success from even the most valiant and well-coordinated attempts at RUF repair. When RUF repair is not feasible, symptom control can often be achieved through fecal and urinary diversion alone. While pelvic exenteration is feasible, it is a very big surgery in a radiated field for a patient population that is typically frail and elderly. Therefore, in our practice, fecal and urinary diversion would be performed first with exenteration reserved for patients who do not have adequate symptom control.

References

1. Rakinic JW, Perry B. Rectourethral and complex fistulas: evaluation and management. In: Steele SR, Hull TL, Hyman N, Maykel JA, Read TE, Whitlow CB, editors. The ASCRS textbook of colon and rectal surgery. 4th ed. Switzerland AG: Springer Nature; 2022. Available from: https://www.ascrsu.com/ascrs/view/ASCRS-Textbook-of-Colon-and-Rectal-Surgery.
2. Rivera R, Barboglio PG, Hellinger M, Gousse AE. Staging rectourinary fistulas to guide surgical treatment. J Urol. 2007;177(2):586–8. https://doi.org/10.1016/j.juro.2006.09.058.
3. Martins FE, Felicio J, Oliveira TR, Martins N, Oliveira V, Palmas A. Adverse features of rectourethral fistula requiring extirpative surgery and permanent dual diversion: our experience and recommendations. J Clin Med. 2021;10(17):4014. https://doi.org/10.3390/jcm10174014. PMID: 34501462; PMCID: PMC8432514
4. Sbizzera M, Morel-Journel N, Ruffion A, Crouzet S, Paparel P, Carnicelli D, Neuville P. Rectourethral fistula induced by localised prostate cancer treatment: surgical and functional outcomes of transperineal repair with Gracilis muscle flap interposition. Eur Urol. 2022;81(3):305–12. https://doi.org/10.1016/j.eururo.2021.09.017. Epub 2021 Oct 20. PMID: 34686386

5. Park KM, Rosli YY, Simms A, Lentz R, Bharadia DR, Breyer B, Hoffman WY. Preventing Rectourethral fistula recurrence with Gracilis flap. Ann Plast Surg. 2022; https://doi.org/10.1097/SAP.0000000000003085. Epub ahead of print. PMID: 35180755
6. Bislenghi G, Verstraeten L, Verlinden I, Castiglione F, Debaets K, Van der Aa F, Fieuws S, Wolthuis A, D'Hoore A, Joniau S. Surgical management of acquired rectourethral fistula: a retrospective analysis of 52 consecutive patients. Tech Coloproctol. 2020;24(9):927–33. https://doi.org/10.1007/s10151-020-02214-9. Epub 2020 Apr 16. PMID: 32301002
7. Zuin M, Ruperto M, Balduino M, Amodeo A, De Zorzi L, Roche B, Pavanello M, Sernagiotto C. Rectal advancement flap plus adipose lipofilling (RAFAL) for the treatment of rectourethral fistulas after radical prostatectomy. Tech Coloproctol. 2019;23(10):1003–7. https://doi.org/10.1007/s10151-019-02078-8. Epub 2019 Sep 18. PMID: 31535239
8. Bergerat S, Rozet F, Barret E, et al. Modified York Mason technique for repair of iatrogenic recto-urinary fistula: 20 years of the Montsouris experience. World J Urol. 2018;36:947–54. https://doi.org/10.1007/s00345-018-2212-z.
9. Dafnis G. Transsphincteric repair of rectourethral fistulas: 15 years of experience with the York Mason approach. Int J Urol. 2018;25(3):290–6. https://doi.org/10.1111/iju.13518. Epub 2018 Jan 11. PMID: 29323430
10. Harris CR, McAninch JW, Mundy AR, Zinman LN, Jordan GH, Andrich D, Vanni AJ, Virasoro R, Breyer BN. Rectourethral fistulas secondary to prostate cancer treatment: management and outcomes from a multi-institutional combined experience. J Urol. 2017;197(1):191–4. https://doi.org/10.1016/j.juro.2016.08.080. Epub 2016 Aug 18. PMID: 27544625
11. Muñoz-Duyos A, Navarro-Luna A, Pardo-Aranda F, Caballero JM, Borrat P, Maristany C, Pando JA, Veloso E. Gracilis muscle interposition for rectourethral fistula after laparoscopic prostatectomy: a prospective evaluation and long-term follow-up. Dis Colon Rectum. 2017;60(4):393–8. https://doi.org/10.1097/DCR.0000000000000763. PMID: 28267006
12. Serra-Aracil X, Labró-Ciurans M, Mora-López L, Muñoz-Rodríguez J, Martos-Calvo R, Prats-López J, Navarro-Soto S. The place of Transanal endoscopic surgery in the treatment of Rectourethral fistula. Urology. 2018;111:139–44. https://doi.org/10.1016/j.urology.2017.08.049. Epub 2017 Sep 12. PMID: 28916253
13. Prabha V, Kadeli V. Repair of recto-urethral fistula with urethral augmentation by buccal mucosal graft and gracilis muscle flap interposition – our experience. Cent European J Urol. 2018;71(1):121–8. https://doi.org/10.5173/ceju.2018.1353. Epub 2017 Dec 8. PMID: 29732218; PMCID: PMC5926628
14. Hanna JM, Turley R, Castleberry A, Hopkins T, Peterson AC, Mantyh C, Migaly J. Surgical management of complex rectourethral fistulas in irradiated and nonirradiated patients. Dis Colon Rectum. 2014;57(9):1105–12. https://doi.org/10.1097/DCR.0000000000000175. PMID: 25101607
15. Voelzke BB, McAninch JW, Breyer BN, Glass AS, Garcia-Aguilar J. Transperineal management for postoperative and radiation rectourethral fistulas. J Urol. 2013;189(3):966–71. https://doi.org/10.1016/j.juro.2012.08.238.
16. Hayden JP, Boysen WR, Kowalik U, Inouye BM, Migaly J, Mantyh CR, Erdmann D, Peterson AC. Outcomes of an algorithmic, multidisciplinary approach to rectourethral fistula repair: a pre- and post-intervention quasi-experimental study. Dis Colon Rectum. 2022; https://doi.org/10.1097/DCR.0000000000002467. Epub ahead of print. PMID: 35507740
17. Hechenbleikner EM, Buckley JC, Wick EC. Acquired Rectourethral fistulas in adults: a systematic review of surgical repair techniques and outcomes. Dis Colon Rectum. 2013;56:374–83. https://doi.org/10.1097/DCR.0b013e318274dc87.
18. Hebert KJ, Naik N, Allawi A, Kelley SR, Behm KT, Viers BR. Rectourethral fistula repair using robotic transanal minimally invasive surgery (TAMIS) approach. Urology. 2021;154:338. https://doi.org/10.1016/j.urology.2021.05.027. Epub 2021 May 30. PMID: 34062165
19. Suhardja TS, Errington B, Khalessi A, Phan-Thien KC. Robotic transanal rectourethral fistula repair-a video vignette. Color Dis. 2021;23(5):1275–6. https://doi.org/10.1111/codi.15557. Epub 2021 Feb 19. PMID: 33527592

20. Kim TD, Gantt G Jr, Kochar K, Marecik S, Park JJ. Rectourethral fistula repair with Endorectal advancement flap and implantation of biologic mesh. Dis Colon Rectum. 2021;64(1):e1. https://doi.org/10.1097/DCR.0000000000001827. PMID: 33306539
21. De Freitas D, Althoff A, Larach S, Atallah S. Robotic transanal minimally invasive surgery for local repair of acquired rectovaginal and rectourethral fistulas – a video vignette. Color Dis. 2019;21(5):610–1. https://doi.org/10.1111/codi.14619. Epub 2019 Apr 4. PMID: 30903727
22. Tseng SI, Huang CW, Huang TY. Robotic-assisted transanal repair of rectourethral fistula. Endoscopy. 2019;51(5):E96–7. https://doi.org/10.1055/a-0826-4220. Epub 2019 Feb 12. PMID: 30754051

Operative vs Non-operative Management of Outlet Obstruction

45

Thomas M. Ward and Liliana G. Bordeiano

Introduction

As with many issues in pelvic floor, the management of outlet obstruction is hotly contested. With such a broad umbrella term as outlet obstruction, we will focus on management of internal intussusception of the rectum in patients with obstructive symptoms for this chapter. There is much debate over whether these patients benefit from intervention, as 20–50% of patients on defecography have asymptomatic internal intussusception, with relatively few (around 2%) going on to develop full-thickness rectal prolapse [1–3]. Difficulty with correlating degree of intussusception to obstructed symptoms has also been found, with increasing grades of internal rectal intussusception not found to correlate with symptoms of constipation [4]. Conversely, patients with radiographically noted internal intussusception are often symptomatic and have an intussusception morphology that differs from that found in asymptomatic volunteers [5]. With such uncertainty, it is unsurprising that a wide range of treatment options for these patients have emerged, ranging from medical therapy alone, to biofeedback and a number of operative interventions.

Search Strategy

A comprehensive literature search of PubMed, Google Scholar and the Cochrane Database of Collected Research was performed to identify all English-language publications from 1990 to 2022 related to outlet obstruction and internal rectal

T. M. Ward · L. G. Bordeiano (✉)
Section of Colon and Rectal Surgery, Division of General and Gastrointestinal Surgery, Department of Surgery, Massachusetts General Hospital, Boston, MA, USA
e-mail: tmward@mgh.harvard.edu; lbordeianou@mgh.harvard.edu

K. Umanskiy, N. Hyman (eds.), *Difficult Decisions in Colorectal Surgery*, Difficult Decisions in Surgery: An Evidence-Based Approach,
https://doi.org/10.1007/978-3-031-42303-1_45

intussusception. Search terms included "rectal intussusception," "rectal outlet obstruction," "outlet obstruction," "internal rectal prolapse," and "obstructed defecation." Studies were excluded if they looked at exclusively external rectal prolapse, lacked adequate follow-up, or looked at outcomes of patients with solely fecal incontinence and outlet obstruction. If a group published similar studies on the same patient cohort, only the most recent study was included. In additional to the systematic literature search, references included in the reviewed papers were additionally searched to find relevant papers (Table 45.1 and 45.2).

Table 45.1 PICO table

Patients	Intervention	Comparator	Outcome
Patients with outlet obstruction, in particular, internal intussusception	Operative management	Non-operative management	Health-related quality of life (HRQOL)

Table 45.2 Study outcomes

Study	Patients	Intervention	Outcome measure	Results	Quality of evidence
Hwang [6]	27 patients with rectal intussusception and constipation	Biofeedback	Symptoms improvement after → = 2 biofeedback sessions	Weekly BMs 2 → 4.1, incompleted evacuation 17 → 9%	Very Low
Ganio [10]	167	Delorme	Functional scores	Improvement in functional scores in majority of patients	Low
Lehur [12]	50	STARR versus Biofeedback	ODS-S	48.1% more patients at 12 months have a halving of their ODS-S in the STARR patients	Moderate
Von Papen [18]	56 with obstructed defecation failing non-operative management	Laparoscopic Resection Rectopexy	Survey at 3–6 months	53% improved constipation, 38% improved incomplete evacuation	Very Low

Table 45.2 (continued)

Study	Patients	Intervention	Outcome measure	Results	Quality of evidence
Consten [20]	677	LVMR	Symptoms and recurrence	74% of patients had subjective symptom improvement. 14% 10-year intussusception recurrence	Low
Franceschilli [22]	100	LVMR with biologic mesh	Symptoms and recurrence	92% subjective improvement. 16% 3-year recurrence	Low
Grossi [23]	28	LVMR	Quality of life scores	PAC-QOL change of −1.3 at 24 weeks, −1.0 at 48 weeks, after surgery	Low

LRR Laparoscopic Resection Rectopexy, *BM* Bowel Movement, *CCCS* Cleveland Clinic Constipation Score, *ODS-S* Obstructed Defecation Syndrome Score, *STARR* Stapled transanal rectal resection, *LVMR* Laparoscopic Ventral Mesh Rectopexy, Patient Assessment of Constipation Quality of Life (PAC-QOL)

Results

Over the past three decades, numerous papers have been published on the topic of internal rectal intussusception and outlet obstruction. The vast majority involve a low number of patients, with inconsistent definitions of what determines a patient to be symptomatic. There have been few randomized trials and limited follow-up in all studies. Furthermore, many studies have poor methodology with limited use of validated quality of life metrics and limited initial screening of patients to determine if the intussusception is the etiology for their symptoms. This has led a paucity of high-quality data to drive clinical decisions. This lack of data is found foremost in studies that examine the first-line treatment for these patients: non-operative therapy. Little to no studies look at medical management alone in this precise patient population, as most study patients with obstructive symptoms did not necessarily have internal rectal intussusception. There have been a few studies looking at biofeedback, such as Hwang et al.'s paper that, in a retrospective fashion, found 27 patients with internal rectal intussusception with constipation who had completed at least two biofeedback sessions. Patients were found to have an improvement in objective measures such as an increase in weekly bowel movements (from 2 to 4.1) and decrease in weekly assisted bowel movements (3.8 to 1.5) [6]. A similar study from Mimura *et. al* looked at 32 women, 38% of who had internal intussusception, with a median follow-up of 10 months after biofeedback sessions. 12% (3 of 25) of patients had resolution of symptoms, with those who still had symptoms, 56% subjectively reporting a small improvement in symptoms and 16% with "a lot" of symptom improvement [7].

The Delorme procedure is an older technique for treatment of internal rectal intussusception with outlet obstruction. Berman published his group's experience in 1990 with the Delorme treating 21 women with three-year follow-up. They found that at three years, 15 of 21 patients (71%) had the majority of their symptoms relieved, with six still having constipation or pressure on defecation [8]. Liberman et al. had a similar study in 2000, where they followed 34 patients with evaluation of subjective symptoms, such as incomplete evacuation, with 76% of patients reporting good symptom relief. There was no statement as to the length of follow-up in the study [9]. Ganio published the largest cohort, looking at 167 patients from 2001 to 2009 who had obstructed defecation and rectal intussusception. It was a more structured study, using the Cleveland Clinic Constipation Score (CCCS), Obstructed Defecation Syndrome Score (ODS-S), and the Patient Assessment of Constipation Quality of Life (PAC-QoL) questionnaire. Of the patients with obstructed defecation, their CCCS and ODS-S decreased from 12.1 to 4.2 and 11.9 to 4.4 respectively ($p < 0.001$). Over 48 of these 167 patients had a greater than 4 years of follow-up [10].

Stapled trans-anal rectal resection (STARR) is another perineal approach that addresses internal rectal intussusception, through a full-thickness resection of rectal tissue [11]. Lehur published a multi-center randomized trial comparing STARR versus 3 months of biofeedback training in patients from 2004–2005. Preoperatively, the patients had to have an ODS-S of at least 7 to enter the trial with intussusception seen on defecography and were followed for 12 months. 50% of the patients in the biofeedback arm withdrew early. For those patients who stayed in the trial, 31 patients had STARR and 19 biofeedback. The Baseline ODS-S went from 16.1 to 4.7 at 12 months in the STARR patients and 14.2 to 10.9 in the biofeedback patients, with a decrease in ODS-S of more than 50% in 81.5% of the STARR patients versus 33% of the biofeedback patients [12]. There have been many additional papers published since STARR's introduction, with a meta-analysis from 2014 looking at 26 publications with a median follow-up of 12 months encompassing 1298 patients. In aggregate, the studies showed an improvement in ODS-S with a decrease by 3.8 (95% CI 3.2–4.5), however, there was a high degree of heterogeneity from the studies suggesting an over-estimation of the improvement [13]. Later publications on the procedure have published on the adverse complications from STARR, including rectovaginal fistulas, accidental rectal closure, and pelvic necrotizing fasciitis [14–16]. Beyond severe complications, longer-term results for STARR have not been durable, as seen in one study where STARR patients' ODS scores, after an initial drop, doubled in-between their 18 and 42 months post-operative evaluation [17].

Abdominal approaches have also been described in the literature to treat internal rectal intussusception. Von Papen published a retrospective review of patients with internal intussusception with obstructed defecation who failed medical and biofeedback treatment for six months who underwent laparoscopic resection with posterior suture rectopexy. Of the 56 patients, follow-up showed that 63% felt their function improved with 53% better constipation [18]. The study was limited by only a three-to-six-month follow-up. The majority of abdominal approach studies over the past two decades have examined the role of using laparoscopic ventral mesh rectopexy [19–21]. Retrospective short-term follow-up studies have shown a general improvement in functional scores such as the CCCS or the Wexner Constipation Score (WCS) [19, 21]. The largest patient cohort comes from a study Consten et al. published in 2015 on a prospectively maintained database of 919 patients who had undergone laparoscopic ventral mesh rectopexy. Of these patients, 677 had internal rectal intussusception. Of those with obstructed defecation, 74% had subjective improvement in their symptoms, although this was not assessed with a standardize scoring system. There was no standard length of follow-up, but using a statistical model, the authors estimated recurrence of the intussusception at five and ten years to be 11.1% and 14.2% respectively [20]. With concerns for permanent mesh, Franceschilli et al. looked at the use of biologic mesh (porcine dermal collagen) in lieu of the standard permanent mesh for rectopexy. In their first 100 cases, patients qualified for an operation if they have a WCS ≥ 5 with rectoanal intussusception. With a median follow-up of 20 months, 92% of patients had their constipation improved with 79% cured. The WCS dropped from 18.4 pre-operatively to 5.4 at one-year follow-up. They additionally found a three-year recurrence of 16% [22]. Grossi et al., using a stepped-wedge randomized controlled trial in patients with internal rectal intussusception and chronic constipation, found improvement in patients at 24 and 48 weeks post-surgery compared to their baseline. The trial aimed to recruit 114 patients but only managed to recruit 28 patients [23]. With the popularization of the robotic platform, one group performed a randomized trial between laparoscopic and robotic ventral mesh rectopexy on 30 patients, 22 of who had internal rectal intussusception, finding similar intra-operative case length, post-operative complication rate, and 3-month magnetic resonance defecography [24].

Recommendations

In patients with obstructive symptoms and internal rectal intussusception who have failed medical therapy, operative treatment could be considered after an appropriate risk-and-benefit discussion with the patient (weak recommendation, low quality of evidence).

If a patient can tolerate a transabdominal operation, minimally invasive ventral mesh rectopexy is the preferred operative approach for patients with internal rectal intussusception and obstructive symptoms (weak recommendation, low quality of evidence).

Personal View

While numerous papers have been published on operative treatment of patients with internal intussusception and obstructed defecation, there still exists a paucity of quality data to guide clinicians in management of this patient population. The data, by-and-large, is retrospective in nature, with a limited number of patients, and limited follow-up. Moreso, inclusion criteria vary widely across all studies, as does the use of validated metrics to assess whether interventions have a true impact on patients' quality of life.

Beyond the data limitations, much difficulty in the assessment of operative intervention on internal rectal intussusception may stem from the obstructive symptoms not arising primarily from the intussusception itself. Rising grades of rectal intussusception have not correlated with worsening constipation, and non-surgical conditions, like Irritable Bowel Syndrome (IBS) and pelvic floor dyssynergia, have a greater impact on the severity of symptoms than intussusception grade [4, 25].

The void of quality data and disputable contribution of internal intussusception to obstructed defecation demands that clinicians, unable to practice evidenced-based medicine, instead rely on the basic guiding principle of *primum non nocere* (first, do no harm). All patients should start with a standardized medical approach with high-fiber diet and ensuring adequate hydration. They should be evaluated with manometry and electromyography (EMG). If evidence of pelvic floor dyssynergia exists, referral to EMG-based biofeedback training should occur. Similarly, if patients are found to have IBS, they should be optimized from a medical standpoint.

In patients who have normal manometry and EMG without IBS, we would then recommend for defecography to assess for intussusception. For those with rectoanal intussusception who failed medical therapy, we would counsel the patient regarding operative management. In particular, we would highlight that the data points towards use of ventral rectopexy as the first-line surgical treatment, as it shows some benefit in short-term follow-up in studies with a limited number of patients. Part of our counseling would highlight the mesh concerns around ventral mesh rectopexy. There have been two larger studies looking at long-term mesh outcomes, with one observational study that showed mesh complications in 4.6% of 919 patients [20]. An additional retrospective review looked at over 2000 patients who had undergone ventral mesh rectopexy and found that 2% of the patients had mesh erosion with 40% necessitating an operation for mesh explantation due to mesh erosion [26].

Going forward, we need to strive to improve our data to provide guidance for surgeons in the treatment of outlet obstruction found in patients with internal intussusception. The numerous publications in this area show that our lack of strong evidence is not for a lack of research effort. Adequate patient enrollment has proven difficult, as has length of follow-up and standardized pre-operative characterization of what truly drives our patients' symptoms. Alternative strategies are needed, with prospective multi-institutional quality improvement registries to track patients' functional outcomes. We have had successful initial efforts at such a registry [27] and encourage others to pursue similar efforts, so that we can start to bring evidence into the treatment of our patients and provide them the data-drive care that they deserve.

References

1. Palit S, Bhan C, Lunniss PJ, Boyle DJ, Gladman MA, Knowles CH, et al. Evacuation proctography: a reappraisal of normal variability. Color Dis. 2014;16(7):538–46.
2. Shorvon PJ, McHugh S, Diamant NE, Somers S, Stevenson GW. Defecography in normal volunteers: results and implications. Gut. 1989;30(12):1737–49.
3. Mellgren A, Schultz I, Johansson C, Dolk A. Internal rectal intussusception seldom develops into total rectal prolapse. Dis Colon Rectum. 1997;40(7):817–20.
4. Hawkins AT, Olariu AG, Savitt LR, Gingipally S, Wakamatsu MM, Pulliam S, et al. Impact of rising grades of internal rectal intussusception on fecal continence and symptoms of constipation. Dis Colon Rectum. 2016;59(1):54–61.
5. Dvorkin LS, Gladman MA, Epstein J, Scott SM, Williams NS, Lunniss PJ. Rectal intussusception in symptomatic patients is different from that in asymptomatic volunteers. Br J Surg. 2005;92(7):866–72.
6. Hwang YH, Person B, Choi JS, Nam YS, Singh JJ, Weiss EG, et al. Biofeedback therapy for rectal intussusception. Tech Coloproctol. 2006;10(1):11–6.
7. Mimura T, Roy AJ, Storrie JB, Kamm MA. Treatment of impaired defecation associated with rectocele by behavioral retraining (biofeedback). Dis Colon Rectum. 2000;43(9):1267–72.
8. Berman IR, Harris MS, Rabeler MB. Delorme's transrectal excision for internal rectal prolapse. Dis Colon Rectum. 1990;33(7):573–80.
9. Liberman H, Hughes C, Dippolito A. Evaluation and outcome of the delorme procedure in the treatment of rectal outlet obstruction. Dis Colon Rectum. 2000;43(2):188–92.
10. Ganio E, Martina S, Novelli E, Sandru R, Clerico G, Realis Luc A, et al. Internal Delorme's procedure for rectal outlet obstruction. Color Dis. 2013;15(3):e144–50.
11. Boccasanta P, Venturi M, Stuto A, Bottini C, Caviglia A, Carriero A, et al. Stapled Transanal rectal resection for outlet obstruction: a prospective, multicenter trial. Dis Colon Rectum. 2004;47(9):1285–97.
12. Lehur PA, Stuto A, Fantoli M, Villani RD, Queralto M, Lazorthes F, et al. Outcomes of stapled transanal rectal resection vs. biofeedback for the treatment of outlet obstruction associated with rectal intussusception and rectocele: a multicenter, randomized, controlled trial. Dis Colon Rectum. 2008;51(11):1611–8.
13. Van Geluwe B, Stuto A, DaPozzo F, Fieuws S, Meurette G, Lehur PA, et al. Relief of obstructed defecation syndrome after stapled Transanal rectal resection (STARR): a meta-analysis. Acta Chir Belg. 2014;114(3):189–97.
14. Gagliardi G, Pescatori M, Altomare DF, Binda GA, Bottini C, Dodi G, et al. Results, outcome predictors, and complications after stapled Transanal rectal resection for obstructed defecation. Dis Colon Rectum. 2008;51(2):186–95.
15. Pescatori M, Gagliardi G. Postoperative complications after procedure for prolapsed hemorrhoids (PPH) and stapled transanal rectal resection (STARR) procedures. Tech Coloproctol. 2008;12(1):7–19.
16. Naldini G. Serious unconventional complications of surgery with stapler for haemorrhoidal prolapse and obstructed defaecation because of rectocoele and rectal intussusception. Color Dis. 2011;13(3):323–7.
17. Madbouly KM, Abbas KS, Hussein AM. Disappointing long-term outcomes after stapled transanal rectal resection for obstructed defecation. World J Surg. 2010;34(9):2191–6.
18. von Papen M, Ashari LHS, Lumley JW, Stevenson ARL, Stitz RW. Functional results of laparoscopic resection rectopexy for symptomatic rectal intussusception. Dis Colon Rectum. 2007;50(1):50–5.
19. Collinson R, Wijffels N, Cunningham C, Lindsey I. Laparoscopic ventral rectopexy for internal rectal prolapse: short-term functional results. Color Dis. 2010;12(2):97–104.
20. Consten ECJ, van Iersel JJ, Verheijen PM, Broeders IAMJ, Wolthuis AM, D'Hoore A. Long-term outcome after laparoscopic ventral mesh rectopexy: an observational study of 919 consecutive patients. Ann Surg. 2015;262(5):742–8.

21. Formijne Jonkers HA, Poierrié N, Draaisma WA, Broeders IAMJ, Consten ECJ. Laparoscopic ventral rectopexy for rectal prolapse and symptomatic rectocele: an analysis of 245 consecutive patients. Color Dis. 2013;15(6):695–9.
22. Franceschilli L, Varvaras D, Capuano I, Ciangola CI, Giorgi F, Boehm G, et al. Laparoscopic ventral rectopexy using biologic mesh for the treatment of obstructed defaecation syndrome and/or faecal incontinence in patients with internal rectal prolapse: a critical appraisal of the first 100 cases. Tech Coloproctol. 2015;19(4):209–19.
23. Grossi U, Lacy-Colson J, Brown SR, Cross S, Eldridge S, Jordan M, et al. Stepped-wedge randomized controlled trial of laparoscopic ventral mesh rectopexy in adults with chronic constipation. Tech Coloproctol. 2022;26(12):941–52.
24. Mäkelä-Kaikkonen J, Rautio T, Pääkkö E, Biancari F, Ohtonen P, Mäkelä J. Robot-assisted vs laparoscopic ventral rectopexy for external or internal rectal prolapse and enterocele: a randomized controlled trial. Color Dis. 2016;18(10):1010–5.
25. Cavallaro PM, Staller K, Savitt LR, Milch H, Kennedy K, Weinstein MM, et al. The contributions of internal intussusception, irritable bowel syndrome, and pelvic floor dyssynergia to obstructed defecation syndrome. Dis Colon Rectum. 2019;62(1):56–62.
26. Evans C, Stevenson ARL, Sileri P, Mercer-Jones MA, Dixon AR, Cunningham C, et al. A multicenter collaboration to assess the safety of laparoscopic ventral Rectopexy. Dis Colon Rectum. 2015;58(8):799–807.
27. Cavallaro PM, Vogler SA, Hyman NH, Ky AJ, Savitt LR, Tyler KM, et al. Preliminary report from the pelvic floor disorders consortium: large-scale data collection through quality improvement initiatives to provide data on functional outcomes after rectal prolapse repair. Dis Colon Rectum. 2021;64(8):986–94.

Part VI

Quality Improvement

46 Is Bowel Prep Necessary for Patients Undergoing Colon Resection?

Kayla Polcari and Benjamin D. Shogan

Introduction

Despite significant advancements in postoperative care of surgical patients through enhanced recovery after surgery (ERAS) pathways and minimally invasive techniques, surgical site infections (SSIs) remain the major contributor to morbidity following colectomy [1]. Although the precise pathogenesis in the development of an SSI remains unclear, direct decontamination of the operative field has long been thought to play a key and causative role. With over 90% of the fecal biomass due to bacteria, stool is densely packed with microorganisms. Given that transection of the bowel can result in spillage of stool, it is not surprising that colorectal surgery continues to account for one of the highest rates of SSI amongst all elective surgeries [2].

Preoperative bowel preparation, first introduced over a half century ago, is designed to prevent postoperative infectious complications by decreasing the high bacterial load in the colon [3]. During its initial development use of a purgative to simply empty the colon of stool was employed. This mechanical bowel preparation (MBP) strategy was thought to improve both ease of bowel manipulation and reduce spillage and subsequent contamination [1, 4]. The addition of non-absorbable oral antibiotics (OAB) emerged in the 1970s with landmark studies by Rosenberg and Nichols, and garnered increased attention in the last decade after several retrospective studies using the American College of Surgeons National Surgical Quality Improvement Program (NSQIP) database suggested improved outcomes with combined MBP and OAB preparation [5–10]. By extension, some have also questioned if OAB alone are sufficient to decontaminate the colon enough to prevent postoperative infections.

K. Polcari · B. D. Shogan (✉)
University of Chicago, Chicago, IL, USA
e-mail: Kayla.Polcari@uchospitals.edu; bshogan@surgery.bsd.uchicago.edu

K. Umanskiy, N. Hyman (eds.), *Difficult Decisions in Colorectal Surgery*, Difficult Decisions in Surgery: An Evidence-Based Approach,
https://doi.org/10.1007/978-3-031-42303-1_46

Despite the theoretical advantage of preoperative colon decontamination and an extensive body of literature, the optimal type of bowel preparation and its efficacy remains controversial. Proponents argue that preoperative decontamination is a proven and safe adjunct to decrease complications, whereas others cite that bowel preparation is associated with dehydration, *Clostridium difficile* infection, and the development of antibiotic resistance. In this chapter, we evaluate the current state of evidence on preoperative bowel preparation and give recommendations to the clinician as to which strategy of preoperative bowel decontamination is most efficacious in preventing complications in patients undergoing colorectal surgery.

Search Strategy

A comprehensive search of PubMed and MEDLINE was performed to identify relevant literature investigating infectious outcomes of patients undergoing elective colectomy as it pertains to preoperative bowel preparation (Table 46.1). The search was limited to English-language articles published between 1970–2022 for which full text versions are available. Study types were limited to clinical trials, randomized controlled trials (RCTs), and meta-analyses. Key search terms included ('colon resection' OR 'colectomy' OR 'colon surgery' OR 'colorectal surgery') AND ('bowel preparation' OR 'preoperative bowel preparation' OR 'mechanical bowel preparation' OR 'oral antibiotics' OR 'PO antibiotics'). Titles and abstracts were reviewed for relevance. Articles pertaining specifically to the pediatric population or those including patients undergoing non-elective surgery were excluded. References of relevant publications were also reviewed.

Table 46.1 PICO table

Patients	Intervention	Comparator	Outcomes
Patients undergoing elective colorectal resection	1. Mechanical bowel preparation (MBP) 2. Oral antibiotic preparation (OAB) 3. Combination of mechanical and oral antibiotic preparation (MOABP)	No bowel preparation (NBP)	Infectious complications (surgical site infection, anastomotic leak)

Results

Mechanical Bowel Preparation Alone

The efficacy of MBP alone has been extensively studied with many RCTs performed over many decades showing no benefit of MBP alone over no bowel preparation (NBP) [11–23]. In 2011, the Cochrane Review released its most recent iteration of recommendations regarding MBP, including 18 trials with a total of 5805 participants allocated to MBP versus NBP. There was no difference in rates of anastomotic leak or wound infection with or without MBP. Similar to previous versions, the authors concluded that MBP alone does not improve outcomes in elective colorectal surgery and is not indicated [24]. Similarly, a meta-analysis of 36 RCTs and observational studies including 21,568 patients conducted by Rollins et al. (2018) demonstrated that MBP did not reduce the incidence of anastomotic leak, SSI, mortality, reoperation, or hospital length of stay (LOS) when compared to NBP [25]. Further, in both the Cochrane Review and the meta-analysis performed by Rollins et al., subgroup analyses of patients receiving solely rectal enemas for decontamination, rather than an oral purgative, did not show any significant benefit over NBP [24, 25]. Most recently, in 2022 Woodfield et al. performed a meta-analysis of 10 high-quality RCTs concluding that MBP did not reduce the incidence of SSI or anastomotic leak compared to NBP [26]. Examination of nationwide data in retrospective review of the ACS-NSQIP database has also shown no benefit of a MBP alone [8–10, 27, 28].

Besides a lack of efficacy, MBP has also been associated with complications. Concerns over possible harm secondary to dehydration and electrolyte disturbances with MBP have been raised [29–31]. One RCT compared healthy patients without baseline renal impairment receiving sodium phosphate versus polyethylene glycol (PEG) bowel preparations. Both groups demonstrated metabolic and electrolyte changes, though the changes were significantly more pronounced with the use of phosphate-based solution [30]. While PEG solutions are preferred, they have been shown to increase postoperative intestinal dysmotility compared to no bowel preparation [32].

Combined Mechanical and Oral Antibiotic Preparation

Comparing MOABP to MBP Alone

The addition of non-absorbable oral antibiotics to MBP (MOABP) was first introduced during a 1971 RCT demonstrating that this combined preparation reduced the incidence of septic complications compared to MBP alone [5]. This was popularized with the advent of the "*Nichols prep*" in 1973, in which the addition of oral neomycin-erythromycin was shown to significantly suppress aerobic and anaerobic growth in colonic contents [6]. Several other early RCTs continued to report improvement in infectious complications with the use of combined MOABP [33–36]. With the development of newer and more potent IV antibiotics in the 1990s, surgeons questioned the role of oral antibiotics. Yet, many RCTs, culminating with a meta-analysis by Bellows et al. (2011), demonstrated that the use of parenteral antibiotics in addition to oral antibiotics was superior to IV alone, with a significant reduction in risk of SSI (RR 0.57, 95% CI 0.43–0.76) [37–39].

More recently, a series of retrospective studies using NSQIP data has been published suggesting that MOABP out-performs MBP alone [7–10]. For example, Koller et al. (2018) found a reduction in SSI (OR 0.49, 95% CI 0.43–0.54), anastomotic leak (OR 0.58, 95% CI 0.48–0.70), postoperative ileus (OR 0.79, 95% CI 0.72–0.87), reoperation (OR 0.69, 95% CI 0.59–0.81), and readmission (OR 0.89, 95% CI (0.80–0.99) with MOABP compared to MBP alone [9]. Many studies have since confirmed the benefits of MOABP over MBP [4, 26, 40–47]. Notably, two studies focusing on the IBD patient population found similar results. Oshima et al. (2013) found a significant reduction in overall SSI with MOABP versus MBP (6.2% vs. 22.4%, p = 0.001) in patients with ulcerative colitis undergoing proctocolectomy and ileal pouch anal anastomosis [48]. Uchino et al. (2019) also found a reduction in incisional SSI from 16.7% to 7.4% (p = 0.01) with the addition of oral antibiotics when examining Crohn's patients undergoing intestinal resection [49].

Comparing MOABP to NBP (Table 46.2)

Dissimilar to MBP alone, the data comparing MOABP to NBP is less extensive and is largely gleaned from retrospective studies using large datasets from quality improvement programs. Cannon et al. (2012) analyzed retrospective prescription data from the Veterans Affairs Surgical Quality Improvement Program (VASQIP) of 9940 patients undergoing elective colorectal resections from 2005–2009 and found that MOABP reduced the incidence of SSI compared to NBP (OR 0.43, 95% CI 0.34–0.55) [50]. In a similar study of 2475 patients in the Michigan Surgical Quality Collaborative (MSQC), Kim et al. (2014) found a significant reduction in superficial, organ space, and overall SSI with use of MOABP compared to NBP [51]. These findings held consistent on a sub-analysis of 957 propensity matched cases.

Several studies interrogating the NSQIP database found similar results. Two analyses of 2012 NSQIP data showed a significantly reduced incidence of SSI and anastomotic leak with MOABP in patients undergoing colorectal resections, with or without stoma creation [8, 27]. Moghadamyeghaneh et al. (2015) examined the same NSQIP data specific to anatomic resections for colon cancer and found that MOABP reduced overall morbidity and superficial SSI for all colectomies, while it only reduced anastomotic leak for left-sided colectomies [28]. Several subsequent studies that sequentially included more patients from more years of NSQIP data repeatedly showed a decreased occurrence of SSI and anastomotic leak with MOABP compared to NBP [7, 9, 10, 52, 53]. Midura et al. (2018) found a reduced incidence of SSI (OR 0.47, 95% CI 0.42–0.53) and anastomotic leak (OR 0.59, 95% CI 0.48–0.73) with MOABP compared to NBP amongst 45,724 patients undergoing elective colectomies from the 2012–2015 NSQIP datasets [53].

MOABP has also been associated with improvements in non-infections complications. On evaluation of secondary outcomes, MOABP reported statistically significant reductions of postoperative ileus, readmission, reoperation, and shorter

Table 46.2 Studies investigating MOABP or OAB alone compared to NBP

Study (year)	Study Design	Intervention (N)	Results (reported as MOABP compared to NBP)	Results (reported as OAB alone compared to NBP)	Quality of Evidence
ACS-NSQIP studies					
Kiran (2015)	Retrospective study using NSQIP 2012 (N = 8442)	MOABP (2324) MBP alone (3822) NBP (2296)	Reduced incidence of SSI (OR 0.40, 95% CI 0.31-0.53) and anastomotic leak (OR 0.57, 95% CI 0.56-0.90)	N/A	Moderate
Scarborough (2015)	Retrospective study using NSQIP 2012 (N = 4999)	MOABP (1494) MBP alone (2322) OAB alone (91) NBP (1092)	Reduced incidence of incisional SSI (OR 0.33, CI 0.23-0.47) and anastomotic leak (OR 0.48, 95% CI 0.32-0.73)	No difference in incisional SSI or anastomotic leak rate	Moderate
Moghada-myeghaneh (2015)	Retrospective study using NSQIP 2012-2013 (N = 5021)	MOABP (1386) MBP alone (2248) OAB alone (117) NBP (1270)	Reduced incidence of superficial SSI for both right- (OR 0.14, 95% CI 0.06-0.33) and left- (OR 0.31, 95% CI 0.18-0.53) sided colectomies; and reduced incidence of anastomotic leak for left-sided colectomies (OR 0.44, 95% CI 0.25-0.78)	No difference in superficial or organ space SSI or anastomotic leak for both right- and left-sided colectomies	Moderate
Garfinkle (2017)	Retrospective study using NSQIP 2012-2014 (N = 40,466)	MOABP (8819) MBP alone (9800) OAB alone (1461) NBP (13219)	Reduced incidence of SSI (OR 0.63, 95% CI 0.45-0.87) and anastomotic leak (OR 0.60, 95% CI 0.34-0.97)	Reduced incidence of SSI (OR, 0.63; 95% CI, 0.45–0.87) and anastomotic leak (OR, 0.60; 95% CI, 0.34–0.97)	Moderate

(continued)

Table 46.2 (continued)

Study (year)	Study Design	Intervention (N)	Results (reported as MOABP compared to NBP)	Results (reported as OAB alone compared to NBP)	Quality of Evidence
Koller (2018)	Retrospective study using NSQIP 2012-2014 (N = 32359)	MOABP (10643) MBP alone (11836) OAB alone (1240) NBP (8640)	Reduced incidence of SSI (OR 0.45, 95% CI 0.40-0.50) and anastomotic leak (OOR 0.53, 95% CI 0.43-0.64)	Reduced incidence of SSI (OR 0.49, 95% CI 0.38-0.64) and anastomotic leak (OR 0.37, 95% CI 0.21-0.67)	Moderate
Midura (2018)	Retrospective study using NSQIP 2012-2015 (N = 45724)	MOABP (16860) MBP alone (15175) OAB alone (1791) NBP (11898)	Reduced incidence of SSI (OR 0.47, 95% CI 0.42-0.53) and anastomotic leak (OR 0.59, 95% CI 0.48-0.73)	Reduced incidence of SSI (OR 0.70, 95% CI 0.55-0.88); no difference in anastomotic leak.	Moderate
Klinger (2019)	Retrospective study using NSQIP 2012-2015 (N = 27804)	MOABP (8855) MBP alone (7617) OAB alone (1374) NBP (5471)	Reduced incidence of SSI (OR 0.39, 95% CI 0.33-0.46) and anastomotic leak (OR 0.53, 95% CI 0.43-0.65)	Reduced incidence of SSI (OR 0.63, 95% CI 0.47-0.83) and anastomotic leak (OR 0.53, 95% CI 0.35-0.79)	Moderate
Others					
Cannon (2012)	Retrospective study using VASQIP	MOABP (3400) MBP alone (3839) OAB alone (723) NBP (1978)	Reduced incidence of SSI (OR 0.43, 95% CI 0.34-0.55)	Reduced incidence of SSI (OR 0.33, 95% CI 0.21-0.50)	Moderate

LOS compared to NBP, though there was mixed evidence regarding its impact on 30-day mortality [7–9, 27, 28, 52]. Importantly, although the NSQIP studies differ slightly in their inclusion criteria and the timeframe for data extraction, they are likely to have significant patient overlap. Further, the use of these retrospective datasets that are heterogenous and often incomplete puts these studies at particular risk for misclassification and selection bias.

Importantly, these studies contributed to a growing body of evidence debunking the concern that preoperative OAB might increase rates of complications, namely postoperative *Clostridium difficile* infection [1, 54]. In fact, several studies suggest that those receiving OAB are actually less likely to develop postoperative *C. difficile* colitis [10, 51, 55]. For example, Kim et al. (2014) found reduced rates of post-colectomy *C. difficile* in the MOABP group compared to NBP (0.5% vs 1.8%, p = 0.01) in a propensity-matched analysis of 957 paired cases [51]. Klinger et al. (2019) also reported a 40% reduction in odds of *C. difficile* infection with use of MOABP (OR 0.60, 95% CI 0.46–0.77) [10]. Other studies show no difference in rates of postoperative *C. difficile* when OAB are used [4, 56].

Few meta-analyses have examined MOABP versus NBP. Rollins et al. (2019), which included 4 cohort studies, found less SSI (RR 0.54, 95% CI 0.43–0.68) and anastomotic leak (RR 0.52, 95% CI 0.45–0.59) with MOABP [4]. Of note, one of the cohort studies included in the meta-analysis included emergent cases with and without resection, which takes it beyond the scope of our review [57]. Mulder et al. (2019) performed a meta-analysis of the NSQIP and VASQIP cohorts, and again showed a reduction in SSI with MOABP compared to NBP (OR 0.42, 95% CI 0.37–0.49) [58]. In a meta-analysis of 38 RCTs, none of which directly compared MOABP to NBP, Toh et al. (2018) indirectly compared these two groups and found a reduction in incisional SSI, organ/space SSI, and overall SSI with MOABP [40]. There was no difference in rates of anastomotic leak between the groups. Likewise, Woodfield et al. (2022) found a reduction in incisional SSI (OR 0.27, 95% CI 0.14–0.54), but not anastomotic leak, with MOABP in a more recent analysis of 10 high-quality RCTs [26].

Finally, in 2019, the first RCT directly comparing MOABP to NBP was published in *The Lancet* [59]. The MOBILE study, conducted by Koskenvuo et al., was a multi-center single-blinded trial in 4 Finish hospitals that randomized 396 patients to either MOABP or NBP prior to their elective colectomies. Contrary to the findings of prior studies, the results indicated that MOABP was not superior to NBP. There was no significant difference detected with regards to either SSI (7% in MOABP group vs 11% in NBP group, p = 0.17) or anastomotic dehiscence (4% in both groups, p = 0.82). There were also no differences in reoperation, readmission, LOS, or 30- or 90-day mortality. In a later subgroup analysis differentiating right versus left colectomy patients, there remained no significant difference in SSI or anastomotic leak [60]. The authors concluded that "current recommendations of using MOABP for colectomies…should be reconsidered." While the results of this investigation are intriguing, several key limitations, including that the study was underpowered and composed primarily of lower risk minimally invasive colectomies, prevent it from completely overturning all of the previously reported benefits of MOABP.

Oral Antibiotic Preparation Alone

Comparing OAB Alone to MOABP

It has been thought that non-absorbable oral antibiotics would only be efficacious in the setting of an empty colon following MBP. To address this, many of the retrospective studies utilizing the VASQIP and NSQIP databases investigated the outcomes in patients given only OAB. Surprisingly, many of those studies found no benefit of MOABP over OAB alone [7, 9, 50]. For example, Cannon et al. (2012) found no significant difference in SSI rates between OAB alone and MOABP cohorts in their VASQIP analysis (8.3% vs 9.2%, p = 0.47) [50]. Garfinkle et al. (2017) and Koller et al. (2018) similarly found no difference in SSI, nor anastomotic leak, ileus, and mortality [7, 9].

On the other hand, others have shown discordant results. Using 2012–2015 NSQIP data of 20,594 patients, 2018 of whom received OAB alone, Kaslow et al. (2018) found a significantly lesser incidence of superficial and organ space SSI, ileus, sepsis, reoperation, mortality, and LOS with MOABP compared to OAB alone [61]. Further, after propensity score matching and inverse probability-weighted regression adjusted analysis, the superiority of MOABP persisted, with 2.2% less total SSI, 2.3% less postoperative ileus, 1.5% less 30-day reoperation, and 0.45-day shorter LOS compared to OAB alone. Given the overall rarity of these events, Kaslow et al. argued that the results are clinically significant and criticized prior NSQIP studies for their comparably smaller sample sizes of patients who received OAB alone, limiting the power of their analyses.

Only two RCTs have directly compared combined MOABP to OAB alone. In an RCT analyzing 380 patients at two Polish centers, Zmora et al. (2003) found no difference in wound infection, anastomotic leak, intra-abdominal abscess, overall infectious complications, LOS, or mortality [62]. Suzuki et al. (2020) later randomized 254 colon cancer patients to receive MOABP versus OAB alone and found no difference in incidence of incisional or organ space SSI [63]. Several meta-analyses have compared MOABP versus OAB alone, all of which found no differences in SSI or anastomotic leak rate between these groups [4, 26, 40, 64]. However, Rollins et al. (2019) did note that those receiving MOABP had significantly lower 30-day mortality (RR 0.58, 95% CI 0.34–0.97) and incidence of post-op ileus (RR 0.83, 95% CI 0.73–0.95) [4]. Together, given the discrepancy in published studies, it currently remains unclear if the addition of MBP to OAB significantly adds to the efficacy of a preop bowel preparation.

Comparing OAB Alone to NBP (Table 46.2)

There is a scarcity of high-quality studies examining OAB alone versus NBP. Amongst numerous retrospective database studies, some demonstrated a reduction in infectious complications with OAB alone [7, 9, 10, 50, 53, 65], while others showed OAB to be no better than NBP [8, 28]. Rollins et al. (2019) found a significant reduction in incidence of overall SSI (RR 0.56, 95% CI 0.38–0.83) with OAB alone over NBP in their analysis combining VASQIP and NSQIP cohorts to include 16,390 patients [4]. Meanwhile, Toh et al. (2018) found no difference in overall SSI, incisional SSI, or anastomotic leak, but did note less organ/space SSI (OR 0.13, 95% CI 0.02–0.55) with OAB compared to NBP on an indirect comparison of RCTs [40].

Other studies have since attempted to clarify this relationship. In an observational pre-post study of 1410 patients in a single Dutch hospital, those undergoing elective colorectal resection after implementation of OAB in 2013 were compared to those whose surgeries occurred in 2012 that received NBP [66]. Results showed a decreased incidence of deep SSI (RR 0.54, 95% CI 0.37–0.78) and anastomotic leak (0.57, 95% CI 0.35–0.90) and a reduced LOS from 8 to 7 days ($p = 0.001$) in the OAB cohort. There was no difference in superficial SSI or *C. difficile* infection between the groups. In a temporal regression analysis, there was an instant decrease in SSI incidence following OAB implementation. However, there was a significantly increased use of minimally invasive techniques in the OAB group, which is well-known to reduce SSI in and of itself, therefore confounding the results.

The only known RCT to directly compare OAB alone to NBP was published by Espin-Basany et al. in 2020 [67]. The ORALEV trial is a multi-center, single-blind RCT, in which a total of 565 patients were randomized to receive either oral ciprofloxacin and metronidazole on the day before surgery or no preparation. The control group had significantly more SSIs (11% vs 5%, $p = 0.013$) and overall complications (28% vs 19%, $p = 0.017$) than those who received OAB. None of the patients receiving OAB preparation developed *C. difficile* or other adverse events. Of note, this trial has been criticized for several key limitations. The primary outcome was a pooled evaluation of overall SSI, and the treatment effect was largely accounted for by reductions in superficial SSI, with independent analyses of deep SSI and anastomotic leak revealing no difference [68, 69]. Further, the OAB regimen was unconventional as it included antibiotics that are readily absorbed in the gastrointestinal tract [70].

Several meta-analyses including the most recent data have all demonstrated decreased SSI with OAB alone compared to NBP, with odds ratios ranging from 0.23 to 0.51 [26, 58, 64]. Ultimately, further high-quality studies are needed to determine if OAB alone are sufficient. Multiple ongoing RCTs aim to provide additional insight [58, 71, 72].

Recommendations

1. **MBP alone is not recommended for patients undergoing elective colorectal resection.**

   Based on overwhelmingly concordant data from high-quality RCTs and multiple meta-analyses, we do not recommend the routine use of MBP alone for preoperative bowel preparation in elective colorectal surgery. *Strength of recommendation: strong.*

2. **Combined MBP with oral antibiotics is recommended for patients undergoing elective colorectal resection.**

   Despite compelling findings in the MOBILE trial that questioned the efficacy of MOABP in reducing infectious complications, there were several important limitations. Based on the entire body of available literature, including multiple RCTs, we recommend the use of combined mechanical and oral antibiotic preparation prior to elective colorectal resections. *Strength of recommendation: moderate.*

3. **Preoperative oral antibiotics alone are only recommended for patients undergoing elective colorectal resection when the use of MBP is precluded.**
   The data supporting OAB alone is less conclusive and of lesser quality. As a whole, the current literature suggests advantages to OAB alone over NBP without any significant harm. Therefore, we recommend the use of preoperative oral antibiotics alone when the use of MBP is precluded, such as in patients with ostomies or obstructions. *Strength of Recommendation: moderate.*

Our recommendations regarding MBP alone and MOABP are in concordance with those from the American Society of Colon and Rectal Surgeons (ASCRS), the ERAS Society, the Society of American Gastrointestinal and Endoscopic Surgeons (SAGES) and the World Health Organization (WHO) [1, 73–75]. Many societal guidelines have not commented on the use of OAB alone as this research is relatively new; the 2018 ASCRS recommendation against use of preoperative oral antibiotics alone was made prior to publication of the Dutch pre-post study or the ORALEV trial [1].

Personal View

The evolution of preoperative bowel preparation over the last half century is fascinating. Initially popularized in the late part of the twentieth century by Nichols and other landmark high-quality RCTs, MOABP fell out of favor as perioperative IV antibiotics became standard of care [6]. With recent NSQIP based studies coupled with new societal guidelines, MOABP has once again become accepted. In fact, an ASCRS survey documented that only 36% of respondents used oral antibiotics in 2010, whereas 83.2% did in 2018 [76, 77].

Why has there been such controversy regarding the use and efficacy of bowel preparation? Even today, 50 years after its introduction, bowel preparations remain empiric and impersonal. In the current era, technology allows us to precisely stage a tumor preoperatively, measure and adjust chemotherapies to circulating tumor cell DNA levels, and treat some patients with metastatic disease with curative intent. Yet, we continue to use a virtually identical bowel preparation as the one introduced in 1973 without any regard to the individual patient's bacterial composition or resistance patterns.

Research over the last decade has cemented the importance of the gut microbiome. Further, there is now an abundance of preclinical and clinical studies that have associated specific microbial changes with the development of anastomotic leak, postoperative ileus, and SSI [78–80]. We have learned that MBP and OAB have individual effects on a patient's microbiome that are dependent upon many variables such as diet, obesity, comorbidities, and prior exposure to antibiotics [81, 82]. While RCTs are designed to control for clinical variables (i.e. age, indication, and type of surgery) there is no current study or technology available that controls for microbial composition – *the precise variable that is being influenced by the bowel*. It therefore stands to reason that decontamination by bowel preparation is beneficial in some patients, whereas in others it allows the emergence of opportunistic pathogens that promote postoperative complications. The very fact that this variable is not controlled for might be the reason for so many discordant studies.

While still a future aim, we are now closer than ever to achieving the ability to measure and individually manipulate one's microbiome to decrease postoperative complications. Until we have this ability when making real-time clinical decisions, the available evidence supports the recommendation of a combined MOABP or OAB only if a MBP is not safe. The heterogeneity of the antibiotic regimens used in the published studies make it impossible to determine a preferred regimen, and we leave this decision up to the individual surgeon based upon regional differences in antibiotic resistance patterns. In future studies, it will be imperative to include culture-level evidence when investigating the relationship between bowel preparation, the microbiome, and surgical site infections.

Recommendations Summary

1. Mechanical bowel preparation alone is not recommended for patients undergoing elective colorectal resection (Strong recommendation).
2. Combined mechanical bowel preparation with oral antibiotics is recommended for patients undergoing elective colorectal resection (Moderate recommendation).
3. Preoperative oral antibiotics alone are only recommended for patients undergoing elective colorectal resection when the use of mechanical bowel preparation is precluded (Moderate recommendation).

References

1. Migaly J, Bafford AC, Francone TD, et al. The American Society of Colon and Rectal Surgeons clinical practice guidelines for the use of bowel preparation in elective colon and Rectal surgery. Dis Colon Rectum. 2019;62(1):3–8. https://doi.org/10.1097/DCR.0000000000001238.
2. Young H, Knepper B, Moore EE, Johnson JL, Mehler P, Price CS. Surgical site infection after colon surgery: National Healthcare Safety Network risk factors and modeled rates compared with published risk factors and rates. J Am Coll Surg. 2012;214(5):852–9. https://doi.org/10.1016/j.jamcollsurg.2012.01.041.
3. Plumley PF. A simple regime for preparation of colon before large-bowel surgery. Br J Surg. 1966;53(5):413–4. https://doi.org/10.1002/bjs.1800530507.
4. Rollins KE, Javanmard-Emamghissi H, Acheson AG, Lobo DN. The role of Oral antibiotic preparation in elective colorectal surgery: a meta-analysis. Ann Surg. 2019;270(1):43–58. https://doi.org/10.1097/SLA.0000000000003145.
5. Rosenberg IL, Graham NG, de Dombal FT, Goligher JC. Preparation of the intestine in patients undergoing major large-bowel surgery, mainly for neoplasms of the colon and rectum. Br J Surg. 2005;58(4):266–9. https://doi.org/10.1002/bjs.1800580408.
6. Nichols RL, Broido P, Condon RE, Gorbach SL, Nyhus LM. Effect of preoperative Neornycin-erythromycin intestinal preparation on the incidence of infectious complications following colon surgery. Ann Surg. 1973;178(4):453–62. https://doi.org/10.1097/00000658-197310000-00008.

7. Garfinkle R, Abou-Khalil J, Morin N, et al. Is there a role for oral antibiotic preparation alone before colorectal surgery? ACS-NSQIP analysis by coarsened exact matching. Dis Colon Rectum. 2017;60(7):729–37. https://doi.org/10.1097/DCR.0000000000000851.
8. Scarborough JE, Mantyh CR, Sun Z, Migaly J. Combined mechanical and oral antibiotic bowel preparation reduces incisional surgical site infection and anastomotic leak rates after elective colorectal resection: an analysis of colectomy-targeted ACS NSQIP. Ann Surg. 2015;262(2):331–7. https://doi.org/10.1097/SLA.0000000000001041.
9. Koller SE, Bauer KW, Egleston BL, et al. Comparative effectiveness and risks of bowel preparation before elective colorectal surgery. Ann Surg. 2018;267(4):734–42. https://doi.org/10.1097/SLA.0000000000002159.
10. Klinger AL, Green H, Monlezun DJ, et al. The role of bowel preparation in colorectal surgery: results of the 2012-2015 ACS-NSQIP data. Ann Surg. 2019;269(4):671–7. https://doi.org/10.1097/SLA.0000000000002568.
11. Miettinen PJR, Laitinen ST, Mäkelä JT, Pääkkönen ME. Bowel preparation with oral polyethylene glycol electrolyte solution vs. no preparation in elective open colorectal surgery. Dis Colon Rectum. 2000;43(5):669–75. https://doi.org/10.1007/BF02235585.
12. Fa-Si-Oen P, Roumen R, Buitenweg J, et al. Mechanical bowel preparation or not? Outcome of a multicenter, randomized trial in elective open colon surgery. Dis Colon Rectum. 2005;48(8):1509–16. https://doi.org/10.1007/s10350-005-0068-y.
13. Bucher P, Gervaz P, Soravia C, Mermillod B, Erne M, Morel P. Randomized clinical trial of mechanical bowel preparation *versus* no preparation before elective left-sided colorectal surgery. Br J Surg. 2005;92(4):409–14. https://doi.org/10.1002/bjs.4900.
14. Burke P, Mealy K, Gillen P, Joyce W, Traynor O, Hyland J. Requirement for bowel preparation in colorectal surgery. Br J Surg. 2005;81(6):907–10. https://doi.org/10.1002/bjs.1800810639.
15. Santos JCM, Batista J, Sirimarco MT, Guimarães AS, Levy CE. Prospective randomized trial of mechanical bowel preparation in patients undergoing elective colorectal surgery. Br J Surg. 2005;81(11):1673–6. https://doi.org/10.1002/bjs.1800811139.
16. Zmora O, Mahajna A, Bar-Zakai B, et al. Is mechanical bowel preparation mandatory for left-sided colonic anastomosis? Results of a prospective randomized trial. Tech Coloproctol. 2006;10(2):131–5. https://doi.org/10.1007/s10151-006-0266-1.
17. Jung B, Påhlman L, Nyström PO, Nilsson E. Multicentre randomized clinical trial of mechanical bowel preparation in elective colonic resection. Br J Surg. 2007;94(6):689–95. https://doi.org/10.1002/bjs.5816.
18. Contant CM, Hop WC, van't Sant HP, et al. Mechanical bowel preparation for elective colorectal surgery: a multicentre randomised trial. Lancet. 2007;370(9605):2112–7. https://doi.org/10.1016/S0140-6736(07)61905-9.
19. Pena-Soria MJ, Mayol JM, Anula R, Arbeo-Escolar A, Fernandez-Represa JA. Single-blinded randomized trial of mechanical bowel preparation for colon surgery with primary intraperitoneal anastomosis. J Gastrointest Surg. 2008;12(12):2103–9. https://doi.org/10.1007/s11605-008-0706-5.
20. van't Sant HP, Weidema WF, Hop WCJ, Lange JF, Contant CME. Evaluation of morbidity and mortality after anastomotic leakage following elective colorectal surgery in patients treated with or without mechanical bowel preparation. Am J Surg. 2011;202(3):321–4. https://doi.org/10.1016/j.amjsurg.2010.10.018.
21. van't Sant HP, Slieker JC, Hop WCJ, et al. The influence of mechanical bowel preparation in elective colorectal surgery for diverticulitis. Tech Coloproctol. 2012;16(4):309–14. https://doi.org/10.1007/s10151-012-0852-3.
22. Mai-Phan AT, Nguyen H, Nguyen TT, Nguyen DA, Thai TT. Randomized controlled trial of mechanical bowel preparation for laparoscopy-assisted colectomy. Asian J Endosc Surg. 2019;12(4):408–11. https://doi.org/10.1111/ases.12671.
23. Platell C, Barwood N, Makin G. Randomized clinical trial of bowel preparation with a single phosphate enema or polyethylene glycol before elective colorectal surgery. Br J Surg. 2006;93(4):427–33. https://doi.org/10.1002/bjs.5274.

24. Güenaga KF, Matos D, Wille-Jørgensen P Mechanical bowel preparation for elective colorectal surgery Cochrane Database Syst Rev Published online September 7, 2011. https://doi.org/10.1002/14651858.CD001544.pub4.
25. Rollins KE, Javanmard-Emamghissi H, Lobo DN. Impact of mechanical bowel preparation in elective colorectal surgery: a meta-analysis. World J Gastroenterol. 2018;24(4):519–36. https://doi.org/10.3748/wjg.v24.i4.519.
26. Woodfield JC, Clifford K, Schmidt B, Thompson-Fawcett M. Has network meta-analysis resolved the controversies related to bowel preparation in elective colorectal surgery? Colorectal Disease Published online 2022. https://doi.org/10.1111/codi.16194.
27. Kiran RP, Murray ACA, Chiuzan C, Estrada D, Forde K. Combined preoperative mechanical bowel preparation with oral antibiotics significantly reduces surgical site infection, anastomotic leak, and ileus after colorectal surgery. Ann Surg. 2015;262. Lippincott Williams and Wilkins:416–23. https://doi.org/10.1097/SLA.0000000000001416.
28. Moghadamyeghaneh Z, Hanna MH, Carmichael JC, et al. Nationwide analysis of outcomes of bowel preparation in colon surgery. J Am Coll Surg. 2015;220(5):912–20. https://doi.org/10.1016/j.jamcollsurg.2015.02.008.
29. Lieberman DA, Ghormley J, Flora K. Effect of oral sodium phosphate colon preparation on serum electrolytes in patients with normal serum creatinine. Gastrointest Endosc. 1996;43(5):467–9. https://doi.org/10.1016/S0016-5107(96)70287-0.
30. Shapira Z, Feldman L, Lavy R, Weissgarten J, Haitov Z, Halevy A. Bowel preparation: comparing metabolic and electrolyte changes when using sodium phosphate/polyethylene glycol. Int J Surg. 2010;8(5):356–8. https://doi.org/10.1016/j.ijsu.2010.04.009.
31. Barish CF, Walker K. Dehydration with bowel purgatives. Am J Gastroenterol. 2006;101:S547–8. https://doi.org/10.14309/00000434-200609001-01437.
32. Yamada T, Kan H, Matsumoto S, et al. Dysmotility by mechanical bowel preparation using polyethylene glycol. J Surg Res. 2014;191(1):84–90. https://doi.org/10.1016/j.jss.2014.03.001.
33. Washington JA, Dearing WH, Judo ES, Elveback LR. Effect of preoperative antibiotic regimen on development of infection after intestinal surgery. Ann Surg. 1974;180(4):567–72. https://doi.org/10.1097/00000658-197410000-00021.
34. Goldring J, Mcnaught W, Scott A, Gillespie G. Prophylactic oral antimicrobial agents in elective colonic surgery. Lancet. 1975;306(7943):997–1000. https://doi.org/10.1016/S0140-6736(75)90289-5.
35. Clarke JS, Condon RE, Bartlett JG, et al. Preoperative oral antibiotics reduce septic complications of colon operations. Ann Surg. 1977;186(3):251–9. https://doi.org/10.1097/00000658-197709000-00003.
36. Matheson DM, Arabi Y, Baxter-Smith D, Alexander-Williams J, Keighley MRB. Randomized multicentre trial of oral bowel preparation and antimicrobials for elective colorectal operations. Br J Surg. 2005;65(9):597–600. https://doi.org/10.1002/bjs.1800650902.
37. Playforth MJ, Smith GMR, Evans M, Pollock AV. Antimicrobial bowel preparation. Dis Colon Rectum. 1988;31(2):90–3. https://doi.org/10.1007/BF02562635.
38. Lewis RT. Oral versus systemic antibiotic prophylaxis in elective colon surgery: a randomized study and meta-analysis send a message from the 1990s. Can J Surg. 2002;45(3):173–80.
39. Bellows CF, Mills KT, Kelly TN, Gagliardi G. Combination of oral non-absorbable and intravenous antibiotics versus intravenous antibiotics alone in the prevention of surgical site infections after colorectal surgery: a meta-analysis of randomized controlled trials. Tech Coloproctol. 2011;15(4):385–95. https://doi.org/10.1007/s10151-011-0714-4.
40. Toh JWT, Phan K, Hitos K, et al. Association of mechanical bowel preparation and oral antibiotics before elective colorectal surgery with surgical site infection: a network meta-analysis. JAMA Netw Open. 2018;1(6):e183226. https://doi.org/10.1001/jamanetworkopen.2018.3226.
41. McSorley ST, Steele CW, McMahon AJ. Meta-analysis of oral antibiotics, in combination with preoperative intravenous antibiotics and mechanical bowel preparation the day before surgery, compared with intravenous antibiotics and mechanical bowel preparation alone to reduce surgical-site infections in elective colorectal surgery. BJS Open. 2018;2(4):185–94. https://doi.org/10.1002/bjs5.68.

42. Anjum N, Ren J, Wang G, et al. A randomized control trial of preoperative Oral antibiotics as adjunct therapy to systemic antibiotics for preventing surgical site infection in clean contaminated, contaminated, and dirty type of colorectal surgeries. Dis Colon Rectum. 2017;60(12):1291–8. https://doi.org/10.1097/DCR.0000000000000927.
43. Hata H, Yamaguchi T, Hasegawa S, et al. Oral and parenteral versus parenteral antibiotic prophylaxis in elective laparoscopic colorectal surgery (JMTO PREV 07–01). Ann Surg. 2016;263(6):1085–91. https://doi.org/10.1097/SLA.0000000000001581.
44. Rybakov E, Nagudov M, Sukhina M, Shelygin Y. Impact of oral antibiotic prophylaxis on surgical site infection after rectal surgery: results of randomized trial. Int J Color Dis. 2021;36(2):323–30. https://doi.org/10.1007/s00384-020-03746-0.
45. Papp G, Saftics G, Szabó BE, et al. Systemic *versus* oral and systemic antibiotic prophylaxis (SOAP) study in colorectal surgery: prospective randomized multicentre trial. Br J Surg. 2021;108(3):271–6. https://doi.org/10.1093/bjs/znaa131.
46. Ghuman A, Kasteel N, Brown CJ, et al. Surgical site infection in elective colonic and rectal resections: effect of oral antibiotics and mechanical bowel preparation compared with mechanical bowel preparation only. Color Dis. 2020;22(11):1686–93. https://doi.org/10.1111/codi.15153.
47. Ambe PC, Zarras K, Stodolski M, Wirjawan I, Zirngibl H. Routine preoperative mechanical bowel preparation with additive oral antibiotics is associated with a reduced risk of anastomotic leakage in patients undergoing elective oncologic resection for colorectal cancer. World J Surg Oncol. 2019;17(1):20. https://doi.org/10.1186/s12957-019-1563-2.
48. Oshima T, Takesue Y, Ikeuchi H, et al. Preoperative oral antibiotics and intravenous antimicrobial prophylaxis reduce the incidence of surgical site infections in patients with ulcerative colitis undergoing IPAA. Dis Colon Rectum. 2013;56(10):1149–55. https://doi.org/10.1097/DCR.0b013e31829f71a0.
49. Uchino M, Ikeuchi H, Bando T, et al. Efficacy of preoperative Oral antibiotic prophylaxis for the prevention of surgical site infections in patients with Crohn disease: a randomized controlled trial. Ann Surg. 2019;269(3):420–6. https://doi.org/10.1097/SLA.0000000000002567.
50. Cannon JA, Altom LK, Deierhoi RJ, et al. Preoperative oral antibiotics reduce surgical site infection following elective colorectal resections. Dis Colon Rectum. 2012;55(11):1160–6. https://doi.org/10.1097/DCR.0b013e3182684fac.
51. Kim EK, Sheetz KH, Bonn J, et al. A statewide colectomy experience: the role of full bowel preparation in preventing surgical site infection. Ann Surg. 2014;259(2):310–4. https://doi.org/10.1097/SLA.0b013e3182a62643.
52. Althumairi AA, Canner JK, Pawlik TM, et al. Benefits of bowel preparation beyond surgical site infection: a retrospective study. Ann Surg. 2016;264(6):1051–7. https://doi.org/10.1097/SLA.0000000000001576.
53. Midura EF, Jung AD, Hanseman DJ, et al. Combination oral and mechanical bowel preparations decreases complications in both right and left colectomy. Surgery (United States). 2018;163(3):528–34. https://doi.org/10.1016/j.surg.2017.10.023.
54. Yeom CH, Cho MM, Baek SK, Bae OS. Risk factors for the development of Clostridium difficile-associated colitis after colorectal cancer surgery. J Korean Soc Coloproctol. 2010;26(5):329–33. https://doi.org/10.3393/jksc.2010.26.5.329.
55. Parthasarathy M, Bowers D, Groot-Wassink T. Do preoperative oral antibiotics increase Clostridium difficile infection rates? An analysis of 13 959 colectomy patients. Color Dis. 2018;20(6):520–8. https://doi.org/10.1111/codi.13926.
56. Sadahiro S, Suzuki T, Tanaka A, et al. Comparison between oral antibiotics and probiotics as bowel preparation for elective colon cancer surgery to prevent infection: prospective randomized trial. Surgery. 2014;155(3):493–503. https://doi.org/10.1016/j.surg.2013.06.002.
57. Mik M, Berut M, Trzcinski R, Dziki L, Buczynski J, Dziki A. Preoperative oral antibiotics reduce infections after colorectal cancer surgery. Langenbeck's Arch Surg. 2016;401(8):1153–62. https://doi.org/10.1007/s00423-016-1513-1.

58. Mulder T, Kluytmans JAJW. Oral antibiotics prior to colorectal surgery: do they have to be combined with mechanical bowel preparation? Infect Control Hosp Epidemiol. 2019;40(8):922–7. https://doi.org/10.1017/ice.2019.157.
59. Koskenvuo L, Lehtonen T, Koskensalo S, et al. Mechanical and oral antibiotic bowel preparation versus no bowel preparation for elective colectomy (Mobile): a multicentre, randomised, parallel, single-blinded trial. Lancet. 2019;394(10201):840–8. https://doi.org/10.1016/S0140-6736(19)31269-3.
60. Koskenvuo L, Lehtonen T, Koskensalo S, et al. Mechanical and oral antibiotic bowel preparation versus no bowel preparation in right and left colectomy: subgroup analysis of Mobile trial. BJS Open. 2021;5(2) https://doi.org/10.1093/bjsopen/zrab011.
61. Kaslow SR, Gani F, Alshaikh HN, Canner JK. Clinical outcomes following mechanical plus oral antibiotic bowel preparation versus oral antibiotics alone in patients undergoing colorectal surgery. BJS Open. 2018;2(4):238–45. https://doi.org/10.1002/bjs5.66.
62. Zmora O, Mahajna A, Bar-Zakai B, et al. Colon and rectal surgery without mechanical bowel preparation a randomized prospective trial. Ann Surg. 2003;237(3):363–7.
63. Suzuki T, Sadahiro S, Tanaka A, et al. Usefulness of preoperative mechanical bowel preparation in patients with colon cancer who undergo elective surgery: a prospective randomized trial using Oral antibiotics. Dig Surg. 2020;37(3):192–8. https://doi.org/10.1159/000500020.
64. Nelson RL, Hassan M, Grant MD. Antibiotic prophylaxis in colorectal surgery: are oral, intravenous or both best and is mechanical bowel preparation necessary? Tech Coloproctol. 2020;24(12):1233–46. https://doi.org/10.1007/s10151-020-02301-x.
65. Atkinson SJ, Swenson BR, Hanseman DJ, et al. In the absence of a mechanical bowel prep, does the addition of pre-operative Oral antibiotics to parental antibiotics decrease the incidence of surgical site infection after elective segmental colectomy? Surg Infect. 2015;16(6):728–32. https://doi.org/10.1089/sur.2014.215.
66. Mulder T, Crolla RMPH, Kluytmans-Van Den Bergh MFQ, et al. Preoperative oral antibiotic prophylaxis reduces surgical site infections after elective colorectal surgery: results from a before-after study. Clin Infect Dis. 2019;69(1):93–9. https://doi.org/10.1093/cid/ciy839.
67. Espin Basany E, Solís-Peña A, Pellino G, et al. Preoperative oral antibiotics and surgical-site infections in colon surgery (ORALEV): a multicentre, single-blind, pragmatic, randomised controlled trial. Lancet Gastroenterol Hepatol. 2020;5(8):729–38. https://doi.org/10.1016/S2468-1253(20)30075-3.
68. Meyer J, Davies J, Buchs NC, Ris F. Preoperative oral antibiotics in colon surgery. Lancet Gastroenterol Hepatol. 2020;5(9):801. https://doi.org/10.1016/S2468-1253(20)30214-4.
69. Lambregts MMC, de Boer MGJ. Preoperative oral antibiotics in colon surgery. Lancet Gastroenterol Hepatol. 2020;5(9):800–1. https://doi.org/10.1016/S2468-1253(20)30244-2.
70. Rollins KE. Bowel preparation in elective colorectal surgery: is mechanical bowel preparation necessary? Lancet Gastroenterol Hepatol. 2020;5(8):712–3. https://doi.org/10.1016/S2468-1253(20)30193-X.
71. Vignaud M, Paugam-Burtz C, Garot M, et al. Comparison of intravenous versus combined oral and intravenous antimicrobial prophylaxis (Combine) for the prevention of surgical site infection in elective colorectal surgery: study protocol for a multicentre, double-blind, randomised controlled clinical trial. BMJ Open. 2018;8(4):e020254. https://doi.org/10.1136/bmjopen-2017-020254.
72. Apte SS, Moloo H, Jeong A, et al. Prospective randomised controlled trial using the REthinking Clinical Trials (REaCT) platform and National Surgical Quality Improvement Program (NSQIP) to compare no preparation versus preoperative oral antibiotics alone for surgical site infection rates in elective colon surgery: a protocol. BMJ Open. 2020;10(7):e036866. https://doi.org/10.1136/bmjopen-2020-036866.
73. Gustafsson UO, Scott MJ, Schwenk W, et al. Guidelines for perioperative care in elective colonic surgery: enhanced recovery after surgery (ERAS®) society recommendations. World J Surg. 2013;37(2):259–84. https://doi.org/10.1007/s00268-012-1772-0.
74. Carmichael JC, Keller DS, Baldini G, et al. Clinical practice guidelines for enhanced recovery after colon and Rectal surgery from the American Society of Colon and Rectal Surgeons

and Society of American Gastrointestinal and Endoscopic Surgeons. Dis Colon Rectum. 2017;60(8):761–84. https://doi.org/10.1097/DCR.0000000000000883.
75. World Health Organization. Global Guidelines for the Prevention of Surgical Site Infection.
76. Markell KW, Hunt BM, Charron PD, et al. Prophylaxis and management of wound infections after elective colorectal surgery: a survey of the American Society of Colon and Rectal Surgeons membership. J Gastrointest Surg. 2010;14(7):1090–8. https://doi.org/10.1007/s11605-010-1218-7.
77. McChesney SL, Zelhart MD, Green RL, Nichols RL. Current U.S. pre-operative bowel preparation trends: a 2018 survey of the American Society of Colon and Rectal Surgeons members. Surg Infect. 2020;21(1):1–8. https://doi.org/10.1089/sur.2019.125.
78. Hyoju SK, Keskey R, Castillo G, et al. A novel nonantibiotic gut-directed strategy to prevent surgical site infections. Ann Surg. 2022;276(3):472–81. https://doi.org/10.1097/SLA.0000000000005547.
79. Shogan BD, Chen J, Duchalais E, et al. Alterations of the rectal microbiome are associated with the development of postoperative ileus in patients undergoing colorectal surgery. J Gastrointest Surg. 2020;24(7):1663–72. https://doi.org/10.1007/s11605-020-04593-8.
80. Shogan BD, Belogortseva N, Luong PM, et al. Collagen degradation and MMP9 activation by enterococcus faecalis contribute to intestinal anastomotic leak. Sci Transl Med. 2015;7(286):286ra68. https://doi.org/10.1126/scitranslmed.3010658.
81. Shobar RM, Velineni S, Keshavarzian A, et al. The effects of bowel preparation on microbiota-related metrics differ in health and in inflammatory bowel disease and for the mucosal and luminal microbiota compartments. Clin Transl Gastroenterol. 2016;7:e143. https://doi.org/10.1038/ctg.2015.54.
82. Gaines S, van Praagh JB, Williamson AJ, et al. Western diet promotes intestinal colonization by collagenolytic microbes and promotes tumor formation after colorectal surgery. Gastroenterology. 2020;158(4):958–970.e2. https://doi.org/10.1053/j.gastro.2019.10.020.

Enhanced Recovery vs. Conventional Perioperative Management

47

Alison Althans and Jennifer Holder-Murray

Introduction

Many colorectal operations can result in extended postoperative hospital stays, significant rates of surgical site infection and other morbidity, poorly controlled perioperative nausea and vomiting, and high costs. The development of minimally invasive surgery, advanced anesthetic techniques, and modern antibiotics provided an opportunity to address some of these pitfalls. However, conventional and non-standardized postoperative management still falls short to improve outcomes and quality of care. Therefore, the idea of utilizing a multimodal approach to address various surgical stressors that drive postoperative morbidity (such as insulin resistance, catabolism, and inflammation/cytokine release) and to improve physiologic homeostasis following surgery was pioneered by Henrik Kehlet in the 1990s [1].

In Kehlet's early attempts at optimizing care, the implementation of preoperative patient counseling, epidural analgesia, early oral nutrition, and early mobilization resulted in a median postoperative length of stay of two days for patients undergoing open sigmoidectomy, a procedure with a typical length of stay of five to ten days at that time [2]. These impressive results launched the development of the Enhanced

A. Althans
Department of Surgery, University of Pittsburgh Medical Center, Pittsburgh, PA, USA
e-mail: althansar@upmc.edu

J. Holder-Murray (✉)
Division of Colon and Rectal Surgery, Department of Surgery, University of Pittsburgh Medical Center, Pittsburgh, PA, USA
e-mail: holdermurrayjm@upmc.edu

K. Umanskiy, N. Hyman (eds.), *Difficult Decisions in Colorectal Surgery*, Difficult Decisions in Surgery: An Evidence-Based Approach,
https://doi.org/10.1007/978-3-031-42303-1_47

Recovery After Surgery (ERAS) Study group, and ongoing efforts to standardize and expand these perioperative principles [3]. Ultimately, numerous studies and systematic reviews have shown that ERAS protocols are associated with reduced length of stay, readmission rates, morbidity, and healthcare costs, as well as improved patient satisfaction in colorectal surgery and other surgical subspecialties [4, 5].

Search Strategy

There are numerous components to ERAS protocols, typically divided into preoperative, perioperative, and postoperative phases. The ERAS Study group released consensus guidelines in 2009, identifying twenty key interventions for optimal perioperative care [6]. An abundance of studies have examined the impact of specific ERAS components (i.e., laparoscopic versus open colectomy, early versus standard enteral feeding), but fewer have looked at implementation of entire ERAS pathways. We therefore set out to highlight randomized, prospective studies comparing the implementation of well-described ERAS protocols, as a whole, to a conventional care pathway for patients undergoing colorectal surgery (Table 47.1).

We began with a search of systematic reviews/meta-analyses to identify landmark randomized control trials, from 1990 (when ERAS was first described) to 2022. The following search terms were utilized: "((randomized) AND (fast track OR enhanced recovery OR eras)) AND (colorectal OR colon OR rectum)". A review of the Cochrane Library and PubMed databases identified the two most recent systematic reviews from 2011 and 2013 that included all patients 18 years or older undergoing elective colorectal surgery [4, 7]. Notably, both of these reviews considered ERAS as the intervention group only if the protocol included seven or more of the components delineated by the ERAS study group consensus guidelines. The randomized trials comparing ERAS to conventional care identified by these reviews are discussed below and summarized in Table 47.2.

Table 47.1 PICO table

Patients	Intervention	Comparator	Outcomes
Patients undergoing colorectal surgery	Enhanced recovery after surgery protocols	Conventional postoperative management	Length of stay, readmission rates, morbidity

Table 47.2 Randomized control trials comparing ERAS to conventional perioperative care

Study	Patients (N) ERAS vs. conventional	Primary hospital length of stay (mean difference ERAS minus conventional)	Readmission (risk ratio ERAS/ conventional)	Total complications (risk ratio ERAS/ conventional)	Major/surgical complications (risk ratio ERAS/ conventional)
Anderson 2003 [27]	14 vs. 11	−3.00 [−4.56, −1.44]	–	0.56 [0.24, 1.29]	1.57 [0.16, 15.16]
Gatt 2005 [28]	19 vs. 20	−2.00 [−2.71, −1.29]	0.26 [0.03, 2.15]	0.63 [0.37, 1.08]	0.45 [0.14, 1.49]
Khoo 2007 [29]	35 vs. 35	−2.00 [−7.64, 3.64]	3.00 [0.33, 27.46]	0.56 [0.29, 1.10]	0.33 [0.04, 3.05]
Muller 2009 [30]	76 vs. 75	−4.00 [5.39, −2.61]	1.48 [0.25, 8.61]	0.43 [0.26, 0.70]	0.56 [0.26, 1.18]
Ionescu 2009 [31]	48 vs. 48	−2.73 [3.96, −1.50]	–	0.55 [0.22, 1.36]	0.71 [0.24, 2.09]
Serclova 2009 [32]	51 vs. 52	−3.00 [−3.92, −2.08]	–	0.45 [0.25, 0.81]	
Van Bree 2011 [33]	36 vs. 35	–	0.47 [0.05, 5.04] (laparoscopic) 0.50 [0.05, 5.04] (open)	0.26 [0.09, 0.77] (laparoscopic) 1.25 [0.65, 2.42] (open)	0.24 [0.03, 1.91] (laparoscopic) 0.60 [0.17, 2.14] (open)
Garcia-Botello 2011 [34]	61 vs. 58	−5.08 [−6.96, −3.20]	1.43 [0.25, 8.23]	0.81 [0.71, 0.91]	0.82 [0.55, 1.22]
Vlug 2011 [35]	193 vs. 207	−1.00 [1.76, −0.24] (laparoscopic) −1.00 [1.76, −0.24] (open)	0.93 [0.32, 2.69] (laparoscopic) 1.05 [0.38, 2.89] (open)	0.98 [0.77, 1.26] (laparoscopic) 1.04 [0.88, 1.22] (open)	1.09 [0.71, 1.67] (laparoscopic) 1.22 [0.88, 1.71] (open)
Ren 2012 [36]	299 vs. 298	−0.90 [−1.23, −0.57]	–	1.03 [0.63, 1.69]	1.17 [0.69, 1.99]
Wang G 2012 [37]	49 vs. 50	-	0.68 [0.12, 3.98]	0.61 [0.24, 1.56]	0.77 [0.18, 3.24]
Wang Q 2012 [38]	40 vs. 38	−1.50 [−1.68, −1.32]	–	0.24 [0.05, 1.05]	0.19 [0.02, 1.55]
Yang 2012 [39]	32 vs. 30	−5.70 [−7.11, −4.29]	–	0.47 [0.20, 1.09]	0.47 [0.04, 4.91]

Results

Ultimately, four studies were included in the 2011 meta-analysis and thirteen in the 2013 meta-analysis. Both studies identified a significant risk reduction in total complications in the ERAS group. The ERAS and conventional care groups were otherwise comparable in primary outcome measures in the 2011 study, which included primary hospital length of stay, readmission rates, total complication rates, and major/surgical complication rates. When using the GRADE methodology to score the quality of evidence to recommend ERAS over conventional care based on each of these primary metrics, each was ranked "low" or "very low" in the earlier analysis. The authors therefore concluded that while ERAS was safe, the evidence quality was too poor to recommend implementing ERAS as the standard of care at that time [4].

These critical comments drove the onset of further randomized control trials and systematic reviews. In contrast to the 2011 study, the 2013 analysis identified a significantly decreased hospital length of stay in the ERAS group; however the groups remained similar in terms of readmission rates and major/surgical complications. Additionally, the quality of evidence for the primary outcomes remained "low" for all primary outcomes other than total hospital stay and readmission rates, which were rated "moderate." This study also looked at time to flatus and stool as secondary outcome measures, and ERAS was superior in both of these metrics (though again, only "moderate" evidence). There were a variety of factors contributing to the overall low quality of evidence for each recommendation, but a major factor inherent to the nature of implementation of a specific perioperative protocol is the inability to blind the surgeon and/or patient.

Review of these randomized trials through meta-analyses suggests that implementation of ERAS protocols is safe, reduces length of stay, and may encourage early return of bowel function (though with limitations with respect to the strength of evidence). While not included as primary outcomes in the aforementioned studies, other important metrics to consider are cost, patient satisfaction and faster recovery of functional outcome. Institutional studies have demonstrated decreased per-patient direct costs on the order of thousands of dollars, when comparing ERAS patients to those receiving conventional care [8]. Rigorous, multi-institutional, cost-effectiveness analysis has also shown ERAS to be associated with shorter hospitalization, decreased resource utilization, and lower societal costs [9]. In addition to being cost-effective when compared to conventional care, the aforementioned studies revealed that patients in ERAS pathways reported higher satisfaction, returned to work sooner, and their caregivers experienced less burden.

Recommendations

Institutional implementation of ERAS protocols for patients undergoing colorectal surgery should be considered in order to decrease hospital length of stay, lower complication rates, minimize healthcare related expenditures, and improve patient satisfaction (Recommendation: strong; Evidence: moderate). There remains significant variation in the components of the ERAS Study group guidelines implemented and in the extent of adherence to described ERAS protocols from institution to institution [10]. However, when buy-in from stakeholders is established and compliance with ERAS protocols is improved, so also are the aforementioned outcomes [11]. By 2021, over 250 hospital units in more than 25 countries have implemented

ERAS protocols via the ERAS Society and ERAS Interactive Audit System, while innumerable more sites have adopted ERAS principles outside of the formal ERAS Society [12].

Personal View

The benefits of ERAS protocols, taken as a whole, have been well demonstrated; both in regards to patient-centered outcomes, as well as healthcare cost and resource minimization. With at least twenty possible elements to include in an ERAS protocol (as delineated by the ERAS Study group consensus guidelines), it can be challenging to determine which of these elements are crucial to improving outcomes and how strong the evidence is behind each element. In 2017, the American Society of Colon and Rectal Surgeons Clinical Practice Guidelines Committee released an updated set of guidelines for ERAS after colorectal surgery [13]. These guidelines described many of the potential components of an ERAS protocol and also graded the evidence for each component. For example, items that were strongly recommended with high-quality evidence include: continuation of clear liquid diet up to two hours before general anesthesia, preemptive multimodal antiemetic prophylaxis to reduce postoperative nausea and vomiting, and utilization of minimally invasive surgical approaches when appropriate. An item that was weakly recommended based upon low-quality evidence and requires further rigorous study was the use of preset admission orders, though this may help in the logistical implementation.

As mentioned above, the many potential elements of these multimodal pathways can also make implementation of and adherence to ERAS pathways daunting. In an attempt to maximize adherence, one institutional study aimed to identify the specific elements in their protocol that were most strongly associated with decreased length of stay [14]. The strongest predictors of decreased length of stay in this study were postoperative components such as no nasogastric tube, early mobilization, early oral nutrition, early removal of epidural catheter, early remove of the urinary catheter, and non-opioid oral analgesia.

It is the author's opinion that while ERAS Society guidelines for colon and rectal surgery describe twenty components of an ERAS protocol, several of the components are nearly universally adopted in Western medicine and can now be considered standard of care. These include components such as antibiotic prophylaxis, venous thromboembolism prophylaxis, the abandonment of nasogastric tubes in the immediate postoperative setting, and the use of minimally invasive surgery when appropriate. Therefore, ERAS pathways in colon and rectal surgery can be simplified in the modern era to seven key components: preoperative counseling, limitation of preoperative fasting, preemptive nausea and vomiting prophylaxis, early postoperative oral nutrition, early postoperative mobilization, opioid sparing multimodal analgesia with the use of neuraxial or peripheral nerve blocks as appropriate, and early urinary catheter removal [15]. Each of these components has important implications for improving recovery but implementation alone often has marginal effects on the broader outcomes of length of stay, complications, and functional recovery.

Also, lack of implementation of other components can be detrimental to isolated implementation of one component (e.g. early urinary catheter removal with primarily opioid analgesia results in higher incidence of urinary retention or early feeding without prophylaxis of nausea and vomiting and high opioid use results in intolerance to enteral nutrition). It has been demonstrated that greater compliance with more components results in greater improvement in outcomes [16]. Therefore, it is imperative that the combination of these core components are implemented and have high adherence for optimal success for an ERAS program as it is the combination of these core components that achieves optimal clinically meaningful outcomes.

In addition to maximizing compliance with these key components, further advances in other elements of broader perioperative care that are not delineated by the ERAS Group guidelines also serve to improve patient care. For example, the practice of prehabilitation has come to the forefront in improving patient-centered outcomes. Prehabilitation programs, built to increase a patient's functional capacity in anticipation of an upcoming surgical stress, have been shown to increase the likelihood that a patient recovers at or above their baseline capacity postoperatively and improve patient-reported quality of life after surgery [17]. Additionally, a 2019 meta-analysis of three prehabilitation trials showed that patients with locally advanced colorectal cancer randomized to prehabilitation before surgery had improved disease free survival when compared to those not undergoing prehabilitation [18]. The impact of prehabilitation programs on patient outcomes and functional status is complementary to that of the more immediate perioperative ERAS components.

Attempts at optimizing other patient medical and lifestyle risk factors are also crucial to mitigating perioperative risk, including correction of malnutrition [19], treatment of anemia [20], smoking cessation [21], and glycemic control [22]. With patients being discharged from the hospital more quickly, it is also important to consider early discharge planning, setting expectations for expected length of stay and additional home care needs following discharge, and provide early ostomy education when applicable in order to minimize readmission rates [23, 24]. Adoption of ERAS and prehabilitation, in addition to achieving these other optimization targets, is an evidence-based strategy to expedite patients' return to baseline health and in turn minimize healthcare costs. Other future directions and areas of interest in ERAS include the implementation of "ultra" fast-track protocols, with select studies reporting outcomes for same-day discharge in patients undergoing minimally invasive colectomy [25, 26].

References

1. Kehlet H. Multimodal approach to control postoperative pathophysiology and rehabilitation. Br J Anaesth. 1997;78(5):606–17.
2. Kehlet H, Mogensen T. Hospital stay of 2 days after open sigmoidectomy with a multimodal rehabilitation programme. Br J Surg. 1999;86(2):227–30.

3. Delaney CP, Fazio VW, Senagore AJ, Robinson B, Halverson AL, Remzi FH. "Fast track" postoperative management protocol for patients with high co-morbidity undergoing complex abdominal and pelvic colorectal surgery. Br J Surg. 2001;88(11):1533–8.
4. Spanjersberg WR, Reurings J, Van Laarhoven CHJM. Fast track surgery versus conventional recovery strategies for colorectal surgery. Cochrane Database Syst Rev. 2011;2:CD007635.
5. Nicholson A, Lowe MC, Parker J, Lewis SR, Alderson P, Smith AF. Systematic review and meta-analysis of enhanced recovery programmes in surgical patients. Br J Surg. 2014;101(3):172–88.
6. Lassen K. Consensus review of optimal perioperative Care in Colorectal Surgery. Arch Surg. 2009;144(10):961.
7. Le Zhuang C, Ye XZ, Zhang XD, Chen BC, Yu Z. Enhanced recovery after surgery programs versus traditional care for colorectal surgery: a metaanalysis of randomized controlled trials. Dis Colon Rectum. 2013;56(5):667–78.
8. Thiele RH, Rea KM, Turrentine FE, et al. Standardization of care: impact of an enhanced recovery protocol on length of stay, complications, and direct costs after colorectal surgery. J Am Coll Surg. 2015;220(4):430–43.
9. Lee L, Mata J, Ghitulescu GA, et al. Cost-effectiveness of enhanced recovery versus conventional perioperative management for colorectal surgery. Ann Surg. 2015;262(6):1026–33.
10. Ahmed J, Khan S, Lim M, Chandrasekaran TV, Macfie J. Enhanced recovery after surgery protocols - compliance and variations in practice during routine colorectal surgery. Color Dis. 2012;14(9):1045–51.
11. Ripollés-Melchor J, Ramírez-Rodríguez JM, Casans-Francés R, et al. Association between use of enhanced recovery after surgery protocol and postoperative complications in colorectal surgery: the postoperative outcomes within enhanced recovery after surgery protocol (power) study. JAMA Surg. 2019;154(8):725–36.
12. Ljungqvist O, De Boer HD, Balfour A, et al. Opportunities and challenges for the next phase of enhanced recovery after surgery: a review. JAMA Surg. 2021;156(8):775–84.
13. Carmichael JC, Keller DS, Baldini G, et al. Clinical practice guidelines for enhanced recovery after colon and rectal surgery from the American Society of Colon and Rectal Surgeons and Society of American Gastrointestinal and Endoscopic Surgeons. Dis Colon Rectum. 2017;60(8):761–84.
14. Bakker N, Cakir H, Doodeman HJ, Houdijk APJ. Eight years of experience with enhanced recovery after surgery in patients with colon cancer: impact of measures to improve adherence. Surg (United States). 2015;157(6):1130–6.
15. Esper SA, Holder-Murray J, Subramaniam K, et al. Enhanced recovery protocols reduce mortality across eight surgical specialties at academic and university-affiliated community hospitals. Ann Surg. 2020;277:101–8.
16. Feng J, Li K, Xu R, et al. Association between compliance with enhanced recovery after surgery (ERAS) protocols and postoperative outcome in patients with primary liver cancer undergoing hepatic resection. J Cancer Res Clin Oncol. 2022;148(11):3047–59.
17. Le Roy B, Selvy M, Slim K. The concept of prehabilitation: what the surgeon needs to know? J Visc Surg. 2016;153(2):109–12. https://doi.org/10.1016/j.jviscsurg.2016.01.001.
18. Trépanier M, Minnella EM, Paradis T, et al. Improved disease-free survival after Prehabilitation for colorectal cancer surgery. Ann Surg. 2019;270(3):493–501.
19. Smith M, Mccall J, Plank L, Herbison G, Soop M, Nygren J. Preoperative carbohydrate treatment for enhancing recovery after elective surgery (review). Cochrane. 2014;8:CD009161.
20. Munting KE, Klein AA. Optimisation of pre-operative anaemia in patients before elective major surgery – why who, when, and how? Anaesthesia. 2019;74:49–57.
21. Thomsen T, Tønnesen H, Møller AM. Effect of preoperative smoking cessation interventions on postoperative complications and smoking cessation. Br J Surg. 2009;96:451–61.
22. Chen E, Nooromid M, Helenowski I, Soper N, Halverson AL. The relationship of preoperative versus postoperative hyperglycemia on clinical outcomes following elective colorectal surgery. Surgery. 2019;166(4):655–62.

23. Jones D, Musselman R, Pearsall E, Mckenzie M, Huang H. Ready to go home? Patients' experiences of the discharge process in an enhanced recovery after surgery (ERAS) program for colorectal surgery. J Gastrointest Surg. 2017;21:1865–78.
24. Chaudhri S, Brown L, Hassan I, Horgan A. Preoperative intensive, community-based vs. tradition stoma education: a randomized, controlled trial. Dis Colon Rectum. 2005;48:504–9.
25. Gignoux B, Gosgnach ÃM, Lanz T, Vulliez A, Blanchet M, Frering ÃV. Short-term outcomes of ambulatory colectomy for 157 consecutive patients. Ann Surg. 2019;270(2):317–21.
26. Curfman KR, Poola AS, Blair GE, et al. The American journal of surgery ambulatory colectomy: a pilot protocol for same day discharge in minimally invasive colorectal surgery. Am J Surg. 2022;224(2):757–60. https://doi.org/10.1016/j.amjsurg.2022.04.039.
27. Anderson ADG, McNaught CE, MacFie J, Tring I, Barker P, Mitchell CJ. Randomized clinical trial of multimodal optimization and standard perioperative surgical care. Br J Surg. 2003;90(12):1497–504.
28. Gatt M, Anderson ADG, Reddy BS, Hayward-Sampson P, Tring IC, MacFie J. Randomized clinical trial of multimodal optimization of surgical care in patients undergoing major colonic resection. Br J Surg. 2005;92(11):1354–62.
29. Khoo CK, Vickery CJ, Forsyth N, Vinall NS, Eyre-brook IA. A prospective randomized controlled trial of multimodal perioperative management protocol in patients undergoing elective colorectal resection for cancer. Ann Surg. 2007;245(6):867–72.
30. Muller S, Zalunardo MP, Hubner M, Clavien PA, Demartines N. A fast-track program reduces complications and length of hospital stay after open colonic surgery. Gastroenterology. 2009;136(3):842–7.
31. Ionescu D, Iancu C, Ion D, et al. Implementing fast-track protocol for colorectal surgery: a prospective randomized clinical trial. World J Surg. 2009;33(11):2433–8.
32. Šerclová Z, Dytrych P, Marvan J, et al. Fast-track in open intestinal surgery: prospective randomized study (clinical trials Gov identifier no. NCT00123456). Clin Nutr. 2009;28(6):618–24.
33. Van Bree S, Vlug M, Bemelman W, et al. Faster recovery of gastrointestinal transit after laparoscopy and fast-track care in patients undergoing colonic surgery. Gastroenterology. 2011;141(3):872–80.
34. García-Botello S, de Lucas RC, Tornero C, et al. Implementation of a perioperative multimodal rehabilitation protocol in elective colorectal surgery. A prospective randomised controlled study. Cirugía Española (English Ed). 2011;89(3):159–66. https://doi.org/10.1016/s2173-5077(11)70021-7.
35. Vlug MS, Wind J, Hollmann MW, et al. Laparoscopy in combination with fast track multimodal management is the best perioperative strategy in patients undergoing colonic surgery: a randomized clinical trial (LAFA-study). Ann Surg. 2011;254(6):868–75.
36. Ren L, Zhu D, Wei Y, et al. Enhanced recovery after surgery (ERAS) program attenuates stress and accelerates recovery in patients after radical resection for colorectal cancer: a prospective randomized controlled trial. World J Surg. 2012;36(2):407–14.
37. Wang G, Jiang ZW, Xu J, et al. Fast track rehabilitation programme enhances functional recovery after laparoscopic colonic resection. Hepato-Gastroenterology. 2012;59(119):2158–63.
38. Wang Q, Suo J, Jiang J, Wang C, Zhao YQ, Cao X. Effectiveness of fast-track rehabilitation vs conventional care in laparoscopic colorectal resection for elderly patients: a randomized trial. Color Dis. 2012;14(8):1009–13.
39. Yang D, He W, Zhang S, Chen H, Zhang C, He Y. Fast-track surgery improves postoperative clinical recovery and immunity after elective surgery for colorectal carcinoma: randomized controlled clinical trial. World J Surg. 2012;36(8):1874–80.

Quality Improvement: Is There a Benefit in Opioid-Sparing Strategies for Management of Postoperative Pain?

48

Allen T. Yu, Alex L. Huang, and Sergey Khaitov

Introduction

Post-operative pain is the most common complaint in surgical patients [1]. Poorly controlled post-operative pain is implicated in many adverse events such as cardiopulmonary complications, opioid overdose, hospital readmissions, prolonged hospital length of stay, and development of chronic pain or opioid addiction [2]. Opioid analgesics have been readily employed since the 1990s, but their rampant use have fueled the recent opioid crisis [3]. Death rates due to opioid overdose have quadrupled since 1999, half of which involve prescription opioids [4]. Of these, a third have been prescribed in the context of a surgical procedure, where many patients received their initial exposure to narcotics [5]. Considering this current state of medicine, it is imperative to pursue opioid-sparing strategies for postoperative analgesia.

For the last two decades, perioperative care protocols pertaining to fast-track recoveries have been explored. Since Engelman et al. described a protocol in 1994 where they saw shorter intensive care unit length of stay, reduction in hospital length of stay (LOS), with comparable rates of morbidity and mortality, multiple studies have established evidence-based perioperative protocols to reduce physiological response to surgical insult [6]. These have culminated as the Enhanced Recovery After Surgery (ERAS) study group [7]. The core elements of the protocol have been expanding since 2001, and the control of post-operative pain has been a main tenant

A. T. Yu (✉) · A. L. Huang · S. Khaitov
Mount Sinai Hospital, New York, NY, USA
e-mail: Allen.Yu@mountsinai.org; alex.huang@mountsinai.org; Sergey.khaitov@mountsinai.org

K. Umanskiy, N. Hyman (eds.), *Difficult Decisions in Colorectal Surgery*, Difficult Decisions in Surgery: An Evidence-Based Approach,
https://doi.org/10.1007/978-3-031-42303-1_48

of the ERAS protocol. Due to the side-effects of opioid analgesics and its negative impact on LOS, the focus has largely shifted towards multimodal analgesia (MMA) and opioid sparing pain management. While there are additional methods to manage pain control such as local anesthetics, regional blocks, or epidural analgesia (EDA) that are invasive, non-opioid analgesics are more pervasive, universal, and generally can be prescribed to the patient upon discharge. In this chapter, we review the literature regarding opioid-sparing management of post-operative pain in colorectal surgery.

Search Strategy

A systematic search of the literature was conducted using MEDLINE, PubMed, Web of Science, and the Cochrane Collaborative to identify articles related to the topic of interest. The initial search included Medical Subject Headings terms, as well as entry terms for relevant interventions and outcomes. Key words included ["colectomy" OR "colon surgery" OR "colorectal surgery"] AND ["pain control" OR "pain"] AND/OR ["perioperative" OR "post-operative" OR "post-surgical" OR "rehabilitation"] AND/OR ["opioid-sparing" OR "multimodal"]. The search was conducted for all dates up to December 2022 and restricted to English language titles. No age limits were applied. Titles and abstracts were screened for inclusion based on relevance. In addition, reference lists of retrieved articles were screened for additional relevant studies. Randomized controlled trials, case control trials, retrospective cohorts, systematic reviews, meta-analyses, reviews, and case reports were considered.

Non-opioid Modes of Analgesia

Gabapentinoids

These include gabapentin and pregabalin, which are GABA analogues and activate presynaptic voltage-gated calcium channel receptors [8]. There is no consensus regarding the choice between the two gabapentinoids; however, meta-analyses and systematic reviews have shown gabapentin to be effective in lowering pain scores [9, 10]. Sedation and respiratory depression are two side effects that are seen with administration of gabapentinoids [11]. Recent data have also shown an association between outpatient opioid related deaths and simultaneous treatment with gabapentin. In light of this, caution must be exercised with the continuation of gabapentin past the perioperative period [12].

Non-steroidal Anti-Inflammatory Drugs

Both non-steroidal anti-inflammatory drugs (NSAIDs) and selective cyclooxygenase-2 (COX-2) inhibitors are effective at improving postoperative pain, and numerous systematic reviews and meta-analyses support their use [13, 14]. However, non-selective NSAIDs have been associated with complications such as anastomotic leaks due to their inhibition of prostaglandin synthesis [15]. Because of this, NSAID use in the perioperative period has largely been controversial and surgeon dependent. A recent large, retrospective, propensity score matched study that included 10,584 patients (1,926 after matching), compared three groups: no NSAIDs, non-selective NSAIDs, and selective COX-2 inhibitors [16]. They found the anastomotic leak rate requiring re-operation to be 1.6%, 3.9%, and 2.4%, respectively, prior to matching, and 2.0%, 3.6%, and 2.0%, after matching. This difference was statistically significant prior to matching ($p < 0.001$), but lost significance after matching ($p = 0.123$).

Acetaminophen

While the complete mechanism for acetaminophen remains to be elucidated, it is well known to be an effective analgesic with a minimal side effect profile [17]. The main safety concern is its dose-dependent hepatotoxicity, and care must be taken not to exceed the recommended maximum daily dose of 4 grams in adults.

Ketamine

Developed as a general anesthetic, ketamine exhibits analgesic and anti-hyperalgesic properties at subanesthetic doses. It is a non-competitive antagonist of the NMDA receptors and also attenuates opioid-induced hyperalgesia [18]. Adverse effects include delirium and nausea at higher doses, but low dose infusion rates can effectively curb the side effects [19, 20]. Interestingly, the studies regarding perioperative ketamine use and opioid reduction have been controversial [21, 22]. As multiple studies use variable bolus and infusion rates, it is possible that the baseline infusion rate for ketamine has not been well established [23].

Results

We have identified over 650 articles from our search. Many were focused on the use of epidural, abdominal plane blocks, and additional neuraxial anesthesia. Recent meta-analyses, retrospective, and prospective studies were included and summarized in Table 48.1 below.

In the early 2000s, as the ERAS protocol began to take hold in multiple institutions, there was a driving force to encourage ambulation, early oral feeding, and balanced analgesia to decrease hospital length of stay and improve patient satisfaction [24]. Opioids were known to decrease bowel function, and early studies focused on using epidural analgesia instead of patient-controlled analgesia and found decreased pain scores and reduced LOS [25, 26]. One of the earlier randomized control trials (RCT) was conducted by Delaney et al. [27], where they implemented

Table 48.1 PICO Table

Patients	Intervention	Comparator	Outcomes
Patients undergoing colorectal surgery	Non-opioid postoperative pain management	Opioid-based postoperative pain management	Pain scores, length of stay, quality of life, postoperative complications, and narcotic use

a controlled rehabilitation with early ambulation and diet (CREAD) protocol. This included the use of scheduled ketorolac every six hours without an epidural, and they found CREAD decreased LOS ($p = 0.022$). Raue et al. [28] and Sim et al. [29] both performed RCTs investigating the efficacy of post-operative valdecoxib, and found significantly faster return of flatus, stool, oral tolerance and decreased length of stay. In addition, Sim et al. found an overall decreased morphine equivalent dose (MED) in the setting of no epidural use, contrary to Raue et al.

As ERAS became more refined and multi-metric, more recent studies have focused on the opioid-sparing aspect of the protocol. Brandal et al. analyzed 383 patients pre-and post ERAS. Their MMA regimen included ketamine for 1 hour in the PACU, regional anesthesia, and scheduled celecoxib and acetaminophen [30]. While 57% of their population was on EDA, they saw a 21% drop in PCA usage ($p < 0.001$, 95% CI 15%–27%). There was a 13 MED decrease ($p < 0.009$, 95% CI 2.4–22.0). Their primary outcome was opioid prescription rate at discharge, which did not decrease significantly. Chapman et al. performed a meta-analysis that included six RCTs involving a total of 563 patients, comparing postoperative pain management using opioid versus NSAIDs [31]. Patient receiving NSAIDs had a faster return of flatus ($p < 0.001$, −17.73 h, 95% CI, −21.26 to −14.19 h), stool ($p < 0.001$, −9.52 h, 95% CI, −14.74 to −4.79 h), and oral tolerance ($p < 0.001$, −12.00 h, 95% CI, −18.01 to −5.99 h). MED was reduced in four studies (average reduction, 12.9–30.0 mg). The incidence of anastomotic leak was similar between groups in most studies and the authors concluded that NSAIDs represent an effective and accessible alternative to opioid analgesia.

The Zaghiyan group from Cedars-Sinai Medical Center performed both a retrospective [32] and prospective [33] study comparing opioid use with MMA, which consists of acetaminophen, gabapentin, and celecoxib. Their retrospective arm contained 161 patients as control and 142 classified as MMA, which was broken into opioid naïve and opioid tolerant groups based on the patient's medication history. In the MMA cohort, they found that there was decreased MED usage and a decrease in pain scores, significant only in opioid naïve patients. Prospectively, they enrolled 30 patients total using the same MMA regimen, and saw decreased MED in the first 48 h (42 mg vs 7.6 mg) and decreased pain score on in the PACU (3.9 vs 2.1). Overall, they did not report a difference in complications, LOS, or incidence of ileus.

Iqbal et al. is similar retrospective study that used the combination of acetaminophen, NSAID, and a gabapentinoid in their ERAS protocol, but also employed the use of an EDA in 96% of the study patients [34]. This well powered study compared 537 opioid vs. 790 MMA patients, and found a drastic decrease in 30 day postoperative narcotic use (2,481 mg vs 31 mg, $p < 0.05$), PCA use (63% vs 0.5%, $p < 0.001$), and reported non-significant pain scores.

Lastly, Yeo et al. performed a non-inferiority RCT comparing PCA or MMA cohort, which consisted of pregabalin, tramadol, and a transversus abdominis plane block (TAP) [35]. The authors concluded that their MMA regimen was non-inferior to a PCA at 24 h and observed decreased times in the PACU. However, the study has a low sample size, includes a TAP block which many previous studies did not employ, and also excluded patients with an ASA class of III and IV.

Study	Patients (opioid vs non-opioid)	Regimen vs. opioids	Results	Quality
Delaney et al. 2003 [27] RCT	33 vs. 31	Ketorolac	Decreased LOS, no no change in pain score, QOL, or readmissions	Moderate quality
Raue et al. 2004 [28] RCT	29 vs 23 EDA	Valdecoxib	Faster return of stool, oral tolerance, decreased LOS	Low quality
Sim et al. 2005 [29] RCT	39 vs. 40	Valdecoxib	Decreased MED, faster return of flatus, stool, oral tolerance, and decreased LOS	Moderate quality
Brandal et al. 2017 [30] Retrospective	194 vs. 189 57% EDA	Celecoxib Ketamine Acetaminophen Regional anesthesia	Decrease in MED usage, PCA usage, no decrease in discharge opioid prescriptions, or pain scores	Moderate quality
Chapman et al. 2019 [31] Meta-analysis	198 vs. 277	Celecoxib/ diclofenac Ketorolac/ morphine Flurbiprofen Valdecoxib	Faster return of flatus, stool, oral tolerance, decreased MED in 4/6 studies.	High quality
Truong et al. 2019 [32] Retrospective	161 vs. 142	Celecoxib Gabapentin Acetaminophen	Decreased MED usage, and decrease in pain scores, significant only in opioid naïve patients	Moderate quality
Mujukian et al. 2020 [33] Prospective	41 vs. 30	Celecoxib Gabapentin Acetaminophen	Decreased MED, improved pain scores, no change in LOS, ileus, or overall complications	Moderate quality
Iqbal et al. 2022 [34] Retrospective	537 vs. 790 96% EDA	Gabapentin Acetaminophen Ibuprofen	Drastic decrease in MED with no change in pain scores	Moderate quality
Yeo et al. 2022 [35] RCT	49 vs. 48	Pregabalin Tramadol TA plane block	Non-inferior to PCA in terms of pain score, decreased remifentanil dose, decreased time in PACU	Moderate quality

Recommendations Based on Data

Given the summary of the literature above, opioid-sparing strategies to treat post-operative pain have the benefit of decreased overall MED, LOS, and return of bowel function. Implementation of these changes in ERAS has helped distribute the adoption of MMA throughout many institutions. While a standard MMA regimen as well as additional adjuncts needs to be established, we recommend that using a combination of one medication per class of analgesic is highly effective in controlling post-operative pain, the most common being gabapentin, acetaminophen, and an NSAID. Patients experience a faster return to the comfort of their homes and decreased medical bills, as well as have a decrease in potential exposure to opioid medications. Prescriptions for opioids have already begun to decrease in the last few years and will continue to do so as the surgical field transitions from opioid-based analgesia to MMA for post-operative pain management.

A Personal View of the Literature

Widespread adoption of the ERAS protocol seems to have numerous benefits in patient outcomes metrics – improved pain scores, return of bowel function and decreased LOS which has been confirmed with numerous studies. Proper patient selection for the ERAS protocol in conjunction with proper patient education appears to be the key for success. Surgeons, administrators, and patients should keep in mind that complications and setbacks are still expected even in patients with the highest protocol compliance rates, but what seems to be the most important in many patients MMA in the setting of ERAS, is to avoid unnecessary exposure to opioids. Based on current literature it appears to be an accomplishable goal in colon and rectal surgery. This is of the utmost importance at the time of the current opioid epidemic.

References

1. Gan TJ. Poorly controlled postoperative pain: prevalence, consequences, and prevention. J Pain Res. 2017;10:2287–98. https://doi.org/10.2147/JPR.S144066.
2. Chou R, et al. Management of postoperative pain: a clinical practice guideline from the American pain society, the American Society of Regional Anesthesia and Pain Medicine, and the American Society of Anesthesiologists' committee on regional anesthesia, executive committee, and administrative council. J Pain. 2016;17(2):131–57. https://doi.org/10.1016/j.jpain.2015.12.008.
3. Rudd RA, Seth P, David F, Scholl L. Increases in drug and opioid-involved overdose deaths - United States, 2010–2015. MMWR Morb Mortal Wkly Rep. 2016;65(50–51):1445–52. https://doi.org/10.15585/mmwr.mm655051e1.
4. Daubresse M, et al. Ambulatory diagnosis and treatment of nonmalignant pain in the United States, 2000–2010. Med Care. Oct 2013;51(10):870–8. https://doi.org/10.1097/MLR.0b013e3182a95d86.

5. Sun EC, Darnall BD, Baker LC, Mackey S. Incidence of and risk factors for chronic opioid use among opioid-naive patients in the postoperative period. JAMA Intern Med. 2016;176(9):1286–93. https://doi.org/10.1001/jamainternmed.2016.3298.
6. Engelman RM, et al. Fast-track recovery of the coronary bypass patient. Ann Thorac Surg. 1994;58(6):1742–6. https://doi.org/10.1016/0003-4975(94)91674-8.
7. Kehlet H, Wilmore DW. Evidence-based surgical care and the evolution of fast-track surgery. Ann Surg. 2008;248(2):189–98. https://doi.org/10.1097/SLA.0b013e31817f2c1a.
8. Patel R, Dickenson AH. Mechanisms of the gabapentinoids and alpha 2 delta-1 calcium channel subunit in neuropathic pain. Pharmacol Res Perspect. 2016;4(2):e00205. https://doi.org/10.1002/prp2.205.
9. Arumugam S, Lau CS, Chamberlain RS. Use of preoperative gabapentin significantly reduces postoperative opioid consumption: a meta-analysis. J Pain Res. 2016;9:631–40. https://doi.org/10.2147/JPR.S112626.
10. Seib RK, Paul JE. Preoperative gabapentin for postoperative analgesia: a meta-analysis. Can J Anaesth. 2006;53(5):461–9. https://doi.org/10.1007/BF03022618.
11. Cavalcante AN, Sprung J, Schroeder DR, Weingarten TN. Multimodal analgesic therapy with gabapentin and its association with postoperative respiratory depression. Anesth Analg. 2017;125(1):141–6. https://doi.org/10.1213/ANE.0000000000001719.
12. Gomes T, Juurlink DN, Antoniou T, Mamdani MM, Paterson JM, van den Brink W. Gabapentin, opioids, and the risk of opioid-related death: a population-based nested case-control study. PLoS Med. 2017;14(10):e1002396. https://doi.org/10.1371/journal.pmed.1002396.
13. Khan JS, Margarido C, Devereaux PJ, Clarke H, McLellan A, Choi S. Preoperative celecoxib in noncardiac surgery: a systematic review and meta-analysis of randomised controlled trials. Eur J Anaesthesiol. Mar 2016;33(3):204–14. https://doi.org/10.1097/EJA.0000000000000346.
14. Straube S, Derry S, McQuay HJ, Moore RA. Effect of preoperative cox-II-selective NSAIDs (coxibs) on postoperative outcomes: a systematic review of randomized studies. Acta Anaesthesiol Scand. 2005;49(5):601–13. https://doi.org/10.1111/j.1399-6576.2005.00666.x.
15. Gorissen KJ, et al. Risk of anastomotic leakage with non-steroidal anti-inflammatory drugs in colorectal surgery. Br J Surg. 2012;99(5):721–7. https://doi.org/10.1002/bjs.8691.
16. Wu CY, Cheng KC, Chen YJ, Lu CC, Lin YM. Risk of NSAID-associated anastomosis leakage after colorectal surgery: a large-scale retrospective study using propensity score matching. Int J Color Dis. 2022;37(5):1189–97. https://doi.org/10.1007/s00384-022-04160-4.
17. Aminoshariae A, Khan A. Acetaminophen: old drug, new issues. J Endod. M2015;41(5): 588–93. https://doi.org/10.1016/j.joen.2015.01.024.
18. De Kock MF, Lavand'homme PM. The clinical role of NMDA receptor antagonists for the treatment of postoperative pain. Best Pract Res Clin Anaesthesiol. 2007;21(1):85–98. https://doi.org/10.1016/j.bpa.2006.12.006.
19. Jouguelet-Lacoste J, La Colla L, Schilling D, Chelly JE. The use of intravenous infusion or single dose of low-dose ketamine for postoperative analgesia: a review of the current literature. Pain Med. 2015;16(2):383–403. https://doi.org/10.1111/pme.12619.
20. Schwenk ES, et al. Adverse drug effects and preoperative medication factors related to perioperative low-dose ketamine infusions. Reg Anesth Pain Med. 2016;41(4):482–7. https://doi.org/10.1097/AAP.0000000000000416.
21. Kafali H, Aldemir B, Kaygusuz K, Gursoy S, Kunt N. Small-dose ketamine decreases postoperative morphine requirements. Eur J Anaesthesiol. 2004;21(11):916–7. https://doi.org/10.1017/s0265021504220282.
22. Katz J, Schmid R, Snijdelaar DG, Coderre TJ, McCartney CJL, Wowk A. Pre-emptive analgesia using intravenous fentanyl plus low-dose ketamine for radical prostatectomy under general anesthesia does not produce short-term or long-term reductions in pain or analgesic use. Pain. 2004;110(3):707–18. https://doi.org/10.1016/j.pain.2004.05.011.
23. Schwenk ES, et al. Consensus guidelines on the use of intravenous ketamine infusions for acute pain management from the American Society of Regional Anesthesia and Pain Medicine, the American Academy of pain medicine, and the American Society of Anesthesiologists. Reg Anesth Pain Med. 2018;43(5):456–66. https://doi.org/10.1097/AAP.0000000000000806.

24. Henriksen MG, Jensen MB, Hansen HV, Jespersen TW, Hessov I. Enforced mobilization, early oral feeding, and balanced analgesia improve convalescence after colorectal surgery. Nutrition. 2002;18(2):147–52. https://doi.org/10.1016/s0899-9007(01)00748-1.
25. Anderson AD, McNaught CE, MacFie J, Tring I, Barker P, Mitchell CJ. Randomized clinical trial of multimodal optimization and standard perioperative surgical care. Br J Surg. 2003;90(12):1497–504. https://doi.org/10.1002/bjs.4371.
26. Gatt M, Anderson AD, Reddy BS, Hayward-Sampson P, Tring IC, MacFie J. Randomized clinical trial of multimodal optimization of surgical care in patients undergoing major colonic resection. Br J Surg. 2005;92(11):1354–62. https://doi.org/10.1002/bjs.5187.
27. Delaney CP, Zutshi M, Senagore AJ, Remzi FH, Hammel J, Fazio VW. Prospective, randomized, controlled trial between a pathway of controlled rehabilitation with early ambulation and diet and traditional postoperative care after laparotomy and intestinal resection. Dis Colon Rectum. 2003;46(7):851–9. https://doi.org/10.1007/s10350-004-6672-4.
28. Raue W, Haase O, Junghans T, Scharfenberg M, Muller JM, Schwenk W. 'Fast-track' multimodal rehabilitation program improves outcome after laparoscopic sigmoidectomy: a controlled prospective evaluation. Surg Endosc. 2004;18(10):1463–8. https://doi.org/10.1007/s00464-003-9238-y.
29. Sim R, Cheong DM, Wong KS, Lee BM, Liew QY. Prospective randomized, double-blind, placebo-controlled study of pre- and postoperative administration of a COX-2-specific inhibitor as opioid-sparing analgesia in major colorectal surgery. Color Dis. 2007;9(1):52–60. https://doi.org/10.1111/j.1463-1318.2006.00998.x.
30. Brandal D, et al. Impact of enhanced recovery after surgery and opioid-free anesthesia on opioid prescriptions at discharge from the hospital: a historical-prospective study. Anesth Analg. 2017;125(5):1784–92. https://doi.org/10.1213/ANE.0000000000002510.
31. Chapman SJ, Garner JJ, Drake TM, Aldaffaa M, Jayne DG. Systematic review and meta-analysis of nonsteroidal anti-inflammatory drugs to improve GI recovery after colorectal surgery. Dis Colon Rectum. 2019;62(2):248–56. https://doi.org/10.1097/DCR.0000000000001281.
32. Truong A, Mujukian A, Fleshner P, Zaghiyan K. No pain, more gain: reduced postoperative opioid consumption with a standardized opioid-sparing multimodal analgesia protocol in opioid-tolerant patients undergoing colorectal surgery. Am Surg. 2019;85(10):1155–8. [Online]. Available: https://www.ncbi.nlm.nih.gov/pubmed/31657314
33. Mujukian A, Truong A, Tran H, Shane R, Fleshner P, Zaghiyan K. A standardized multimodal analgesia protocol reduces perioperative opioid use in minimally invasive colorectal surgery. J Gastrointest Surg. Oct 2020;24(10):2286–94. https://doi.org/10.1007/s11605-019-04385-9.
34. Iqbal A, Aijaz N, Hughes SJ, Tan SA, Read TE. The impact of a narcotic-sparing enhanced recovery protocol on postoperative narcotic use following colectomy. Dis Colon Rectum. 2022; https://doi.org/10.1097/DCR.0000000000002292.
35. Yeo J, et al. Comparison of the analgesic efficacy of opioid-sparing multimodal analgesia and morphine-based patient-controlled analgesia in minimally invasive surgery for colorectal cancer. World J Surg. 2022;46(7):1788–95. https://doi.org/10.1007/s00268-022-06473-5.

What Can Be Done to Prevent Readmission After Ileostomy Formation?

49

Sonja Boatman, Julia Kohn, and Elliot Arsoniadis

Introduction

As of 2016, 120,000 patients annually undergo some type of ostomy creation per year [1]. Ileostomy is used in multiple contexts: after total colectomy or abdominoperineal resection; defunctioning/diverting loop ileostomy (DLI) to protect new anastomoses in low anterior resection (LAR), ileal pouch-anal anastomosis (IPAA), or surgery for acute diverticulitis; and as an emergency procedure in the setting of anastomotic leak. High rates of readmission after ileostomy creation are noted, sometimes up to 30% [2, 3]. A substantial portion of these are due to high output, which can cause dehydration and resulting renal injury, electrolyte imbalances, and peristomal skin breakdown [4]. One systematic review and meta-analysis of readmission after ileostomy creation identified a 20% all-cause 30-day readmission rate, with dehydration being a primary contributor; another meta-analysis identified multiple associated variables, including diabetes, hypertension, diuretic use, renal disease, age, BMI, and IPAA creation [5, 6]. A large study using NSQIP data to examine risk factors for all-cause readmission after ileostomy found preoperative renal disease and postoperative renal insufficiency to be risk factors [7]. These studies identify key targets for reducing post-ileostomy readmission, with intersections between high ileostomy output, dehydration, and renal dysfunction.

Authors Sonja Boatman and Julia Kohn are equally contributed to this chapter.

S. Boatman · J. Kohn · E. Arsoniadis (✉)
Division of Colon and Rectal Surgery, University of Minnesota, Minneapolis, MN, USA
e-mail: arson001@umn.edu

K. Umanskiy, N. Hyman (eds.), *Difficult Decisions in Colorectal Surgery*, Difficult Decisions in Surgery: An Evidence-Based Approach,
https://doi.org/10.1007/978-3-031-42303-1_49

Since the previous edition of this text, there has been further research into understanding and modifying causes of hospital readmission after ileostomy creation. By addressing these factors, patient health and quality of life can be improved, and healthcare resource utilization can be reduced, which is critical in the setting of increasing costs and decreasing availability.

Search Strategy

A PubMed database search was performed to identify all studies relevant to readmission after ileostomy creation, in English, of adults who underwent colorectal surgery. The search period was between January 1, 2017 and August 1, 2022. This timepoint was chosen to continue from the previous edition of this chapter in 2017, which found only three articles with low-quality evidence. Search terms were "readmission" and "ileostomy," "ostomy," or "stoma." Titles and abstracts of each article were reviewed to include those discussing ileostomy-focused interventions were included.

Patient population	Interventions	Comparison	Outcomes studied
Adults with newly created ileostomy in the setting of colorectal surgery	Patient education Antimotility regimens Early reversal or initial avoidance Close outpatient care: calls, follow-up visits, IV fluids	Routine postoperative care	Readmission

Results

Early ileostomy Reversal (GRADE Criteria: Low Quality Evidence) (Table 49.1)

Early ileostomy closure has been suggested as a strategy to decrease stoma-associated complications, thereby lowering readmission rates. The evidence for its impact is limited, with four studies found in the literature review [8–11]. Danielsen et al. (2017) [8] conducted a multicenter randomized controlled trial (RCT) that examined early (8–13 days, n = 55) vs. late (>12 weeks, n = 57) ileostomy closure after LAR with total mesorectal excision (TME) for rectal cancer. Patients in the early reversal group experienced fewer overall complications in the 12-month follow-up period, with a mean 1.2 vs. 2.9 ($P < 0.0001$) complications in the early vs. late closure cohorts. The mean number of stoma-related complications, including skin irritation, ulceration, leakage, and high-volume output, was also lower in the early group (0.3 vs. 1.25, $P < 0.0001$). Of note, this trial did not include readmission rates as an endpoint. However, in a follow-up cost analysis that found a mean

Table 49.1 Summary of the data

Author, Year	Intervention	Outcome	GRADE
Danielsen 2017	Early (8–13 days) vs. late (> 12 weeks) stoma closure (RCT)	Fewer complications with early closure, no comment on readmission rates	Moderate
Shaffer 2017	Post-discharge home nursing care with step-down monitoring and education protocol (single-center pilot)	Reduced readmissions; reduced cost of readmissions	Low
Yin 2017	Time to stoma closure (retrospective, single-institution)	More complications associated with shorter time interval to stoma closure, no comment on readmission rates	Very low
Abdalla 2018	Early (< 6 months) vs. late (> 6 months) ileostomy closure (retrospective, single-institution)	Fewer complications with early stoma closure, no difference in readmission rates	Low
Blok 2018	Highly selective diversion after total mesorectal excision (ambispective single-center cohort study)	Decrease in stoma-related complications and total 1-year admission days (including admission for stoma closure)	Low
Chen 2018	Scoring system to predict readmission with dehydration (trained on NSQIP data) with recommended interventions	Model performed appropriately on NSQIP test cohort, but not validated in a prospective patient cohort	Low
Migdanis 2018	Outpatient oral isotonic hydration solution (RCT)	Decreased electrolyte/renal function abnormalities and reduced readmission rate in oral hydration group	Moderate
Chapman 2019	Temporary diversion to prevent anastomotic leak in sphincter-sparing proctectomy (retrospective matched cohort study using state database)	Incidence of anastomotic leak unchanged; diverted patients had higher risk of readmission and reintervention	Moderate
Park 2019	Cost analysis of RCT by Danielsen et al.	Increased readmission rate and associated cost in late closure group	Moderate
Alqahtani 2020	Risk calculator for readmission with dehydration (model trained on ACS-NSQIP data)	Performed appropriately on NSQIP test cohort; not validated in a prospective patient cohort	Low
Augestad 2020	Telemedicine vs. in-person follow-up with wound and stoma nurses (RCT)	Decreased readmission rate and travel burden, no improvement in quality of life	Low
Borsuk 2021	Mandatory outpatient IVF hydration (retrospective, single-institution study)	Reduced dehydration-related complications and readmissions after protocol implementation, no difference in overall readmissions	Low

(continued)

Table 49.1 (continued)

Author, Year	Intervention	Outcome	GRADE
Chang 2020	Morbidity assessment in ileostomy patients vs. colectomy only (retrospective propensity-matched cohort; NSQIP data)	Ileostomy status did not reduce mortality but was associated with higher NSQIP morbidity	Moderate
Fearn 2020	App-linked "smart" ostomy bag with output tracking and telehealth access (observational study)	Lower rates of readmission and ED visits	Very low
Mesli 2021	Use of lanreotide in addition to antidiarrheal agents for high-output stoma (prospective, multicenter RCT)	No difference with addition of lanreotide (trial prematurely stopped due to low enrollment)	Very low
Santamaria 2021	Follow-up nutrition consult after discharge (single-center, ambispective cohort study)	Reduced readmissions in the nutrition group; cost-effective intervention	Low
Eid 2022	Stepwise additions of service-specific PA, standardized rehydration protocol, nursing staff education, inpatient fiber supplementation (single-center QI project)	Reduced readmissions by 50% (addition of PA had greatest effect: 27.5% reduction)	Moderate
Ho 2022	Partially hydrolyzed guar gum (PHGG) to reduce stoma output (prospective cross-sectional pilot study)	Significantly reduced volume of ileostomy output and thicker consistency	Low
Hsu 2022	Use of HOS protocol, home health care, and scripted patient calls (retrospective institutional database review)	Decrease in readmissions vs. NSQIP data	Low
Nizum 2022	Use of an ostomy care pathway (meta-analysis)	Implementation may improve patient satisfaction, length of stay, and readmission rates	Moderate
Smithson 2022	App with reminders, educational content, daily postoperative health checks (non-randomized cohort study)	Decreased length of stay	Very low

HOS high-output stoma, *RCT* randomized controlled trial

difference of $4060 per patient in favor of the early closure group, readmission was a major contributor to increased cost in the late closure group [9]. They observed doubling of readmissions in the late closure group (49% vs. 24%) within 12 months.

The retrospective study by Yin et al. (2017) included 66 patients who underwent LAR with TME and defunctioning stoma for rectal cancer; 28 received ileostomy and 38 received transverse colostomy [10]. The authors found higher post-reversal complication rates in patients with earlier stoma closure, with an average 121 days prior to closure in patients who developed complications compared to 169 days in those without. In multivariate analysis, stoma closure before 110 days had a 6.31 odds ratio of postoperative complications. Notably, the authors did not differentiate between colostomy and ileostomy reversal in their analyses and readmission rate was not assessed in relation to time to stoma closure. Abdalla and Scarpinata (2018) conducted a retrospective study examining the effect of early (<6 months, n = 25) and late (>6 months, n = 50) ileostomy reversal on readmission and complication rates [11]. The mean number of complications was elevated in the late closure group (0.66 vs. 0.33 for early, P = 0.04), but there was no difference in 30-day readmission rate (16% early vs. 14% late, P > 0.05).

Overall, the results of these studies must be taken with caution, given considerable variation in timing of ileostomy reversal and definitions of "early" and "late" stoma closure, and conflicting results regarding complications and readmission. The decision to elect for early ileostomy closure should involve patient-centered discussion weighing individual patient factors.

Outpatient Intravenous and Oral Hydration (GRADE Criteria: Low to Moderate Quality Evidence)

Outpatient intravenous fluid (IVF) and oral rehydration protocols have been implemented to reduce hospital readmissions due to high ileostomy output-related dehydration [12, 13]. Borsuk et al. (2021) conducted a retrospective review of ileostomy creation outcomes during a period of sporadic at-home IVF hydration (n = 119) compared to a subsequent period of mandatory at-home IVF (n = 122) [12]. Their endpoints included dehydration, hospital readmission, and emergency department (ED) visits. The protocol entailed discharge with midline catheter and daily 1 L 0.9% sodium chloride boluses for 5 days, with continuation of daily boluses until ileostomy output fell below 1200 mL/day. Dehydration occurred in 15% of the sporadic group and 7.4% in the protocol group (P = 0.028), and related readmissions were reduced from 11% (sporadic) to 3.3% (protocol; P = 0.01). However, all-cause incidence of ED visits (26% vs. 29%, P = 0.68) and hospital readmissions (29% vs. 25%, P = 0.29) remained the same between groups. Thus, while outpatient IVF hydration reduced dehydration-specific readmission, it did not impact overall readmissions due to other ileostomy-related complaints.

Migdanis et al. (2018) performed a RCT assigning patients to an oral rehydration protocol (n = 39) or no intervention (n = 41) after rectosigmoid resection with DLI [13]. Protocol patients were instructed to drink 1 L/day of oral isotonic hydration solution for 40 days after hospital discharge. Throughout the study period, control patients had significantly lower serum sodium, higher creatinine, and more readmissions for electrolyte abnormalities and dehydration compared to the intervention group (24% vs. 0%, P < 0.01). All-cause 30-day readmission was also higher in the control patients vs. the rehydration group (29% vs. 10%, P = 0.02).

Antimotility Therapy (GRADE Criteria: Low Quality Evidence)

Studies on preventing post-ileostomy readmissions often mention the use of antimotility agents without formally assessing their use. Hsu et al. (2022) studied a stepwise regimen in 80 patients, to be started if tolerating diet and with ostomy output over 1000 mL/day: loperamide with fiber, then Lomotil, then cholestyramine, with outpatient IV rehydration if high output persisted [14]. All-cause and dehydration-related readmissions were reduced (8.75% vs. historical national cohort rate of 20.1%) with this plan. Another study piloted the use of partially hydrolyzed guar gum fiber (PHGG) to reduce ileostomy output, with higher PHGG intake associated with significantly lower stoma output on discharge (371 mL vs. 477 mL, $p = 0.004$), although the study only included 32 patients [15]. An additional trial attempted the use of lanreotide plus an antimotility regimen to improve ileostomy output, but this was stopped for funding reasons before any effect was observed [16].

Patient-Centered Interventions (GRADE Criteria: Low Quality Evidence)

Multiple patient-centered interventions to facilitate ostomy care have been assessed, including in-hospital teaching, standardized protocols, and outpatient check-ins. A systematic review by Nizum and Jacob (2022) indicated that standardized ostomy care pathways may improve patient satisfaction, length of stay, and readmission rates [17]. They especially noted perioperative education and post-hospital follow-up as helpful. Santamaría et al. (2021) instructed patients on identifying dehydration via a post-discharge nutrition consultation [18]. This process was cost-effective and demonstrated a lower rate of readmission for high-output stoma (28.6% pre- to 10.3% post-implementation). A U.S. teaching hospital with a rural patient population improved their readmission rate from 29% to 14% with stepwise changes [19]. They hired a physician assistant to maintain continuity of care for all colorectal surgery patients, given the frequent rotation of residents through the service. They also initiated a standardized oral rehydration protocol tailored to patient-documented intake and output, and they trained nursing and unit staff on fiber supplementation for patients with high ileostomy output. Shaffer et al. (2017) initiated mandatory visiting nurse support for patients with new ileostomies, with decreasing visit frequency only if patients remained without symptoms of dehydration [20]. They found a non-significant decrease in readmission rate (20.8% to 8.7%, $p = 0.1$), and total hospital readmission cost decreased by 89% in new ileostomy patients. Additionally, telemedicine has been used to reach patients in remote locations who otherwise might lack access to close follow-up for stoma care. Augestad et al. (2020) saw no increase in readmission rates when follow-up was primarily via telemedicine, suggesting an effective alternative when in-person care is difficult to access [21].

Fearn et al. (2022) proposed the use of a "smart" ostomy device to record output volume and connect with patients and the provider team via a smartphone app and an online portal [22]. They saw a 15% readmission rate but were limited by cohort size ($n = 14$) and a lack of institutional readmission data prior to app implementation. Likewise, Smithson et al. (2022) used an app-based patient education and check-in system, which they found to aid timely discharge without increasing readmission rates [23]. However, 2/3 of eligible patients refused enrollment in the app, calling into question the effectiveness of an intervention when few patients want to, or can, use it.

Scoring systems to identify new ileostomy patients at highest risk for early dehydration-related readmission have been proposed [24, 25]. These models incorporate factors including age, gender, ASA class and comorbidities, tobacco use, underlying diagnosis, procedure performed, whether surgery was elective, operative time, length of stay, and major morbidity at index admission. These calculators could help target additional education and resource-intensive interventions like outpatient IVF or home care towards those at highest risk.

Avoidance of ileostomy Creation (GRADE Criteria: Low to Moderate Quality Evidence)

Perhaps the most effective means of preventing early readmission after ileostomy is to avoid ileostomy creation. At a single institution in the Netherlands, a shift from routine to highly selective DLI at the time of TME reduced 1-year readmission, reintervention, and hospital days [26]. This difference was mostly attributed to the lack of readmission for ileostomy reversal, although they also demonstrated a significant reduction in complications, including high-output stoma, without increased pelvic sepsis or mortality. However, the transition to highly selective ileostomy use was simultaneous with their adoption of transanal TME, which affected their ability to interpret risk of anastomotic leak. Chang et al. (2020) described a propensity-matched retrospective analysis of NSQIP data, in which patients receiving colectomy with DLI compared to colectomy alone had increased readmissions (18.2% vs 11%, $P < 0.01$) and renal failure (3.2% vs 0.9%, $P < 0.01$), but no improvement in 30-day mortality [27]. They concluded that the morbidity of ileostomy may outweigh its benefits. In another retrospective study using a matched cohort of proctectomy patients with vs. without DLI, there was no difference in the incidence of anastomotic leak (4.5% diverted vs. 4.3% undiverted patients), but 90-day readmission (including 16.4% for acute kidney injury and 9.8% for dehydration) and non-elective reintervention were significantly more likely in diverted patients, with associated higher healthcare costs [28]. They concluded there was no benefit of routine diversion for all comers, although it may be beneficial in specific patients.

Recommendations Based on the Data

There is a growing body of evidence around ileostomy-specific interventions for preventing readmission and reducing complications. However, the quality of available data is low to moderate at best. Patient-focused education should be implemented preoperatively, in hospital, and after discharge, given the complexity and risk of morbidity after ileostomy creation. Instruction on measuring ileostomy output, identifying signs of dehydration, and self-care with antimotility agents and oral rehydration should be repeated and reinforced with patients throughout their operative course (strong recommendation in favor of education; no recommendation can be made as to optimal method of education delivery). There is sparse evidence regarding protocolized outpatient IVF and oral hydration pathways in newly formed ileostomates. Protocol-based home oral hydration is low risk and the benefits against dehydration-associated complications are intuitive; it would be reasonable to incorporate this into clinical practice (weak recommendation in favor). However, outpatient IV hydration carries the potential for volume-status derangements among patients with pre-existing cardiac, pulmonary, or renal co-morbidities and requires an indwelling venous catheter with an inherent risk for infection (weak recommendation against). There should be easy access to a colorectal care team for patients to communicate their concerns, with flexibility in the approach depending on the resources available in the community, potentially including telemedicine and/or home nursing visits (weak recommendation in favor). There is insufficient evidence surrounding the use of app-based interventions, and no recommendation can be made here. Early ileostomy reversal may reduce complications, readmissions, and healthcare costs, but the existing literature is inconsistent and no recommendation can currently be made on optimal timing of ileostomy reversal. Ultimately, this should be tailored to the individual patient at the surgeon's judgment. The decision to create a diverting ileostomy should likewise be individualized, rather than being routine practice for colectomy or high rectal anastomoses (weak recommendation in favor).

Personal View of the Data

Our practice includes a service-specific advanced practice provider to assist with continuity of care despite rotating residents and fellows, a preoperative outpatient visit with an ostomy nurse for site marking and education, and postoperative in-hospital visits with ostomy nurses for appliance and ostomy teaching. No patient is discharged with ileostomy output higher than 1.2 L over 24 hours and until they have an antimotility medication regimen as needed to maintain appropriate output. Lisinopril is stopped. On discharge, patients receive a graduated cylinder, are instructed to keep a daily log of ileostomy output, and are given standardized written instruction on diet and oral rehydration, including a solution recipe and recommended commercial brands. Instructions also include 24-hour contact information for the colorectal surgery team and immediate at-home interventions for high output. Patients receive a phone call from a colorectal clinic nurse coordinator within one week and an in-person clinic visit with a colorectal advanced practice provider within two weeks of discharge.

Despite the very real toll that ileostomy complications, especially dehydration and renal injury, cause patients, providers, and the healthcare system, there are few randomized large-scale studies providing high-quality evidence to implement readmission-preventing protocols. However, some generalizations can be made via large, retrospective, multi-site studies, which also suggest areas to inform further inquiry. First, the most effective way to prevent ileostomy complications is to not create an ileostomy. Data suggest that ileostomies once enshrined in colorectal surgical "dogma" (i.e. after low rectal anastomosis or ileal pouch creation) may not prevent post-surgical complications and may contribute to worse outcomes. Larger, multi-site, and well-organized studies are necessary to provide further guidance on patient populations where DLI formation can be avoided. These studies will have to be well executed with definitive results in order to change such a strongly held practice within the culture of colorectal surgery.

In many instances, ileostomy formation cannot be avoided. There is no data-supported gold standard for post-ileostomy care. However, some common-sense approaches should be incorporated into every new ileostomate's care. Fundamentally important aspects of this pathway include education and communication. Education regarding ileostomy care should begin, when able, in the preoperative setting. We have found the preoperative ostomy nurse visit to be highly instructive and helpful. Other interventions may include web or app-based teaching modules and/or joining online ostomy support groups. Continued education as the patient recovers from surgery and adjusts to life with an ileostomy should continue while in hospital and upon discharge. Postoperative communication with patients following ileostomy formation is paramount and is most essential during the 30-day window following surgery. Regular "check-ins" with new ileostomates via in-person visits, telemedicine, or phone calls should be scheduled as part of routine care. These "check-ins" allow clinic staff the opportunity to assess ostomy output and success with pouching, and can help circumvent difficulties in this initial period.

We encourage active investigation into these issues. Although we have provided some general guidelines, the best way to implement these interventions and how to address different populations must be elucidated. We encourage investigators to partner with experts in implementation science to develop thoughtful interventions as well as studies to evaluate and report their findings. We further encourage future investigators to engage patients early in the process of protocol development and evaluation. Although the population of patients "pre" ileostomy formation may be difficult to define, those who have undergone this procedure (either planned or unplanned) likely have an important story to tell those seeking to help their future counterparts. This important qualitative aspect should not be discounted, but rather become a focal point of future endeavors to reduce complications following ileostomy formation.

References

1. McGee MF. Stomas. JAMA. 2016;315(18):2032.
2. Loria A, Melucci A, Speranza J, Cellini C, Salloum R, Temple LK, et al. Acute kidney injury is a common and significant complication following ileostomy formation. Color Dis. 2022;24(1):102–10.
3. Van Butsele J, Bislenghi G, D'Hoore A, Wolthuis AM. Readmission after rectal resection in the ERAS-era: is a loop ileostomy the Achilles heel? BMC Surg. 2021;21(1):267.
4. Ouro S, Ferreira MP, Albergaria D, Maio R. Loop ileostomy in rectal cancer surgery: factors predicting reversal and stoma related morbidity. Langenbeck's Arch Surg. 2021;406(3):843–53.

5. Vogel I, Shinkwin M, van der Storm SL, Torkington J, Cornish PJ, Tanis R, et al. Overall readmissions and readmissions related to dehydration after creation of an ileostomy: a systematic review and meta-analysis. Tech Coloproctol. 2022;26(5):333–49.
6. Liu C, Bhat S, Sharma P, Yuan L, O'Grady G, Bissett I. Risk factors for readmission with dehydration after ileostomy formation: a systematic review and meta-analysis. Color Dis. 2021;23(5):1071–82.
7. Kim NE, Hall JF. Risk factors for readmission after ileostomy creation: an NSQIP database study. J Gastrointest Surg. 2021;25(4):1010–8.
8. Danielsen AK, Park J, Jansen JE, Bock D, Skullman S, Wedin A, et al. Early closure of a temporary ileostomy in patients with rectal cancer: a multicenter randomized controlled trial. Ann Surg. 2017;265(2):284–90.
9. Park J, Angenete E, Bock D, Correa-Marinez A, Danielsen AK, Gehrman J, et al. Cost analysis in a randomized trial of early closure of a temporary ileostomy after rectal resection for cancer (EASY trial). Surg Endosc. 2020;34(1):69–76.
10. Yin TC, Tsai HL, Yang PF, Su WC, Ma CJ, Huang CW, et al. Early closure of defunctioning stoma increases complications related to stoma closure after concurrent chemoradiotherapy and low anterior resection in patients with rectal cancer. World J Surg Oncol. 2017;15(1):80.
11. Abdalla S, Scarpinata R. Early and late closure of loop ileostomies: a retrospective comparative outcomes analysis. Ostomy Wound Manage. 2018;64(12):30–5.
12. Borsuk DJ, Studniarek A, Marecik SJ, Park JJ, Kochar K. Protocol-based intravenous fluid hydration for newly created ileostomies decreases readmissions secondary to dehydration. Am Surg. 2021;87(6):897–902.
13. Migdanis A, Koukoulis G, Mamaloudis I, Baloyiannis I, Migdanis I, Kanaki M, et al. Administration of an oral hydration solution prevents electrolyte and fluid disturbances and reduces readmissions in patients with a diverting ileostomy after colorectal surgery: a prospective, randomized. Control Trial Dis Colon Rectum. 2018;61(7):840–6.
14. Hsu AT, Crawford TC, Zhou X, Safar B, Efron J, Atallah C, et al. Decreasing readmissions after ileostomy creation through a perioperative quality improvement program. Dis Colon Rectum. 2022;65(8):e797–804.
15. Ho CY, Majid HA, Jamhuri N, Ahmad AF, Selvarajoo TA. Lower ileostomy output among patients with postoperative colorectal cancer after being supplemented with partially hydrolyzed guar gum: Outcome of a pilot study. Nutrition. 2022;103–104:111758.
16. Mesli Y, Holterbach L, Delhorme JB, Zaher L, Ortega-Deballon P, Deguelte S, et al. Is Lanreotide really useful in high output stoma? Comparison between Lanreotide to conventional antidiarrheal treatment alone. J Investig Surg. 2021;34(12):1312–6.
17. Nizum N, Jacob G. Systematic review of ostomy care pathways. Adv Skin Wound Care. 2022;35(5):290–5.
18. Santamaria MM, Villafranca JJA, Abiles J, Ruiz FR, Navarro PU, Goitia BT. Impact of a nutrition consultation on the rate of high output stoma-related readmission: an ambispective cohort study. Sci Rep. 2021;11(1):16620.
19. Eid MA, Oliver BJ, Goldwag JL, Gray PJ, Shaw RD, Henkin JR, et al. Reducing new ileostomy readmissions in a rural health care setting: a quality improvement initiative. Dis Colon Rectum. 2022;65(7):928–35.
20. Shaffer VO, Owi T, Kumarusamy MA, Sullivan PS, Srinivasan JK, Maithel SK, et al. Decreasing hospital readmission in ileostomy patients: results of novel pilot program. J Am Coll Surg. 2017;224(4):425–30.
21. Augestad KM, Sneve AM, Lindsetmo RO. Telemedicine in postoperative follow-up of STOMa PAtients: a randomized clinical trial (the STOMPA trial). Br J Surg. 2020;107(5):509–18.
22. Fearn RI, Gorgun E, Sapci I, Mehta SN, Dinh B, Yowell QV, et al. Improved 30-day surgical outcomes in ostomates using a remote monitoring and care management program: an observational study. Dis Colon Rectum. 2020;63(12):e581–e6.
23. Smithson M, McLeod MC, Theiss L, Shao C, Kennedy G, Hollis R, et al. Ileostomy patients using patient engagement technology experience decreased length of stay. J Gastrointest Surg. 2022;26(3):635–42.

24. Alqahtani M, Garfinkle R, Zhao K, Vasilevsky CA, Morin N, Ghitulescu G, et al. Can we better predict readmission for dehydration following creation of a diverting loop ileostomy: development and validation of a prediction model and web-based risk calculator. Surg Endosc. 2020;34(7):3118–25.
25. Chen SY, Stem M, Cerullo M, Canner JK, Gearhart SL, Safar B, et al. Predicting the risk of readmission from dehydration after ileostomy formation: the dehydration readmission after ileostomy prediction score. Dis Colon Rectum. 2018;61(12):1410–7.
26. Blok RD, Stam R, Westerduin E, Borstlap WAA, Hompes R, Bemelman WA, et al. Impact of an institutional change from routine to highly selective diversion of a low anastomosis after TME for rectal cancer. Eur J Surg Oncol. 2018;44(8):1220–5.
27. Chang YW, Davenport D, Dugan A, Patel JA. Significant morbidity is associated with proximal fecal diversion among high-risk patients who undergo colectomy: a NSQIP analysis. Am J Surg. 2020;220(4):830–5.
28. Chapman WC Jr, Subramanian M, Jayarajan S, Makhdoom B, Mutch MG, Hunt S, et al. First, do no harm: rethinking routine diversion in sphincter-preserving rectal cancer resection. J Am Coll Surg. 2019;228(4):547–56. e8

50 Do Bundles Help to Reduce Surgical Site Infections and Improve Safety?

Traci L. Hedrick

PICO Table

Patients	Intervention	Comparator	Outcome
Patients undergoing colorectal surgery	Surgical Site Infection Prevention Bundle	No Surgical Site Infection Prevention Bundle	Surgical Site Infection

Search Strategy

A comprehensive literature search of Cochrane Database of Collected Research, MEDLINE, EMBASE, and PubMed was performed to identify all the English-language publications using the following keywords: "Colorectal Surgery" or "colorectal" or "colon" or "rectum", "Surgical wound infection" or "infection" "wound healing" or "surgical site infection"or "surgical wound infection" or "SSI" or "Patient care bundles" or "bundle" or "checklist" or "surgical site infection bundle" or "SSI bundle". Studies conducted during the last 10 years were included while studies including pediatric patients were excluded. Supplementary cascading searches were performed on the reference lists of recent systematic reviews and guidelines related to the prevention of SSI.

T. L. Hedrick (✉)
Chief, Division of General Surgery, Department of Surgery, University of Virginia Health, Charlottesville, VA, USA
e-mail: Th8q@uvahealth.org

K. Umanskiy, N. Hyman (eds.), *Difficult Decisions in Colorectal Surgery*, Difficult Decisions in Surgery: An Evidence-Based Approach,
https://doi.org/10.1007/978-3-031-42303-1_50

Results

The term "bundle" as it pertains to quality improvement first emerged in the early 2000's to describe a collection of scientifically proven elements (usually three to five) that, when initiated together, were associated with greater clinical improvements than when initiated individually. Although this concept could be applied in any scenario, it gained the most traction within the context of healthcare-associated infection prevention [1]. Since that initial description, there has been a plethora of research, ranging in quality from single institution retrospective studies to prospective randomized controlled trials and clinical practice guidelines dedicated to the use of SSI prevention bundles in colorectal surgery.

Several meta-analyses demonstrate that implementation of SSI prevent bundles are associated with reduced SSI rates [2–4]. In one of the largest studies to date, SSI prevention bundles were associated with greater than 40% reduction in the incidence of SSI following colorectal surgery as compared with standard care [3]. In contrast to the initial description of care bundles, recent literature suggest that quality improvement is tied to increasing number of bundle elements (≥ 11 elements associated with lowest reported SSI rates) [3]. The composition of bundle elements is heterogenous including but not limited to fascial closure trays, change of gloves prior to wound closure, use of antimicrobial sutures and wound protectors, mechanical bowel prep with oral antibiotics, negative pressure wound dressing in contaminated wounds, and preoperative chlorhexidine showers.

The Centers of Disease Control and Prevention (CDC), National Institute of Health and Care Excellence (NICE), World Health Organization (WHO), and the American College of Surgeons in concert with the Surgical Infection Society have published guidelines on the prevention of SSI which provide an overview of the evidence for varying individual bundle elements [5–9].

Assuring successful implementation and ongoing maintenance of the bundle is equally important as the composition of specific bundle elements. This relies on active communication, involvement of front-line providers in the development of standard work, and constant provision of compliance data to reinforce the importance of bundle application.

Recommendations

A surgical site infection prevention bundle should be employed to reduce surgical site infection following colorectal surgery. Grade of Recommendation: Strong recommendation based on moderate-quality evidence.

Personal View

Colorectal surgery may not be glamorous, but it is ubiquitous. Unlike some other procedures which may only be performed at quaternary referral centers, most hospitals in the U.S. perform colon surgery, regardless of their size and affiliation. Additionally, the incidence of surgical site infection following colorectal surgery is relatively high and carries significant morbidity [10]. Thus, colon SSI is seen as a valuable quality metric to reliably compare across a wide variety of institutions. The Centers for Medicare and Medicaid Services (CMS) requires acute-care hospitals to report colon SSI outcomes in order to receive full CMS reimbursement as part of the Inpatient Prospective Payment System (IPPS). As such, efforts to reduce colon SSI are a central focus for many hospital-wide quality improvement initiatives throughout the U.S.

SSI prevention quality improvement efforts obviously require a rigorous commitment to always providing the best possible evidenced-based care, such as the use of an SSI prevention bundle. However, it also requires a full understanding of the metrics being measured and how they are reported. Currently, the key CMS metric for IPPS, known as "Complex 30-Day colon SSI", includes in-plan, inpatient colon (COLO) procedures in adult (≥ 18 years of age) patients. It does not include superficial SSI, but rather deep incisional and organ/space SSIs with an event date within 30 days of the procedure. The data is collected through the National Healthcare Safety Network (NHSN) and includes all patients having any of the procedures included in the NHSN COLO procedure category. It is important to note that a wide variety of procedures fall under the NHSN COLO category, for example open and minimally invasive colectomy, colostomy creation/revision/reversal, small bowel resection, and (somewhat surprisingly) removal of transplanted intestinal allograft. A full listing of the respective COLO procedures can be found on the NHSN website (https://www.cdc.gov/nhsn/pdfs/pscmanual/9pscssicurrent.pdf).

If the patient has a *documented* infection present at the time of surgery (PATOS), any subsequent infection that they may develop within the same anatomical space after surgery is not included in the SSI report from CMS. However, there are strict criteria which must be documented within the narrative portion of the operative report to meet the PATOS definition. Examples that indicate evidence of infection include but are not limited to "abscess, infection, purulence/pus, phlegmon, or feculent peritonitis". Verbiage that would NOT be considered evidence of infection present at the time of surgery per NHSN include "colon perforation, contamination, necrosis, gangrene, fecal spillage, murky fluid, or inflammation". As a real-world example, consider a patient who underwent sigmoid colectomy for "perforated sigmoid colon". Within the operative report narrative description, there is mention of a "feculent cavity" with a "colon that was clearly perforated". The surgeon states that they "did not do an anastomosis given the contamination" and "left the skin open because the wound was frankly contaminated". Because the words 'abscess, infection, purulence/pus, phlegmon, or feculent peritonitis' were not mentioned within the narrative portion of this operative report, the case was not coded as having an infection present at the time of surgery. When the patient subsequently developed a postoperative abscess, this was counted as a colon SSI within NHSN.

Other data points that may be miscoded within an administrative database are wound classification and elective versus emergency status [11]. It is important to note that, within NHSN, any SSI is attributed to the patient's most recent procedure. This becomes relevant in the case of an unstable patient presenting with an abdominal catastrophe whose abdomen is left open and taken to the intensive care unit. When that patient has been stabilized and is brought back to the OR for abdominal closure and colostomy creation, any subsequent SSI will be attributed to this procedure. If this procedure is coded as a "clean" procedure, or an "elective" procedure, this will obviously have significant implications on risk adjustment for this critically ill patient. These scenarios exemplify that attention to documentation and coding are nearly as important as actual quality-based initiatives, such as SSI prevention bundles, in assuring the lowest possible institutional rate of colon SSI.

In general, SSI prevention bundle elements can be categorized into preoperative, intraoperative and postoperative groups. Important preoperative elements that are generally supported by a majority of published guidelines are glycemic control, mechanical bowel preparation with oral antibiotics, smoking cessation, treatment of malnutrition, and chlorohexidine bathing [5–9]. Intraoperative factors include the use of minimally invasive surgery when appropriate, normothermia, clippers for hair removal, intravenous prophylactic antibiotics, avoidance of hypotension, air leak testing of left sided anastomoses, antimicrobial sutures, wound protectors, and negative pressure wound therapy for high-risk contaminated wounds. Postoperative management should follow Enhanced Recovery principles which have been demonstrated in multiple studies to reduce the rate of SSI in colorectal surgery [12, 13].

Table 50.1 outlines my current institutional colon SSI prevention bundle. There are obviously many other successful examples throughout the literature which may contain slightly different protocol elements [14, 15]. Some elements are widely accepted across multiple guidelines while others are a bit more controversial and will depend on local practice.

It is my personal belief that the actual individual bundle components (assuming they are reasonable and evidenced-based) are not as important as the standardization process itself in improving surgical outcomes. By bringing a multidisciplinary group of stakeholders together to collaborate and standardize practice around a shared quality improvement goal, outcome improvement is likely to follow. This does rely on sustained efforts to ensure compliance with bundle elements and regular provision of compliance and outcome data with frontline staff. It also requires continual appraisal of current literature to incorporate latest evidenced-based practice.

Table 50.1 University of Virginia's Institutional Surgical Site Infection Prevention Bundle

Preoperative
Malnutrition screening
Glycemic control
Optimizing chronic medical conditions
Mechanical bowel preparation with oral antibiotics
Chlorhexidine bathing
Smoking cessation
Preoperative warming
Enhanced Recovery Protocol
Intraoperative
Minimally invasive surgery
Indocyanine green angiography and air-leak test for left sided anastomoses
Meticulous technique to minimize blood loss
Clippers for hair removal
Antibiotic coated sutures
Double gloving
Change gloves prior to closure
Separate fascial closure tray
Avoidance of hyperglycemia
Drain avoidance
Wound irrigation with aqueous iodine in high risk contaminated wounds
Negative pressure wound therapy in high risk contaminated wounds
Alcohol-based skin prep
IV Antibiotic prophylaxis
Normothermia
Wound Protector
Postoperative
Hyperoxygenation
Early Discharge
Minimize volume overload
Glycemic control
Handwashing
Enhanced Recovery protocol

References

1. Ruscitti LE, Puro V. The use of bundles in clinical practice. Infez Med. 2008;16:121–9.
2. Tanner J, Padley W, Assadian O, Leaper D, Kiernan M, Edmiston C. Do surgical care bundles reduce the risk of surgical site infections in patients undergoing colorectal surgery? A systematic review and cohort meta-analysis of 8,515 patients. Surgery. 2015;158:66–77.
3. Pop-Vicas AE, Abad C, Baubie K, Osman F, Heise C, Safdar N. Colorectal bundles for surgical site infection prevention: a systematic review and meta-analysis. Infect Control Hosp Epidemiol. 2020;41:805–12.
4. Zywot A, Lau CSM, Stephen Fletcher H, Paul S. Bundles prevent surgical site infections after colorectal surgery: meta-analysis and systematic review. J Gastrointest Surg. 2017;21:1915–30.
5. Leaper D, Rochon M, Pinkney T, Edmiston CE. Guidelines for the prevention of surgical site infection: an update from NICE. Infect Prev Pract. 2019;1:100026.

6. Ban KA, Minei JP, Laronga C, Harbrecht BG, Jensen EH, Fry DE, Itani KMF, Dellinger EP, Ko CY, Duane TM. Executive summary of the American College of Surgeons/surgical Infection society surgical site Infection Guidelines-2016 update. Surg Infect. 2017;18:379–82.
7. Berrios-Torres SI, Umscheid CA, Bratzler DW, Leas B, Stone EC, Kelz RR, Reinke CE, Morgan S, Solomkin JS, Mazuski JE, Dellinger EP, Itani KMF, Berbari EF, Segreti J, Parvizi J, Blanchard J, Allen G, Kluytmans J, Donlan R, Schecter WP, Healthcare Infection Control Practices Advisory C. Centers for Disease Control and Prevention guideline for the prevention of surgical site Infection, 2017. JAMA Surg. 2017;152:784–91.
8. Leaper DJ, Edmiston CE. World Health Organization: global guidelines for the prevention of surgical site infection. J Hosp Infect. 2017;95:135–6.
9. Ruiz-Tovar J, Boermeester MA, Bordeianou L, Chang GJ, Gorgun E, Justinger C, Lawson EH, Leaper DJ, Mahmoud NN, Mantyh C, McGee MF, Nfonsam V, Rubio-Perez I, Wick EC, Hedrick TL, Colorectal Delphi Facilitating G. Delphi consensus on intraoperative technical/surgical aspects to prevent surgical site infection after colorectal surgery. J Am Coll Surg. 2022;234:1–11.
10. Hedrick TL, Sawyer RG. Surgical infections. Surg Clin North Am. 2014;94:xvii–xviii.
11. Turrentine FE, Giballa SB, Shah PM, Jones DR, Hedrick TL, Friel CM. Solutions to intraoperative wound classification miscoding in a subset of American College of Surgeons National Surgical Quality Improvement Program patients. Am Surg. 2015;81:193–7.
12. Thiele RH, Rea KM, Turrentine FE, Friel CM, Hassinger TE, McMurry TL, Goudreau BJ, Umapathi BA, Kron IL, Sawyer RG, Hedrick TL. Standardization of care: impact of an enhanced recovery protocol on length of stay, complications, and direct costs after colorectal surgery. J Am Coll Surg. 2015;220:430–43.
13. Albert H, Bataller W, Masroor N, Doll M, Cooper K, Spencer P, Winborne D, Zierden EM, Stevens MP, Scott M, Bearman G. Infection prevention and enhanced recovery after surgery: a partnership for implementation of an evidence-based bundle to reduce colorectal surgical site infections. Am J Infect Control. 2019;47:718–9.
14. Schlick CJR, Huang R, Brajcich BC, Halverson AL, Yang AD, Kreutzer L, Bilimoria KY, McGee MF, Illinois Surgical Quality Improvement C. Unbundling bundles: evaluating the Association of Individual Colorectal Surgical Site Infection Reduction Bundle Elements on Infection rates in a statewide collaborative. Dis Colon Rectum. 2022;65:1052–61.
15. McGee MF, Kreutzer L, Quinn CM, Yang A, Shan Y, Halverson AL, Love R, Johnson JK, Prachand V, Bilimoria KY, Illinois Surgical Quality Improvement C. Leveraging a comprehensive program to implement a Colorectal surgical site Infection reduction bundle in a statewide quality improvement collaborative. Ann Surg. 2019;270:701–11.

Part VII

Technique

51 Total Mesorectal Excision for Rectal Cancer: Top Down or Bottom Up?

Natalie F. Berger and Patricia Sylla

Introduction

Colorectal cancer is projected to be diagnosed in 153,020 individuals in the United States this year [1]. While incidence rates have declined in those 65 and older, they have remained stable in those 50–64 and have increased by 2% yearly in adults less than 50 years of age [1]. These younger patients are more likely to present with more advanced and more aggressive disease than older patients [2].

Locally advanced rectal cancers are treated with neoadjuvant chemotherapy and/or radiation followed by surgical resection, unless a complete clinical response is demonstrated. While we stand at the advent of complete neoadjuvant treatment and a trend towards increased adoption of non-operative management, surgery remains the cornerstone of current treatment. The goal of surgical management of rectal cancer is to achieve margins that are histologically free from tumor (R0 resection) with sphincter preservation when possible. The gold standard technique to achieve this is called total mesorectal excision (TME). TME is indicated for the treatment of

Disclosure Statements:
Dr. Berger has nothing to disclose.
Dr. Sylla serves as a consultant for Ethicon, Medtronic, Olympus, Stryker, Safeheal, RedDress and GI Windows.

N. F. Berger
Department of Surgery, NYU Langone Hospital, New York, NY, USA
e-mail: natalie.berger@nyulangone.org

P. Sylla (✉)
Department of Colon and Rectal Surgery, Mount Sinai Hospital, New York, NY, USA
e-mail: patricia.sylla@mountsinai.org

K. Umanskiy, N. Hyman (eds.), *Difficult Decisions in Colorectal Surgery*, Difficult Decisions in Surgery: An Evidence-Based Approach,
https://doi.org/10.1007/978-3-031-42303-1_51

rectal cancers that cannot be treated with local excision, including cT1 cancers with unfavorable histology, cT2 cancers, and locally advanced (cT3/cT4 N+) cancers after neoadjuvant treatment.

TME involves sharp dissection directly above the endopelvic fascia along the avascular presacral plane with en-bloc resection of the primary tumor, mesorectum, and lymphatics. TME was traditionally performed through a transabdominal or "top down" approach, which evolved from open to laparoscopic, and most recently, to robotic-assisted surgery. Following the development of minimally invasive transanal techniques, a new hybrid technique to address distal rectal tumors in patients with hostile pelvises was developed. Drs. Patricia Sylla and Antonio Lacy performed the first hybrid transanal total mesorectal excision (taTME) in 2010 [3]. At centers of expertise, this has rapidly evolved to become the preferred approach for distal rectal cancers in patients with challenging anatomy and when sphincter preservation is not only desired but deemed oncologically feasible.

This chapter will outline the indications, benefits, and challenges of taTME relative to traditional, abdominal TME. A review of the largest and most robust studies comparing these methods was undertaken, with a focus on postoperative, oncologic, and functional outcomes. We will conclude with recommendations on how to select the appropriate surgical approach for an individual patient with rectal cancer.

Patient population	Intervention	Comparator	Outcomes Studied
Patients with rectal cancer	TME	Transabdominal (open, lap, robotic) TME vs. taTME	Clinical, pathological, and functional outcomes

Top Down (Low Anterior Resection)

The transabdominal approach can be undertaken through three methods: open, laparoscopic (LapTME), and robotic (R-TME). In the setting of malignancy, the first step of each of these procedures involves high ligation of the inferior mesenteric artery to ensure adequate node harvest. The left colon is then mobilized medial-to-lateral and the inferior mesenteric vein is ligated near the tail of the pancreas. The splenic flexure is routinely taken down and the rectum is mobilized. Dissection of the mesorectum is continued down until the pelvic floor is reached and an adequate distal margin below the tumor is established. This dissection is especially challenging in the narrow male pelvis and in patients with significant visceral obesity. The specimen is then typically extracted through the abdominal wall, either through a low midline or Pfannenstiel incision, and a stapled colorectal or coloanal anastomosis is constructed, usually with a diverting loop ileostomy.

Randomized controlled trials (RCTs) have shown oncologic equivalence between the three transabdominal approaches to TME. The multicenter RCTs COLOR II, CLASICC, and COREAN found comparable outcomes between LapTME and open TME in overall survival (OS), disease-free survival (DFS), and recurrence rates [4–6]. The ALaCaRT and ACOSOG Z6051 trials, however, failed to show noninferior pathologic outcomes between laparoscopic and open TME [7, 8]. ACOSOG Z6051 also showed no difference in long-term oncologic outcomes including DFS and recurrence between techniques [9]. Two single center RCTs from China and South Korea from Tang et al. and Kim et al., respectively, and the multicenter international ROLARR trial showed equivalent short-term oncologic outcomes between LapTME and R-TME in terms of TME quality, resection margins, and the number of harvested lymph nodes [10–12]. One multicenter RCT from China by Feng et al., conversely, found significantly fewer positive circumferential margins (CRM) in the R-TME group [13]. Tang et al. additionally demonstrated long-term oncologic equivalence with similar rates of 2-year OS and 2-year DFS between LapTME and R-TME [11] .

Minimally invasive approaches to TME are currently preferred over open TME when technically feasible, as they have been shown to have higher rates of sphincter preservation, reduced short-term and long-term morbidity, and improved postoperative recovery including improved analgesia, earlier mobilization, and shorter length of hospital stay [14–16]. This chapter will therefore focus on the comparison between LapTME and R-TME to taTME.

The main challenge encountered by the transabdominal approaches to TME is the ability to obtain adequate visualization to conduct the mesorectal dissection in patients with challenging anatomy; a narrow pelvis and visceral fat pose technical barriers to this dissection. This is demonstrated through the high rates of conversion from laparoscopic to open approach in the COLOR II, CLASICC, ALaCaRT, and ACOSOG trials, which range from 9–34% [4, 5, 7, 8]. Of note, the COREAN trial had a conversion rate of just 1%, however, the median BMI of 24.08 was significantly lower than the median in Western trials [6]. Relatively high conversion rates were also seen in the ROLAAR trial, with 8.1% of operations converted from robotic to open [12]. Dissection into the lower pelvis for tumors 5 cm or less from the anal verge is particularly challenging with higher rates of abdominoperineal resection (APR). In a population-based study involving 20,959 patients from the Netherlands, sphincter preservation was only achieved in 29.3% of patients with low rectal tumors [17]. The main limitation of top-down TME, therefore, is that even in experienced hands, rates of conversion and APR are high due to technical challenges.

Bottom Up (taTME)

Transanal endoscopic surgery was pioneered by Dr. Gerhard Buess in the 1980s for the full-thickness resection of middle or upper rectal lesions that were inaccessible through transabdominal approaches and to facilitate sphincter preservation in lower rectal tumors. Dr. Buess developed the rigid transanal endoscopic microsurgery (TEM) platform, which could achieve pneumorectum through CO2 insufflation. Visualization with the platform takes place through either direct binocular view or projection onto a screen. Since then, multiple rigid and soft platforms have been developed, as well as platforms developed specifically for transanal minimally invasive surgery (TAMIS), in which conventional laparoscopic instruments can be used.

At a time where natural orifice transluminal endoscopic surgery (NOTES) was being explored with the first reports of transgastric cholecystectomy, gastrojejunostomy, and splenectomy being published in 2006 [18–20], transanal NOTES was facilitated by the use of transanal endoscopic platforms. Reports of transanal NOTES procedures on animal models and human cadavers included transanal colectomies and proctosigmoidectomies soon followed [21, 22]. In 2010, Sylla et al. published the first clinical case of transanal NOTES rectosigmoid resection, for rectal cancer, a procedure later renamed taTME [3]. Since then, taTME has been performed in over 40 countries worldwide.

TaTME can be performed with either one or two teams. The abdominal phase involves the same initial steps as transabdominal TME, beginning with vascular control, followed by mobilization of the splenic flexure and dissection along the TME plane. Once exposure becomes too challenging, the transanal phase begins. This is started with partial or complete intersphincteric resection (ISR) for very low rectal tumors or tumors at or below the anorectal ring to achieve a negative distal margin. Pursestring closure of the rectum below the tumor is then performed. Pneumorectum is then established and full-thickness proctotomy is made below the pursestring. Circumferential transanal TME dissection is continued with identification and preservation of the neurovascular bundle anteriolaterally, and pelvic plexus laterally. Through combined transanal and transabdominal dissection, peritoneal entry is achieved and the TME specimen is extracted. The anastomosis is carried out either through handsewn anastomosis or with a double pursestring with a circular stapler. A diverting loop ileostomy is created depending on the surgeon's assessment.

Although the majority of taTME-specific oncologic data are derived from retrospective single-center and multicenter series reporting 2–3 year oncologic outcomes, oncologic results from series with greater than 200 patients are comparable to those reported in the laparoscopic groups from the COLOR II and ACOSOG clinical trials. Local recurrence rates following taTME range from 3.1–6.2% [23–25], similar to the 5% and 4.6% rates reported in COLOR II and ACOSOG trials, respectively [4, 8]. The largest international taTME registry from 2021 with 2803 patients and a median followup of 24 months similarly found a 2-year local recurrence rate of 4.8% [26]. Two-year DFS and OS reported from the largest taTME studies are also similar to the Lap-TME clinical trials. DFS at 2 years was reported in the largest case series at 81–89.3% [23–25], from the international taTME database at 77% [26], and at 79.5% in the ACOSOG trial [8]. OS was reported between 90–95.7% in the largest taTME trials [23–25], 92% in the international taTME database [26], and 86.7% at 3 years in the COLOR II trial [4]. These findings are further supported by the recently published RCT comparing LapTME to taTME by Serra-Aracil which found no statistically significant difference between groups in local recurrence rates (6.1% vs. 1.8%; p = 0.3), DFS (89.8% vs. 89.1%; p = 1), or OS (79.6% vs. 87.3%; p = 3) [27]. Longer-term data will be published from ongoing RCTs including the phase II multicenter North American clinical trial (NCT03144765), the COLOR III trial, and the GRECCAR 11 trial [28–30].

Specific indications for taTME for rectal cancer include both patient and tumor adverse characteristics that may be mitigated by using a transanal approach [31]. These include male sex (with narrow and deep pelvis), visceral obesity and BMI > 30, and enlarged prostate. Tumor-related factors include neoadjuvant radiation (which can distort tissue planes) and low rectal tumors where R0 resection and sphincter salvage are threatened.

TaTME-specific complications include higher rates of urethral injury and CO2 embolism. An international retrospective analysis of urethral injuries that occurred during taTME reported that 51% of the injuries occurred during a surgical team's first 8 taTME cases, while the remaining occurred between the 12th and 101st case [32]. The authors concluded that the risk of injury during the surgeon's early learning curve could be reduced by increased proctoring and that injuries that occurred later were likely due to high case complexity and could be reduced with more strict case selection. Another unique challenge in taTME is a higher incidence of CO2 embolism, which has been reported to have an incidence of 0.4% based on data from international registries [33]. A recent review by Zhu et al. identified accidental vascular injury from anatomical distortion, patent vessels remaining open during pneumopelvis, and cyclic billowing from pneumatic instability, as unique causes of CO2 embolism during taTME [34].

Top Down vs. Bottom Up

Search Strategy

A comprehensive literature search using PubMed was performed to identify articles that compared LapTME and/or R-TME to taTME. Key search terms included "laparoscopic TME," "robotic TME," "taTME," "oncologic outcomes," and "functional outcomes." Studies were excluded if they did not directly compare taTME to a transabdominal approach. All RCTs and cohort studies with greater than 90 patients that compare LapTME to taTME are included in Table 51.1. As there are currently no published findings from RCTs comparing R-TME to taTME, data from all cohort studies and meta-analyses with greater than 80 patients are included in Table 51.3. To compare functional outcomes, all available studies comparing taTME to LapTME and/or R-TME were identified and included in Table 51.2.

Results

LapTME vs. taTME

Four RCTs [27, 35–38] and ten cohort studies [38–47] with at least 90 patients that compared clinical and pathologic outcomes between LapTME and TaTME were included. Patient and tumor characteristics of these studies were all similar after propensity score or case matching with the exception of lower tumors observed in

Table 51.1 RCTs & cohort studies with >90 Patients Comparing LapTME to TaTME

Study	Liu et al. 2023 [37]	Serra-Aracil et al 2022 [27]	Zeng et al. 2022 [57]	Hol et al. 2021 [47]	Ye et al. 2020 [45]	de Lacy et al. 2020 [44]	Alhanafy et al. 2020 [46]	Zeng et al. 2019 [38]	Detering et al. 2019 [42]	Sparreboom et al. 2019 [43]	Chen et al. 2018 [40]	Persiani et al. 2018 [41]	Denost et al. 2018 & 2014 [35, 36]	Chen et al. 2016
Study Type	Prospective RCT	Prospective RCT	Retrospective, Case-Matched Cohort	Retrospective, Propensity Score Matched Cohort	Retrospective, Propensity Score Matched Cohort	Retrospective Cohort	Retrospective, Propensity Score Matched Cohort	Prospective RCT	Retrospective, Propensity Score Matched Cohort	Prospective, Propensity Score Matched Cohort	Retrospective Cohort	Retrospective, Propensity Score Matched Cohort	Prospective RCT	Prospective, Matched Case-Control
Level of Evidence	1b	1b	2b	2b	2b	2b	2b	1b	2b	2b	2b	2b	1b	3b
Country	China	Spain	China	Netherlands	China	Spain & Netherlands	South Korea	China	Netherlands	Belgium & Netherlands	Taiwan	Italy	France	China & Taiwan
Years	2016–2021	2015–2021	2014–2017	2015–2017	2014–2019	2011–2018	2014–2017	2016–2018	2015–2017	2015–2017	2008–2019	2007–2017	2008–2012	2013–2015
Patients (top vs. bottom)	545 vs. 544	57 vs. 59	208 vs. 104	108 vs. 108	70 vs. 70	366 vs. 344	202 vs. 202	133 vs. 128	396 vs. 396	48 vs. 48	64 vs. 39	46 vs. 46	50 vs. 50	76 vs. 28
Follow-Up (months)	-	39	-	-	20 vs. 18	61.1 vs. 28.4	34	-	-	0.9	37.5 vs. 17.5	-	60.2	-
Clinical outcomes														
Conversion Rate	Comparable	20% vs 1.8% (p = 0.003)	3.4% vs. 0%, p = 0.057	–	Comparable	–	Comparable	Comparable	8.6% vs. 1.5%; p < 0.001	Comparable	Comparable	19.6% vs. 0%; p = 0.002	Comparable	Comparable
ISR	8.8% vs. 14.9%; p = 0.002	–	–	–	–	–	–	Comparable	–	–	–	–	Comparable	–
APR	Comparable	4% vs. 0%; p not calculated	–	41.4% vs. 24.6%; p < 0.001	–	–	–	11.1% vs. 1%; p not calculated	–	–	–	–	Comparable	–

Anastomotic Leak	Comparable	Comparable	Comparable	–	Comparable	–	Comparable	–	Comparable	Comparable	Comparable	Comparable	Comparable	–
30-Day Mortality	-	Comparable	Comparable	–	–		–	Comparable	–	–	Comparable	–	Comparable	–
Pathologic outcomes														
Completeness of TME	Comparable	88% vs. 100% (p = 0.03)	Comparable	–	Comparable	Comparable	Comparable	Comparable	–	–	–	Comparable	Comparable	–
CRM Distance (mm)	Comparable	Comparable	–	–	–	7.5 (6–10) vs. 10 (10–12); p = 0.0131	–	–	–	–	Comparable	–	Comparable	–
CRM Involvement	Comparable	Comparable	Comparable	–	Comparable	16.2% vs. 9.5%; p = 0.0038	Comparable	Comparable	Comparable	Comparable	–	Comparable	18% vs. 4%; p = 0.025	–
DRM Distance (mm)	Comparable	Comparable	1.9 ± 1.3 vs. 1.4 ± 0.9; p = 0.001	–	–	Comparable	–	Comparable	–	–	Comparable	Overall: 15 (5–40) vs. 25 (5–60); p < 0.001, Low: 12 (5–40) vs. 20 (5–45); p < 0.006, Middle: 17 (5–40) vs. 30 (5–60); p < 0.001	Comparable	1.5 ± 0.9 vs. 2.4 ± 1.2; p = 0.000
DRM Involvement	Comparable	Comparable	Comparable	–	–	Comparable	Comparable	Comparable	–	Comparable	–	–	–	–

(continued)

Table 51.1 (continued)

Study	Liu et al. 2023 [37]	Serra-Aracil et al 2022 [27]	Zeng et al. 2022 [57]	Hol et al. 2021 [47]	Ye et al. 2020 [45]	de Lacy et al. 2020 [44]	Alhanafy et al. 2020 [46]	Zeng et al. 2019 [38]	Detering et al. 2019 [42]	Sparre-boom et al. 2019 [43]	Chen et al. 2018 [40]	Persiani et al. 2018 [41]	Denost et al. 2018 & 2014 [35, 36]	Chen et al. 2016
Lymph Node Yield	Compa-rable	Comparable	Comparable	–	Compa-rable	14 (14–15) vs. 15 (15–16); p = 0.0133	Compa-rable	Compa-rable	Comparable	–	Compa-rable	–	Compa-rable	Comparable
Overall Survival	–	Comparable	Comparable	–	–	Comparable	Compa-rable	–	–	–	Compa-rable	–	Compa-rable	–
Disease Free Survival	–	Comparable	Comparable	–	–	Overall: Compa-rable, Sphincter-Preserving: p = 0.033, TaTME improved	Compa-rable	–	–	–	Compa-rable	–	Compa-rable	–
Overall Recur-rence	–	–	–	–	Compa-rable	–	–	–	Comparable	–	–	–	Compa-rable	–
Local Recur-rence	–	Comparable	Comparable	–	Compa-rable	9.6% vs. 3.6%; p = 0.001	Compa-rable	–	Comparable	–	Compa-rable	–	Compa-rable	–
Distant Recur-rence	–	Comparable	–	–	Compa-rable	–	–	-	Comparable	–	–	–	–	–

Table 51.2 Functional outcomes: LapTME, Robotic TME, TaTME

Study	Miura et al. 2022 [56]	Grass et al. 2021 [65]	Ha et al 2021 [55]	Foo et al. 2020 [54]	Bjoern et al. 2020 [53]	Rubinkiewicz et al. 2019 [52]	Veltcamp Helbach et al. 2019 [51]	Dou et al. 2019 [50]	Bjoern et al. 2018	Pontallier et al. 2016
Study Type	Prospective, Cohort	Prospective, Cohort	Retrospective, Propensity-Score Matched Cohort	Retrospective, Propensity-Score Matched Cohort	Prospective, Cohort	Prospective, Cohort	Prospective, Cohort	Retrospective, Cohort	Prospective, Cohort	Prospective, Cohort
Level of Evidence	2b	2b	2b	2b	2b	2b	2b	2b	2b	2b
Years	2016–2020	2014–2018	2014–2017	2016–2018	2011–2017	2013–2017	2010–2012	2016–2017	2010–2017	2008–2012
Country	Japan	Germany & Italy & Taiwan	South Korea	China	Denmark	Poland	Netherlands	China	Denmark	France
Top-Down Approach	Robotic & Laparoscopic	Robotic	Laparoscopic	Laparoscopic	Laparoscopic	Laparoscopic	Laparoscopic	Laparoscopic	Laparoscopic	Laparoscopic
Patients	33 vs. 11 vs. 8	55 vs. 85	44 vs. 42	35 vs. 35	12 vs. 36	23 vs. 23	27 vs. 27	53 vs. 54	36 vs. 49	34 vs. 38
Quality of life										
ED-5D-3L	–	–	–	–	–	–	Comparable	–	–	–
EORTC-QLQ C30	–	–	Comparable	–	–	–	Comparable	–	Emotional Functioning: 93.51 vs. 87.07; p = 0.041, Diarrhea: 4.62 vs. 17.68; p = 0.009	–

(continued)

Table 51.2 (continued)

Study	Miura et al. 2022 [56]	Grass et al. 2021 [65]	Ha et al 2021 [55]	Foo et al. 2020 [54]	Bjoern et al. 2020 [53]	Rubinkiewicz et al. 2019 [52]	Veltcamp Helbach et al. 2019 [51]	Dou et al. 2019 [50]	Bjoern et al. 2018	Pontallier et al. 2016
EORTC-QLQ C29	–	–	–	–	–	–	Fecal Incontinence: 16.7 ± 26 vs. 33.3 ± 25; p = 0.032	–	Buttock Pain: 2.77 vs. 14.28; p = 0.011, Taste: 4.16 vs. 0; p = 0.047	–
EORTC-QLQ-CR38	–	–	Comparable	–	–	–	–	–	–	–
Fecal function										
mFIQL	Comparable	–	–	–	–	–	–	–	–	–
Manometry (mean) *Resting Pressure* *Squeeze Pressure*	–	–	Comparable Comparable	–	Comparable Comparable	–	–	–	–	
LARS	Comparable	4.3 ± 2.2 vs. 9.8 ± 1.5, p = 0.038	13 (0–22.5) vs. 25 (15–32); p < 0.001, Comparable after multivariate analysis (OR 2.3 (0.79–6.72); p = 0.127)	3 months: 32 vs. 37; p = 0.045, 6 months: Comparable, 12 months: Comparable	Comparable	Comparable	Comparable	Total: Comparable, Clustering of Stools: 45.3% vs. 68.5%; p = 0.019	Total: Comparable, Urgency LaTME<TaTME; p = 0.032, Clustering of stools LaTME< TaTME; p = 0.017	Comparable

Study	2022 [56]	2021 [65]	[55]	2020 [54]	2020 [53]	2019 [52]	[51]	2019 [50]	Bjoern et al. 2018	et al. 2016
FISI	–	–	Comparable	–	–	–	–	–	–	–
Wexner	Comparable	Compa-rable	–	3/6/12 months: Comparable	–	Compa-rable	–	–	–	Comparable
Urinary function										
ICIQ-MLUTS/ ICQ-FLUTS	–	13.8 ± 4.9 vs. 1.8 ± 5.8, p = 0.038, Compa-rable	–	–	–	–	–	–	–	–
IPSS ***Severe IPSS***	Comparable Comparable	Compa-rable	Comparable	–	–	–	Comparable	–	Comparable	Comparable
Sexual function										
IIEF/FSFI	–	Compa-rable/ Compa-rable	–	–	–	–	–	–	–	Overall: Comparable/ Comparable, Sexual Activity: 39% vs. 71%; p = 0.02

the taTME groups in both studies by Chen et al. ($p = 0.022$, $p < 0.01$) and a higher proportion of patient receiving neoadjuvant therapy in the LapTME group in Sparreboom et al. ($p = 0.041$) [39, 40, 43]. Eight cohort studies [48–55] that compared functional outcomes in LapTME to taTME and one cohort study [56] that compared LapTME, R-TME, and TaTME were included.

Postoperative Outcomes

The rate of conversion to open procedure was significantly higher in the LapTME group in every study in which a significant difference between operative approach was observed. Conversion rates in these studies ranged from 3.4%–20% for LapTME and 0–1.7% for taTME [27, 38, 41, 42]. Anastomotic leak rate and 30-day mortality were comparable between techniques across all studies.

Patients who received taTME were more likely to have a sphincter-saving resection and were less likely to have APR. In Zeng et al., rates of ISR were similar between groups with 3.8% in the taTME group and 3.3% in the LapTME group, however, 1% of patients in the taTME group had APR while 11.1% had APR in the LapTME group [57]. Hol et al. found significantly higher rates of APR at LapTME centers compared to taTME centers: 33.3% vs. 10.2%; $p < 0.001$ [47]. In the RCT by Serra-Aracil et al., 2 of the 11 patients in the LapTME group who were converted to open underwent APR compared to none in the taTME group (4% vs. 0%) [27]. This finding is further supported with level 1b evidence from Liu et al., which reported significantly higher ISR rates in the taTME group (14.9% vs. 8.8%; $p = 0.002$) [37]. In contrast, the RCT by Denost et al. found comparable rates of ISR and APR between taTME and LapTME (60% vs. 65%; $p = 0.685$) [35].

Three studies reported results relative to perioperative recovery. TaTME was associated with improved outcomes including significantly shorter time to first flatus ($p < 0.001$, $p = 0.001$), first oral intake ($p < 0.001$, $p = 0.001$), ambulation ($p = 0.001$), and foley removal ($p = 0.007$) [37, 39, 41], relative to LapTME. Chen et al. also reported that taTME patients had a shorter time to adjuvant chemotherapy relative to LapTME patients($p = 0.003$) [39].

The length of hospital stay, reoperation, postoperative complications, severity of complications (Clavien-Dindo), and readmission rates were comparable between groups in most studies. Alhanfy et al. showed significantly more surgical site infections in LapTME compared to taTME (1.5% vs. 1%; $p = 0.0007$), however this study appears to be an outlier [46]. While Alhanfy et al. found no significant difference in Clavien-Dindo (CD) grade of complications between groups overall, on subgroup analysis of tumors <5 cm from the anal verge, they found significantly more severe complications (CD III, IV) in patients who had received LapTME compared to taTME (11.9% vs. 1.7%; $p = 0.0366$) [46].

Oncologic Outcomes

Pathologic outcomes between groups were comparable overall between LapTME and taTME, although variation in several outcomes did arise, particularly in studies with level 2b evidence. In the RCT by Serra-Aracil et al., taTME was found to have a significantly higher rate of complete TME specimen (100% vs. 88%; $p = 0.03$), however, there was no difference between groups in the three other RCTs [27]. Positive CRM were observed at a significantly higher rate in the LapTME group in the Denost et al. RCT (18% vs. 4%; p = 0.025) and the cohort study by de Lacy et al. (16.2% vs. 9.5%; p = 0.0038) [36, 44]. Chen et al. and Persiani et al. reported a greater length of distal radial margin (DRM) in the taTME group (2.4 ± 1.2 vs. 1.5 ± 0.9; p = 0.000, 25 (5–60) vs. 15 (5–40); p < 0.001) [39, 41]. In contrast, the Zeng et al. RCT found a significantly longer DRM in the LapTME group (1.9 ± 1.3 vs. 1.4 ± 0.9; p = 0.001) [38]. Length of CRM, DRM involvement, lymph node yield, OS, DFS, overall recurrence, local recurrence, and distant recurrence were comparable in all studies with the exception of the cohort study from de Lacy et al., which found significantly greater CRM length in the taTME group (10 (10–12) vs. 7.5 (6–10); p = 0.0131), significantly greater lymph node yield in the taTME group (15 (15–16) vs. 14 (14–15); p = 0.0133), comparable DFS overall but improved DFS in the taTME group in patients who had undergone sphincter-sparing procedures (HR = 0.78; 95% CI, 0.62–0.98; p = 0.033) [44].

Functional Outcomes

Nine cohort studies compared functional outcomes between patients who underwent LapTME vs. taTME. Three of these studies assessed quality of life using the ED-5D-3L, EORTC-QLQ-C29, C30, and/or CR38 questionnaires. The overall scores measured in each of these studies were comparable between groups. All categories were comparable between groups for the EORTC-QLQ C30 across three studies except for worsened emotional functioning and increased diarrhea reported in the taTME group by Bjoern et al. (87.07 vs. 93.51; p = 0.041, 17.68 vs. 4.62p = 0.009, respectively) [49]. For the EORTC-QLQ-C29, worse fecal incontinence was reported in the taTME group by Veltcamp et al. (33.3 ± 25 vs. 16.7 ± 26; p = 0.032), and worse buttock pain in the taTME group by Bjoern et al. (14.28 vs. 2.77.; p = 0.011,) [49, 51]. All other outcomes in the EORTC-QLQ-C29 questionnaire [49], and outcomes in the ED-5D-3L and EORTC-QLQ-CR38, which were assessed in a single study, were comparable between the groups [51, 55].

With regards to anorectal function, anorectal manometry, Modified Fecal Incontinence Quality of Life score (mFIQL), Fecal Incontinence Severity Index (FISI), and Wexner scores were comparable between LapTME and taTME across all studies. Total LARS score was comparable at 1 year postoperatively in all nine studies, however, taTME patients reported worse clustering of stools in the study by Dou et al. (68.5% vs. 45.3%; p = 0.019), Bjoern et al. (p = 0.017) and worse urgency in the study by Dou et al. (p = 0.032) [49, 50]. Urinary function was comparable between the groups across all studies [48, 49, 51, 55, 56]. Sexual function was assessed in only one study, with comparable International Index of Erectile Function (IIEF) and Female Sexual Function Index (FSFI) scores between groups [48]. Pontallier et al., however, reported that a significantly greater proportion of patients in the taTME group remained sexually active following surgery (71% vs. 39%; p = 0.02). On multivariate analysis, LapTME was the only risk factor associated with loss of sexual activity (OR 3.49; 1.02–11.97; p = 0.047) [48].

R-TME vs. taTME

Six retrospective cohort studies with at least 80 patients comparing postoperative and oncologic outcomes between patients undergoing R-TME and taTME were included [47, 58–62]. Two meta-analyses were also included; Butterworth et al., which included RCTs, prospective, and retrospective cohort and case-control studies that assessed R-TME, taTME, and studies that compared the two approaches, with a total of 5326 patients and Ryan et al. which only included data from RCTs with a total of 2286 patients [63, 64]. Patients were younger and had significantly lower tumors in the R-TME group in Shin et al. ($p < 0.001$, $p = 0.004$, respectively) [58]. Patients had significantly more cN0 disease in the taTME group and more advanced disease (N+) in the R-TME group in both Lee et al. and Buan et al. ($p < 0.001$ in both studies) [59, 62]. Tumors were significantly larger in the R-TME group in Law et al.($p = 0.031$) [60]. All other patient and tumor characteristics between groups were comparable. One study compared functional outcomes between R-TME and taTME [65].

Postoperative Outcomes

The conversion rate to open approach was comparable between groups in all the cohort studies where it was measured, and in the meta-analysis by Butterworth et al. [58–61, 64]. Anastomotic leak rate was comparable between R-TME and taTME in four cohort studies and both meta-analyses [58–60, 62–64]. Thirty-day mortality was reported by two cohort studies and both meta-analyses and was comparable between groups [59, 60, 63, 64]. Intraoperative complications were comparable in two cohort studies [47, 60], and were significantly fewer in the taTME group than in the R-TME group in Hol et al. (27.8% vs. 42.6%; $p = 0.023$) [47].

Buan et al. was the only study to compare recovery times in the immediate postoperative period between the groups. They reported significantly shorter time to return of bowel function in the taTME group (2 (1–7) vs. 3 (1–5); $p = 0.013$), and fewer patients requiring stays in the high dependency unit or ICU follow taTME compared to R-TME (38.2% vs. 73.7%; $p = 0.010$) [62]. Time to first oral intake and ambulation were comparable between groups [62].

Length of stay, postoperative complications, and severity of postoperative complications were comparable between groups across every study in which they were reported. Hol et al. reported a lower rate of post-op ileus in the taTME group (9% vs. 25%; $p = 0.003$) [47], however Shin et al., Lee et al., Buan et al., and the meta-analysis by Ryan et al. all reported similar rates between groups [58, 59, 62, 63]. Re-operation rate was reported by three studies and was comparable across all groups [59, 60, 62]. Readmission rate was reported by Buan et al. and was significantly higher in the taTME group than the R-TME group (0% vs. 19%; $p = 0.006$) [62].

Oncologic Outcomes

Oncologic outcomes were largely comparable between studies; Shin et al., Lee et al., Law et al., Hol et al., Butterworth et al. and Ryan et al. reported comparable rates of TME specimen completeness, CRM and DRM involvement and lymph node yield (before subgroup analyses) [47, 58–60, 63, 64]. Perez et al. reported longer CRM in the R-TME groups (19 (12–49) vs. 12 (5–20); $p < 0.001$), however, all the other studies found no significant differences between groups [61]. The DRM was reported to be longer in the R-TME group in Perez et al. (31 (19–45) vs. 19 (8–30); $p = 0.007$) and Butterworth et al. (26.2 (23.5–28.8) vs. 21 (18.3–23.6); $p = 0.007$). Conversely, Buan et al. found the DRM length to be longer in the taTME group (16.5 (2–72) vs. 25 (3–100); $p = 0.021$) as did Lee et al. in their sub-analysis of low rectal tumors (9.6 ± 10.3 vs. 12.2 ± 10.2; $p = 0.033$) [59]. CRM margin involvement was comparable between surgical approaches in five cohort studies and the two meta-analyses [47, 58–60, 62], with the exception of the subgroup analysis of pT3-T4 tumors by Buan et al., that reported significantly higher rate of positive margins in the R-TME group(18.2% vs. 0%; $p = 0.012$) [62].

The only studies that have reported data on survival and recurrence between groups are the cohort study by Buan et al. and the meta-analysis by Ryan et al. Ryan et al. found comparable outcomes between groups in OS, DFS, overall recurrence, local recurrence, and distant recurrence [63]. In Buan et al., OS was comparable overall between groups, however in a subanalysis of pT3–4 tumors, survival was significantly longer in the taTME group (21.4 (1.27–69.6) vs. 37.5 (3.5–57.1); $p = 0.046$) [62]. DFS was significantly longer in the taTME group in both the overall group (15.7 (1–69.6) vs. 25.9 (0.8–57.1); $p = 0.049$) and after sub-analysis of pT3–4 tumors (11.1 (1.0–69.6) vs. 25.9 (0.8–57.1); $p = 0.017$) [62]. Similar to Ryan et al., Buan et al. found no differences overall or in sub-analyses of disease recurrence [62].

Functional Outcomes

Two studies compared functional outcomes between taTME and R-TME (Table 51.3). Miura et al. studied anorectal outcomes using the Wexner score, Low Anterior Resection Syndrome score (LARS), and mFIQL score and urinary function using the International Prostate Symptom Score (IPSS) in 33 patients who underwent R-TME and 11 patients who underwent taTME. Although no statically significant differences were observed between the groups (which is likely the result of small sample size), there was a trend towards better functionality scores for all anorectal functional measures and a smaller percentage of scores in the severe range: 75% (vs. 51.5%) of taTME patients had severe-range Wexner scores, 100% (vs. 78.8%) had severe-range LARS scores, and 62.5% (vs. 30.3%) had severe range mFIQL scores. The median IPSS score was the same for each group and severe was observed in 6.1% of patients in the R-TME group and 0% of patients in the taTME group ($p = 1.00$) [56].

Grass et al. is currently the largest study comparing functional outcomes between 55 R-TME and 85 taTME patients. Anorectal function was assessed using the LARS and Wexner scores, urinary function was assessed using the ICIQ-MFLUTS/FLUTS and IPSS, and sexual function was assessed using the IIEF and FSFI [65]. LARS scores were significantly worse in the taTME group (9.8 ± 1.5 vs. 4.3 ± 2; $p = 0.038$), while Wexner scores were comparable between groups. Male urinary function was significantly worse in the R-TME group with a greater median ICIQ-MLUTS score (13.8 ± 4.9 vs. 1.8 ± 5.8, $p = 0.038$). Female urinary function and sexual function for both sexes were comparable [65].

Table 51.3 Cohort studies and meta-analyses with >80 patients comparing robotic TME to TaTME

Study	Butterworth et al. 2021 [64]	Ryan et al. 2021 [63]	Hol et al. 2021 [47]	Buan et al. 2021 [62]	Shin et al. 2020 [58]	Lee et al. 2019 [59]	Law et al. 2018 [60]	Perez et al. 2018 [61]
Study Type	Meta-Analysis	Meta-Analysis	Retrospective, Propensity Score Matched Cohort	Retrospective, Cohort	Retrospective, Cohort	Retrospective, Case-Matched Cohort	Retrospective, Propensity Score Matched Cohort	Retrospective, Cohort
Level of Evidence	3a	1a	2b	2b	2b	2b	2b	2b
Country	Multiple	Multiple	Netherlands	Singapore	South Korea	USA, Canada, South Korea, Spain	China	Germany
Years	2011–2019	2006–2018	2015–2017	2015–2020	2008–2018	2011–2017	2008–2017	2013–2016
Follow-Up (months)			-	23.3 (1.27–69.6) vs. 29.1 (3.50–57.1)	-	-	-	-
Patients (top vs. bottom)	3939 vs. 1387	388 vs. 178	108 vs. 108	38 vs. 42	212 vs. 94	370 vs. 226	40 vs. 40	60 vs. 55
Clinical outcomes								
Conversions	Comparable		-	–	Comparable	Comparable	Comparable	Comparable
Anastomotic Leak	Comparable	Comparable	–	Comparable	Comparable	Comparable	Comparable	–
30-Day Mortality	Comparable	Comparable	–	–	–	Comparable	Comparable	–
Pathologic outcomes								
Completeness of TME	Comparable	Comparable	Comparable	–	Comparable	Comparable	–	Comparable
CRM Distance (mm)	–	–	Comparable	Comparable	-	19 (12–49) vs. 12 (5–20); $p < 0.001$	–	Comparable

CRM Involvement	Comparable	Comparable	Comparable	Comparable, T3-T4: 18.2% vs. 0%; p = 0.012	Comparable	Comparable	Comparable	-
DRM Distance (mm)	26.2 (23.5–28.8) vs. 21 (18.3–23.6); p = 0.007	Comparable	–	16.5 (2–72) vs. 25 (3–100); p = 0.021, T3-T4: comparable	Comparable	Comparable overall and for mid-rectal tumors, 9.6 ± 10.3 vs. 12.2 ± 10.2; p = 0.033 for low rectal tumors	Comparable	31 (19–45) vs. 19 (8–30); p = 0.007
DRM Involvement	–	–	–	–	Comparable	Comparable	-	–
Lymph Node Yield	Comparable	Comparable	–	–	–	Comparable	Comparable	Comparable
Overall Survival (months)	–	Comparable	–	Comparable, T3-T4: 21.4 (1.27–69.6) vs. 37.5 (3.5–57.1); p = 0.046	-	–	–	–
Disease Free Survival (months)	–	Comparable	–	15.7 (1–69.6) vs. 25.9 (0.8–57.1); p = 0.049, T3-T4: 11.1 (1.0–69.6) vs. 25.9 (0.8–57.1); p = 0.017	–	–	–	–
Overall Recurrence	–	Comparable	–	Comparable	–	–	–	–
Local Recurrence	–	Comparable	–	Comparable	–	–	–	–
Distant Recurrence	–	Comparable	–	Comparable	–	–	–	–

Recommendation

Patients in need of TME for rectal cancer can be offered treatment through transabdominal (top down) or transanal (bottom up) approaches. TaTME offers unique advantages relative to transabdominal approaches including decreased risk of conversion to open surgery compared to LapTME and increased rate of sphincter preservation. TaTME is particularly useful in patients with challenging anatomy and should be reserved for use in these groups as taTME does not offer a significant benefit over transabdominal approaches in tumors above the peritoneal reflection or in those with favorable anatomy.

1. Patients with low rectal cancers and those with mid rectal cancers and a hostile body habitus should be considered for treatment with taTME when performed at experienced centers. (Grade of recommendation: Weak recommendation based on moderate quality evidence, 2A)

Personal View

- TaTME is a clinically and oncologically safe alternative to transabdominal approaches to TME that offers unique benefits including decreased conversion rates and increased sphincter preservation.
- TaTME should be reserved for patients with mid-rectal tumors and challenging anatomy including narrow pelvis, visceral obesity, and enlarged prostate, and patients with tumors 4–6 cm from the anal verge, just above or abutting the anorectal ring.
- RCTs comparing taTME to LapTME and R-TME that focus on functional outcomes should be pursued to aid in future decision making.

References

1. Siegel RL, Wagle NS, Cercek A, Smith RA, Jemal A. Colorectal cancer statistics, 2023, vol. 73. CA: A Cancer Journal for Clinicians; 2023. p. 233–54.
2. Read B, Sylla P. Aggressive Colorectal Cancer in the Young. Clin Colon Rectal Surg. 2020;33(5):298–304.
3. Sylla P, Rattner DW, Delgado S, Lacy AM. NOTES transanal rectal cancer resection using transanal endoscopic microsurgery and laparoscopic assistance. Surg Endosc. 2010;24(5):1205–10.
4. Bonjer HJ, Deijen CL, Abis GA, Cuesta MA, van der Pas MH, de Lange-de Klerk ES, et al. A randomized trial of laparoscopic versus open surgery for rectal cancer. N Engl J Med. 2015;372(14):1324–32.
5. Green BL, Marshall HC, Collinson F, Quirke P, Guillou P, Jayne DG, et al. Long-term follow-up of the Medical Research Council CLASICC trial of conventional versus laparoscopically assisted resection in colorectal cancer. Br J Surg. 2013;100(1):75–82.
6. Park JW, Kang SB, Hao J, Lim SB, Choi HS, Kim DW, et al. Open versus laparoscopic surgery for mid or low rectal cancer after neoadjuvant chemoradiotherapy (COREAN trial): 10-year

follow-up of an open-label, non-inferiority, randomised controlled trial. Lancet Gastroenterol Hepatol. 2021;6(7):569–77.

7. Stevenson AR, Solomon MJ, Lumley JW, Hewett P, Clouston AD, Gebski VJ, et al. Effect of laparoscopic-assisted resection vs open resection on pathological outcomes in rectal cancer: The ALaCaRT randomized clinical trial. JAMA. 2015;314(13):1356–63.
8. Fleshman J, Branda M, Sargent DJ, Boller AM, George V, Abbas M, et al. Effect of laparoscopic-assisted resection vs open resection of stage II or III rectal cancer on pathologic outcomes: The ACOSOG Z6051 randomized clinical trial. JAMA. 2015;314(13):1346–55.
9. Fleshman J, Branda ME, Sargent DJ, Boller AM, George VV, Abbas MA, et al. Disease-free survival and local recurrence for laparoscopic resection compared with open resection of stage II to III rectal cancer: Follow-up results of the ACOSOG Z6051 randomized controlled trial. Ann Surg. 2019;269(4):589–95.
10. Kim MJ, Park SC, Park JW, Chang HJ, Kim DY, Nam BH, et al. Robot-assisted versus laparoscopic surgery for rectal cancer: a phase II open label prospective randomized controlled trial. Ann Surg. 2018;267(2):243–51.
11. Tang B, Gao GM, Zou Z, Liu DN, Tang C, Jiang QG, et al. Efficacy comparison between robot-assisted and laparoscopic surgery for mid-low rectal cancer: a prospective randomized controlled trial. Zhonghua Wei Chang Wai Ke Za Zhi. 2020;23(4):377–83.
12. Jayne D, Pigazzi A, Marshall H, Croft J, Corrigan N, Copeland J, et al. Effect of robotic-assisted vs conventional laparoscopic surgery on risk of conversion to open laparotomy among patients undergoing resection for rectal cancer: The ROLARR randomized clinical trial. JAMA. 2017;318(16):1569–80.
13. Feng Q, Yuan W, Li T, Tang B, Jia B, Zhou Y, et al. Robotic versus laparoscopic surgery for middle and low rectal cancer (REAL): short-term outcomes of a multicentre randomised controlled trial. Lancet Gastroenterol Hepatol. 2022;7(11):991–1004.
14. Gong J, Shi DB, Li XX, Cai SJ, Guan ZQ, Xu Y. Short-term outcomes of laparoscopic total mesorectal excision compared to open surgery. World J Gastroenterol. 2012;18(48):7308–13.
15. Ng SS, Lee JF, Yiu RY, Li JC, Hon SS, Mak TW, et al. Laparoscopic-assisted versus open total mesorectal excision with anal sphincter preservation for mid and low rectal cancer: a prospective, randomized trial. Surg Endosc. 2014;28(1):297–306.
16. Zhou ZG, Hu M, Li Y, Lei WZ, Yu YY, Cheng Z, et al. Laparoscopic versus open total mesorectal excision with anal sphincter preservation for low rectal cancer. Surg Endosc. 2004;18(8):1211–5.
17. Koëter T, de Nes LCF, Wasowicz DK, Zimmerman DDE, Verhoeven RHA, Elferink MA, et al. Hospital variation in sphincter-preservation rates in rectal cancer treatment: results of a population-based study in The Netherlands. BJS Open. 2021;5(4):zrab065.
18. Kantsevoy SV, Hu B, Jagannath SB, Vaughn CA, Beitler DM, Chung SS, et al. Transgastric endoscopic splenectomy: is it possible? Surg Endosc. 2006;20(3):522–5.
19. Bergström M, Ikeda K, Swain P, Park PO. Transgastric anastomosis by using flexible endoscopy in a porcine model (with video). Gastrointest Endosc. 2006;63(2):307–12.
20. Pai RD, Fong DG, Bundga ME, Odze RD, Rattner DW, Thompson CC. Transcolonic endoscopic cholecystectomy: a NOTES survival study in a porcine model (with video). Gastrointest Endosc. 2006;64(3):428–34.
21. Sylla P, Willingham FF, Sohn DK, Gee D, Brugge WR, Rattner DW. NOTES rectosigmoid resection using transanal endoscopic microsurgery (TEM) with transgastric endoscopic assistance: a pilot study in swine. J Gastrointest Surg. 2008;12(10):1717–23.
22. Telem DA, Han KS, Kim MC, Ajari I, Sohn DK, Woods K, et al. Transanal rectosigmoid resection via natural orifice translumenal endoscopic surgery (NOTES) with total mesorectal excision in a large human cadaver series. Surg Endosc. 2013;27(1):74–80.
23. Kang L, Chen YG, Zhang H, Zhang HY, Lin GL, Yang YC, et al. Transanal total mesorectal excision for rectal cancer: a multicentric cohort study. Gastroenterol Rep (Oxf). 2020;8(1):36–41.
24. Roodbeen SX, Spinelli A, Bemelman WA, Di Candido F, Cardepont M, Denost Q, et al. Local recurrence after transanal total mesorectal excision for rectal cancer: a multicenter cohort study. Ann Surg. 2021;274(2):359–66.

25. Perdawood SK, Kroeigaard J, Eriksen M, Mortensen P. Transanal total mesorectal excision: the Slagelse experience 2013–2019. Surg Endosc. 2021;35(2):826–36.
26. Roodbeen SX, Penna M, van Dieren S, Moran B, Tekkis P, Tanis PJ, et al. Local recurrence and disease-free survival after transanal total mesorectal excision: results from the international TaTME registry. J Natl Compr Cancer Netw. 2021;19(11):1232–40.
27. Serra-Aracil X, Zarate A, Bargalló J, Gonzalez A, Serracant A, Roura J, et al. Transanal versus laparoscopic total mesorectal excision for mid and low rectal cancer (Ta-LaTME study): multicentre, randomized, open-label trial. Br J Surg. 2022;110:150–8.
28. Sylla P Multicenter Phase II Study of Transanal TME (taTME) ClinicalTrials.gov: NIH; 2023 [Available from: https://clinicaltrials.gov/ct2/show/NCT03144765.
29. Deijen CL, Velthuis S, Tsai A, Mavroveli S, de Lange-de Klerk ES, Sietses C, et al. COLOR III: a multicentre randomised clinical trial comparing transanal TME versus laparoscopic TME for mid and low rectal cancer. Surg Endosc. 2016;30(8):3210–5.
30. Lelong B, de Chaisemartin C, Meillat H, Cournier S, Boher JM, Genre D, et al. A multicentre randomised controlled trial to evaluate the efficacy, morbidity and functional outcome of endoscopic transanal proctectomy versus laparoscopic proctectomy for low-lying rectal cancer (ETAP-GRECCAR 11 TRIAL): rationale and design. BMC Cancer. 2017;17(1):253.
31. McFadgen HL, Farooq AO. Indications and technical considerations for transanal total mesorectal excision. Dis Colon Rectum. 2022;65(8):958–61.
32. Sylla P, Knol JJ, D'Andrea AP, Perez RO, Atallah SB, Penna M, et al. Urethral injury and other urologic injuries during transanal total mesorectal excision: an international collaborative study. Ann Surg. 2021;274(2):e115–e25.
33. Dickson EA, Penna M, Cunningham C, Ratcliffe FM, Chantler J, Crabtree NA, et al. Carbon dioxide embolism associated with transanal total mesorectal excision surgery: a report from the international registries. Dis Colon Rectum. 2019;62(7):794–801.
34. Zhu Y, Wang W, Liu D, Zhang H, Chen L, Li Z, et al. Carbon dioxide embolism during transanal total mesorectal excision: case report and literature review. Front Surg. 2022;9:873964.
35. Denost Q, Adam JP, Rullier A, Buscail E, Laurent C, Rullier E. Perineal transanal approach: a new standard for laparoscopic sphincter-saving resection in low rectal cancer, a randomized trial. Ann Surg. 2014;260(6):993–9.
36. Denost Q, Loughlin P, Chevalier R, Celerier B, Didailler R, Rullier E. Transanal versus abdominal low rectal dissection for rectal cancer: long-term results of the Bordeaux' randomized trial. Surg Endosc. 2018;32(3):1486–94.
37. Liu H, Zeng Z, Zhang H, Wu M, Ma D, Wang Q, et al. Morbidity, mortality, and pathologic outcomes of transanal versus laparoscopic total mesorectal excision for rectal cancer short-term outcomes from a multicenter randomized controlled trial. Ann Surg. 2022;277(1):1–6.
38. Zeng Z, Luo S, Chen J, Cai Y, Zhang X, Kang L. Comparison of pathological outcomes after transanal versus laparoscopic total mesorectal excision: a prospective study using data from randomized control trial. Surg Endosc. 2020;34(9):3956–62.
39. Chen CC, Lai YL, Jiang JK, Chu CH, Huang IP, Chen WS, et al. Transanal total mesorectal excision versus laparoscopic surgery for rectal cancer receiving neoadjuvant chemoradiation: a matched case-control study. Ann Surg Oncol. 2016;23(4):1169–76.
40. Chen YT, Kiu KT, Yen MH, Chang TC. Comparison of the short-term outcomes in lower rectal cancer using three different surgical techniques: Transanal total mesorectal excision (TME), laparoscopic TME, and open TME. Asian J Surg. 2019;42(6):674–80.
41. Persiani R, Biondi A, Pennestrì F, Fico V, De Simone V, Tirelli F, et al. Transanal total mesorectal excision vs laparoscopic total mesorectal excision in the treatment of low and middle rectal cancer: a propensity score matching analysis. Dis Colon Rectum. 2018;61(7):809–16.
42. Detering R, Roodbeen SX, van Oostendorp SE, Dekker JT, Sietses C, Bemelman WA, et al. Three-year nationwide experience with transanal total mesorectal excision for rectal cancer in The Netherlands: a propensity score-matched comparison with conventional laparoscopic total mesorectal excision. J Am Coll Surg. 2019;228(3):235–44.e1.

43. Sparreboom CL, Komen N, Rizopoulos D, van Westreenen HL, Doornebosch PG, Dekker JWT, et al. Transanal total mesorectal excision: how are we doing so far? Color Dis. 2019;21(7):767–74.
44. de Lacy FB, Roodbeen SX, Ríos J, van Laarhoven J, Otero-Piñeiro A, Bravo R, et al. Three-year outcome after transanal versus laparoscopic total mesorectal excision in locally advanced rectal cancer: a multicenter comparative analysis. BMC Cancer. 2020;20(1):677.
45. Ye J, Tian Y, Li F, van Oostendorp S, Chai Y, Tuynman J, et al. Comparison of transanal total mesorectal excision (TaTME) versus laparoscopic TME for rectal cancer: a case matched study. Eur J Surg Oncol. 2021;47(5):1019–25.
46. Alhanafy MK, Park SS, Park SC, Park B, Kim MJ, Sohn DK, et al. Early experience with transanal total mesorectal excision compared with laparoscopic total mesorectal excision for rectal cancer: a propensity score-matched analysis. Dis Colon Rectum. 2020;63(11):1500–10.
47. Hol JC, Burghgraef TA, Rutgers MLW, Crolla R, van Geloven NAW, Hompes R, et al. Comparison of laparoscopic versus robot-assisted versus transanal total mesorectal excision surgery for rectal cancer: a retrospective propensity score-matched cohort study of short-term outcomes. Br J Surg. 2021;108(11):1380–7.
48. Pontallier A, Denost Q, Van Geluwe B, Adam JP, Celerier B, Rullier E. Potential sexual function improvement by using transanal mesorectal approach for laparoscopic low rectal cancer excision. Surg Endosc. 2016;30(11):4924–33.
49. Bjoern MX, Nielsen S, Perdawood SK. Quality of life after surgery for rectal cancer: a comparison of functional outcomes after transanal and laparoscopic approaches. J Gastrointest Surg. 2019;23(8):1623–30.
50. Dou R, Sun W, Luo S, Hou Y, Zhang C, Kang L. Comparison of postoperative bowel function between patients undergoing transanal and laparoscopic total mesorectal excision. Zhonghua Wei Chang Wai Ke Za Zhi. 2019;22(3):246–54.
51. Veltcamp Helbach M, Koedam TWA, Knol JJ, Velthuis S, Bonjer HJ, Tuynman JB, et al. Quality of life after rectal cancer surgery: differences between laparoscopic and transanal total mesorectal excision. Surg Endosc. 2019;33(1):79–87.
52. Rubinkiewicz M, Zarzycki P, Witowski J, Pisarska M, Gajewska N, Torbicz G, et al. Functional outcomes after resections for low rectal tumors: comparison of Transanal with laparoscopic Total Mesorectal excision. BMC Surg. 2019;19(1):79.
53. Bjoern MX, Perdawood SK. Manometric assessment of anorectal function after transanal total mesorectal excision. Tech Coloproctol. 2020;24(3):231–6.
54. Foo CC, Kin Ng K, Tsang JS, Siu-Hung Lo O, Wei R, Yip J, et al. Low anterior resection syndrome after transanal total mesorectal excision: a comparison with the conventional top-to-bottom approach. Dis Colon Rectum. 2020;63(4):497–503.
55. Ha RK, Park SC, Park B, Park SS, Sohn DK, Chang HJ, et al. Comparison of patient-reported quality of life and functional outcomes following laparoscopic and transanal total mesorectal excision of rectal cancer. Ann Surg Treat Res. 2021;101(1):1–12.
56. Miura T, Sakamoto Y, Morohashi H, Suto A, Kubota S, Ichisawa A, et al. Robotic surgery contributes to the preservation of bowel and urinary function after total mesorectal excision: comparisons with transanal and conventional laparoscopic surgery. BMC Surg. 2022;22(1):147.
57. Zeng Z, Liu Z, Luo S, Liang Z, Huang L, Ruan L, et al. Three-year outcomes of transanal total mesorectal excision versus standard laparoscopic total mesorectal excision for mid and low rectal cancer. Surg Endosc. 2022;36(6):3902–10.
58. Shin JK, Kim HC, Yun SH, Park YA, Cho YB, Huh JW, et al. Comparison of transanal total mesorectal excision and robotic total mesorectal excision for low rectal cancer after neoadjuvant chemoradiotherapy. Surg Endosc. 2021;35(12):6998–7004.
59. Lee L, de Lacy B, Gomez Ruiz M, Liberman AS, Albert MR, Monson JRT, et al. A multicenter matched comparison of transanal and robotic total mesorectal excision for mid and low-rectal adenocarcinoma. Ann Surg. 2019;270(6):1110–6.
60. Law WL, Foo DCC. Comparison of early experience of robotic and transanal total mesorectal excision using propensity score matching. Surg Endosc. 2019;33(3):757–63.

61. Perez D, Melling N, Biebl M, Reeh M, Baukloh JK, Miro J, et al. Robotic low anterior resection versus transanal total mesorectal excision in rectal cancer: A comparison of 115 cases. Eur J Surg Oncol. 2018;44(2):237–42.
62. Buan JLB, So WZ, Lim XC, Chong CS. Outcomes of robotic low anterior resection versus transanal total mesorectal excision for rectal cancer. BJS Open. 2021;5(5):zrab079.
63. Ryan OK, Ryan ÉJ, Creavin B, Rausa E, Kelly ME, Petrelli F, et al. Surgical approach for rectal cancer: a network meta-analysis comparing open, laparoscopic, robotic and transanal TME approaches. Eur J Surg Oncol. 2021;47(2):285–95.
64. Butterworth JW, Butterworth WA, Meyer J, Giacobino C, Buchs N, Ris F, et al. A systematic review and meta-analysis of robotic-assisted transabdominal total mesorectal excision and transanal total mesorectal excision: which approach offers optimal short-term outcomes for mid-to-low rectal adenocarcinoma? Tech Coloproctol. 2021;25(11):1183–98.
65. Grass JK, Persiani R, Tirelli F, Chen CC, Caricato M, Pecorino A, et al. Robotic versus transanal total mesorectal excision in sexual, anorectal, and urinary function: a multicenter, prospective, observational study. Int J Color Dis. 2021;36(12):2749–61.

Intracorporeal vs Extracorporeal Anastomosis for Right Colectomy

52

Henry J. Lujan and Victor Maciel

Minimally invasive surgery was introduced to colorectal surgery in 1991 with the original reports of laparoscopic colectomy [1]. This represented a radical change and part of an evolution in how colorectal surgery would be performed that has advanced to robotics. The robotic approach was introduced to colorectal surgery in 2002 [2]. Upgrades in the robotic platform have finally resulted in the increased adoption of minimally invasive techniques by colorectal surgeons [3].

Laparoscopic colorectal surgery has been around for over 30 years and has seen a relatively slow overall adoption and with the most common anastomotic techniques being extracorporeal. However, as a few surgeons became more familiar with and mastered minimally invasive suturing techniques, intracorporeal anastomosis became possible. From the minimally invasive approach to right colectomy has emerged the option of creating an anastomosis in an extracorporeal fashion or intracorporeal fashion. Similarly, the adoption of intracorporeal techniques has been slow to realization for most surgeons.

Laparoscopic intracorporeal anastomosis is considered an advanced technique and possibly the most technically challenging maneuver in minimally invasive colorectal surgery. It is considered so challenging that it has limited the application to expert surgeons with advanced skill sets. For those surgeons that were able to safely introduce intracorporeal anastomosis into their practices, there were perceived short-term advantages to this approach. However, robotics has introduced a stable platform with surgeon-controlled HD 3D visualization and advanced

H. J. Lujan (✉)
Jackson South Medical Center, Colon and Rectal Surgery, Miami, FL, USA
e-mail: Henry.Lujan@jhsmiami.org

V. Maciel
Allegheny General Hospital / St. Vincent Hospital, Colon and Rectal Surgery, Pittsburgh, PA, USA

K. Umanskiy, N. Hyman (eds.), *Difficult Decisions in Colorectal Surgery*, Difficult Decisions in Surgery: An Evidence-Based Approach,
https://doi.org/10.1007/978-3-031-42303-1_52

instrumentation that facilitates difficult tasks like intracorporeal suturing. Thus, with robotic right colectomy, intracorporeal anastomosis became the norm compared to laparoscopic right colectomy where extracorporeal remained and continues to be more common than intracorporeal.

With increasing publications suggesting advantages of intracorporeal anastomosis (ICA) over extracorporeal anastomosis (ECA), specifically in right colectomy (a common and key procedure in colon and rectal surgery) arises the great debate: Which is better?

PICO table

P	I	C	O
Patients requiring right colectomy	Right colectomy with intracorporeal anastomosis	Right colectomy with extracorporeal anastomosis	Outcomes: Operative time Conversion rate Complications Anastomotic leak Return of bowel function Length of stay Incision length Hernia

Search Strategy

A comprehensive literature search of PubMed, Cochrane Database of Systematic Reviews, MEDLINE was performed on 11/6/2022, to identify all the English-language publications related to intracorporeal versus extracorporeal anastomosis in right colectomy in the last 13 years.

The search prompts were (intracorporeal OR extracorporeal) AND anastomosis AND "right colectomy". Limits: Case Reports, Clinical Study, Clinical Trial, Comparative Study, Evaluation Study, Guideline, Meta-Analysis, Multicenter Study, Observational Study, Practice Guideline, Randomized Controlled Trial, Review, Systematic Review, in the last 13 years, English, Adult: 19+ years.

Studies were excluded if they did not directly contrast extracorporeal anastomosis to intracorporeal anastomosis in right colectomy, or if they failed to measure the studied variables. The references of the included studies were reviewed to identify additional studies. A total of 75 studies were identified and reviewed. Individual studies were discarded because they were of low and very low quality and were included in systematic reviews and meta-analysis. Four randomized, controlled trials (RCTs) were identified along with a meta-analysis of the 4 RCTs which were of moderate to high quality. Summary tables of the systematic reviews, meta-analyses, and RCTs were created, and recommendations are based on the studies found in the tables.

Results

Although not all studies addressed all the same outcomes of interest, there were enough outcomes in common that a few generalizations can be concluded. The main outcomes evaluated by most studies include operative time (OT), conversion rate, return of bowel function, length of stay (LOS), complications, anastomotic leak, incision length, and incisional hernia. Table 52.1. represents a summary of the meta-analysis that reviewed studies that directly compared ECA to ICA in right colectomy. Table 52.2. is a summary of the 4 available RCTs and the meta-analysis by Hajibandeh et al. [4] that combined the results of these trials. All the studies in Table 52.1. excluded robotic colectomy except Emile [5] [2019]. Only Van Oostendorp [6] [2017] included robotic cases but excluded studies that were totally robotic. Similarly, all 5 studies in Table 52.2. excluded robotics. In other words, the results presented in this chapter are based almost exclusively on laparoscopic right colectomy with intracorporeal anastomosis data. The literature contains moderate to high quality data for laparoscopic right colectomy with extracorporeal and intracorporeal anastomosis and is why these particular studies were chosen. Our conclusion for each outcome is stated below:

Table 52.1 Summary of meta-analysis that reviewed studies that directly compared ECA to ICA in right colectomy

Study	Number or patients	Measured outcome	Favors	Quality of evidence
Selvy (2020) [7]	3699	Operative time Conversion rate Complications Anastomotic leak Return of bowel function Length of stay Incision length Hernia	ICA Comparable Comparable Comparable ICA ICA N/A ICA	Moderate
Feroci (2013) [8]	425	Operative time Conversion rate Complications Anastomotic leak Return of bowel function Length of stay Incision length Hernia	Comparable N/A Comparable Comparable ICA ICA Comparable N/A	Moderate
Emile (2019) [5]	4450	Operative time Conversion rate Complications Anastomotic leak Return of bowel function Length of stay Incision length Hernia	Comparable ECA ECA ECA Comparable ICA ICA ECA	Moderate

(continued)

Table 52.1 (continued)

Study	Number or patients	Measured outcome	Favors	Quality of evidence
Ricci (2017) [9]	1717	Operative time Conversion rate Complications Anastomotic leak Return of bowel function Length of stay Incision length Hernia	Comparable Comparable ICA Comparable ICA ICA N/A ICA	Moderate
Wu (2017) [10]	1957	Operative time Conversion rate Complications Anastomotic leak Return of bowel function Length of stay Incision length Hernia	Comparable Comparable Comparable Comparable ICA ICA ICA Comparable	Moderate
Van Oostendorp (2017) [6]	1492	Operative time Conversion rate Complications Anastomotic leak Return of bowel function Length of stay Incision length Hernia	Comparable N/A ICA Comparable ICA ICA N/A N/A	Moderate
Cirocchi (2013) [11]	945	Operative time Conversion rate Complications Anastomotic leak Return of bowel function Length of stay Incision length Hernia	N/A N/A N/A Comparable ICA N/A ICA N/A	Moderate
Milone (2015) [12]	512	Operative time Conversion rate Complications Anastomotic leak Return of bowel function Length of stay Incision length Hernia	Comparable comparable ICA comparable ICA Comparable N/A N/A	Low

ICA Intracorporeal anastomosis, *ECA* Extracorporeal anastomosis, *N/A* Not available

Operative Times

Comparable. No data on OT was available in one meta-analysis. No study favored ECA. Operative times favored ICA in only one study and were comparable in 6.

Conversion Rates

Comparable. Conversion rates were comparable in 4 studies, favored ECA in only one study and no data was available in three studies. No study found better conversion rates for ICA.

Complications

Slightly favor ECA. In other words, studies tend to show fewer complications with ICA. Complications were comparable in 3 studies, favored ICA in 4 and ECA in only one. No conclusion reported in 1 study.

Anastomotic Leak

Comparable. The anastomotic leak rates were comparable in 6 studies. Only one study found fewer leaks with ECA.

Return of Bowel Function

Favors ICA, most studies show quicker return of bowel function with ICA. Return of bowel function was measured by return to flatus or first bowel movement and was often reported by day or hour at several points during the postoperative period. For example, return to bowel function was 1.5 days for ICA compared to 1.8 days for ECA ($p < 0.0001$) by Cleary et al. Authors concluded that return of bowel function was quicker with ICA in 7 studies and comparable in 1.

Length of Stay

Favor ICA. Length of stay was shorter for ICA in 6 studies and no data regarding length of stay was reported in 2 studies. No studies showed shorter length of stay with ECA.

Table 52.2 Summary of the four available RCTs and the meta-analysis of these RCTs

study	Patients (N) IC vs EC.	Measured outcome	Favors	Quality of evidence
Vignali (2016) [13]	30 vs 30	Operative time Conversion rate Complications Anastomotic leak Return of bowel function Length of stay Incision length Hernia	ECA Comparable Comparable ECA ICA Comparable ICA N/A	High
Mari (2018) [15]	30 vs 30	Operative time Conversion rate Complications Anastomotic leak Return of bowel function Length of stay Incision length Hernia	Comparable Comparable ECA ICA ICA N/A N/A N/A	High
Bollo(2020) [14]	69 vs 70	Operative time Conversion rate Complications Anastomotic leak Return of bowel function Length of stay Incision length Hernia	ECA N/A ICA Comparable ICA ICA ICA N/A	High
Allaix (2019) [16]	70 vs 70	Operative time Conversion rate Complications Anastomotic leak Return of bowel function Length of stay Incision length Hernia	Comparable ICA Comparable Comparable ICA Comparable Comparable Comparable	High
Hajibandeh (2020) [4]	199 vs 200	Operative time Conversion rate Complications Anastomotic leak Return of bowel function Length of stay Incision length Hernia	Comparable Comparable Comparable Comparable Comparable ICA ICA N/A	High

ICA Intracorporeal anastomosis, *ECA* Extracorporeal anastomosis, *N/A* Not available, *Vs* Versus

Incision Length

Favor ICA, most studies show shorter incisions with ICA. Three studies reported shorter incision lengths for ICA, one reported comparable length between ICA and ECA, 4 studies did not include data on incision lengths.

Incisional Hernia

Not enough long-term data but possibly favor ECA, in other words fewer hernias are seen with ICA. Incisional hernia rates were reported in only 4 studies. 2 favored ICA, 1 favored ECA, and one reported comparable incidence of incisional hernias.

Randomized Controlled Trials

Table 52.2. is a summary of the 4 randomized, controlled trials (RCTs) [13–16] and the meta-analysis of these same 4 studies by Hajibandeh et al. [4] All the RCT had small numbers but represent the highest level of data available.

Operative Times

Comparable. In regard to operative times (OT) Vignali [13] compared 30 ECA versus 30 ICA and shorter operative times were seen for EC anastomosis, however, in the meta-analysis by Hajibandeh, OTs were comparable across all 4 studies [4].

Conversion Rates

Comparable. Conversion rates were comparable across all studies.

Return of Bowel Function

Favor ICA, return of bowel function is quicker with ICA. Return of bowel function favored ICA in 3 of the 4 RCTs and ileus was addressed by the meta-analysis and favored ICA in the same 3 of 4 RCTs.

Length of Stay

Favor ICA, Length of stay was shorter for ICA in 3 studies and in the meta-analysis.

Incision Length

Favor ICA, Incision lengths were shorter for ICA in 2 studies, one reported comparable lengths and one did not report on data on incision lengths.

Incisional Hernia

Comparable. Only one study reported on incisional hernia and found no statistically significant differences between ICA and ECA.

Recommendations Based on the Data

Over the past two decades, most studies comparing extracorporeal anastomosis to intracorporeal anastomosis for right colectomy have been based on retrospective, small series, or observational studies and, thus, of very low quality or low-quality data. More recently, 4 prospective, randomized controlled trials (RCT) and a meta-analysis of the same 4 RCT has shed some light on the perceived advantages of ICA and improved the level of evidence on the topic [4, 13–16]. For the most part, the RCT and meta-analysis have supported the results of lower quality studies.

Intracorporeal anastomosis is associated with short term benefits. Specifically, ICA has shorter incisions, quicker return of bowel function, shorter LOS, and possibly fewer minor complications. These benefits also seem to be mostly related to smaller incisions that can be placed lower in the abdomen resulting in fewer extraction site complications. Furthermore, because the anastomosis tends to require less manipulation of the bowel and its mesentery faster return of bowel function occurs, possibly less ileus and thus shorter LOS. (Evidence: Moderate; Recommendation: Moderate).

Some points are worthy of noting. For robotic right colectomy unlike with laparoscopic right colectomy, the norm is to perform ICA. In some ways, laparoscopic ICA is limited to highly skilled surgeons with advanced skill sets and intracorporeal suturing skills. High-quality data for robotic right colectomy with ICA is lacking in the literature. However, the robotic outcomes in available observational and comparative studies are similar to the results presented in the tables and studies reviewed in this chapter [17]. Secondly, Enhanced recovery after surgery (ERAS) protocols and enhanced recovery like practices probably varied significantly between studies. The increasing adoption of ERAS by medical institutions in the past decade has possibly influenced the results of some factors like length of stay which are common measures used to evaluate the advantages and disadvantages of anastomotic techniques. The uneven adoption of the ERAS protocols should be considered when interpreting the purported benefits of ICA.

Personal View of the Data

I had the good fortune of doing my Colon and Rectal Fellowship in 1996 with one of the pioneers in laparoscopic colectomy, Dr. Sergio Larach at the Colon and Rectal Clinic of Orlando in Orlando, Florida and when laparoscopic colectomy was in its early years. The following year I joined a Colon and Rectal Surgery practice in Miami, Florida. Dr. Moises Jacobs and Dr. Gustavo Plasencia were my senior partners, pioneers in laparoscopic colon surgery as well and who founded one of the first Fellowships in Minimally Invasive Surgery in the United States. Since the introduction of minimally invasive surgery to colectomy in the early 1990s by these same surgeons, laparoscopic and later robotic approaches to colectomy have brought about radical changes in surgical techniques. At the start of this revolution, the most common anastomotic techniques were extracorporeal. As a few surgeons became more familiar with and mastered minimally invasive suturing techniques, intracorporeal anastomosis became possible. However, the adoption of intracorporeal techniques has been slow to realization for most surgeons. Robotics likely accelerated the conversion to intracorporeal anastomosis specifically in right colectomy because it facilitated intracorporeal suturing and made this skill set available to even more surgeons. Previously, the slow adoption was likely due to the perceived difficulty with suturing in a closed space, the feeling of lack of control, and the concern for risk of intra-abdominal infection.

When I learned laparoscopic right colectomy, it was done almost exclusively with ECA. Although we dabbled in ICA for right colectomy on a few occasions, it was felt to be too technically demanding and not worth the effort. In addition, there were fears of contamination or spillage that might occur from colotomy or enterotomy, and concerns about that the anastomosis could not be made to be air and watertight without handling it under direct view as opposed to via a camera and monitor. Historically, we had been taught as a general surgical principle, the notion that the anastomosis is the critical aspect of the case and should be done in our hands, under direct view, and under dexterous control to ensure no technical errors would occur.

To my knowledge, there were few if any surgeons performing ICA for right colectomy in the late 1990s or early 2000s except for maybe Dr. Morris Franklin [18] who touted its routine use. Laparoscopic ICA is still considered by many to be the most technically challenging maneuver in laparoscopic colectomy and limited its broad adoption. My own experience with laparoscopic courses, surgical society meetings, case observations, and proctoring reinforced this general attitude towards ICA. Most surgeons either lacked the skill set or feared this specific maneuver and thus performed ECA [3].

In 2009, I was trained in robotic colectomy. I performed 2 robotic right colectomies with ECA and then adopted ICA and have almost abandoned the ECA for right colectomy. It was such an immediate and natural transition that I have to credit robotics for making it possible. In fact, when ICA became my routine, our practice began performing ICA in laparoscopic right colectomy more frequently. Then, with the advent of barbed suture, ICA became the preferred technique not only for robotic surgery but for laparoscopic right colectomy as well. The barbed suture allowed for the easy and consistent closure of the common enterotomy in an iso-peristaltic side-to-side ileocolic anastomosis. The iso-peristaltic side-to-side ileocolic anastomosis remains the most commonly performed type of ICA. Thus, using the robot taught me how to perform the ICA so we could safely apply the technique in our laparoscopic cases.

I believe the robot and its 3D HD visualization, the stable platform with surgeon-controlled camera, and ability to suture in a controlled and precise manner was the key to adopting ICA. It took away the fear and instilled confidence in me to perform the anastomosis safely and consistently. The anastomosis, which for laparoscopic cases I considered difficult and tricky at times because of the technical challenges of working through a small incision (especially in obese patients with thick abdominal walls or patients with short mesenteries) became the easiest, most reliable, and reproducible portion of the procedure when performed intracorporeally. In fact, I found when teaching the procedure to residents and fellows, it was the first part of a right colectomy that I turned over to them to complete independently. I had less worry about allowing a trainee to perform the anastomosis than to do a medial to lateral dissection!

The isoperistaltic side-to-side anastomosis is the only ICA we perform for right colectomy. Because of natural orientation of the terminal ileum mesentery and the standardized port placement (especially for the stapler) used for minimally invasive colectomy, it is very consistent and reproducible. In our hands, we have leak rates below the published rates commonly quoted for right colectomy. Our extraction sites are smaller, specimen lengths longer, fewer complications, and hernia rates less than for ECA. Operative times are longer, however, all other outcomes including return of bowel function, LOS, lymph node harvest, conversion rates, and readmissions are comparable [3].

Interestingly, when you review the robotic literature on ICA for right colectomy, it is almost exclusively with ICA. That was not the case until recently with laparoscopic right colectomy data which was almost exclusively with ECA. In the last 10 years there has been a sudden increase in publications with laparoscopic right colectomy and ICA. Several authors have attributed this due to an increased ability of dedicated laparoscopic surgeons; this technique has gained popularity and interest as testified by the several meta-analyses comparing ICA vs. ECA published in the literature in the last 10 years [3, 5–8, 10, 11, 18].

This was my journey to ICA and by no means do I want to claim that the above-mentioned observations were in any way the only journey or even an important one. There are so many great surgeons who deserve much more credit and recognition. And although many of them can be found in the references listed below, there are many great contributors to minimally invasive surgery and ICA that are not mentioned.

I perform ICA because it is technically less challenging in my hands and with my skill set (especially in the obese patient) whether laparoscopic or robotic. Furthermore, extraction sites are smaller and easier to protect, because the only manipulation on the extraction site wound is the wound protector briefly to remove the specimen. Therefore, wound complications such as wound infection and hernia are likely less. The data suggest that short term benefits are associated with ICA. I suspect that long-term outcomes are similar except for less extraction site hernias. Long-term, ICA is likely equivalent to ECA for the patient. However, I can confidently say that once a surgeon performs ICA, it is very unlikely he will continue to perform ECA with any regularity.

Finally, when comparing laparoscopic right colectomy with ICA to robotic right colectomy with ICA, similar efficacy, safety, and outcomes are seen. The procedure is longer with the robot but with some possible clinical advantages. Future studies may show that, in obese and other technically challenging patients, robotics facilitates resection of a longer, consistent specimen with less mesentery trauma that can be extracted through smaller incisions. Furthermore, the anastomosis can be created in a more reliable, reproducible, and easier manner than with standard laparoscopy. Future studies could address whether robotic ICA is more reliable than laparoscopic ICA. In any event, the minimally invasive surgeon that practices colon and rectal surgery should have intracorporeal anastomosis in their armamentarium.

References

1. Jacobs M, Verdeja JC, Goldstein HS. Minimally invasive colon resection (laparoscopic colectomy). Surg Laparosc Endosc. 1991;1(3):144–50.
2. Weber PA, et al. Telerobotic-assisted laparoscopic right and sigmoid colectomies for benign disease. Dis Colon Rectum. 2002;45(12):1689–94;discussion 1695-6
3. Lujan HJ, et al. Advantages of robotic right colectomy with intracorporeal anastomosis. Surg Laparosc Endosc Percutan Tech. 2018;28(1):36–41.
4. Hajibandeh S, et al. Meta-analysis of randomised controlled trials comparing intracorporeal versus extracorporeal anastomosis in laparoscopic right hemicolectomy: upgrading the level of evidence. Updat Surg. 2021;73(1):23–33.
5. Emile SH, et al. Intracorporeal versus extracorporeal anastomosis in minimally invasive right colectomy: an updated systematic review and meta-analysis. Tech Coloproctol. 2019;23(11):1023–35.
6. van Oostendorp S, et al. Intracorporeal versus extracorporeal anastomosis in right hemicolectomy: a systematic review and meta-analysis. Surg Endosc. 2017;31(1):64–77.
7. Selvy M, et al. Intra-versus extracorporeal anastomosis in laparoscopic right colectomy: a meta-analysis of 3699 patients. Int J Color Dis. 2020;35(9):1673–80.
8. Feroci F, et al. Intracorporeal versus extracorporeal anastomosis after laparoscopic right hemicolectomy for cancer: a systematic review and meta-analysis. Int J Color Dis. 2013;28(9):1177–86.
9. Ricci C, et al. A critical and comprehensive systematic review and meta-analysis of studies comparing intracorporeal and extracorporeal anastomosis in laparoscopic right hemicolectomy. Langenbeck's Arch Surg. 2017;402(3):417–27.
10. Wu Q, et al. Intracorporeal versus extracorporeal anastomosis in laparoscopic right colectomy: a systematic review and meta-analysis. J Laparoendosc Adv Surg Tech A. 2017;27(4):348–57.
11. Cirocchi R, et al. Intracorporeal versus extracorporeal anastomosis during laparoscopic right hemicolectomy - systematic review and meta-analysis. Surg Oncol. 2013;22(1):1–13.
12. Milone M, et al. Intracorporeal versus extracorporeal anastomosis. Results from a multicentre comparative study on 512 right-sided colorectal cancers. Surg Endosc. 2015;29(8):2314–20.

13. Vignali A, et al. Extracorporeal vs. Intracorporeal ileocolic stapled anastomoses in laparoscopic right colectomy: an interim analysis of a randomized clinical trial. J Laparoendosc Adv Surg Tech A. 2016;26(5):343–8.
14. Bollo J, et al. Randomized clinical trial of intracorporeal versus extracorporeal anastomosis in laparoscopic right colectomy (IEA trial). Br J Surg. 2020;107(4):364–72.
15. Mari GM, et al. Intracorporeal anastomosis reduces surgical stress response in laparoscopic right hemicolectomy: a prospective randomized trial. Surg Laparosc Endosc Percutan Tech. 2018;28(2):77–81.
16. Allaix ME, et al. Intracorporeal or extracorporeal ileocolic anastomosis after laparoscopic right colectomy: a double-blinded randomized controlled trial. Ann Surg. 2019;270(5):762–7.
17. Cleary RK, et al. Intracorporeal and extracorporeal anastomosis for robotic-assisted and laparoscopic right colectomy: short-term outcomes of a multi-center prospective trial. Surg Endosc. 2022;36(6):4349–58.
18. Franklin ME Jr, et al. Laparoscopic right hemicolectomy for cancer: 11-year experience. Rev Gastroenterol Mex. 2004;69(Suppl 1):65–72.

53 Anastomotic Leak Management Following Low Anterior Resections

Sarah Choi and Kyle G. Cologne

Introduction

Anastomotic leaks commonly occur after low anterior resections (LAR) and are among the most feared complications encountered by surgeons. Although, overall mortality rates remain low (~2%) following LAR, one-third of all postoperative deaths occur in patients with an anastomotic leak [5]. Anastomotic leaks also result in increased rates of patient morbidity, longer hospital stays, higher costs of hospitalizations, increased risk of permanent stomas, and poor anorectal function (increased frequency, urgency, incontinence, and incomplete evacuation) [1–3, 6, 7]. Despite an extensive amount of literature addressing risk factors and methods of prevention, anastomotic leaks following low anterior resections continue to occur [4].

Anastomotic leak is a difficult subject with innumerable definitions. A proposed definition for an anastomotic leak has been described as "a leak of luminal contents from a surgical join between two hollow viscera" [8]. In 2010, the International Study Group of Rectal Cancer defined it as a "defect of the intestinal wall at the anastomotic site leading to a communication between the intra- and extraluminal component" and developed a grading system based on clinical management once a leak was diagnosed. Grade A leaks are those managed expectantly, Grade B leaks are those requiring a therapeutic intervention but not necessarily a re-operation, and Grade C leaks are those that require a re-operation [9].

It is well recognized that the urgency and invasiveness with which a leak is managed depends on the severity of the leak as determined by the hemodynamic

S. Choi · K. G. Cologne (✉)
Division of Colon and Rectal Surgery, Department of Surgery, Keck School of Medicine, University of Southern California, Los Angeles, CA, USA
e-mail: Sarah.Choi@med.usc.edu; Kyle.Cologne@med.usc.edu

K. Umanskiy, N. Hyman (eds.), *Difficult Decisions in Colorectal Surgery*, Difficult Decisions in Surgery: An Evidence-Based Approach,
https://doi.org/10.1007/978-3-031-42303-1_53

stability of the patient, location of the anastomosis (intraperitoneal vs extraperitoneal), and size of the anastomotic defect. Smaller, contained leaks in clinically stable patients can be managed expectantly while larger ones need percutaneous drainage or re-operative intervention for proximal diversion or drainage of uncontrolled sepsis. A high clinical suspicion and expedited diagnosis is paramount in proper management of an anastomotic leak.

Management of an Anastomotic Leak

Anastomotic leaks can present in various ways and timeframes, from a subtle and insidious manner weeks after an operation to excruciating abdominal pain with hemodynamic instability and diffuse peritonitis often days after an operation. Abnormal vital signs (fever, tachycardia, hypotension, tachypnea, etc.) and laboratory values (leukocytosis, elevated C-reactive protein or procalcitonin, etc.) as well as derangements in cardiorespiratory, gastrointestinal, or urinary systems may be the first signs of a leak and expedited diagnostic work-up is warranted, but are also non-specific and thus make diagnosis difficult.

Patients with hemodynamic instability with a high clinical suspicion for anastomotic leak should be taken back immediately to the operating room regardless of the location or size of anastomotic defect, with the aim of controlling life-threatening sepsis. Fluid resuscitation and intravenous antibiotics should be initiated prior to the operating room. The abdomen should be washed out and the anastomosis resected with creation of an end stoma, with or without a mucous fistula. In selective cases, if the patient is hemodynamically stable during the operation and intraoperative findings show no gross spillage of stool or bowel ischemia, a resection and re-anastomosis with proximal diversion may be considered.

In contrast, subclinical leaks, found incidentally on imaging studies, are managed with observation regardless of the location of the leak. The nuances of managing the different size and location of anastomotic leaks in a hemodynamically stable patient will be discussed below.

Intraperitoneal Anastomotic Leaks

Due to the location of the anastomosis, intraperitoneal leaks often present with generalized or localized peritonitis and present earlier than extraperitoneal leaks that present insidiously in a delayed fashion due to lack an innervated peritoneal surface [10]. A leak after a low anterior resection is particularly challenging due to nature of a very short rectal stump and requirement of likely a pull-through and hand-sewn coloanal anastomosis if the anastomosis were to be resected with creation of an end stoma [11].

Intraperitoneal leaks in patients that are hemodynamically stable can be diagnosed by radiological imaging (CT scan with oral/rectal contrast or water-soluble contrast enema (WSCE)) or by digital rectal exam for low colorectal or coloanal anastomoses. If imaging shows an uncontained free-flowing leak into the abdomen, a trip to the operating room for washout and exploration of the anastomosis is necessary. For patients with high-risk for another leak such as those who are septic, hypotensive, malnourished, or diagnosed with inflammatory bowel disease, an operation with resection and creation of an end stoma is recommended. For larger anastomotic defects (described as >1 cm or > 1/third of the circumference) or with ischemic appearing ends of the bowel, a resection with re-anastomosis and proximal diversion may help restore gastrointestinal continuity while promote healing of the anastomosis [10]. For smaller anastomotic defects (<1 cm or < 1/3rd of the circumference), a primary suture repair of the anastomosis with primary diversion may be feasible. If no anastomotic defect can be identified or if a phlegmon is present preventing exploration of the anastomosis due to the risk of causing more harm, a proximal diverting ostomy or placement of drains may be required. In all scenarios the use of copious irrigation to washout the abdomen as well as the placement of perianastomotic drains is imperative in controlling sepsis.

For intraperitoneal leaks that are contained, intravenous antibiotics and drainage of the fluid collections are key principles in management. For large abscesses (>3 cm) that are contained, a CT guided drainage procedure should be performed after discussion with the interventional radiologist regarding the feasibility of the procedure [12]. For smaller abscesses (<3 cm), intravenous antibiotics alone may treat the leak [13]; however, aspiration of the abscess may be another option depending on the accessibility of the fluid collection. For patients that do not improve despite drainage or are unable to get their large abscess drained, an operation should be strongly considered for intraoperative assessment of the anastomosis and operative management similar to those with an uncontained leak.

PICO table

Patients	Interventions	Comparator	Outcome
Patients with low pelvic anastomotic leaks	Surgical trans-anal drainage	Interventional Radiology percutaneous drainage	Resolution of sepsis

Search Strategy

A comprehensive literature search of Cochrane database, MEDLINE, and PubMed was performed to identify English-language publications related to treatment of anastomotic leaks in colorectal surgery. Relevant studies published between 1945 and December 2022 were identified with key search terms including the following: "anastomotic leak", "proctectomy", "rectal cancer", "treatment", "management", "transanal", and "low anterior resection". Exclusion criteria included studies primarily focusing on risk factors or prevention of anastomotic leaks as well as those discussing other types of anastomoses (ileocolic, colo-colonic) and treatment options (endoluminal vacuum therapy).

Study	Patients (N) Trans-anal drainage vs. percutaneous drainage	Need for additional procedures due to failure	Quality of Evidence
Creavin [19]	2 vs. 24	0 vs 2 (8.3%)	Low
Vu [20]	2 vs. 9	0 vs. 3 (33%)	Low
Kirat [21]	53 vs. 18	13 (24.5%) vs. 3 (17%)	Low
Blumetti [22]	1 vs. 32	1 (100%) vs. 12 (37.5%)	Low

Personal View

For extraperitoneal leaks that are contained, intravenous antibiotics and drainage of the fluid collections are key principles in management, identical to that of intraperitoneal leaks. For large abscesses (>3 cm) that are contained and those that are in continuity with the leak but remains extraperitoneal, a drainage procedure should be performed. For smaller contained abscesses (<3 cm), intravenous antibiotics alone may resolve the infection.

Patients requiring drainage procedure for a low pelvic anastomotic leak can undergo either surgical placement of a trans-anal drain or a percutaneous drain placement by Interventional Radiology for adequate sepsis control. Only a few studies have compared the two methods of sepsis control with no significant differences found comparing the rates of failure. For surgically placed drains, an exam under anesthesia (EUA), with or without a flexible sigmoidoscopy, to drain the abscess trans-anally or trans-anastomotically can be completed. Some may elect to place a small drain (Red rubber Robinson catheter or Malecot catheter) into the abscess cavity to facilitate continued drainage and shrinkage of the tract while others may elect to open up the anastomotic defect with a finger or instrument to facilitate drainage via the anal canal [14].

Things to consider in terms of choosing the appropriate approach may be guided by the location of the leak (need for transrectal, transgluteal, transabdominal drain) as well as feasibility of outpatient management (need for return to OR for exchange). Additional things to consider include complications associated with each procedure including formation of fistula, bleeding, infection, and drain site pain for percutaneous drains and need for multiple EUAs or flexible sigmoidoscopies +/− sedation and general anesthesia for surgically placed drains.

For extraperitoneal leaks that already have a proximal diverting ostomy, management depends on whether the anastomotic leak presents as clinical or subclinical leak. For leaks that present symptomatically with signs of peritonitis or sepsis or radiologically with findings of an abscess, management is as described above. For leaks that are subclinical and found incidentally on imaging (usually done prior to discussion for diverting stoma reversal), management will depend on location of the leak. For intraperitoneal subclinical leaks with proximal diversion, continued observation (with or without intravenous antibiotics) and re-imaging in 6 to 8 weeks intervals up to 6 months is acceptable [10]. If the leak persists on imaging at 6 months or an anastomotic stricture is identified via WSCE, a surgical revision of anastomosis would be necessary. For extraperitoneal subclinical leaks with proximal diversion, management depends on the size of the chronic sinus tract. If small (<1 cm), the sinus tract is not a contraindication for proximal diverting ostomy reversal [10]. If large (>1 cm), a flexible catheter may be placed through the cavity and downsized every 3 to 4 weeks to facilitate closure of the cavity [6].

Newer Interventions for Anastomotic Leaks

Newer advancements aiming to salvage the anastomoses have been developed and used in management of low colorectal anastomotic leaks, especially for those who have already been proximally diverted. These newer approaches have variable success rates and should be individualized to the patient and the clinical situation.

The endosponge is an endoscopically placed sponge placed through the anastomotic defect and into the abscess cavity and connected to a negative pressure vacuum drainage system. This method was first described in Germany in 2008 and showed successful treatment in 29 out of 34 patients with a mean duration of therapy of 34 days and requiring an average of 11 exchanges and downsizing of the sponge [15]. Proponents of the endosponge treatment feel that the sponge not only stents open the anus and allows for unobstructed drainage of the cavity but also facilitates decreased size of the cavity over time [16]. Despite FDA approval and experience of use in Europe, the endosponge vacuum device is not manufactured in the United States.

Endoscopic stenting has also been described in managing anastomotic leaks. The stents (covered or self-expandable metal) can only be placed across an end-to-end anastomosis and requires the distal extent of the stent to be at least 5 cm above anal verge [17]. Stent migration is a major complication of this method and despite its success seen in limited studies, may limit their use in most situations.

Lastly, endoscopic clips have been described as an endoscopic treatment method for anastomotic leaks. The over-the-scope clips are larger and allow for full thickness closure of a defect less than 1.5 cm in size and without an associated abscess cavity [18]. A smaller series showed success in 86% of 14 leaks treated using this method with 2 with diverting stomas at the time of clip placement. This method may be limited by its strict criteria for use but can be one option to manage anastomotic leaks.

Conclusion

Anastomotic leaks continue to occur despite newer techniques to try to prevent them such as intraoperative assessment of blood supply using Indocyanine Green (ICG) intravenously and performing an intraoperative leak test. Therefore, it is paramount to maintain a high clinical suspicion for an anastomotic leak and manage them appropriately depending on the severity of the leak, often determined by the patient's hemodynamic status as well as the size and location of the defect. Expeditious diagnosis and management of the leak as described in this chapter will help minimize the potential increased morbidity and mortality of this dreaded complication.

References

1. Lindgren R, Hallböök O, Rutegård J, Sjödahl R, Matthiessen P. What is the risk for a permanent stoma after low anterior resection of the rectum for cancer? A six-year follow-up of a multicenter trial. Dis Colon Rectum. 2011;54:41–7.
2. Ogilvie JW Jr, James W, Dietz DW, Stocchi L. Anastomotic leak after restorative proctosgmoidectomy for cancer: what are the chances of a permanent ostomy? Int J Color Dis. 2012;27:1259–66.
3. Nesbakken A, Nygaard K, Lunde OC. Outcome and late functional results after anastomotic leakage following mesorectal excision for rectal cancer. Br J Surg. 2001;3:400–4.
4. Paun BC, Cassie S, MacLean AR, Dixon E, Buie WD. Postoperative complications following surgery for rectal cancer. Ann Surg. 2010;251(5):807–18.
5. Snijders HS, Wouters MW, van Leersum NJ, Kolfschoten NE, Henneman D, de Vries AC, Tollenaar RA, Bonsing BA. Meta-analysis of the risk for anastomotic leakage, the postoperative mortality caused by leakage in relation to the overall postoperative mortality. Eur J Surg Oncol. 2012;38:1013–9.
6. Hallbook O, Sjodahl R. Anastomotic leakage and functional outcome after anterior resection of the rectum. Br J Surg. 1996;83(1):60–2.
7. Makela JT, Kiviniemi H, Litnen S. Risk factors for anastomotic leak after left-sided colorectal resection with rectal anastomosis. Dis Colon Rectum. 2003;46:653–60.
8. Peel AL, Taylor EW. Proposed definitions for the audit of postoperative infection: a discussion paper. Surgical infection study group. Ann R Coll Surg Engl. 1991;73:385–8.
9. Rahbari NN, Weitz J, Hohenberger W, et al. Definition and grading of anastomotic leakage following anterior resection of rectum: a proposal by the international study group of rectal cancer. Surgery. 2010;147(3):339–51.
10. Phitayakorn R, Delaney CP, Reynolds HL, Champagne BJ, Heriot AG, Neary P, Senagore AJ. Standardized algorithms for management of anastomotic leaks and related abdominal and pelvic abscesses after colorectal surgery. World J Surg. 2008;32(6):1147–56.
11. Umanskiy K, Hyman N. Anastomotic complications. In: The ASCRS textbook of colon and rectal surgery. Springer; 2016. p. 161–71.
12. Siewart B, Tye G, Kruskal J, et al. Impact of CT-guided drainage in the treatment of diverticular abscess: size matters. AJR Am J Roentgenol. 2006;186:680–868.
13. Kumar RR, Kim JT, Haukoos JS, et al. Factors affecting the successful management of intra-abdominal abscess with antibiotics and the need for percutaneous drainage. Dis Colon Rectum. 2006;49:183–9.
14. Sirosi-Gigurere E, Boulanger-Gobeil C, Bouchard A, et al. Transanal drainage to treat anastomotic leaks after low anterior resection for rectal cancer: a valuable option. Dis Colon Rectum. 2013;56(5):586–92.
15. Weidenhagen R, Gruetzner KU, Wiecken T, Spelsberg F, Jauch KW. Endoscopic vacuum-assisted closure of anastomotic leakage following anterior resection of the rectum: a new method. Surg Endosc. 2008;22:1818–25.
16. Blumetti K, Abcarian H. Management of low colorectal anastomotic leak: preserving the anastomosis. World J Gastrointest Surg. 2015;7(12):378–83.
17. DiMaio CJ, Dorfman MP, Gardner GJ, Nash GM, Schattner MA, Markowitz AJ, Chi DS, Gerdes H. Covered esophageal self-expandable metal stents in the nonoperative management of postoperative colorectal anastomotic leaks. Gastrointest Endosc. 2012;76:421–35.

18. Arezzo A, Verra M, Reddavid R, Cravero F, Bonino MA, Morino M. Efficacy of the over-the-scope clip (OTSC) for treatment of colorectal postsurgical leaks and fistulas. Surg Endosc. 2012;26:3330–3.
19. Creavin B, Ryan ÉJ, Kelly ME, Moynihan A, Redmond CE, Ahern D, et al. Minimally invasive approaches to the management of anastomotic leakage following restorative rectal cancer resection. Color Dis. 2019;21(12):1364–71.
20. Vu L, Penter C, Platell C. Long-term significance of an anastomotic leak in patients undergoing an ultra-low anterior resection for rectal cancer. ANZ J Surg. 2019;89:1291–5.
21. Kirat HT, Remzi FH, Shen B, Kiran RP. Pelvic abscess associated with anastomotic leak in patients with ileal pouch-anal anastomosis (IPAA): transanastomotic or CT-guided drainage? Int J Color Dis. 2011;26(11):1469–74.
22. Blumetti J, Chaudhry V, Cintron JR. Management of anastomotic leak: lessons learned from a large colon and rectal surgery training program. World J Surg. 2014;38(04):985–91.

Colorectal Anastomosis Construction: Is there a Benefit to a Reservoir?

54

Matthew Z. Wilson and David B. Stewart

Introduction

Given the rectum serves as a reservoir for flatus and stool, allowing deferral of the urge to defecate until an opportune moment, it is understandable that clinical data has suggested that removal of part or all of the rectum will result in altered bowel habits. These alterations can vary from increased frequency, to fractionated and/or segmented bowel movements, to urgency and fecal incontinence [1, 2]. More recently, these symptoms have noted to occur concurrently as a functional abnormality referred to as low anterior resection syndrome (LARS), which can represent a chronic condition of altered intestinal function [3, 4]. To minimize some of these complaints, especially those related to frequency and incontinence, surgeons have adapted anastomotic techniques that are purported to improve postoperative function compared to a straight colorectal or coloanal anastomosis [5, 6]. In part, the acknowledgement that the colon is not as distensible as the rectum and that it does not have a function that mimics the accommodation response observed in anorectal physiology, was the motivation behind the development of colonic reservoirs (Table 54.1.) Deciding on whether to create a colonic reservoir requires an assessment of preoperative continence and an evidence-based understanding of the magnitude and duration of improvement in function attributable to the additional time and effort of creating a reservoir.

M. Z. Wilson (✉)
Dartmouth Hitchcock Medical Center, Geisel School of Medicine at Dartmouth, Division of Colon and Rectal Surgery, Lebanon, NH, USA
e-mail: Matthew.z.wilson@hitchcock.org

D. B. Stewart
Southern Illinois University School of Medicine, SIU Department of Surgery, Springfield, IL, USA
e-mail: dstewart52@siumed.edu

K. Umanskiy, N. Hyman (eds.), *Difficult Decisions in Colorectal Surgery*, Difficult Decisions in Surgery: An Evidence-Based Approach,
https://doi.org/10.1007/978-3-031-42303-1_54

Table 54.1 PICO table

Patients	Intervention	Comparator	Outcome
Patients requiring sphincter-sparing rectal resections for benign or malignant disease	Low and extended low anterior resections with colorectal or coloanal anastomosis involving a colonic reservoir	Low and extended low anterior resections with the creation of a straight colorectal or coloanal anastomosis	Quality of life related to intestinal function

Search Strategy

A literature search of the Cochrane database, EMBASE, MEDLINE, and PubMed was undertaken to identify all English-language publications related to colorectal and coloanal anastomotic techniques that involved a colonic reservoir and that included an assessment of functional outcomes. Key search terms included "colorectal," "low anterior resection," "colonic reservoir," "colonic J-pouch," "coloplasty," and "functional outcomes." All studies written in English, with no limitations on publication date, were eligible for inclusion; all studies provided functional outcomes, at minimum, with some studies comparing quality of life between different reconstruction techniques. If multiple studies were included from the same institution, only the most recent study was included in this review.

Results

A larger body of literature is available for colonic J-pouches (CJP) than for the transverse coloplasty (TC). For the CJP, the majority of studies provide less than 2 years of follow-up, with these data suggesting a lower incidence of incontinence, urgency, and frequency compared to a straight anastomosis (SA). A smaller number of studies provide follow-up as far as 5 years from reconstruction, suggesting that the improved functional outcomes are durable. The best functional outcomes for CJP occur with coloanal anastomoses or anastomoses involving the extraperitoneal rectum. Since CJPs involving the mid and proximal rectum are associated with emptying difficulties, a SA is recommended for these scenarios.

When comparing earlier descriptions of CJP to later descriptions, larger reservoirs (8-cm to 12-cm) were associated with complaints of difficult evacuation and constipation. Subsequent evaluations have confirmed that a pouch length of up to 6-cm provides superior functional results compared to larger pouches.

CJP does not appear to be associated with a higher incidence of anastomotic leaks; there is limited data suggesting that leak rates may be lower than with SA, though this data often does not control for the presence of a diverting stoma. (Table 54.2.)

Technical limitations to the creation of a CJP include visceral adiposity and narrow pelvic dimensions, and from these circumstances came the TC, touting the benefits of a CJP but without the difficulties with evacuation. Most of the data for

Table 54.2 Results

Study	Patients (n)	Outcome Measure	Results (CJP *vs* SA)	Quality of Evidence
Zaman et al	1712 *vs* 1581 (CJP *vs* SA)	Anastomotic Complications *Leak* *Stricture* SSI and Sepsis Functional Outcomes *Frequency* *Urgency* *Anti-Diarrheal Usage* *Incontinence*	8.1% *vs* 12.3% Comparable Comparable Favor CJP (MD 1.44) Favor CJP (MD 2.7) Favor CJP (MD 3.85) Comparable	Moderate
Brown et al	245 *vs* 228 (SA vs CJP) 79 *vs* 79 (CJP vs TC)	Anastomotic Complications *Leak* SA *vs* CJP TC *vs* CJP Functional Outcome *(8-18months)* SA vs CJP *Frequency* *Urgency* *Fecal Incontinence Score* *Incomplete Evacuation* *Anti-Diarrheal Use* TC *vs* CJP *Frequency* *Urgency* *Fecal Incontinence Score* *Incomplete Evacuation* *Anti-Diarrheal se*	Favor CJP (OR 0.71) Favor CJP (OR 2.37) Favor CJP Favor CJP Comparable Comparable Favor CJP Comparable Favor TC Comparable Comparable Comparable	High

Note: MD "mean difference" degree to which one approach is favored over the comparator

TC involves comparisons with a SA, given that TC is often utilized when CJP is not technically feasible.

Recommendations

The majority of coloanal and distal colorectal anastomoses constructed in the United States are SA; as such, while the creation of a colonic reservoir is an option, it cannot currently be described as a requirement. A colonic reservoir is an option for distal colorectal or coloanal anastomoses, and among the options, a CJP is the preferred reservoir when the colon and pelvis can accommodate this conduit. The functional outcomes, compared to SA, are superior, at least in the first 2 years following creation; while there is evidence that these results may be durable as far as 5 years from surgery, the consistency of these results after 2 years remains less certain than short-term results. The benefit of TC remains uncertain, since the majority of the available data suggest that functional outcomes are inferior to CJP but not superior to SA, which suggests that TC provides no benefit but requires additional effort compared to SA.

Personal View

The authors of this chapter infrequently utilize colonic reservoirs for patients who are older and/or have preoperative complaints of urgency, frequency, or partial fecal incontinence, who require a distal colorectal or a coloanal anastomosis and who are highly motivated to avoid a permanent stoma. When a colonic reservoir is planned, it is virtually always a CJP, given the lack of consensus that TC is superior to either CJP or an SA. The questions regarding durability of improved function with CJP, coupled with the additional time and the technical challenges in certain patients, are reasons that most of our anastomoses are SA.

Our standard CJP is no larger than a 6-cm reservoir, which can be created with no more than two applications of a 75-mm linear-cutting stapler. A colotomy is created at the apex of the pouch, allowing introduction of the linear-cutting stapler, with the option of introducing the anvil for an end-to-end anastomotic stapling device. These techniques are analogous to those used for creating a J-pouch ileoanal anastomosis.

Our practice is to reserve CJPs for anastomoses within 6-cm of the anal verge, both to avoid complaints of difficult evacuation and given that retaining longer lengths of rectum obviates the benefit of a CJP.

References

1. Quezada-Diaz FF, Elfeki H, Emmertsen KJ, et al. Comparative analysis of the memorial Sloan Kettering bowel function instrument and the low anterior resection syndrome questionnaire for assessment of bowel dysfunction in rectal cancer patients after low anterior resection. Color Dis. 2021;23(2):451–60.
2. Temple LK, Bacik J, Savatta SG, et al. The development of a validated instrument to evaluate bowel function after sphincter-preserving surgery for rectal cancer. Dis Colon Rectum. 2005;48(7):1353–65.
3. Emmertsen KJ, Laurberg S. Low anterior resection syndrome score: development and validation of a symptom-based scoring system for bowel dysfunction after low anterior resection for rectal cancer. Ann Surg. 2012;255(5):922–8.
4. Croese AD, Lonie JM, Trollope AF, Vangaveti VN, Ho YH. A meta-analysis of the prevalence of low anterior resection syndrome and systematic review of risk factors. Int J Surg. 2018;56:234–41.
5. Zaman S, Mohamedahmed AYY, Ayeni AA, et al. Comparison of the colonic J-pouch versus straight (end-to-end) anastomosis following low anterior resection: a systematic review and meta-analysis. Int J Color Dis. 2022;37(4):919–38.
6. Brown CJ, Fenech DS, McLeod RS. Reconstructive techniques after rectal resection for rectal cancer. Cochrane Database Syst Rev. 2008;2008(2):Cd006040.

Management of the Unhealed Perineal Wound After Proctectomy

55

Vitaliy Poylin and Mohammad Abbass

Introduction

Abdominoperineal resection (APR) is the surgical standard for low rectal cancers when sphincter salvage is not [1]. Other indications for abdominoperineal resection include inflammatory bowel disease, proctectomy in the setting of poor sphincter function, and salvage surgery for persistent or recurrent cancer. [2, 6] Common use of peri operative chemoradiation and wider excisions increase the chances of wound complications, thereby making it an issue that needs to be considered proactively in every patient undergoing APR. [7] In addition to a diminished quality of life, these complications can lead to prolonged hospital stays, delayed oncologic treatments, worsening quality of life and increased healthcare costs [5].

An unhealed perineal wound is classified as a persistent perineal sinus (PPS) if it lasts for greater than 6 months following surgery [8]. The incidence of unhealed wounds and PPS vary in the literature, but overall are reported to be between 30–70% with higher rates reported for inflammatory bowel disease [9, 10]. As many as 33% of cases of PPS have not healed by 1 year, and chronic PPS becomes increasingly unlikely to heal spontaneously without aggressive intervention. [11]

V. Poylin (✉)
Division of Gastrointestinal Surgery Northwestern Medicine, Feinberg School of Medicine, Chicago, IL, USA

Northwestern University Feinberg School of Medicine, Northwestern Medical Group, Chicago, IL, USA
e-mail: vitaliy.poylin2@nm.org

M. Abbass
Division of Gastrointestinal Surgery Northwestern Medicine, Feinberg School of Medicine, Chicago, IL, USA
e-mail: mohammad.abbass@nm.org

K. Umanskiy, N. Hyman (eds.), *Difficult Decisions in Colorectal Surgery*, Difficult Decisions in Surgery: An Evidence-Based Approach,
https://doi.org/10.1007/978-3-031-42303-1_55

In the case of PPS, the size of the defect may dictate whether conservative or aggressive treatment strategies would be more appropriate.

Multiple risk factors have been associated with increased risk of perineal wound infections including diabetes mellitus, tobacco use, malnutrition, and obesity [2, 4, 6, 8]. Since most of these surgeries are scheduled well ahead of time, it is important to address as many of these factor as possible prior to operating. Patients with inflammatory bowel disease, particularly Crohn's disease, present a challenge [3, 10, 11]. In the setting of proctectomy for perineal Crohn's Disease, one should assess for the presence of any new or ongoing enteric fistulas and large areas of inflammation that could prohibit local wound healing [3].

In order to determine optimal treatment for unhealed perineal wounds and PPS, it is important to understand the anatomical predisposition created following pelvic exenteration and radical extirpations of the anorectum. The pelvic cavity is bound anteriorly by the urogenital organs (in the female the uterus, cervix and vagina and in the male the prostate, seminal vesicles, and bladder), bound posterolaterally by the coccyx, sacrum and the two ischia, and bound superiorly by the pelvic peritoneum. [8, 12] These well-defined landmarks are generally immobile, except for possibility of mobilizing and retroflexing the uterus over the pelvic inlet. The postoperative pelvic vacancy leads to an intrinsic susceptibility for postoperative fluid collections. Bacterial contamination can result in secondary infection of this fluid, abscesses, inflammation, and fibrosis. These processes actively hinder further healing and can progress to perineal sepsis.

Several methods are available to treat non healing perineal wounds after they develop as well as methods used preventively. These vary significantly and include expectant wound care, vacuum assisted devices, placement of the implants as well as various tissue allografts. All carry a balance of risks and benefits along with often significant costs. Several of the most effective treatment strategies have addressed the anatomical defect left following proctectomy, with the goal to further close the pelvic space. However, all treatments have potential drawbacks, and an honest discussion has to be had with the patient about pros and cons of available approaches. This chapter will review the alternative methods utilized to promote healing and closure of the perineal sinus.

PICO table

Patient population	Intervention	Comparator	Outcome
Patients with unhealed perineal wounds/PPS following proctectomy	Surgical advancement flap	Non-operative strategy/local wound care	Primary perineal wound healing

Literature Search Strategy

All studies evaluating the management of perineal wounds following proctectomy were considered for inclusion. Inclusion was not restricted to study design and all types of studies (retrospective vs. prospective, randomized vs. non-randomized, observational, etc.) were eligible for consideration. Studies were identified via search of the Pubmed database (1991–2022) with the following MeSH terms: "post-operative complications", "perineum", and "wound healing". The results were then evaluated for relevancy to the topic, and citation lists of relevant papers were reviewed for further references. All papers were evaluated for the quality of their evidence and recommendations via the GRADE approach (Grades of Recommendation, Assessment, Development, and Evaluation). Papers were classified in quality as high, moderate, low, or very low based on multiple factors including methodology, consistency, precision of results, and directness of the evidence given [13].

Non-operative Strategies

Perineal wounds allowed to heal by secondary intentions has been a historic standard. Although usually successful, can result prolonged wound healing, in some cases taking close to a year after surgery. [7] Conservative approaches for the management of the unhealed perineal wound include local wound care, topical medications and antibiotics, chemical debridement agents, and negative pressure wound therapy. Important factors to consider for optimizing wound healing include nutritional status, blood supply, and immune function as well as patient's wishes and consideration for any further treatment that is needed.

Ongoing infection and the presence of fibrinous exudate or devitalized tissue will impair wound healing. Removal of devitalized tissue, necrotic material and fibrinous exudate will augment the healing process. The removal of such devitalized tissues via surgical debridement and control of any localized sepsis has been shown to accelerate healing.

Debridement

Debridement refers to the surgical removal of devitalized tissue and fibrinous material, with the goal to promote the growth of the underlying healthy tissue. Debridement is often required even when other treatment methods are planned and is often a first step undertaken for non-healing wounds. Various forms of debridement include sharp debridement, biological debridement, chemical debridement, mechanical debridement, enzymatic debridement, and autolytic debridement [14]. Sharp debridement, typically using a scalpel or scissors can be performed either in the operating room or at the bedside, depending on the extent of the wound debridement and the patient's pain control. The wet-to-dry dressing, frequently applied within the realm of postsurgical care, utilizes both mechanical and autolytic debridement. Comparisons of modern dressings (alginates, hydrocolloids, polyurethane foam, silicone foam) to traditional gauze dressings seem to suggest a modest improvement in wound healing with modern dressings, though these studies have been criticized for small sample sizes and methodological flaws [14].

Local Antibiotic Agents

Ongoing infection is a risk factor for developing PPS and delayed wound healing. Presence of sepsis and significant local infection may require systemic antibiotics and is beyond the scope of this chapter. Use of local antibiotics have been attempted over time as a logical treatment option to control the infection and promote wound healing, but results have been disappointing. There are multiple delivery agents for local antibiotics, including sponges, fleeces, injections, and beads. Some agents appear to work by space filling potential rather than anti-bacterial properties [15]. A study by Gruessner et al. found that gentamicin absorbable fleeces used following APR reduced postoperative wound infection to 6% compared to 21% of controls, but this did not translate into a statistically significant improvement in rates of wound healing [15]. However, a large multicenter randomized control trial comparing gentamicin-collagen fleeces following APR to standard care failed to demonstrate any reduction in perineal wound complications [16].

Currently, there is a lack of evidence to recommend use of local antibiotic agent to aid perineal wound healing.

Negative Pressure Wound Therapy

Vacuum-assisted closure (VAC) are increasingly common tool used for difficult surgical wounds to expedite the secondary intention healing process. Its proposed mechanism decreases bacterial colonization within the wound, as well as tissue edema and wound tension while increasing blood flow to the wound area [17]. Further, the device may confer benefit by creating a mechanical stimulus at the wound site, stimulating neo-angiogenesis, and enhancing granulation tissue production. The tight seal associated with the VAC equipment additionally prevents exogenous contamination between dressings. Although familiarity and insurance coverage made VAC dressing use is more common, its use for treatment of perineal wounds and sinuses remains limited. One of the main issues is maintaining the tight seal required for use of this device on perineum, where the anatomy is affected by both contours effects of ambulation.

Few studies examine effects of VAC dressing on the perineum. Study by Walma et al. of 171 patients reported no significant improvement after abdominoperineal resection [18]. On the other hand a meta-analysis by Cahill et al. reported decreases in perineal wound complications, but study was limited by selection bias and heterogeneity [17].

Currently, negative pressure wound therapy can be recommended in selected patients as either a bridge to a definitive procedure such as advancement flap or as primary treatment. However, the failure rate and long-term durability of this approach remains a significant issue.

Hyperbaric Oxygen Therapy

The use of hyperbaric oxygen therapy has demonstrated improved efficacy in healing difficult and chronic wounds. A small case series (13 patients) of Crohn's patients showed improvement with Hyperbaric Oxygen Therapy [19]. Another study by Chan et al. combined the use of hyperbaric oxygen with the use of myocuteneous flaps and reported healing in all four patients, who all had a history of multiple previous procedures [20].

Use of hyperbaric oxygen seems to be promising, but data is still lacking. In addition, this therapy is not widely available and insurance coverage varies, thereby further limiting its use.

Operative Strategies

Surgery continues to be the most aggressive, yet most reliable way to close perineal defects. This remains true in both prophylactic and therapeutic settings. However, these procedures are morbid in themselves and may be significantly limited by anatomy and other patient factors. Overall, flaps should be considered with patients with expected large perineal defect (dead space as well as large skin opening) and chronically infected pelvis/perineum. Other considerations include use of radiation, especially at larger doses, and suboptimal nutrition. These factors can affect not only flap healing, but more significantly, they have an adverse effect on primary closure. Prior to any additional operative intervention it is critical to evaluate patient anatomy, patient surgical risk factors, and patient care goals.

Omental Pedicle Grafts

The significant anatomical vacancy left following proctectomy leaves a space that can fill with fluid and become infected. One strategy is the use of omental pedicle grafts to fill the defect. Technically this can be accomplished via creation of a vascular pedicle (typically based off the right or left gastro-epiploic vessels), with pelvic delivery via either a retrocolic or paracolic approach. This graft can typically be performed with a minimally invasive approach and is not as time-intensive or invasive as other autologous tissue grafts. There are two systematic review and meta-analysis on the subject, looking at roughly similar studies and number of patients. A report by Devaney et.al included older studies and reported improvement in outcomes. On the other hand, a study by Blok et al. looking at studies since 2000 only, and at the time of original operation, reported no improvement in perineal wound healing and there was an associated higher rate of hernia [21].

Currently, omental flaps can be considered as part of the prevention/treatment algorithm, but not as a standalone strategy.

Wide Excision and Split Thickness Skin Grafts

Use of split thickness skin grafts after debridement and wide excision can be less morbid, mainly due to lesser impact on the donor site. Technically less challenging when compared to other flaps, it can suffer from the same issues as VAC therapy with limitations of perineal contours and effects of ambulation. It can also only address reasonably superficial wounds. However, in selected patients these can be an effective treatment. McLeod et al. reported healing in five of nine patients with this technique in a small case series [22].

Meshes and Biological Implants

Advancement flaps can be morbid and often require considerable technical expertise. It has been proposed that the use of meshes can mitigate, if not fully avoid, perineal issues. However, the current data suggests minimal beneficial effects of biologic meshes on perineal wound healing. Musters et al. in a randomized control trial of biologic meshes vs primary closure showed no significant difference in wound healing, although at a 5 year follow up, there were fewer perineal hernias in the mesh group [23, 24]. Similarly, in meta-analysis by Zaheer et al., there was no difference in perineal wound healing, but slightly decreased chances of perineal hernia [25]. While synthetic meshes can overcome some of the issues related to hernias, concerns with placing them into infected field (for treatment) or contaminated field (during primary procedure) remain with few studies available to make meaningful conclusions.

Gracilis Muscle Flap

The gracilis muscle flap is performed with a longitudinal incision in the medial thigh to harvest a gracilis muscle vascular pedicle (from the medial circumflex femoral artery), and subsequently transposing the pedicle to the perineal defect. [12] The loss of gracilis muscle, either unilaterally or bilaterally, does not cause significant functional limitations. This advancement flap is most successful when the sinus to be filled is relatively narrow. It has been shown to be effective in cancer as well as inflammatory bowel disease patients, but the number of patients remains small [26].

Rectus Abdominus Myocutaneous Flap

The rectus abdominus muscle (RAM) flap is the most commonly used flap for perineal closure. It can be harvested in various configurations including vertical harvest (VRAM), transverse approach (TRAM), and oblique orientation (Taylor's Flap) with a pedicle derived from the superior or inferior epigastric arteries. Advantages to this flap include its availability within the operative field and its ability to be harvested extra peritoneally. It can provide substantial bulk when a large pelvic defect needs to be closed. Flaps can, however, limit surgical approaches to the primary problem – done mostly open, it may change the operation from minimally invasive to open, leading to well describe issues associated with open abdominal procedures. Robotic harvesting of the rectus abdominus have been well described but is not widely utilized. RAM flaps remain very successful in both treatment of perineal defects as well as prophylaxis during primary procedure. Harries et al. reported outcomes of 178 VRAM's with overall only 2.3% failure, however, there was significant associated morbidity with 22.5% perineal wound dehiscence and 10.1% need for re-operation in addition to prolonged length of stay [27]. Similarly, a systematic review by Radwan et al. showed an overall high morbidity of 27%, but with a flap loss of only 1.8%. [28] A major potential drawback of rectus abdominus muscle use in the setting of colorectal surgery is the loss of potential sites for ostomy creation. Other potential donor site morbidity include the possibility of ventral hernias at the donor site due to weakening of the abdominal wall, which may be ameliorated with propylene mesh placement at the procurement site. Overall, RAM flaps are very successful in treating and prevention of perineal wounds, but remain to be morbid and requires careful discussion [29].

Intervention	References	Study design	GRADE of evidence	Summary of recommendations
Debridement and curettage	Lewis et al. (2001) [14]	Review and metanalysis	Moderate	Some modern dressings (i.e., hydrocolloid, alginate, and foam dressings) may improve secondary intention wound healing compared to traditional gauze, however many trails suffered from methodological flaws and may be prone to bias.
Local antibiotic agents	Collin et al. (2013) [16]	Multicenter RCT (7 hospitals, n = 102)	High	No significant differences in perineal wound healing were noted between those who received local gentamicin-collagen and those who did not.
Negative pressure (VAC) wound therapy	Cahill et al. (2018) [17]	Systemic review 5 articles, n-169	Moderate	VAC therapy appears to be a useful adjunct to speed perineal wound healing by secondary intention.
Hyperbaric oxygen	Lansdorp et al. (2020) [19]	Case series (n = 13)	Very low	Hyperbaric oxygen therapy, appears to be a safe treatment modality for Crohn's patients with persistent perineal wounds

Intervention	References	Study design	GRADE of evidence	Summary of recommendations
Omental pedicle grafts	Blok et al. (2020) [21]	Review and metanalysis (14 studies, n-1894)	Moderate	Omental mobilization, transfer, and buttressing of primary perineal repair following protectomy did not affect perineal wound healing and increased likelihood of perineal hernia
Gracilis muscle flap	Menon et al. (2005) [12]	Case series (n = 17)	Low	A gracilis transposition is relatively simple operation with minimal morbidity useful for superficial sinuses not requiring much bulk.
Rectus Abdominus muscle (RAM) flap	Radwan et al. (2021) [28]	Systematic review, 65 studies,(n-1827)	Moderate	RAM flaps, when compared to primary closure alone, had a significantly lower rate of perineal wound infections but associated with significant morbidity.
Pudendal flap	Bodinet al. (2015) [30]	Case series (n - 6)	Very low	Advantages to this flap include less donor site morbidity, rich blood supply, immediate proximity to wound, and complete supra-fascial procurement.
Gluteus maximus flap	Jackisch et al. (2022) [31]	Retrospective cohort (n – 107)	Moderate	Modified gluteal maximus flaps (V-Y) provide good wound related outcomes with moderate morbidity
Biologic mesh implants	Zaheer et al. (2021) [25]	Systematic review	Moderate	Use of biologic mesh provides no improvement in perineal wound short term healing, but may decrease chances of hernia long term

Pudendal Flaps

Flaps derived from branches of the internal pudendal artery have been reported with success in the literature, under various names such as pudendal flaps, lotus flaps, gluteal fold flaps, and Singapore flaps [32]. Advantages include effective coverage and healing without muscle harvesting or decrease in function, the option for unilateral or bilateral flaps, and improved cosmesis (as the flaps are procured from within the gluteal fold). When APR is performed in the prone position, no repositioning is required. Only small case series are available, but they demonstrate overall good outcomes and low chances of complications [30, 32].

Gluteus Maximus Flap

The gluteus maximus flap is a local flap which provides ample tissue for filling the desired defect, and can be performed in either a bilateral or unilateral fashion. This strategy provides a bulky and reliable flap immediately adjacent to the wound site. Classic gluteal flaps that include large portions of the muscle provide great coverage and filling of the large defect with low chances of wound complications. The loss of gluteus maximus function, however, can be very morbid and can affect gait and balance, and are associated with high levels of pain while seated [33].

More recently, various alternations of this techniques are being utilized with V-Y perforator flaps gaining popularity. Although they gather less tissue and may not close defects deep in the pelvis, they work very well for wound coverage. They avoid the need to enter the abdomen and can be easily combined with a minimally invasive approach. These flaps can be employed in association with primary procedure in preventive fashion (especially if primary procedure is finished prone) and as a treatment option for non-healing wound [31, 34].

Personal View of the Data

Perineal wound issues after proctectomy are common and result in significant morbidity for patients after surgery. Multiple strategies have been employed and range greatly in their complexity and cost. Although none of the strategies seems to be superior, one thing is clear – all have its potential benefits, significant drawbacks, and are often associated with limited data to support them.

One of the main decision points currently is whether to consider advancements flap at the time of primary surgery or early in the treatment of wound issues as they arise. Available data supports that approach (**** which approach- you just mentioned two of them****). This approach is not without significant issues including added short and long term morbidity of the flaps, longer operating room time, and complexity of scheduling.

There are many patient and disease specific factors that must be considered when determining which approach to take. It is important to assess the impact of the unhealed wound on patients' quality of life to determine the most appropriate treatment. Other factors include nutritional consideration, patient anatomy, the chance of needing further intervention, availability of technical expertise, and resources. All put together, these decisions require thorough discussion with family and involved providers prior to proceeding.

For small wounds, with a minimal impact on the patient, debridement of any devitalized tissue is needed. Depending on the size of the remaining defect, local wound care and healing by secondary intention may be all that is necessary. Negative pressure wound therapy or hyperbaric oxygen may be useful adjunct to speed secondary intention healing.

For large sinuses, excision with an autograft may be necessary to close the space. Rectus abdominus and modified gluteus maximus are the main autologous grafts to be considered at the moment. Multiple factors must be taken into account when choosing a flap for your patient as mentioned above.

Finally, evaluation of the current evidence makes it clear that there are many promising and innovative therapies in this field, but with only minimal evidence to support. There is a need for high quality, large randomized trials to improve the strength of current recommendations. Until that time, controversies in treatment strategy will remain and management is based on anecdotal evidence.

References

1. Miles WE. A method of performing abdomino-perineal excision for carcinoma of the rectum and of the terminal portion of the pelvic colon (1908). CA Cancer J Clin. 1971;21(6):361–4. https://doi.org/10.3322/canjclin.21.6.361.
2. Foster JD, Tou S, Curtis NJ, et al. Closure of the perineal defect after abdominoperineal excision for rectal adenocarcinoma – ACPGBI position statement. Color Dis. 2018;20(Suppl 5):5–23. https://doi.org/10.1111/codi.14348.
3. Li W, Stocchi L, Elagili F, Kiran RP, Strong SA. Healing of the perineal wound after proctectomy in Crohn's disease patients: only preoperative perineal sepsis predicts poor outcome. Tech Coloproctol. 2017;21(9):715–20. https://doi.org/10.1007/s10151-017-1695-8.
4. Althumairi AA, Canner JK, Gearhart SL, et al. Risk factors for wound complications after abdominoperineal excision: analysis of the ACS NSQIP database. Color Dis. 2016;18(7):O260–6. https://doi.org/10.1111/codi.13384.
5. Hassel K, Andersson K, Koinberg IL, Wennstrom B. Postoperative wound infections after a proctectomy – patient experiences. Int J Qual Stud Health Well-being. 2016;11:30393. https://doi.org/10.3402/qhw.v11.30393.
6. Curran T, Poylin V, Nagle D. Real world dehiscence rates for patients undergoing abdominoperineal resection with or without myocutaneous flap closure in the national surgical quality improvement project. Int J Color Dis. 2016;31(1):95–104. https://doi.org/10.1007/s00384-015-2377-5.
7. Poylin V, Curran T, Alvarez D, Nagle D, Cataldo T. Primary vs. delayed perineal proctectomy-there is no free lunch. Int J Color Dis. 2017;32(8):1207–12. https://doi.org/10.1007/s00384-017-2790-z.
8. Lohsiriwat V. Persistent perineal sinus: incidence, pathogenesis, risk factors, and management. Surg Today. 2009;39(3):189–93. https://doi.org/10.1007/s00595-008-3846-z.
9. Asplund D, Prytz M, Bock D, Haglind E, Angenete E. Persistent perineal morbidity is common following abdominoperineal excision for rectal cancer. Int J Color Dis. 2015;30(11):1563–70. https://doi.org/10.1007/s00384-015-2328-1.
10. Yamamoto T, Mylonakis E, Keighley MR. Omentoplasty for persistent perineal sinus after proctectomy for Crohn's disease. Am J Surg. 2001;181(3):265–7. https://doi.org/10.1016/s0002-9610(01)00561-x.
11. Chau A, Prodeau M, Sarter H, et al. Persistent perineal sinus after abdominoperineal resection. Langenbeck's Arch Surg. 2017;402(7):1063–9. https://doi.org/10.1007/s00423-017-1619-0.
12. Menon A, Clark MA, Shatari T, Keh C, Keighley MR. Pedicled flaps in the treatment of nonhealing perineal wounds. Color Dis. 2005;7(5):441–4. https://doi.org/10.1111/j.1463-1318.2005.00838.x.
13. Guyatt G, Gutterman D, Baumann MH, et al. Grading strength of recommendations and quality of evidence in clinical guidelines: report from an american college of chest physicians task force. Chest. 2006;129(1):174–81. https://doi.org/10.1378/chest.129.1.174.

14. Lewis R, Whiting P, ter Riet G, O'Meara S, Glanville J. A rapid and systematic review of the clinical effectiveness and cost-effectiveness of debriding agents in treating surgical wounds healing by secondary intention. Health Technol Assess. 2001;5(14):1–131. https://doi.org/10.3310/hta5140.
15. Gruessner U, Clemens M, Pahlplatz PV, et al. Improvement of perineal wound healing by local administration of gentamicin-impregnated collagen fleeces after abdominoperineal excision of rectal cancer. Am J Surg. 2001;182(5):502–9. https://doi.org/10.1016/s0002-9610(01)00762-0.
16. Collin A, Gustafsson UM, Smedh K, Pahlman L, Graf W, Folkesson J. Effect of local gentamicin-collagen on perineal wound complications and cancer recurrence after abdominoperineal resection: a multicentre randomized controlled trial. Color Dis. 2013;15(3):341–6. https://doi.org/10.1111/j.1463-1318.2012.03196.x.
17. Cahill C, Fowler A, Williams LJ. The application of incisional negative pressure wound therapy for perineal wounds: a systematic review. Int Wound J. 2018;15(5):740–8. https://doi.org/10.1111/iwj.12921.
18. Walma MS, Burbach JP, Verheijen PM, Pronk A, van Grevenstein WM. Vacuum-assisted closure therapy for infected perineal wounds after abdominoperineal resection. A retrospective cohort study. Int J Surg. 2016;26:18–24. https://doi.org/10.1016/j.ijsu.2015.12.009.
19. Lansdorp CA, Buskens CJ, Gecse KB, D'Haens GR, Van Hulst RA. Wound healing of metastatic perineal Crohn's disease using hyperbaric oxygen therapy: a case series. United European Gastroenterol J. 2020;8(7):820–7. https://doi.org/10.1177/2050640620934915.
20. Chan XH, Koh CE, Glover M, Bryson P, Travis SP, Mortensen NJ. Healing under pressure: hyperbaric oxygen and myocutaneous flap repair for extreme persistent perineal sinus after proctectomy for inflammatory bowel disease. Color Dis. 2014;16(3):186–90. https://doi.org/10.1111/codi.12500.
21. Blok RD, Hagemans JAW, Klaver CEL, et al. A systematic review and meta-analysis on omentoplasty for the management of abdominoperineal defects in patients treated for cancer. Ann Surg. 2020;271(4):654–62. https://doi.org/10.1097/SLA.0000000000003266.
22. McLeod RS, Palmer JA, Cohen Z. Management of chronic perineal sinuses by wide excision and split-thickness skin grafting. Can J Surg. 1985;28(4):315–6. 318
23. Musters GD, Klaver CEL, Bosker RJI, et al. Biological mesh closure of the pelvic floor after extralevator abdominoperineal resection for rectal cancer: a multicenter randomized controlled trial (the BIOPEX-study). Ann Surg. 2017;265(6):1074–81. https://doi.org/10.1097/SLA.0000000000002020.
24. Blok RD, Sharabiany S, Stoker J, et al. Cumulative 5-year results of a randomized controlled trial comparing biological mesh with primary perineal wound closure after extralevator abdominoperineal resection (BIOPEX-study). Ann Surg. 2022;275(1):e37–44. https://doi.org/10.1097/SLA.0000000000004763.
25. Zaheer Ahmad N, Abbas MH, Al-Naimi N, Parvaiz A. Meta-analysis of biological mesh reconstruction versus primary perineal closure after abdominoperineal excision of rectal cancer. Int J Color Dis. 2021;36(3):477–92. https://doi.org/10.1007/s00384-020-03827-0.
26. Rius J, Nessim A, Nogueras JJ, Wexner SD. Gracilis transposition in complicated perianal fistula and unhealed perineal wounds in Crohn's disease. Eur J Surg. 2000;166(3):218–22. https://doi.org/10.1080/110241500750009311.
27. Harries RL, Radwan RW, Dewi M, et al. Outcomes following immediate vertical rectus abdominis Myocutaneous (VRAM) flap-based perineal reconstruction following resectional surgery for pelvic malignancies. World J Surg. 2021;45(7):2290–7. https://doi.org/10.1007/s00268-021-06044-0.
28. Radwan RW, Tang AM, Harries RL, Davies EG, Drew P, Evans MD. Vertical rectus abdominis flap (VRAM) for perineal reconstruction following pelvic surgery: a systematic review. J Plast Reconstr Aesthet Surg. 2021;74(3):523–9. https://doi.org/10.1016/j.bjps.2020.10.100.
29. Proctor MJ, Westwood DA, Donahoe S, et al. Morbidity associated with the immediate vertical rectus abdominus myocutaneous flap reconstruction after radical pelvic surgery. Color Dis. 2020;22(5):562–8. https://doi.org/10.1111/codi.14909.

30. Bodin F, Dissaux C, Seigle-Murandi F, Dragomir S, Rohr S, Bruant-Rodier C. Posterior perineal reconstructions with "supra-fascial" lotus petal flaps. J Plast Reconstr Aesthet Surg. 2015;68(1):e7–12. https://doi.org/10.1016/j.bjps.2014.10.028.
31. Jackisch J, Jackisch T, Roessler J, et al. Tailored concept for the plastic closure of pelvic defects resulting from extralevator abdominoperineal excision (ELAPE) or pelvic exenteration. Int J Color Dis. 2022;37(7):1669–79. https://doi.org/10.1007/s00384-022-04196-6.
32. Sinna R, Qassemyar Q, Benhaim T, et al. Perforator flaps: a new option in perineal reconstruction. J Plast Reconstr Aesthet Surg. 2010;63(11):e766–74. https://doi.org/10.1016/j.bjps.2010.07.012.
33. Haapamaki MM, Pihlgren V, Lundberg O, Sandzen B, Rutegard J. Physical performance and quality of life after extended abdominoperineal excision of rectum and reconstruction of the pelvic floor with gluteus maximus flap. Dis Colon Rectum. 2011;54(1):101–6. https://doi.org/10.1007/DCR.0b013e3181fce26e.
34. Kokosis G, Phillips BT, Soo J, et al. Modified V-Y fasciocutaneous flap reconstruction after abdominoperineal resection in irradiated patients prevents wound dehiscence and associated complications: a retrospective analysis and benchtop confirmation. Ann Plast Surg. 2019;82(2):218–23. https://doi.org/10.1097/SAP.0000000000001672.

Gender Affirmation Procedure: What Are the Reconstructive Options?

56

Paulo Vitor Barreto Guimaraes, Omer Raheem, and Ervin Kocjancic

Introduction

It is estimated that approximately 0.2 to 0.6% of the adult population are transgender worldwide [1] whom can present with various degrees of gender dysphoria – a discrepancy between biological sex and gender identity. The transitioning process is non-binary and varies in different stages of a patient's life. By definition, the genital affirming procedures can be divided into masculinizing and feminizing procedures for the trans male and trans female population respectively. For trans males, masculinizing procedures include Metoidioplasty and Phalloplasty. However, for trans females, feminizing procedures include simple orchiectomy, penectomy, and configuration of a vulva (vuolvoplasty) or a full-depth neo vagina (Vaginoplasty). Different surgical techniques have been described to create a neovagina in trans female patients, like penile inversion vaginoplasty [2, 3]. Moreover, various skin flaps or grafts have been utilized, such as full-thickness skin graft vaginoplasty [4], and pudendal tight flaps [5]. One of the most frequent complications of skin vaginoplasties is the stenosis of the neovagina, which can be prevented with daily neovaginal dilation. In recurrent neovagina stenosis or vaginal skin loss, surgical revision is often indicated with intestinal or peritoneal vaginoplasty with lower rates of vaginal stenosis and longer vaginal depth [6, 7, 8]. In this chapter, we provide a comprehensive review of the published literature pertaining to intestinal vaginoplasty in

P. V. B. Guimaraes · O. Raheem
Department of Urology, University of Chicago, Chicago, IL, USA
e-mail: oraheem@bsd.uchicago.edu

E. Kocjancic (✉)
Department of Urology, University of Chicago, Chicago, IL, USA

Reconstructive Urology and Trans Health, Chicago, IL, USA
e-mail: ekocjancic@bsd.uchicago.edu

K. Umanskiy, N. Hyman (eds.), *Difficult Decisions in Colorectal Surgery*, Difficult Decisions in Surgery: An Evidence-Based Approach,
https://doi.org/10.1007/978-3-031-42303-1_56

transgender patients with particular focus on functional, sexual and complications outcomes.

Search Strategy

A comprehensive literature search of the Cochrane Database, Pubmed, LILACS, and Scielo was performed to collect published data in English language specifically related to intestinal vaginoplasty outcomes – pertaining to functional, sexual, and complication outcomes over the past 10 years (from 2012 to 2022). Key search terms included "vaginoplasty and intestinal", "vaginoplasty and bowel", and "outcomes". Exclusion criteria were non-transgender studies, case reports, descriptive technique, review articles, and editor letters. We carefully screened and cross referenced the included studies in this review to make sure all studies met inclusion criteria.

Results

Despite the growth of transgender affirming surgeries, there has been paucity of published data pertaining to functional, sexual and complication outcomes following vaginoplasty utilizing various bowel segments. Moreover, most of these studies often limited with inherited bias, lower quality and non-validated questionnaire designated to evaluate this unique at-risk population. Nevertheless, recently, studies have recognized this limitation and utilized validated instruments for the description of their outcomes [9–12], such as the Female Sexual Function Index (FSFI) – considered the gold standard for the assessment of sexual function in cis women. The FSFI is a 19-item, self-report questionnaire which measure female sexual function based in sexual desire, arousal, orgasm, pain, and satisfaction, and scores of ≤26.55 can identify relevant sexual dysfunction [13]. Nonewithstanding, it is critical to mention that FSFI questionnaire has not been studied or validated in transgender women, making its validity and/or reproducibility a significant concern.

Our review selected 12 studies after analyses of inclusion criteria. Ten of these papers described the outcomes in trans patients submitted to intestinal vaginoplasty, and two of the studies compared outcomes of intestinal vaginoplasty vs perineal full-thickness skin graft vaginoplasty, and sigmoid vs penile inversion outcomes. Studies describing outcomes of intestinal vaginoplasty are listed in Table 56.1.

Evidence Synthesis for this Review

Conflicting evidence exists in relation to offering an intestinal vaginoplasty instead of conventional technique such as penile inversion vaginoplasty. Undoubtedly, this confusing opinion largely stems from lack of convincing large studies demonstrating superior safety and improved outcomes in this at-risk population. Conventionally,

Table 56.1 Intestinal vaginoplasty studies

Study	Patients (n)	Technique	Complications	Outcomes	Conclusion	Quality of evidence
Bouman [26] (2016)	31	Sigmoid. Observational. Survey study.	Not described	Life satisfaction 8.0 (median) Subjective happiness scale 5.6 (mean) Functionality 8 of 10 (median) Esthetics 8 of 10 (median) FSFI 26 ± 6.8	Satisfactory functional and esthetic results	Low
Bouman [8] (2016)	42	Primary vaginoplasty with the sigmoid. Observational. Prospective descriptive study.	Short-term (< 30 days): Death (necrotizing fasciitis) (n = 1) Anastomotic leakage (n = 1) Bleeding (n = 2) Long-term (> 30 days) Introital stenosis (n = 6) Mucosal prolapse (n = 1)	Vaginal depth 16.3 ± 1.5 cm	Sigmoid vaginoplasty seems to have a similar complication rate as other types of elective laparoscopic colorectal surgery.	Low
Garcia [16] (2020)	22	Right colon. Observational. Retrospective descriptive study.	Short-term (< 30 days): Ileocecal pedicle injury (n = 1) Bladder injury (n = 1) SBO/ ileus (n = 3) Long-term (> 30 days): Neovagina prolapse (n = 5) Stenosis (n = 4) Diversion neovaginitis (n = 3)	100% related satisfaction with the neovagina function and appearance.	Laparoscopic right colon has several advantages over the use of the sigmoid or ileum.	Low

(continued)

Table 56.1 (continued)

Study	Patients (n)	Technique	Complications	Outcomes	Conclusion	Quality of evidence
Marinque [10] (2017)	15	Transverse colon Observational. Retrospective descriptive study.	Narrowing introitus (n = 1) Excessive secretion in the first month (n = 1)	Length 15 cm Width 2.8 cm FSFI 28.6 (24–31) FGSIS 20.0 ± 4.5	Valuable alternative with good results and low complication	Low
Morison [18] (2015)	83	Sigmoid Observational. Retrospective descriptive study.	Protrusion of corpus spongiosum (n = 13) Prolapse (n = 2) Stenosis (n = 18) Recto vaginal fistula (n = 2)	Dyspareunia in 13 of 34 patients who answered Of 21 patients who answered, all reported high satisfaction	The procedure is safe and effective and should be offered for primary vaginoplasty.	Low
Mukai [6] (2019)	18	Sigmoid Observational. Retrospective descriptive study.	Anastomotic leak (n = 1) Neovaginal prolapse (n = 2)	Not described	Reliable technique in the Japanese population	Low
Ozkan [11] (2018)	43 (9 trans)	Sigmoid (left in ischemic state and denervated) Observational. Retrospective descriptive study.	Partial necrosis (n = 1) Hematoma (n = 2)	"Good esthetic" in all patients FSFI (n = 15): 14 of them above 26.5	Vaginal reconstruction performed using rectosigmoid colon with Nerve excision from the pedicle and temporary ischemia seems to Be a reasonable option.	Low
Salgado [7] (2018)	12	Primary sigmoid vaginoplasty Observational. Retrospective descriptive study.	Ileus (n = 2) Bladder laceration (n = 1) Deep venous thrombosis (n = 1) Death (n = 1): Pulmonary embolism Vaginal stenosis at introitus (n = 2)	Neovaginal depth 13.9 ± 2.0 cm All patients reported satisfaction with the depth and pleasurable sensation	Reliable technique for primary vaginoplasty to patients with penis <11.4 cm	Low

Van der Sluis [12] 2016	24	Sigmoid (n = 23) and Ileal (n = 1) Observational. Retrospective descriptive study.	Neovaginal necrosis (n = 1) Introitus stenosis (n = 13) Fistula (n = 3) Prolapse (n = 3)	Median depth 15.5 cm [12 – 20] 9 patients answered: QoL: 27.1 ± 2.1 FSFI: 5 patients above 26.55 AHPFSW: 8.3 ± 2.3 FGSIS: mean score from 2.9 to 3.1 in all items	Although surgical corrections were frequently necessary, women reported satisfaction.	Low
Van der Sluis [15] 2018	32 (27 trans)	Ileal Observational. Retrospective descriptive study.	Recto neovaginal fistula (n = 1) Introital stenosis (n = 4)	Neovagina depth 13.2 ± 3.1 cm	Ileal vaginoplasty appears to have similar complication rates to sigmoid vaginoplasty	Low

FSFI Female Sexual Function Index, *FGSIS* Female Genital Self-Image Scale, *SBO* Small Bowel Obstruction, *QoL* Quality of Life, *AHPFSW*, Amsterdam Hyperactive Pelvic Floor Scale for Women intestinal vaginoplasty can be offered in revision and redo complex cases. Although, primary intestinal vaginoplasty has been advocated in select cases there is a shortage native skin tissue to perform a penoscrotal or penile inversion vaginoplasty, early adoption of puberty blocker hormonal treatment or generally in subjects with a reduced penile length [7, 8]. This proposition is based on the potential advantages intestinal vaginoplasty – albeit non-validated – can provide particularly, lower neovagina stenosis rates, forgoing vaginal lubrications and/or dilators use.

Functional and Sexual Outcomes

Functional/Neovaginal Length Outcomes

Usually, the authors have very similar conclusions: the intestinal approach to vaginoplasty presents good results regarding functional and aesthetic with low rates of complication [9, 10, 14]. Although, various bowel segments such as ileum [15], transverse colon [10], sigmoid [7, 8], and right sided colon [16] have been utilized in the creating of intestinal vaginoplasty, it is agreed upon that sigmoid colon is the most widely used bowel segment for the creation of neovagina [7, 8].

In relation to neovaginal length following intestinal vaginoplasty, the reported results are encouraging, with mean results varying from 13.2cm[15] to 16.3 cm[8]. A study by Van der Sluis et al. compared the outcomes of laparoscopic intestinal vaginoplasty (21 patients) with perineal full-thickness skin graft vaginoplasty (32 patients) [17] and found significant difference in the neovaginal length after intestinal vaginoplasty compared with full-thickness skin graft vaginoplasty (15.9 ± 1.4 cm vs 12.5 ± 2.8 cm respectively) ($p < 0.01$). Additionally, Van der Sluis's study showed no significant difference in the rectal perforation rate, but there is significant difference in operative times (intestinal vaginoplasty 191 min vs full-thickness skin graft vaginoplasty 131 min) ($p < 0.01$).

Van der Sluis described in one of his studies a measure to indicate hypertonic pelvis, the Amsterdam Hyperactive Pelvic Floor Scale for Women (AHPFSW), in this study 2 patients relate a score greater than eleven [12], which can indicate hypertonicity and can be related to dyspareunia but there is no evidence to support this correlation in transgender women after bowel vaginoplasty.

Sexual Outcomes

In relation to satisfaction outcomes following intestinal vaginoplasty, most of the studies used generic evaluation to describe post operative satisfaction rates and all of them describe that patients have "good satisfaction" with bowel vaginoplasty [11, 16, 18]. Interestingly, the studies that used the FSFI questionnaire to evaluate the sexual function found good results. Marinque et al. and Van der Sluis et al. described that all the patients had normal sexual function based on their respective FSFI scores [10, 12]. Additionally, Oskan et al. found that 14 from 15 patients had an FSFI above 26.5 – which is considerate normal. These results are in accordance with Schardein et al., who described up to 80% of sexual function satisfaction after vaginoplasty (regardless of the technique) [19].

In 2019, a study by Di Summa et al. published in Journal of Sexual Medicine compared penile inversion vaginoplasty (30 patients) to sigmoid colon vaginoplasty (13 patients), showed higher satisfactory, pleasure and orgasmic rates. 63% vs 54% of patients had vaginal and/or clitoral pleasure following sigmoid colon vaginoplasty and penile inversion vaginoplasty respectively [20]. Summary of data is listed in Table 56.2.

Complications

Neovaginal Stenosis

Neovaginal stenosis is considered the most common complication following intestinal vaginoplasty. Many of these patients are dissatisfied and often required revision or redo vaginoplasty procedures with concomitant use of neovaginal dilators to mitigate the risk restenosis [7, 10, 12, 16, 18]. Di Summa et al. also compared complications of penile inversion vaginoplasty to sigmoid colon vaginoplasty [20]. The results showed PI group had higher rate of neovaginal stenosis at 43% compared to only 30% stenosis located at introitus in the sigmoid group.

Bouman et al. also described occurrence of stenosis limited at introitus in 14% after primary sigmoid vaginoplasty [8]. Morrison et all, the study with the biggest number of patients (n = 83) described a prolapse incidence of 21% using sigmoid [18] while Marinque et al. related only 1 narrowing introitus from 15 patients submitted a vaginoplasty with transverse colon [10].

Fistulas

The same study comparing stenosis in PI versus Sigmoid vaginoplasty shows results about rectovaginal fistula – the number of rectovaginal fistulae was higher in the sigmoid group. Claes et al. describe that this complication is more common in secondary (revision) vaginoplasty, usually when we use bowel to rebuild the vagina [14]. Another systematic review about intestinal vaginoplasty outcomes report fistulas as complications in 7 from 31 studies included [21]. In our review, three different authors related occurrence of fistula in their studies with incidence between 2% and 12% as described in Table 56.1.

Bleeding and Infection

Bleeding and infection are complications less related in the published studies, often resolve without major sequalae [7, 8, 11]. Exceedingly rare, in one patient, mortality related to severe sepsis secondary to necrotizing fasciitis was reported [8].

Neovaginal Discharge and Malodor

One of the advantages of intestinal vaginoplasty is the natural lubrication secondary to the mucosa production. However, this excessive mucus secretion can lead to an excessive mucosal discharge in some patients, sometime associated with dissatisfaction and malodorous discharge. In most cases, this mucosal discharge is reduced after 3 to 4 months following intestinal vaginoplasty [6].

Table 56.2 Functional outcomes and complications comparing penile inversion vs sigmoid [20]

					Patient satisfaction (28 patients answered: 20 Penile Inversion and 8 Sigmoid)				
	Patients (n)	Vaginal stenosis	Vulvar partial necrosis	Rectovaginal fistula	Aesthetic	Functional Result	Easy of Orgasm	Location of Orgasm	Pain during Intercourse
Sigmoid (secondary vaginoplasty)	13	4 introitus stenosis	1	2	Unsatisfaction (n = 2)	No patient unsatisfied	All the patients achieved	Vaginal and clitoral in 63% after the surgery	Median answer: occasionally
Penile inversion	30	13	3	1	Unsatisfaction (n = 1)	Unsatisfaction (n = 4)	Never achieved (n = 4)	Clitoral in 54%	Median answer: occasionally

Neovaginal Prolapse

Another related complication is neovaginal prolapse, however, the definition used to describe this condition is not well standardized. After penile inversion vaginoplasty, around 0–5% of patients have presented neovaginal prolapse [22]. Regarding to intestinal vaginoplasty, studies included in our review show an incidence from 2 to 20% [6, 16, 18], with limited definitions and diagnosis.

Intestinal Complications

Not surprisingly, intestinal related complication can also be encountered following interesting vaginoplasty such as anastomotic leak, bowel ileus, bowel obstruction, and colitis [6, 8, 16, 18]. Often these complications can be managed conservatively in similar fashion to other colorectal surgery complications [11, 16, 18, 15, 8, 12, 17, 20].

Recommendations

The utilization of intestinal segments in secondary vaginoplasty appears to be viable and safe option in trans female patients who had developed surgical complications following primary vaginoplasty such as neovaginal stenosis. Various surgical approaches and grafts can be chosen for better outcomes pertaining to intestinal vaginoplasty (ileal, colonic, or sigmoid). Reported outcomes appear to be promising in terms of functional, and sexual outcomes [10–12], depth of the vaginal canal [17, 19], and quality of life [12]. Additionally, some patients may benefit from using intestinal techniques in primary vaginoplasty setting when penoscrotal skin shortage or reduced skin qualities encountered for vaginoplasty by a skin graft [8].

Personal View

Gender affirming surgery has been proven to be the most successful treatment for treating gender dysphoria and significantly improving the quality of life of these patients [23]. If the patient has enough skin in the genital area to implement a traditional technique to construct a neovagina, like penile inversion vaginoplasty and skin grafts and in the absence of consensus guideline regarding the gold standard technique for vagioplasty [9], we do recommend entertaining an alternative surgical approach with intestinal vaginoplasty in either primary or secondary/revision setting given available reported evidence regarding its safety, acceptable functional and sexual outcomes and lower complications rates following the procedures [22, 24].

Management of primary vaginoplasty complications can be challenging and require specialized centers with multidisciplinary experts. In case of focal neovaginal stenosis, a more conservative approach like neovaginal dilations or scar tissue removal can be a safe option. Otherwise, significant and functional vaginal tissue loss can be more involved and require surgical revision often achieved secondary intestinal vaginoplasty. The use of the intestinal bowel is useful to achieve a good neovaginal depth, has less tendency to total stenosis (less need for long-term dilators), and proper lubrification [22, 25, 6]. Notwithstanding the advantages, using the intestine in vaginoplasty may increase the risk of secondary bowel related complications like an anastomotic leak, bowel ileus or obstruction, and risk of colitis, excessive mucus production [9, 21].

It is paramount to mention that the overall evidence for published studies is of a low level [2]. Despite this, some studies described intestinal vaginoplasty have shown higher rate of satisfaction after the procedures. Schardein et al. describes overall 80% of satisfaction with sexual function after vaginoplasty regardless of the technique and 60–80% satisfaction with the vaginal canal depth [19].

Finally, and while there is limited published evidence regarding the long-term functional, sexual and complications outcomes following vaginoplasty, it is critical to design well conducted studies reporting and comparing outcomes in prospective randomized studies (level 1 evidence) where patients satisfaction, outcomes, and complications are end-points.

PICO table

Patient	Intervention	Comparator	Outcomes
Trans Female patients.	Surgical treatment with bowel vaginoplasty.	How effective are the different surgical procedures of intestinal vaginoplasty.	Surgical results and complications Patient satisfaction, Quality of Life, and FSFI.

References

1. Joseph A, Cliffe C, Hillyard M, Majeed A. Gender identity and the management of the transgender patient: A guide for non-specialists. J R Soc Med 110:144–152. Preprint at (2017) https://doi.org/10.1177/0141076817696054.
2. Dunford C, Bell K, Rashid T. Genital reconstructive surgery in male to female transgender patients: a systematic review of primary surgical techniques, complication profiles, and functional outcomes from 1950 to present day. Eur Urol Focus 7:464–471. Preprint at (2021) https://doi.org/10.1016/j.euf.2020.01.004.
3. Shoureshi P, Dugi D. Penile inversion vaginoplasty technique. Urol Clin N Am 46:511–525 Preprint at (2019) https://doi.org/10.1016/j.ucl.2019.07.006.
4. Hage J, Karim R. Abdominoplastic secondary full-thickness skin graft vaginoplasty for male-to-female transsexuals. Plast Reconstr Surg. 1988;101:1512–5.
5. Selçuk CT, Evsen MS, Özalp B, Durgun M. Reconstruction of vaginal agenesis with pudendal thigh flaps thinned with liposuction. J Plast Reconstr Aesthet Surg. 2013;66:e246–50.
6. Mukai Y, et al. Laparoscopic rectosigmoid colon vaginoplasty in male-to-female transsexuals: experience in Japan. Acta Med Okayama. 2019;73:205–11.
7. Salgado CJ, Nugent A, Kuhn J, Janette M, Bahna H. Primary sigmoid vaginoplasty in transwomen: technique and outcomes. BioMed Res Int 2018 Preprint at (2018) https://doi.org/10.1155/2018/4907208.

8. Bouman MB, et al. Primary total laparoscopic sigmoid vaginoplasty in transgender women with penoscrotal hypoplasia: a prospective cohort study of surgical outcomes and follow-up of 42 patients. Plast Reconstr Surg. 2016;138:614e–23e.
9. Bouman MB, et al. Intestinal vaginoplasty revisited: a review of surgical techniques, complications, and sexual function. J Sex Med. 2014;11:1835–47.
10. Manrique OJ, et al. Gender-confirmation surgery using the pedicle transverse colon flap for vaginal reconstruction: a clinical outcome and sexual function evaluation study. Plast Reconstr Surg. 2018;141:767–71.
11. Özkan Ö, et al. Vaginal reconstruction with the modified rectosigmoid colon: surgical technique, long-term results and sexual outcomes. J Plast Surg Hand Surg. 2018;52:210–6.
12. van der Sluis WB, et al. Long-term follow-up of transgender women after secondary intestinal Vaginoplasty. J Sex Med. 2016;13:702–10.
13. Meston CM, Freihart BK, Handy A B, Kilimnik CD, Rosen RC. Scoring and interpretation of the FSFI: what can be learned from 20 years of use? J Sex Med. 17:17–25 Preprint at (2020) https://doi.org/10.1016/j.jsxm.2019.10.007.
14. Claes KEY, Pattyn P, D'Arpa S, Robbens C, Monstrey SJ. Male-to-female gender confirmation surgery: intestinal vaginoplasty. Clin Plast Surg. 45:351–360 Preprint at (2018) https://doi.org/10.1016/j.cps.2018.03.006.
15. van der Sluis WB, et al. Ileal vaginoplasty as vaginal reconstruction in transgender women and patients with disorders of sex development: an international, multicentre, retrospective study on surgical characteristics and outcomes. BJU Int. 2018;121:952–8.
16. Garcia MM, et al. Use of right colon vaginoplasty in gender affirming surgery: proposed advantages, review of technique, and outcomes. Surg Endosc. 2021;35:5643–54.
17. van der Sluis WB, Bouman MB, Buncamper ME, Mullender MG, Meijerink WJ. Revision vaginoplasty: a comparison of surgical outcomes of laparoscopic intestinal versus perineal full-thickness skin graft vaginoplasty. Plast Reconstr Surg. 2016;138:793–800.
18. Morrison SD et al. Long-term outcomes of rectosigmoid neocolporrhaphy in male-to-female gender reassignment surgery. Plast Reconstr Surg. 136:386–394 Preprint at (2015) https://doi.org/10.1097/PRS.0000000000001459.
19. Schardein JN, Nikolavsky D. Sexual functioning of transgender females post-vaginoplasty: evaluation, outcomes and treatment strategies for sexual dysfunction. Sex Med Rev. 10:77–90 Preprint at (2022) https://doi.org/10.1016/j.sxmr.2021.04.001.
20. di Summa PG et al. Colic-based transplant in sexual reassignment surgery: functional outcomes and complications in 43 consecutive patients. J Sex Med. 16:2030–2037 (Elsevier B.V., 2019).
21. Georgas K, Belgrano V, Andreasson M, Elander A, Selvaggi G. Bowel vaginoplasty: a systematic review. J Plast Surg Hand Surg. 52:265–273 Preprint at (2018) https://doi.org/10.1080/2000656X.2018.1482220.
22. Hontscharuk R, Alba B, Hamidian Jahromi A, Schechter L. Penile inversion vaginoplasty outcomes: Complications and satisfaction. Andrology. 9:1732–1743 Preprint at (2021) https://doi.org/10.1111/andr.13030.
23. Lindqvist EK, et al. Quality of life improves early after gender reassignment surgery in transgender women. Eur J Plast Surg. 2017;40:223–6.
24. Horbach SER, et al. Outcome of Vaginoplasty in male-to-female Transgenders: a systematic review of surgical techniques. J Sex Med. 2015;12:1499–512.
25. Bustos SS et al. Complications and atient-reported outcomes in transfemale vaginoplasty: an updated systematic review and meta-analysis. Plast Reconstr Surg Glob Open. Preprint at (2021) https://doi.org/10.1097/GOX.0000000000003510.
26. Bouman MB, et al. Patient-reported esthetic and functional outcomes of primary total laparoscopic intestinal vaginoplasty in transgender women with penoscrotal hypoplasia. J Sex Med. 2016;13:1438–44.

Index

K. Umanskiy, N. Hyman (eds.), *Difficult Decisions in Colorectal Surgery*, Difficult Decisions in Surgery: An Evidence-Based Approach,
https://doi.org/10.1007/978-3-031-42303-1

Q

R